MANUAL OF CLINICAL PROBLEMS IN OBSTETRICS AND GYNECOLOGY
WITH ANNOTATED KEY REFERENCES

MANUAL OF CLINICAL PROBLEMS IN OBSTETRICS AND GYNECOLOGY
WITH ANNOTATED KEY REFERENCES

EDITED BY

MICHEL E. RIVLIN, M.D.
Assistant Professor, Department of Obstetrics and Gynecology, University of Mississippi School of Medicine; Director, Junior Medical Students' Program in Obstetrics and Gynecology, University of Mississippi Medical Center, Jackson

JOHN C. MORRISON, M.D.
Professor, Department of Obstetrics and Gynecology, University of Mississippi School of Medicine; Director, Division of Maternal-Fetal Medicine, University of Mississippi Medical Center, Jackson

G. WILLIAM BATES, M.D.
Associate Professor, Department of Obstetrics and Gynecology, University of Mississippi School of Medicine; Director, Division of Reproductive Endocrinology, University of Mississippi Medical Center, Jackson

Foreword by Winfred L. Wiser, M.D.
Professor, Department of Obstetrics and Gynecology, University of Mississippi School of Medicine; Chairman, Department of Obstetrics and Gynecology, University of Mississippi Medical Center, Jackson

LITTLE, BROWN AND COMPANY   BOSTON

To our wives, Jane, Rita, and Susanne

CONTENTS

FOREWORD

This outstanding teaching volume in obstetrics and gynecology is unique in its approach to providing in-depth information in simple readable fashion about major topics in the specialty. The list of authors demonstrates a variety of qualified teachers and practitioners with the ability to provide critical information in a succinct but forceful manner. The annotated references following each topic are invaluable to medical students and residents as well as to the busy practicing physician.

Michel E. Rivlin is a dedicated, highly competent teacher who constantly strives to uncover improved vehicles for learning. This volume demonstrates his interest in providing better patient care through an improved method of learning.

Winfred L. Wiser

The purpose of this manual is to provide a concise review of common clinical problems in obstetrics and gynecology with pertinent references from the literature. Comments on each reference either indicate why it was chosen or are used to amplify a particular aspect of the clinical situation. It is therefore advantageous to read both the text and the annotated bibliography.

The book is intended to serve the student, resident, and practitioner in several respects. First, it is designed as a rapid reference in the management of current clinical problems on the wards or in the office. Second, it should serve as a convenient guide to the preparation of clinical case or grand round presentations. Lastly, it may be used as a short, easily assimilated review prior to undertaking National Board, FLEX, or college examinations.

Dr. John Morrison, Director of the Division of Maternal-Fetal Medicine at the University of Mississippi, edited the obstetric section. He and his contributors present a contemporary view of the discipline but acknowledge and present older and perhaps more conservative approaches to the vexing clinical problems so commonly encountered in this fascinating field.

Dr. G. William Bates, Director, Division of Reproductive Endocrinology and Director of the Residency Training Program at the University of Mississippi, edited the endocrine and infertility sections. He and his contributors provide a clear, easily understood approach to a field that many students have traditionally regarded as being both difficult and complex.

During the past five years I have functioned both as a student and as a teacher. As a student, I successfully completed the FLEX and American Board of Obstetrics and Gynecology examinations. As a teacher, I am Director of the Junior Medical Students' Program in Obstetrics and Gynecology at the University of Mississippi. In compiling this volume, I have attempted to produce the book I would like to have had available to me in both these capacities.

I would like to thank Dr. Winfred Wiser for writing the foreword and for placing the facilities of his department at our disposal in preparing this book. Kathy O'Brien of Little, Brown and Company provided useful criticism and seemingly endless patience. I would also like to acknowledge the work of Margaret Taylor, who transferred the book contents to the word processor, thus simplifying the inevitable revisions. Above all, my thanks are due to Donna Welch, whose secretarial alchemy transmuted the schoolwall graffiti of the original draft to the neat sentences and paragraphs of the final copy.

M. E. R.

CONTRIBUTING AUTHORS

THOMAS N. ABDELLA, M.D.
E. H. Crump Women's Hospital and Perinatal Center; University of Tennessee College of Medicine, Memphis

GARLAND D. ANDERSON, M.D.
E. H. Crump Women's Hospital and Perinatal Center; University of Tennessee College of Medicine, Memphis

G. WILLIAM BATES, M.D.
University of Mississippi Medical Center; University of Mississippi School of Medicine, Jackson

FRANK H. BOEHM, M.D.
Vanderbilt University Medical Center; Vanderbilt University School of Medicine, Nashville, Tennessee

SISTER CLARICE CARROLL, M.S.N.
University of Mississippi Medical Center; University of Mississippi School of Medicine, Jackson

RICHARD O. DAVIS, M.D.
University of Alabama in Birmingham Medical Center; University of Alabama School of Medicine, Birmingham

STAVROS G. DOUVAS, M.D.
University of Mississippi Medical Center; University of Mississippi School of Medicine, Jackson

MARY F. HAIRE, R.N.
Vanderbilt University Medical Center; Vanderbilt University School of Medicine, Nashville, Tennessee

BRUCE A. HARRIS, M.D.
University of Alabama in Birmingham Medical Center; University of Alabama School of Medicine, Birmingham

JOHN F. HUDDLESTON, M.D.
University of Alabama in Birmingham Medical Center; University of Alabama School of Medicine, Birmingham

WILLIAM F. HUGGINS, M.D.
University of Alabama in Birmingham Medical Center; University of Alabama School of Medicine, Birmingham

JEFFERY LIPSHITZ, M.B.Ch.B., M.R.C.O.G.
E. H. Crump Women's Hospital and Perinatal Center; University of Tennessee College of Medicine, Memphis

JOHN A. LUCAS III, M.D.
Obstetrics and Gynecology, Doctors Hospital, Mobile, Alabama

JACK McCUBBIN, M.D.
E. H. Crump Women's Hospital and Perinatal Center; University of Tennessee College of Medicine, Memphis

G. RODNEY MEEKS, M.D.
University of Mississippi Medical Center; University of Mississippi School of Medicine, Jackson

JOHN C. MORRISON, M.D.
University of Mississippi Medical Center; University of Mississippi School of Medicine, Jackson

FERYAL R. RAHMAN, M.D.
King Faisal Specialist Hospital and Research Centre, Riyadh, Saudi Arabia

JANE B. RIVLIN, M.S.N.
University of Mississippi Medical Center; University of Mississippi School of Nursing, Jackson

MICHEL E. RIVLIN, M.D.
University of Mississippi Medical Center; University of Mississippi School of Medicine, Jackson

ABRAHAM RUBIN, M.D.
Michael Reese Hospital and Medical Center; The University of Chicago, The Pritzker School of Medicine, Chicago, Illinois

BAHA M. SIBAI, M.D.
E. H. Crump Women's Hospital and Perinatal Center; University of Tennessee College of Medicine, Memphis

ERIC R. STRASBURG, M.B., F.R.C.O.G.
Cleveland Metropolitan General Hospital; Case Western Reserve University School of Medicine, Cleveland, Ohio

J. TATE THIGPEN, M.D.
University of Mississippi Medical Center; University of Mississippi School of Medicine, Jackson

JAMES B. UNGER, M.D.
University of Mississippi Medical Center; University of Mississippi School of Medicine, Jackson

MARC VATIN, M.D.
Columbia Hospital for Women; George Washington University School of Medicine and Health Sciences, Washington, D.C.

MENDLEY A. WULFSOHN, M.D.
Mount Sinai Medical Center; Mount Sinai School of Medicine of the City University of New York, New York

MANUAL OF CLINICAL PROBLEMS IN OBSTETRICS AND GYNECOLOGY

WITH ANNOTATED KEY REFERENCES

Notice

The indications and dosages of all drugs in this manual have been recommended in the medical literature and conform to the practices of the general medical community. The medications described do not necessarily have specific approval by the Food and Drug Administration for use in the diseases and dosages for which they are recommended. The package insert for each drug should be consulted for use and dosage as approved by the FDA. Because standards for usage change, it is advisable to keep abreast of revised recommendations, particularly those concerning new drugs.

OBSTETRICS

HEMORRHAGE IN PREGNANCY

Abortion is the termination of pregnancy before the fetus is capable of extrauterine life, generally considered to be prior to the twentieth week of gestation, or the conceptus achieving a mass of 500 g or a crown-rump length of 18 cm. The incidence of spontaneous abortion (also called miscarriage) has been estimated at 10%–20% of all pregnancies. The most common cause of fetal death is an abnormality of the conceptus, probably occurring in between 50% and 80% of abortions. Malformations of the conceptus can be caused by such conditions as defective implantation of a normal trophoblast, maternal viral infections, chromosomal abnormalities or ingestion of cytotoxic agents.

Chromosomally abnormal fetuses account for approximately 35% of these abortions. Two situations exist among the parents of chromosomally abnormal abortuses. In most instances the couple is chromosomally normal and the abortuses' abnormalities occur in a random and sporadic fashion. In a small percentage of cases, one member of the couple is a carrier of a balanced translocation; offspring of these parents may be repeatedly aborted.

Other factors implicated include acute maternal bacterial infections, chronic maternal cardiac and renovascular disease, and maternal endocrine disorders. Some investigators have noted a higher incidence of toxoplasmosis, herpes simplex, cytomegalovirus, T-strain mycoplasma, and *Listeria monocytogenes* among these patients.

Uterine developmental abnormalities and cervical incompetence may cause midtrimester abortions. These disorders are often amenable to surgical correction (metroplasty, cervical cerclage).

Abortion is said to be "threatened" when a pregnant woman experiences uterine bleeding. Pain, if present at all, is minimal. The cervix will be found to be closed and uneffaced. Differential diagnosis includes ectopic pregnancy and trophoblastic disease. Pregnancy tests and ultrasound are helpful for diagnosis and prognosis. Management is limited to explaining the pathologic process and the prognosis to the patient. She is advised that there is no increase in fetal congenital anomalies when such pregnancies continue. Bed rest has not been shown to be beneficial and need not be recommended.

An abortion is inevitable when bleeding is accompanied by pain and dilatation of the internal os. The abortion is incomplete when products of conception protrude through the cervix. In pregnancies of 14 or less weeks, suction and/or sharp curettage is performed. In pregnancies of more than 14 weeks, abortion is expedited by administration of intravenous oxytocin. The abortion is termed *complete* when the uterus is empty.

The term *missed abortion* is applied when the conceptus dies but is not passed. Diagnosis is confirmed by a negative pregnancy test and real time ultrasonography. If the conceptus is retained more than 4 weeks, there is a risk of disseminated intravascular coagulation (DIC). The uterus should therefore be evacuated once appropriate clotting studies are obtained.

Although any abortion may become infected septicemia usually follows criminal interference. The organisms are commonly aerobic and anaerobic, occurring in mixed culture. Generally these are gram-negative bacilli, most commonly *Escherichia coli* and *Bacteroides fragilis*, and gram-positive cocci, particularly enterococcus and beta hemolytic streptococcus. Other important organisms are *Clostridium perfringens* and *Clostridium tetanus*.

The infection may be localized to the products of conception, or there may be a spreading endometritis with parametritis, salpingo-oophoritis, peritonitis, septic thrombophlebitis, and septicemia. Other major complications include renal failure, septic shock, uterine perforation, and disseminated coagulopathy.

Rapid resuscitation; adequate antibiotic therapy (penicillin, gentamicin, and clindamycin in severe cases); and evacuation of the uterus, usually within 12 hours of admission, or laparotomy, or both; and hysterectomy when appropriate, will minimize morbidity and mortality.

Women having three or more consecutive abortions are usually defined as being habitual aborters. The causes of the abortions are similar to those mentioned previously for spontaneous miscarriage. A full workup is called for, but, in fact, the risk of further abortion is still only 25%–30%.

An induced abortion is an elective termination of a pregnancy prior to viability. The indications may be therapeutic or at the patient's request. In 1977 in the United States there were 1,079,430 legal abortions, an abortion ratio of 325 per thousand live births.

The earliest intervention is "menstrual regulation," which consists of aspiration of the endometrium within 14 days of a missed menstrual period when pregnancy has been confirmed by serum radioimmunoassay.

After 6 weeks of gestation, dilatation of the cervix is required for evacuation of the uterus. The procedure of dilatation and suction curettage for termination of first trimester pregnancies is usually performed under paracervical block as an outpatient procedure. The uterine contents must always be sent for histologic examination to rule out ectopic pregnancy or trophoblastic disease. Complications include cervical laceration and uterine perforation, possibly accompanied by intraabdominal hemorrhage and bowel injury. These complications must be immediately and adequately treated.

Second-trimester pregnancy terminations are more difficult, more dangerous, and usually require admission to the hospital. They are commonly brought about by the intraamniotic instillation of prostaglandin F_{2a}, or hypertonic saline or urea solutions. More recently, prostaglandin E_2 vaginal suppositories and intramuscular 15 methyl prostaglandin F_{2a} have also been used. Labor may be supplemented by the use of intravenous oxytocin once the membranes have ruptured. Hypertonic saline infusion may lead to hypernatremia or diffuse coagulopathy in rare instances; prostaglandin appears to be marginally safer.

Dilatation and evacuation may also be performed between the twelfth and twentieth week, provided it is performed by surgeons skilled in the procedure. The operation is facilitated by the use of laminaria (placed in the cervical canal some hours beforehand, they swell up with fluid, passively dilating the cervix), large dilators, and intraamniotic urea to produce fetal demise and maceration. The patient is spared a prolonged induction delivery interval.

Induction of abortion is safest when performed at a period of gestation of less than 9 weeks. Death to case rate increases by approximately 40%–60% with each week of delay after the eighth week. Hysterotomies and hysterectomies carry a relatively high morbidity and mortality and should be avoided in the absence of specific indications.

Although rates for immediate and delayed complications from legal abortions are low, the potential long-term effects of abortion on subsequent fertility await final evaluation. Some studies suggest a higher spontaneous abortion rate and an increased perinatal morbidity and mortality for pregnancies that occur subsequent to elective vaginal terminations of pregnancy.

Incidence

1. Miller, J. F., et al. Fetal loss after implantation. *Lancet* 1:544, 1980.
   A prospective study employing beta-specific subunit human chorionic gonadotropin pregnancy-testing demonstrated an incidence of 43%.

Etiology

2. Stenchever, M. A., et al. Cytogenetics of habitual abortion and other pregnancy wastage. *Am. J. Obstet. Gynecol.* 127:143, 1977.
   The most common abnormalities in abortuses are autosomal trisomy, x-monosomy, and polyploidy.
3. Daling, J. R., Spadoni, L. R., and Emanuel, I. Role of induced abortion in secondary infertility. *Obstet. Gynecol.* 57:59, 1981.
   A retrospective review of 105 patients with secondary infertility after induced abortions were compared to a like group of controls. A trend toward a higher risk in the former group was found but it was not statistically significant when related to secondary infertility.
4. McDonald, I. A. Incompetence of the cervix. *Aust. N.Z. J. Obstet. Gynaecol.* 18:34, 1978.
   Diagnosis of the incompetent cervix is unfortunately somewhat subjective.
5. Stenchever, M. A. Genetic clues to reproductive wastage. *Cont. Ob/Gyn.* 17:37, 1981.
   The author reviews the multitude of genetic clues regarding early reproductive wastage. A nice summary is given of chromosomal abnormalities as they apply to repetitive abortions.

Threatened Abortion

6. Editorial. Vaginal bleeding in early pregnancy. *Br. Med. J.* 1:470, 1980.
   Perinatal morbidity is increased in approximately 40% of patients whose pregnancy continues.
7. Goldzieher, J. W. Double-blind study of progestin in habitual abortion. *J.A.M.A.* 188:561, 1964.
   Progestin replacement is not therapeutic in threatened abortion.

Septic Abortion

8. Chow, A. W., Marshall, J. R., and Guze, L. B. A double-blind comparison of clindamycin with penicillin plus chloramphenicol in treatment of septic abortion. *J. Infect. Dis.* 135:535, 1977.
   Clindamycin alone was less effective than penicillin with chloramphenicol.
9. Duff, P. Pathophysiology and management of septic shock. *J. Reprod. Med.* 24:109, 1980.
   Good general review.

Habitual Abortion

10. Stenchever, M. A. Managing habitual abortion. *Contrib. Gynecol. Obstet.* 16:23, 1980.
    A comprehensive review of etiology, diagnosis, and possible treatments.

Induced Abortion

11. Bracken, M. B. Psychosomatic aspects of abortion: Implications for counseling. *J. Reprod. Med.* 19:265, 1977.
    Adequate counseling is vital.
12. Lauersen, N. H., et al. A new abortion technique: Intravaginal and intramuscular prostaglandin. *Obstet. Gynecol.* 58:96, 1981.

Abortion using a suppository and intramuscular injection of methylated prostaglandin was successful in inducing abortion in 80 of 81 women. Not only did the new method have high accuracy but there was a reduced number of side effects.

13. Burnett, L. S., Wentz, A. C., and King, T. M. Techniques of pregnancy termination—Part II. *Obstet. Gynecol. Surv.* 29:6, 1974.
    Review of all the methods.

14. Methods of midtrimester abortion. *ACOG Tech. Bull.* No. 56, December, 1979.
    Modern methods.

15. Freiman, S. M., and Wulff, G. J. L., Jr. Management of uterine perforation following elective abortion. *Obstet. Gynecol.* 50:647, 1977.
    An emergency that often causes confusion.

16. Grimes, D. A., et al. Midtrimester abortion by dilatation and evacuation—a safe and practical alternative. *N. Engl. J. Med.* 296:1141, 1977.
    Unacceptable in many institutions because of adverse emotional and psychological reactions encountered in many staff members.

17. Richardson, J. A., and Dixon, G. Effects of legal termination on subsequent pregnancy. *Br. Med. J.* 1:1303, 1976.
    After a vaginal termination, there is considerable risk to a subsequent pregnancy, according to this article.

18. Grimes, D. A., and Gates, W., Jr. Complications from legally-induced abortion. *Obstet. Gynecol. Surv.* 34:177, 1979.
    A comprehensive review.

(Think) Ectopic Pregnancy

An ectopic gestation refers to an implantation of the fertilized ovum in an abnormal site. In over 95% of cases this site is tubal, although implantation may also occur elsewhere in the uterus (cornua, cervix, in a rudimentary horn); in the ovary; or, via secondary attachment, in the broad ligament (intraligamentary) or anywhere in the peritoneal cavity (abdominal pregnancy).

The incidence varies with the population studied and should properly be based on the conception rate (live births plus abortions) rather than on live births alone. In practice, however, the latter is the measure used, and rates, while variable, average 1%–1½%. Most patients are in their twenties and of low parity.

The incidence appears to be increasing, and the increase seems to be related to factors leading to infertility. Chronic endosalpingitis is the most common factor; the therapy for the infection may have increased the incidence rather than diminished it by means of partial healing, after which a semifunctional tube is left. The intrauterine device (IUD) is associated with a 1 in 23 incidence of ectopic pregnancy if pregnancy occurs. This may simply be due to protection afforded against intrauterine pregnancy, so that there is no real increased incidence, or, infection related to the IUD may be a factor. Surgical procedures on the tubes related to sterilization or infertility also predispose to ectopic gestation, as does a history of previous ectopic pregnancies.

The anatomic site of implantation affects the pathophysiology and the clinical outcome. Implantation is usually ampullary, no decidua is present, and the tubal musculature cannot contain a gestation of any size, usually resulting in external rupture or less often, internal rupture with tubal abortion. Hemorrhage may be diffuse or be contained in a hematocele. Isthmic pregnancy may rupture externally into the peritoneal cavity or into the broad ligament (broad ligament hematoma). Internal rupture with abortion is uncommon. Interstitial pregnancy (rudimentary horn pregnancy is similar) may rupture externally into the abdominal cavity or internally into the uterine cavity. Hemorrhage is heavy because of the greater vascularity, and, because the wall is thicker, pregnancy is often more advanced.

Cervical pregnancy is rare, and histologic proof of nidation below the internal os is necessary for the diagnosis. Bleeding is heavy, and the condition is usually diagnosed during attempted curettage of an "abortion."

Ovarian pregnancy may follow primary or secondary implantation. Four criteria need to be fulfilled for the diagnosis: the tube must be intact, ovarian tissue must be present in the sac wall, the pregnancy site must be connected to the uterus, and the fetal sac must be in the region of the ovary.

Abdominal pregnancy may be primary but is usually by secondary implantation on serosal surfaces. While fetal growth to viability may occur, the fetus often dies before the onset of spurious labor, probably due to poor placental circulation. Fetal membranes separate the fetus from the peritoneal cavity and the lie is usually abnormal. After death the fetus may calcify (lithopedian) or undergo fat degeneration (adipocere). Intraligamentary pregnancy is the rarest; implantation is extraperitoneal, and the pregnancy may progress to viability.

Irregular bleeding or relative amenorrhea, or both, is the first symptom in 40% of patients with ectopic gestation. In 25%, pain is the first symptom. The mechanism of the bleeding is unclear, while pain results from tubal distention and peritonism caused by bleeding. Generalized bleeding may cause shoulder pain, fainting, and shock. Abdominal pain, unilateral or generalized, is present in 99% of ectopic gestations. Physical examination reveals adnexal tenderness in 97% of cases, though an adnexal mass is present in only 70%. The uterus is somewhat enlarged in about 25% and, rarely, a decidual cast may have been passed. Pyrexia is uncommon. Hypovolemic shock is usually present in patients with hemoperitoneum.

With an ectopic pregnancy the white cell count may be elevated, the hematocrit is dependent on the degree of blood loss, and the serum pregnancy test is invariably positive. Pelvic ultrasound is a valuable diagnostic tool, although it is less useful before 7 weeks in establishing the presence of an intrauterine sac. If the patient has had a diagnostic curettage, a decidual reaction is present in 60%, while 9% exhibit the Arias-Stella reaction. The remainder may show any phase of the cycle. In doubtful cases laparoscopy may be called for; the most valuable diagnostic test, however, is culdocentesis, which reveals nonclotting blood in up to 95% of cases. X-ray is useful only in patients with suspected abdominal pregnancy in whom the diagnosis is made if fetal parts are seen behind the maternal spine.

The differential diagnosis includes pelvic inflammatory disease, intrauterine pregnancy (with or without abortion), and ovarian lesions (particularly a ruptured corpus luteum). In particular, bleeding from a hemorrhagic corpus luteum may mimic an ectopic pregnancy in all respects and may only be differentiated at laparoscopy.

Early laparotomy is essential in the treatment of ectopic gestation. Hypovolemia must be corrected with blood transfusion, taking great care to avoid fluid overload. Surgery may be radical (removal of tube) or conservative (tubal repair), depending on the circumstances. If the patient desires further children, some form of tubal repair may be performed, especially if there has been no rupture. Salpingectomy is called for if further pregnancy is not desired. If the patient is in good condition and further pregnancy is not desired, hysterectomy may be the procedure of choice, especially if other pathology is present. In deciding on conservative surgery, the incidence of recurrence must be considered: with conservative surgery the incidence is probably 10%–15% and is not much different with radical surgery.

The surgical management of ectopic gestations, other than tubal, differs to some extent. Interstitial pregnancies may be shelled out and the defect repaired or hysterectomy may be necessary. Patients with abdominal pregnancies should be operated on when the diagnosis is made, or, occasionally, operation can be delayed until the fetus is mature. After fetal delivery, the placenta can be removed rarely, and in most cases it should be left in situ. Cervical pregnancy is complex since the placenta is often accreta. Packing of the cervix and uterus after digital removal may achieve hemostasis, but hysterectomy is often necessary.

Prognosis with ectopic gestation is dependent on early recognition. If the physician "thinks ectopic," the outlook is excellent. Failure to do so contributes to maternal mortality. The maternal mortality rate with ectopic gestation is similar to that for repeat cesarean section, about 0.1%.

A convenient rule of thumb as regards the prognosis for further pregnancy is as follows: "Of ten ectopics, five will have intrauterine pregnancies, two-thirds of these will have babies (high abortion rate), and one will have another ectopic." This situation may be improved by the rising incidence of diagnosis of unruptured ectopic pregnancies and by the increasing use of conservative surgery, including microsurgical techniques, follow-up laparoscopy, and intraoperative and postoperative medications.

Reviews

1. Breen, J. L. A 21 year survey of 654 ectopic pregnancies. *Am. J. Obstet. Gynecol.* 106:1004, 1970.
   An older paper in which 80% of the ectopic pregnancies reported were already ruptured.
2. Helvacioglu, A., Long, E. M., and Yang, S. Ectopic pregnancy: An eight-year review. *J. Reprod. Med.* 22:87, 1979.
   A recent report in which only 48% of the pregnancies reported in 313 women had ruptured.

Etiology

3. Hallatt, J. G. Ectopic pregnancy associated with the intrauterine device: A study of seventy cases. *Am. J. Obstet. Gynecol.* 125:754, 1976.
   The IUD was removed or replaced in 50% of the women 1 to 8 weeks before surgery.
4. Hallatt, J. G. Repeat ectopic pregnancy: A study of 123 consecutive cases. *Am. J. Obstet. Gynecol.* 122:520, 1975.
   Nine percent of 1330 women who had had ectopic pregnancies experienced repeat tubal pregnancies.
5. Walton, S. M. A survey of tubal ectopic pregnancy, with particular reference to cases following sterilization. *Aust. N.Z. J. Obstet. Gynaecol.* 18:266, 1978.
   Pregnancy rate of 0.25%–2% follows tubal sterilization. About one-third of these pregnancies will be extrauterine.
6. Ory, H. W., and The Women's Health Study. Ectopic pregnancy and intrauterine contraceptive devices: New perspectives. *Obstet. Gynecol.* 57:137, 1981.
   In a cooperative multicenter study, the relationship of the intrauterine

device to ectopic pregnancy was studied. The use of the IUD, based on this study, did not play a role in the genesis of ectopic pregnancy.

7. Kallenberger, D. A., et al. Ectopic pregnancy: A 15-year review of 160 cases. *South. Med. J.* 71:758, 1978.
   There was a significant correlation between the incidence of ectopic pregnancy and the incidence of gonorrhea.

Epidemiology
8. Beral, V. An epidemiological study of recent trends in ectopic pregnancy. *Br. J. Obstet. Gynaecol.* 82:775, 1975.
   An increasing incidence of ectopic pregnancy appeared to be related to IUD use but not to tubal infection. Progestogen-only contraceptives, induced abortion, and tubal surgery may be factors, but there is insufficient available data to confirm or support this.

Diagnosis
9. Schwartz, R. O., and Di Pietro, D. L. Beta-HCG as a diagnostic aid for suspected ectopic pregnancy. *Obstet. Gynecol.* 56:197, 1980.
   Positive radioimmunoassay (RIA) for serum beta-subunit of human chorionic gonadotropin (HCG) with a low level of HCG for the period of gestation, is highly suggestive of ectopic pregnancy. A negative RIA excludes the diagnosis.
10. Maklad, N. F., and Wright, C. H. Grey scale ultrasonography in the diagnosis of ectopic pregnancy. *Radiology* 126:221, 1978.
    The ultrasonic signs and criteria are outlined; diagnostic accuracy was 92%.
11. Pelosi, M. A., D'Amico, R. J., and Goldstein, P. J. Improved accuracy in the clinical diagnosis of ectopic pregnancy by the simultaneous use of pelvic ultrasonography and a radioreceptor assay of human chorionic gonadotropin. *Surg. Gynecol. Obstet.* 149:538, 1979.
    The combination of the hormone assay with ultrasound is of great value in the early diagnosis of ectopic cyesis.
12. Esposito, J. M. The laparoscope: An aid in the diagnosis of the intact ectopic gestation. *J. Reprod. Med.* 9:158, 1972.
    Reference 4 of this article, recommending peritoneoscopy in the differential diagnosis of ectopic gestation, is dated 1937.
13. Brenner, P. F., Roy, S., and Mishell, D. R. Ectopic pregnancy. A study of 300 consecutive surgically treated cases. *J.A.M.A.* 243:673, 1980.
    In a series of 300 patients with ectopic gestations, culdocentesis was performed on all and was positive in 95%. Hematocrit value on the culdocentesis specimens was greater than 15% in 97% of the samples taken.

Rare Forms of Extrauterine Gestation
14. Radman, H. M. Abdominal pregnancy: Pathogenesis, diagnosis, and treatment. *South. Med. J.* 71:670, 1978.
    The management of the placenta forms the crux of the problem once the diagnosis is established. In general, the placenta is usually best left in situ.
15. Orr, J. E., et al. False negative oxytocin challenge test associated with abdominal pregnancy. *Am. J. Obstet. Gynecol.* 133:108, 1979.
    The inability to induce uterine contractions with oxytocin or prostaglandin is highly suggestive of extrauterine gestation.
16. Nelson, R. M. Bilateral internal iliac artery ligation in the cervical pregnancy. Conservation of reproductive function. *Am. J. Obstet. Gynecol.* 134:145, 1979.
    Hysterectomy is the standard therapy for this rare ectopic gestation. This

paper presents an alternative therapy that was successfully employed in two patients.

17. Evans, M. I., et al. The intrauterine device and ovarian pregnancy. *Fertil. Steril.* 32:31, 1979.
Spiegelberg's criteria for ovarian pregnancy were met by three patients with IUDs in one year. This brought the number of such cases reported to 50. Nevertheless, a cause and effect relationship has yet to be established.

Treatment

18. Harralson, J. D., Van Nagell, J. R., and Roddick, J. W. Operative management of ruptured tubal pregnancy. *Am. J. Obstet. Gynecol.* 115:995, 1973.
The classic surgical management of ectopic gestation is salpingectomy. In this paper, 15% of the patients were treated by hysterectomy, the indications for which included pelvic inflammatory disease and sterilization.

19. Bukovsky, I., et al. Conservative surgery for tubal pregnancy. *Obstet. Gynecol.* 53:709, 1979.
Improved diagnostic methods have led to earlier diagnosis, and conservative surgical procedures, particularly salpingostomy, are now employed for patients with poor reproductive histories.

20. De Cherney, A., and Kase, N. The conservative surgical management of unruptured ectopic pregnancy. *Obstet. Gynecol.* 54:451, 1979.
Pregnancy rates following conservative and radical surgery were similar; nevertheless, salpingostomy is recommended for unruptured ampullary pregnancies.

Prognosis

21. May, W., Miller, J., and Greiss, F. Maternal deaths from ectopic pregnancy in the South Atlantic region, 1960 through 1976. *Am. J. Obstet-Gynecol.* 132:140, 1978.
All medical practitioners and health care providers need to join with their "Ob-Gyn" colleagues in "thinking ectopic."

Gestational Trophoblastic Neoplasms

Gestational trophoblastic neoplasms (GTN) range from the generally benign hydatidiform mole (1 in 1200 pregnancies) through the locally infiltrating invasive mole (1 in 12,000 pregnancies) to the highly malignant choriocarcinoma (1 in 40,000 pregnancies). The incidence of GTN is independent of age, race, or parity but is much higher in underdeveloped countries, particularly in the Orient (1 in 125 pregnancies).

The hydatidiform mole is characterized grossly by a grapelike appearance due to cystic swelling of the placental villi. Three characteristic microscopic features distinguish the molar pregnancy: stromal edema, absent villus vasculature, and trophoblastic proliferation. It is not possible to predict on histopathology alone which moles will persist or which will develop malignant changes.

The invasive mole (chorioadenoma destruens) is distinguished by local invasion of the myometrium, sometimes to the extent of perforation. Occasionally metastasis will occur.

Choriocarcinoma is an epithelial tumor of syncytiotrophoblast and cytotrophoblast. It is preceded by molar pregnancy in about 50% of cases, follows term pregnancy in about 25%, and follows abortion or ectopic pregnancy in a further 25%. Approximately 5% of moles progress to choriocarcinoma. The gross appearance is characteristically dark red and hemorrhagic. Histology demonstrates sheets or foci of trophoblast with absent villus structure. Trophoblastic tissue produces human chorionic gonadotropin (HCG). The amount produced correlates with the amount of tissue present. Radioimmunoassay of the beta-chain of HCG distinguishes the substance from pituitary luteinizing hormone. Since histopathology is often equivocal, gonadotropin excretion is crucial to diagnosis and management, especially in identifying the 15%–20% of hydatidiform moles that will persist after curettage.

Hydatidiform mole may be complete or partial; in the latter instance it may be associated with a separate normal pregnancy. Clinically, in some 45% of patients uterine size is large for gestational age, in 38% it is smaller, and in 16% it is normal size. Vaginal bleeding, which is the most common presenting feature, may be slight or heavy. Spontaneous abortion generally occurs by the seventeenth to twenty-eighth week. High levels of HCG result in theca-lutein cyst formation, with resultant marked ovarian enlargement in some 15%–25% of cases. Preeclampsia is encountered in 10%–15% of cases. Hyperemesis and lower abdominal pain are also frequently encountered. Molar vesicles may be passed vaginally.

The diagnosis is suspected in the absence of fetal parts or heart tones in a uterus of a size in which these would be expected to be present. The differential diagnosis includes threatened or missed abortion. Ultrasound is highly reliable in establishing the diagnosis by picking up multiple echoes in a "honeycomb" pattern, demonstrating the absence of fetal activity, and outlining ovarian cysts if present.

Management of the molar pregnancy is usually by uterine evacuation by dilatation and suction curettage (D and C). Occasionally, hysterotomy may be necessary in a uterus over 20 weeks size, but this procedure appears to be associated with an increased chance of malignancy. Hysterectomy may be the treatment of choice if further childbearing is not a factor. Hemorrhage, infection, perforation, and pulmonary edema are the major complications of therapy. The role of pitocin and/or prostaglandin evacuation of the uterus is controversial due to fear of dissemination of disease.

After evacuation, management is dependent on beta-subunit HCG titers. In 75% of cases, tests are negative by 40 days after the therapeutic procedure. Of patients with positive tests at 56 days after, 50% have trophoblastic disease. Reelevation or plateauing of the titer is evidence of persistent disease. The tests are repeated every 2 weeks together with clinical evaluation of uterine and ovarian involution. Evidence of persistent disease or metastasis is an indication for treatment with chemotherapy. Routine prophylactic chemotherapy seems too hazardous since in 80% of patients disease remits without therapy. Contraception is essential during this period since an intercurrent pregnancy would greatly complicate follow-up and treatment. A confirmatory titer is obtained 1 month after the first negative (under 5 mIU/ml) test. Titers are then repeated every 3 months for 1 year. After a year of negative follow-up, pregnancy is allowed if desired.

Malignant trophoblastic disease may be diagnosed on curettage for irregular bleeding after pregnancy, or the tumor may be deep in the myometrium or be metastatic only. On rare occasions, disease may present years after the antecedent pregnancy. The common sites for metastasis are lung (75%), vagina, liver, brain, and bowel, although unexplained metastases in any area may be due to trophoblastic disease; HCG titers should always be obtained in patients with unexplained urinary, gastrointestinal, or pulmonary bleeding, as well as for central nervous system tumors or atypical pelvic malignancies.

The disease is staged as nonmetastatic (confined to uterus) or metastatic by chest x-ray, liver and brain scan, intravenous pyelogram, and any further tests that may be indicated by the findings in the individual patient. Liver, renal, and bone marrow baseline studies are obtained because chemotherapy is especially toxic to these systems.

Patients with metastatic disease are further classified into low- and high-risk groups. The high-risk group includes patients with cerebral or hepatic metastases, those with disease following term pregnancy, patients with failure of prior chemotherapy, those with initial serum HCG titer over 40,000 mIU/ml, or those having a duration of symptoms of over 4 months.

Single agent chemotherapy is used for nonmetastatic and low-risk metastatic disease. Multiple-agent combined chemotherapy is used in the high-risk group. The most common single agents employed are actinomycin D and methotrexate. The standard combined therapy is methotrexate, actinomycin D, and chlorambucil (MAC).

Treatment must be aggressive, with close observation and control of drug toxicity, if optimal results are to be obtained. Drug effects are predictable and not idiosyncratic. During treatment courses daily blood counts and chemistries are obtained. Therapy is suspended for white cell counts under 3000, platelets under 100,000, or significant changes in renal or hepatic function. Generally, 5-day courses are given with 7 to 10 days between each. Oral contraception is used for pituitary suppression for at least 1 year.

Consideration is given to altering drug therapy if HCG levels plateau or rise, or if metastases increase in size or number. Therapy is stopped when clinical evidence of disease, as monitored by weekly pelvic examinations and chest x-rays, is absent and three normal consecutive weekly HCG levels are obtained. All high-risk cases should receive from one to three chemotherapy courses after titers become negative.

Surgery may be indicated for severe hemorrhage, uterine infection, or urinary tract obstruction. Hysterectomy is also useful in patients who do not desire more children, since less chemotherapy may be required thereafter. In this instance the surgery is generally performed during the first course of chemotherapy.

Radiotherapy is used as adjunctive treatment for patients with cerebral or hepatic metastases. Whole-organ irradiation decreases the incidence of hemorrhage.

Patients who have responded to therapy require HCG titers to be checked every 2 weeks for 3 months, then every month for 3 months, followed by every 2 months for 6 months, and thereafter every 6 months for life. Pregnancy is contraindicated for a year.

Prognosis in low-risk cases is excellent, with cure rates up to 98% and retained fertility in 90% of those desiring further pregnancies; nor is there an increased incidence of congenital anomalies in these children. In high-risk cases the cure rate is 50%–80% if managed in specialized centers.

Reviews

1. Surwit, E. A., and Hammond, C. B. Gestational Trophoblastic Neoplasia. In R. M. Pitkin and F. J. Zlatnick (Eds.), *1980 Year Book of Obstetrics and Gynecology.* Chicago: Year Book, 1980.
   Summarizes the experience of the Southeastern Regional Trophoblastic Disease Center at Duke University.
2. Management of gestational trophoblastic neoplasia. *ACOG Tech. Bull.* No. 59, December, 1980.
   Patients with poor-prognosis disease are probably best treated in regional trophoblastic disease centers.

Diagnosis

3. Woodward, R. M., Filly, R. A., and Callen, P. W. First trimester molar pregnancy: Nonspecific ultrasonographic appearance. *Obstet. Gynecol.* 55:31S, 1980.
   Three cases of early molar pregnancy did not exhibit characteristic ultrasound features.
4. Berkowitz, R. S., et al. Pretreatment curettage—A predictor of chemotherapy response in gestational trophoblastic neoplasia. *Gynecol. Oncol.* 10:39, 1980.
   Worsened trophoblastic histology in pretreatment curettings was associated with the necessity for multiple courses of chemotherapy.
5. Berkowitz, R. S., Goldstein, D. P., and Bernstein, M. R. Laparoscopy in the management of gestational trophoblastic neoplasms. *J. Reprod. Med.* 24:261, 1980.
   Helpful in diagnosing unsuspected uterine perforation, abdominal metastases, and ovarian cyst complications.

Pathology

6. Kuhn, R. J. P., Long, A. R., and Fortune, D. W. Choriocarcinoma coexistent with intrauterine pregnancy. *Aust. N.Z. J. Obstet. Gynaecol.* 20:94, 1980.
   Reviews the literature (30 cases) regarding presentation, pathogenesis, and survival.
7. Federschneider, J. M., et al. Natural history of recurrent molar pregnancy. *Obstet. Gynecol.* 55:457, 1980.
   Reviews literature and adds 7 cases. None of the patients had normal pregnancies after two consecutive moles.
8. Nisula, B. C., and Taliadouros, G. S. Thyroid function in gestational trophoblastic neoplasia. Evidence that the thyrotropic activity of chorionic gonadotropin mediates the thyrotoxicosis of choriocarcinoma. *Am. J. Obstet. Gynecol.* 138:77, 1980.
   HCG has intrinsic thyroid-stimulating activity, and 3% of patients with GTN exhibit hyperthyroidism.
9. Vassilakos, P., Riotton, G., and Kajii, T. Hydatidiform mole: Two entities. *Am. J. Obstet. Gynecol.* 127:167, 1977.
   Moles may be complete (diploid, usually XX, androgenetic in origin, no fetal development) or partial (fetus at some stage, triploid).
10. Yamashita, K., et al. Human lymphocyte antigen expression in hydatidiform mole: Androgenesis following fertilization by a haploid sperm. *Am. J. Obstet. Gynecol.* 135:597, 1979.
    Moles develop from an egg fertilized by a haploid sperm that duplicates its own chromosomes after meiosis.

Management

11. Berkowitz, R. S., et al. Methotrexate with citrovorum factor rescue. Reduced chemotherapy toxicity in the management of gestational trophoblastic neoplasms. *Cancer* 45:423, 1980.
    Alternating folinic acid with methotrexate reduced the incidence of hepatic and/or hematologic toxicity to 4%, and no patients developed skin rash or marked alopecia. This may be the best therapy for all but poor-prognosis patients.
12. Twiggs, L. B., Morrow, C. P., and Schlaerth, J. B. Acute pulmonary complications of molar pregnancy. *Am. J. Obstet. Gynecol.* 135:189, 1979.
    Acute respiratory distress developed in 12 of 128 patients after evacuation of a mole; 7 of the 12 required chemotherapy thereafter. This complication may be related to trophoblastic emboli.

13. Hammond, C. B., Weed, J. C., Jr., and Currie, J. L. The role of operation in the current therapy of gestational trophoblastic disease. *Am. J. Obstet. Gynecol.* 136:844, 1980.
Wound healing or postoperative complications do not appear to be adversely affected by chemotherapy.

Poor-Prognosis Disease

14. Surwit, E. A., and Hammond, C. B. Treatment of metastatic trophoblastic disease with poor prognosis. *Obstet. Gynecol.* 55:565, 1980.
Usual criteria for marrow function must be temporized. Aggressive multiagent chemotherapy with transfusions, antibiotics, total parenteral nutrition, and intensive medical management are essential for improved survival in these high-risk patients who usually show marked immunosuppression after prolonged treatment.

15. Grumbine, F. C., et al. Management of liver metastasis from gestational trophoblastic neoplasia. *Am. J. Obstet. Gynecol.* 137:969, 1980.
Suggests the use of selective hepatic artery occlusion and simultaneous multiagent chemotherapy.

16. Weed, J. C., Jr., and Hammond, C. B. Cerebral metastatic choriocarcinoma: Intensive therapy and prognosis. *Obstet. Gynecol.* 55:89, 1980.
Recommends use of computerized axial tomogram (CAT) scan for diagnosis and follow-up.

17. Miller, J. M., Jr., Surwit, E. A., and Hammond, C. B. Choriocarcinoma following term pregnancy. *Obstet. Gynecol.* 53:207, 1979.
These authors feel that post-term gestation choriocarcinoma tends to metastasize more extensively and is less responsive to chemotherapy.

18. Bagshawe, K. D. Choriocarcinoma: Can we afford to cure cancer? *Ann. R. Coll. Surg. Engl.* 60:36, 1978.
Bagshawe's multiagent regimes employ up to seven chemotherapeutic agents in an attempt to maximize response while minimizing toxicity.

Placenta Previa

Placenta previa is defined as trophoblastic implantation on the lower uterine segment that obstructs the presenting part prior to or during labor. The nomenclature regarding placenta previa is confusing. In total placenta previa the placenta covers the entire internal cervical os. On the other hand, partial placenta previa describes the situation in which only a portion of the internal cervical os is covered. The percentage of cervix covered can change, depending on the dilatation of the cervix. Finally, marginal or low-lying placenta previa is a condition in which the leading edge of the placenta reaches the internal cervical os but does not encroach on any part of it. Another term for the low-lying variety may be *lateral placenta previa*. The only practical value of this classification is that vaginal delivery can occur in all but the total placenta previa, although it is less likely to do so if a large amount of internal os is covered.

Most reviews quote an incidence of placenta previa ranging from 1 in 100 to 1 in 250, and it is much more common in multiparas than in those with low parity. Parity is seen as the most common etiology of placenta previa in that the endometrium in the fundal region has been scarred by previous implantation and the fertilized egg searches for a more favorable location for nidation. In addition, if the placenta is quite large (as in multiple gestation or with syphilis or Rh disease) it may cover a larger area of the uterus, including the cervix; in these cases it is viewed as an adaptation phenomenon. Associated but not necessarily etiologic factors include prematurity, uterine or fetal anomalies, abnormal presentations, and other abnormalities of the placenta such as succenturiate lobes.

The most common clinical manifestation is significant but painless vaginal bleeding in the third trimester, particularly around the thirty-fourth week. This is the time when the placenta previa is most likely to be disturbed by the thinning of the lower uterine segment. The initial bleeding episode is usually limited and, while it may be substantial in amount, it is seldom enough to produce maternal shock or fetal compromise. The physical examination of the fundal area reveals the uterus to be nontender and soft. Usually on Leopold maneuvers the presenting part is not engaged and the fetus usually presents in a breech, oblique, or transverse lie. Although the bleeding that accompanies placenta previa is usually painless, about a quarter of the patients who have it will experience concomitant spontaneous labor, while 10% will show some evidence of placental abruption. Uterine irritability or firmness suggests an abruption. The differential diagnosis should include abruptio placentae, genital lacerations, excessive show, cervical lesions, nongenital bleeding (rectum or bladder), and blood dyscrasias.

The diagnostic procedures that are available should be preceded by adequate preparation with regard to blood replacement. Three to four units of packed red blood cells should be crossmatched and available, while a large bore intravenous catheter should be initiated to allow intravenous fluid replacement. The most important thing to determine before any invasive procedure is performed is the maturity of the fetus. If by history and physical examination the patient is near term (>37 weeks), the appropriate direct intervention steps such as examination in the operating theater can be undertaken. On the other hand, if there is a question about the maturity or the gestational age of the fetus (<37 weeks) or the gestational age is known to be premature, less invasive forms of diagnosis are carried out. This initial division of management assumes, as it will be in most cases, that extensive hemorrhage is not continuing.

The most common diagnostic tool is real time ultrasonography (USG). It is noninvasive and can be performed in the labor suite without moving the patient. Advantages include its assessment of placental location, documentation of fetal maturity (by biparietal diameter), and location of fluid for amniocentesis. Disadvantages of USG relate to its nonspecificity in delineating the marginal placenta previa and the estimate of fetal maturity, which is ± 3 weeks. Amniography, in which 30–50 cc of radiopaque dye (Conray, Renograffin-60) can be injected into the amniotic sac, can also be used to outline the placenta. It is important that, if one uses amniography, the megulamine dyes should be used so that the sodium content will not be so high as to initiate labor. Additionally, soft tissue x-ray has been utilized, but it is not very accurate. Placental localization using radioactive iodinated albumin or technetium can also be performed. While isotopes are not generally used during pregnancy, these actually provide less radiation to the fetus than simple soft tissue radiography. Arteriography, while accurate, is time-consuming and very complicated for both mother and fetus. Thermography has been used but like isotope scans is very difficult to interpret, particularly if the placenta is posterior.

Once the diagnosis is established, therapy for placenta previa is performed on the basis of fetal maturation in an attempt to yield the maximum of fetal time in utero combined with the minimum of maternal risk. Next, the patient is approached with a simple speculum exam to rule out any vaginal or cervical lesions. If fetal immaturity has been documented and no extensive hemorrhage is present, "expectant management" is by far the most salient choice. In many centers, a two- to threefold decrease in perinatal mortality has been obtained by the conservative management when the fetus was not mature. On the other hand, if there is a question of fetal immaturity, an amniocentesis should be performed and conservative management maintained until the results are known. In cases of fetal immaturity, bedrest (until the bleeding ceases) and then gradual ambulation is the rule. In many cases, several weeks to months in gestational age can be gained with simple modified bedrest in the hospital and, in some cases, at home. Repeat episodes of bleeding during the conservative management of these patients, particularly to the point of continued transfusions, often force the clinician's hand toward an operative delivery.

In cases in which aggressive therapy is called for (continued bleeding or documented maturity), abdominal delivery or a double set-up examination is necessary. In the double set-up exam, the blood is ready and the scrub nurse and anesthesiologist are standing by while the patient is examined in an operating room. A sterile speculum examination is done to rule out other genital lesions. If the digital examination of the cervix reveals cervical dilatation, and if the placenta previa is not central, the vertex may be guided into the pelvis, the membranes ruptured, and vaginal delivery attempted by use of either spontaneous labor or pitocin. On the other hand, fetal maturity being assured, if the double set-up reveals a total placenta previa or a large degree of placenta previa, then cesarean section is the mode of delivery of choice.

If cesarean section is the option taken, the low vertical uterine incision should be the choice since a transverse incision would usually find the lower uterine segment not fully developed and covered with placenta. The fetus may sustain an enormous amount of blood loss during the operative procedure if the placental area is incised; and it may suffer from acute asphyxia due to placental shunting. Likewise, the incisional area may not heal as rapidly and certainly the lower uterine segment forms a nidus for infection. Therefore, the early use of therapeutic antibiotics for 3 to 5 days (prior to surgery through the postpartum period) is recommended. In addition, since there is no contractile force in the lower uterine segment to reduce postpartum bleeding, lifesaving hysterectomy or ligation of internal iliac arteries occasionally is mandatory for massive hemorrhage.

The outlook for both mother and baby in placenta previa is extremely good. The maternal death rate is said to be less than 1 per 1000 and almost all of these are due to complications of placenta previa, such as infection or intolerable hemorrhage with placenta increta or percreta. The outcome for the fetus is likewise very bright in uncomplicated cases in which the diagnosis and management is undertaken with skill. On the other hand, if there is uncontrollable hemorrhage, concomitant placental separation, improper timing and/or method of delivery, then the outlook for the fetus can be quite grim. This particular medical problem underscores the need for the team approach to perinatal care. There must be close cooperation between the obstetric, neonatal, and anesthesia personnel in the management of such patients.

Review

1. Hibbard, L. T. Placenta Previa. In J. J. Sciarra (Ed.), *Gynecology and Obstetrics*. Hagerstown, Md.: Harper & Row, 1979. Vol. 2.
   A very clinical review of the etiology, diagnosis, and management aspects of placenta previa.

2. Pritchard, J. A., and MacDonald, P. C. *Williams Obstetrics.* New York: Appleton-Century-Crofts, 1976. P. 416.
   An in-depth assessment of the subject, including 72 references.
3. Tatum, H., and Mule, J. Placenta previa: A functional classification and a report on 408 cases. *Am. J. Obstet. Gynecol.* 46:118, 1952.
   A report on the nomenclature of placenta previa, one that is still used today. Also, there is discussion of over 400 cases and their management.
4. Crenshaw, C. Placenta previa: A survey of twenty years experience with improved perinatal survival by expectant therapy and cesarean delivery. *Obstet. Gynecol. Surv.* 28: 461, 1973.
   One of the best papers demonstrating the improved perinatal survival by expectant management and abdominal delivery compared with the previous management plans.

Etiology
5. Iffy, L. Contributions to the etiology of placenta previa. *Am. J. Obstet. Gynecol.* 50:969, 1962.
   A complex and classic paper regarding the etiology of placenta previa. The attractive feature of each etiologic factor is explored in depth.
6. Tremewan, R. N., Chandra, M., and Duff, G. B. The mid-trimester low lying placenta: A prospective study. *N.Z. Med. J.* 92:151, 1980.
   This study demonstrates that although the percentage of low-lying placenta previas during the midtrimester is very high, it is reduced by placental migration (growth of the uterine fundus) as pregnancy progresses.
7. Ballas, S., et al. Midtrimester placenta previa: Normal or pathologic finding. *Obstet. Gynecol.* 54:12, 1979.
   The mechanics behind placental migration are detailed. The significance of the midtrimester placenta previa is discussed.
8. Brenner, W. E., Edelman, D. A., and Hendricks, C. H. Characteristics of patients with placenta previa and results of "expectant management." *Am. J. Obstet. Gynecol.* 132:180, 1978.
   One hundred and eighty-five patients with placenta previa were studied. Higher portions of these patients were multiparous, were older, had had previous abortions, and were carrying male fetuses or twins. Rate of prematurity, antepartum and intrapartum fetal death, neonatal death, congenital abnormality and low Apgar scores in the neonate were higher among patients who had placenta previa.
9. Naeye, R. L., et al. Placenta previa. Predisposing factors and effects on the fetus and surviving infants. *Obstet. Gynecol.* 52:521, 1978.
   The perinatal death associated with placenta previa is 73 per 100,000 births. The frequency of death increased with short maternal stature, increasing parity, prior preterm deliveries, and prior perinatal death. More male infants died than females, and the infants had a pattern of fetal growth retardation characteristic of undernutrition. Long-term physical growth and psychomotor development were normal except for a small increase in neurologic abnormalities.
10. Wexler, P., and Gottesfeld, K. R. Second trimester placenta previa. An apparently normal placentation. *Obstet. Gynecol.* 50:706, 1977.
    Placental positions in 214 patients undergoing genetic amniocentesis were reviewed. Low-lying placenta, or placenta previa, may be a normal variant in early pregnancy. Parity 4 or more, but not age, correlated with an increased incidence of partial or total placenta previa, but not with a low-lying placenta.

Complications
11. Macafee, C. H. G., et al. Maternal and fetal mortality in placenta previa. *J. Obstet. Gynaecol. Br. Commonw.* 69:203, 1962.

An overall review of the maternal and neonatal statistics as regards placenta previa. Suggestions for improvement in management are outlined.

12. Neri, A., et al. Impact of placenta previa on intrauterine fetal growth. *Isr. J. Med. Sci.* 16:429, 1980.
These authors indicate that placenta previa may be a frequent cause of intrauterine growth retardation although it definitely contributes to premature infants in general.

13. Jouppila, P., et al. Vaginal bleeding in the last two trimesters of pregnancy. A clinical and ultrasonic study. *Acta Obstet. Gynecol. Scand.* 58:461, 1979.
A review of 97 cases of vaginal bleeding during the second and third trimesters of pregnancy is presented. The perinatal mortality was 11%, and the rate of premature delivery was 23% compared to 22% and 35% respectively, in cases of recurrent bleeding. Placenta previa of some degree was the most common definite etiologic factor behind the bleeding.

14. Collins, M., O'Brien, P., and Tabrah, N. Placenta previa percreta with bladder invasion. *J.A.M.A.* 240:1749, 1978.
First reported in 1900, placenta percreta is a rare but potentially catastrophic obstetric condition, with a high incidence of fetal death and maternal morbidity and mortality. Reported is a case of placenta previa percreta with bladder invasion that resulted in massive hemorrhage and prolonged shock.

Diagnosis

15. Knox-Macaulay, H. H., Smith, O. A., and Scott, A. [131]I isotope placentography: Simple counting equipment in obstetric practice. *Int. J. Gynaecol. Obstet.* 18:136, 1980.
This article outlines a simplified method of using isotopes in placentography.

16. Wexler, P., and Gottesfeld, K. R. Early diagnosis of placenta previa. *Obstet. Gynecol.* 54:231, 1979.
The methods of early diagnosis of placenta previa are explored; principally, ultrasound is used.

17. Rizos, N., et al. Natural history of placenta previa ascertained by diagnostic ultrasound. *Am. J. Obstet. Gynecol.* 133:287, 1979.
The use of diagnostic ultrasound in following the progress of placenta previas diagnosed early in pregnancy is detailed by the authors. An excellent review of the possible etiologies of placenta previa are also given.

18. Honor'e, E., and Frederiksen, P. B. Placenta scintigraphy using markers of the uterine cervix and pelvic skeleton. *Acta Radiol.* (Stockh.) 20:111, 1979.
The modality of placental scintigraphy is outlined. Although it is not widely used, it may prove useful in some cases.

19. Edelstone, E. I., et al. Placenta localization by ultrasound. *Clin. Obstet. Gynecol.* 20:285, 1977.
A review of various aspects of placentography by ultrasound, namely, the scanning techniques currently utilized and the indications for their use in the antepartum period.

20. Sand, H., et al. Ultrasonic diagnosis of placenta praevia. *Acta Obstet. Gynecol. Scand.* 56:109, 1977.
The ultrasound diagnosis during the last trimester correlated with the findings at delivery in most cases.

21. Mittelstaedt, C. A., et al. Placenta previa: Significance in the second trimester. *Radiology* 131:465, 1979.

A prospective study of 98 patients to determine the risk of a second trimes-
ter placenta previa remaining until term. The overall incidence of a
second trimester placenta previa persisting until term was 8.8%.

22. Kurjak, A., and Barsie, B. Changes of placental site diagnosed by repeated ultrasonic examination. *Acta Obstet. Gynecol. Scand.* 56:161, 1977.
Midpregnancy ultrasound in 67 patients showed placenta previa. Repeat
scans demonstrated placental migration in 63 of the 67 patients.

Management

23. Cotton, D. B., et al. The conservative aggressive management of
placenta previa. *Am. J. Obstet. Gynecol.* 137:687, 1980.
the most up-to-date reference indicating the various management tech-
niques available for placenta previa. An excellent review of previous treat-
ment regimens is offered.
24. Hill, D. J., and Beischer, N. A. Placenta previa without antepartum
haemorrhage. *Aust. N.Z. J. Obstet. Gynaecol.* 20:21, 1980.
A large number of patients with placenta previa do not have hemorrhage
until late in pregnancy or during early labor. A warning is given against
frequent pelvic exams in which the cervix is invaded in the last trimester,
even in the absence of bleeding.

Abruptio Placentae

Abruptio placentae is the premature separation of the normally implanted
placenta. The etiology of placental abruption remains obscure, although
pregnancy-induced or chronic hypertension occurs in 47% of patients with
abruption. Many investigators also find high parity to be associated with
abruptio placentae, while trauma, unusually short umbilical cord, uterine
anomaly, or uterine tumors are occasionally implicated. Sudden uterine decompression, as may occur with the release of hydramnios or following delivery of the first fetus in multiple gestations, may also lead to premature
separation of the placenta. Furthermore, experimental obstruction of the inferior vena cava and ovarian vein has been reported to produce placental abruption, but this has not been proved clinically. Finally, folic acid deficiency
has been reported to have an etiologic role in placental abruption, but this
hypothesis has been carefully examined and there is no evidence to support
it.

Women with a history of a spontaneous abortion are more likely to suffer
later abruptio placentae. The patient who has had an abruptio placentae is
10 to 15 times more likely to have a recurrence. Of all pregnancies 3.5% are
associated with third trimester bleeding; nearly one-third of these are due to
abruptio placentae, for an incidence of 0.49%–1.29% of deliveries, depending
upon the diagnostic criterion. In significant cases, some of the bleeding from
the placental abruption usually insinuates itself between the membranes
and the uterus, escapes through the cervix, and appears as vaginal bleeding.
Less often, the blood does not escape externally but remains between the
placental abruption and uterine wall. This concealed hemorrhage is a much
greater maternal hazard as the extent of the hemorrhage is not appreciated.
The amount of vaginal bleeding bears no relation to the degree of placental
separation.

Abruptio placentae is initiated by hemorrhage into the decidua basalis.
Consequently the process in its earliest stage consists of the development of a

decidual hematoma that leads to separation, compression, and ultimate destruction of the portion of the placenta adjacent to the separation. Since the uterus is still distended by the products of conception, it is unable to contract and compress the torn vessels supplying the placental site.

The clinical findings of a placental abruption are abdominal pain (which may be variable in intensity), vaginal bleeding, hypertonic contractions, uterine tenderness, absence of fetal heart sounds, and variable evidence of hypovolemia. Oliguria, caused by inadequate renal perfusion, is frequently observed in these circumstances. Many deviations from this typical picture occur. In concealed hemorrhage there is no vaginal bleeding, but uterine rigidity and tenderness is likely to be pronounced. Unless the majority of the placenta has been separated, the fetal heart tones are usually audible. The mild forms of abruptio are more common and more difficult to recognize clinically. It is necessary to rule out placenta previa and other causes of bleeding by clinical inspection and sonographic study. Hematoma of the rectus muscles, degeneration of fibroids, twisted ovarian cyst, appendicitis, or any acute abdominal emergency must be considered in the differential diagnosis.

Abruptio placentae has complications that affect the fetus as well as the mother. Fetal loss is high, ranging from 25%–50% in abruptio placentae, and accounts for 15%–20% of all perinatal deaths. Disseminated intravascular coagulopathy (DIC) occurs in approximately 30% of patients with abruptio placentae. The mechanism of DIC in placental abruption is due to the release of tissue thromboplastin into the circulation. The coagulation system is activated by the latter. This results in the conversion of prothrombin into thrombin. Thrombin, in turn, cleaves fibrinogen into fibrin monomer, which polymerizes to form an unstable gel. Fibrin monomer is then converted into fibrin by Factor XIII. The coagulation process activates the fibrinolytic system by conversion of the plasminogen into plasmin, and proteolytic enzymes digest both fibrinogen and fibrin. These fibrin degradation products also interfere with normal blood coagulation. Clinically, the patients with DIC may manifest heavy uterine bleeding and/or spontaneous bleeding from extragenital sites such as bladder, nose, or venous punctures.

Renal failure occurs in 1%–3% of patients and is usually reversible unless there is delayed or incomplete treatment of hypovolemia. The precise cause of renal damage that may be associated with placental abruption is not clear. It might be due to vasospasm within the kidney secondary to hypovolemia; adequate blood replacement therefore plays an important role in its prevention.

In the severe form of placental abruption (uteroplacental apoplexy or Couvelaire uterus), widespread extravasation of blood often takes place into the uterine musculature and beneath the uterine serosa. Such effusion of blood is also seen occasionally beneath the tubal serosa in the connective tissue of the broad ligament and in the substance of the ovary, as well as in the peritoneal cavity. The incidence of postpartum hemorrhage is increased in patients with placental abruption and may be due to coagulation defects.

The hemorrhage and the hypovolemia due to abruptio placentae demands immediate treatment. Administration of fluids intravenously, packed red cells, fresh frozen plasma, or platelets may be required. The use of whole blood is unusual since it must be less than 12 hours old or it will not suffice. The amount transfused will be determined by the patient's response. Urine flow should be kept to at least 30 cc per hour. In case of oliguria, the central venous pressure (CVP) should be monitored and more fluid administered. Since the CVP measurement might not detect early pulmonary congestion, the patient must also be observed for other signs, especially dyspnea, cough, and rales in the chest. During the time period in which blood is to be replaced, the status of the fetus should be evaluated.

There has been much controversy regarding timing and method of delivery in placental abruption. It has been felt by many that delivery should be accomplished within 6 hours of the onset of abruption. However, there is some evidence that maternal results are not related to time elapsing until delivery but rather to the adequacy of treatment of blood loss. If abruption appears to be mild and there is no fetal distress, most advocate induction of labor with amniotomy and oxytocin with a view toward vaginal delivery, resorting to cesarean birth if fetal or maternal condition deteriorates or labor does not begin in a reasonable length of time. In the severe form, if the baby is alive, cesarean section should be done immediately in order to maximize fetal survival. If there is no evidence of fetal life, vaginal delivery is preferred unless hemorrhage is so brisk that it cannot be successfully managed by means of blood replacement, or there are other obstetric complications that contraindicate vaginal delivery. If vaginal delivery is not possible, it may be necessary to perform an abdominal procedure even if the infant is dead or in the face of DIC. In all cases, intensive management of each patient will result in the best outcome.

Review
1. Preucell, R. W., Lavin, J. P., and Colman, R. W. Placental Abruption and Premature Separation. In J. J. Sciarra (Ed.), *Gynecology and Obstetrics*. Hagerstown, Md.: Harper & Row, 1980. Vol. 2.
   A very complete review of placental abruption, its causes, and its treatment.

Etiology
2. Goujard, J., et al. Maternal smoking, alcohol consumption, and abruptio placentae. *Am. J. Obstet. Gynecol.* 130:738, 1978.
   Recent paper emphasizes the possible etiologic role of maternal smoking in fetal death caused by abruptio placentae.
3. Patterson, M. E. L. The aetiology and outcome of abruptio placentae. *Acta Obstet. Gynecol. Scand.* 58:31, 1979.
   The incidence of abruptio placentae was 0.55%, the recurrence rate was 5.6%, and the perinatal mortality was 35%.
4. Pritchard, J. A. Genesis of severe placental abruption. *Am. J. Obstet. Gynecol.* 108:24, 1970.
   The author details the clinical and laboratory studies frequently found in cases of severe placental separation. Management techniques and methods of follow-up are listed.

Clinical Features
5. Lundberg, J. Diagnosis of abruptio placentae by ultrasound. *Lancet* 1:806, 1971.
   The author details the mechanism of diagnosis of placental abruption by the use of ultrasound and suggests methods of management.

Complications
6. Notelovitz, M., et al. Painless abruptio placentae. *Obstet. Gynecol.* 53:270, 1979.
   The abruption of a posteriorly inserted placenta that is severe enough to cause fetal death differs from the usual clinical presentation of abruptio placentae. It is characterized only by vaginal bleeding and backache. The uterus is invariably nontender, relaxes well between contractions. Fetal mortality is high.
7. Sher, G. Pathogenesis and management of uterine inertia complicating

abruptio placentae with consumption coagulopathy. *Am. J. Obstet. Gynecol.* 129:164, 1977.

Hemorrhagic diathesis due to consumption coagulopathy occurs in about 10% of cases of abruptio placentae. Approximately 1 in 5 of these patients presents with failure to progress in labor due to uterine inertia.

8. Blair, R. G. Abruption of the placenta. *J. Obstet. Gynaecol. Br. Commonw.* 80:242, 1973.

In 189 cases of abruption of the placenta, there was one maternal death with a perinatal loss of 55%.

Management

9. Sher, G. A rational basis for the management of abruptio placentae. *J. Reprod. Med.* 21:123, 1978.

A fibrinolytic inhibitor has been used to stop the lysis and enhance the anticoagulation effects of fibrin degradation products. Management protocols are introduced.

10. Knad, D. R. Abruptio placentae: An assessment of the time and method of delivery. *Obstet. Gynecol.* 52:625, 1978.

Analysis of 388 cases of abruptio placentae indicated that 75% of fetal deaths occurred more than 90 minutes after admission to the hospital, and almost 70% of all perinatal mortality occurred in infants who were delivered more than 2 hours after the time of diagnosis.

11. Lunan, C. B. The management of abruptio placentae. *J. Obstet. Gynaecol. Br. Commonw.* 80:120, 1973.

In 379 cases studied perinatal mortality was 38%. They advocate intensive fetal monitoring and readiness to do cesarean section in most patients with abruptio placentae.

12. Golditch, I. M., and Boyce, E. Management of abruptio placentae. *J.A.M.A.* 212:288, 1970.

One hundred and thirty cases were studied and the authors' recommendation is for vaginal delivery after amniotomy and oxytocin stimulation in mild cases. In moderate and severe cases, if vaginal delivery is not imminent, the viable fetus probably will not survive unless cesarean section is performed as soon as possible.

13. Muldoon, M. J. The use of central venous pressure monitoring in abruptio placentae. *J. Obstet. Gynaecol. Br. Commonw.* 76:225, 1969.

The advantages of monitoring the central venous pressure in patients with abruptio placentae are detailed. Case management presentations are given.

14. Sher, G. Trasylol in the management of abruptio placentae with consumption coagulopathy and uterine inertia. *J. Reprod. Med.* 25:113, 1980.

Forty patients with abruptio placentae complicated by intrauterine fetal demise and consumptive coagulopathy were treated with Trasylol intravenously. All but 1 patient so treated improved.

Essential Hypertension

Hypertension is one of the most common medical complications of pregnancy and has a reported incidence of 6%–30%. One-third to one-half of these patients are women with essential hypertension. When the mean arterial pressure is greater than 90 mm Hg during the second trimester, there is a significant increase in the rate of stillbirths, preeclampsia, and small for gestational age (SGA) infants. Overall perinatal mortality is reported to be 8%–15% but is even higher with superimposed preeclampsia. Differentiating between chronic essential hypertension complicating pregnancy and pregnancy-induced hypertension (PIH) can be very difficult. All obstetric patients experience a decrease in blood pressure in the second trimester because the placenta is a low resistance system in parallel with the mother's circulation. Women with moderate chronic hypertension may therefore have normal blood pressure recordings if first seen during midpregnancy. In late pregnancy, however, when the blood pressure rises to prepregnancy levels, the hypertension may be erroneously attributed to acute PIH.

The diagnosis of preexisting hypertension is secure only if it is confirmed prior to pregnancy or if the patient demonstrates elevated blood pressure prior to the twentieth week of gestation. Essential hypertension is also suspected, in retrospect, in the patient who receives the diagnosis of PIH but in whom there is persistent hypertension postpartum. Although unproved, it is possible that latent hypertension is unmasked by pregnancy. Clues that favor the diagnosis of chronic preexisting hypertension include: (1) hypertension associated with chronic diseases such as diabetes mellitus, renal disease, and collagen diseases; (2) abnormal optic fundi (hemorrhages or exudates); and (3) abnormal renal function tests (BUN greater than 20 mg/dml or plasma creatinine greater than 1 mg/dml).

In addition to essential hypertension, other chronic causes of elevated blood pressure must be considered. Conditions such as vascular abnormalities (renal vascular disease, coarctation of aorta), endocrinopathies (diabetes mellitus, pheochromocytoma, hyperaldosteronism), and renal disease (glomerulonephritis, pyelonephritis, collagen disease with renal involvement, polycystic disease) should be included in the differential diagnosis. A flank bruit is suggestive of renovascular hypertension, whereas coarctation of the aorta can be detected by comparing arterial pressures in upper and lower extremities and by palpating in femoral arteries.

The greatest threat of chronic essential hypertension to the obstetric patient is the increased prevalence of superimposed PIH. Although a diastolic pressure of 95 or more has been shown to increase the risk of fetal death, it is the development of superimposed PIH that jeopardizes the mother. The three common signs are: accelerating hypertension, onset or worsening of proteinuria, and edema. The diagnosis can be based on one sign if it is severe but is more secure if at least two signs are present. The sudden presence of headaches, visual disturbance, tremulousness, or epigastric pain often means impending convulsion.

Accurate documentation of gestational age is extremely important in the management of the pregnant woman with hypertension. In addition to the risk of superimposed preeclampsia, many of the fetuses in these women will be SGA. An early correlation of uterine size and menstrual dates and documentation of first documented fetal heart tones by fetoscope are all significant data. Because of the increased incidence of SGA infants, serial ultrasonography should be performed in these women. Growth retardation in the fetus is more common in patients with chronic hypertension than in patients with PIH. Serial measurements of fundal height, progressive increases in estimated fetal weight, and appropriate increments in maternal weight are indications of fetal growth.

Initial evaluation of the pregnant woman with essential hypertension should include careful examination of optic fundi and renal evaluation by checking a 24-hour urine sample for protein and creatinine clearance. In addition, a chest x-ray and electrocardiogram are appropriate if the hypertension has been longstanding or there is any question of heart disease. Because of the high mortality rate in pregnant women with undiagnosed pheochromocytoma, a screening urine metanephrine should be done in women with severe hypertension.

Ideally, women of childbearing age who have chronic hypertension should be counseled *before* they become pregnant. This is not always possible. A patient with chronic hypertension and a past episode of severe PIH or eclampsia has at least a 50% chance of recurrent PIH, while the normotensive patient with a past history of severe PIH or eclampsia has only a one in four chance of recurrence. Unfortunately, the next episode is often more severe and occurs at an earlier stage of pregnancy.

Management of pregnancy complicated by essential hypertension is controversial. The only point of universal agreement is restriction of physical activity. In addition to increased bed rest, the hypertensive gravida should limit household duties, shopping, and exercise. Often neglected is dietary counseling. While sodium may exacerbate hypertension, its restriction may decrease placental perfusion. The appropriate diet does not exceed 2 g sodium or 5 g table salt. Most patients with mild to moderate hypertension will not require medication during pregnancy. One of the major unresolved questions in management is whether there is autoregulation of uterine blood flow in the human. If there is no autoregulation, placental perfusion will vary directly with maternal arterial pressure, in which case a reduction in blood pressure might be detrimental to the fetus. On the other hand, if autoregulation of uterine blood flow is present, reduction of blood pressure to "normal" would present no problem. European obstetricians have been more aggressive in their treatment of women with chronic hypertension by attempting to maintain diastolic blood pressure in the range of 80–90 mm Hg. In the United States, most centers have not given antihypertensive medication for diastolic blood pressure under 100 mm Hg, and some centers do not institute therapy until diastolic blood pressure exceeds 110 mm Hg.

Two management questions frequently arise: What is the agent of choice, and what course is proper for the pregnant patient who is already on an established antihypertensive regimen? Alpha methyldopa (Aldomet) is the oral medication of choice. The customary initial dose is 750 mg/day. This may be increased to a total of 3 g daily. Occasionally it is necessary to add oral hydralazine to maintain a diastolic pressure in the 90–100 range. Lower pressures are not desirable because of possible adverse effects on placental perfusion. It is emphasized that medications are *not* prescribed for the patient with suspected PIH, but rather for the chronic hypertensive patient whose diastolic pressure exceeds 100–110. Diuretics are contraindicated in pregnancy—except in the rare patient with pulmonary edema or congestive heart failure. Diuretics acutely reduce placental blood flow (as measured by placental clearance of dehydroisoandrosterone sulfate). Evidence also suggests that the chronic use of diuretics reduces birth weight of infants while making maternal pancreatitis more likely. Electrolyte disturbances, fetal thrombocytopenia, and neonatal jaundice are also well-established consequences of diuretic therapy. Most authorities discontinue maintenance diuretics when pregnancy is discovered. Oral methyldopa and hydralazine can be continued. Until more evidence is accumulated, propranolol and other beta blockers are best discontinued.

Fetal surveillance is important in the woman with chronic hypertension. In addition to serial ultrasonography, a weekly nonstress test (NST) or contraction stress test (CST) should be performed. In women with mild hypertension antepartum fetal heart rate tests should be started at 34 weeks of gestation. In women with severe hypertension, a history of previous stillbirths, or suspicion of an SGA fetus these tests should be initiated at 28 to 32 weeks.

Timing of delivery is a crucial question in all high-risk pregnancies. This decision is easy when the fetus is mature and the cervix is favorable for induction; even with mild hypertension, there is no benefit from procrastination. A well-monitored induction of labor is indicated. When there is evidence of superimposed PIH or if severe intrauterine growth retardation is suspected, it is necessary to deliver the infant prior to 37 weeks. In this situation, it is comforting that maternal hypertension is associated with accelerated maturation of fetal lungs. After 32 to 34 weeks gestation, the risk of severe respiratory distress syndrome in the neonate diminishes when compared to newborns who are products of normal pregnancies of similar duration. When superimposed pregnancy-induced hypertension occurs, convulsions should be prevented by use of magnesium sulfate and any severe hypertension (systolic greater than 160, diastolic greater than 110) should be controlled with intravenous hydralazine. Once superimposed PIH is established, delivery is the only cure. Induction of labor with oxytocin is recommended unless an obstetric indication necessitates cesarean birth.

Reviews

1. Davidson, J. M., and Lindheimer, M. D. Hypertension and Pregnancy. In J. J. Sciarra and R. Depp (Eds.), *Gynecology and Obstetrics*. Hagerstown, Md.: Harper & Row, 1977. Vol. 3.
   Recent 20-page overview of hypertension complicating pregnancy.
2. Gant, N. F., and Worley, F. J. *Hypertension in Pregnancy*. New York: Appleton-Century-Crofts, 1980.
   An excellent book-length review of both basic science and clinical management. Includes a critical analysis of major topics on this subject.
3. Roberts, J. M., and Perloff, D. L. Hypertension and the obstetrician-gynecologist. *Am. J. Obstet. Gynecol.* 127:316, 1977.
   Concise review of hypertensive problems of the female patient.

Physiology and Pathophysiology

4. Chesley, L. C. The renin-angiotensin system in pregnancy. *J. Reprod. Med.* 15:173, 1975.
   For the student seeking basic science understanding of the renin-angiotensin-aldosterone system in pregnancy.
5. Marx, J. L. Natriuretic hormone linked to hypertension. *Science.* 212:1255, 1981.
   The author proposed that excess salt in the diet may produce hypertension by releasing a natriuretic hormone into the blood stream. The effect of this mechanism is outlined.
6. Page, E. W., and Christianson, R. The impact of mean arterial pressure in the middle trimester upon the outcome of pregnancy. *Am. J. Obstet. Gynecol.* 125:740, 1976.
   Presents a simple formula for calculating the mean arterial pressure and demonstrates that perinatal mortality increases as the mean arterial pressure increases.

7. Gant, N. F., et al. Metabolic clearance rate of dehydroisoandrosterone sulfate: V. Studies of essential hypertension complicating pregnancy. *Obstet. Gynecol.* 47:319, 1976.
   This paper reports progressive decrease of clearance of dehydroisoandrosterone sulfate several weeks prior to onset of accelerated hypertension.
8. Gant, N. F., Madden, J. D., and Sitteri, P. K. The metabolic clearance rate of dehydroisoandrosterone sulfate: III. The effect of thiazide diuretics in normal and future preeclamptic pregnancies. *Am. J. Obstet. Gynecol.* 123:159, 1975.
   The metabolic clearance of dehydroisoandrosterone sulfate (a reflection of uteroplacental perfusion) is dramatically decreased during diuretic therapy.

Diagnosis

9. Roach, C. J. Renovascular hypertension in pregnancy. *Obstet. Gynecol.* 42:857, 1973.
   A case report and general review of renovascular hypertension as a complication of pregnancy.

Management

10. Lieb, S. M., et al. Nitroprusside-induced hemodynamic alterations in normotensive and hypertensive pregnant sheep. *Am. J. Obstet. Gynecol.* 139:925, 1981.
    The treatment of severe hypertension with sodium nitroprusside was studied in pregnant ewes. This agent was shown to reduce hypertension and the reduction in blood pressure was shown to increase uterine blood flow.
11. Gluck, L., and Kolovich, M. V. Lecithin/sphingomyelin [L/S] ratios in amniotic fluid in normal and abnormal pregnancy. *Am. J. Obstet. Gynecol.* 115:539, 1973.
    In patients with hypertension as a complication of pregnancy, amniotic fluid L/S is usually 2 : 1 or more by the thirty-third week of gestation. Maternal hypertension appears to accelerate lung maturation.
12. Berkowitz, R. L. Anti-hypertensive drugs in the pregnant patient. *Obstet. Gynecol. Surv.* 35:191, 1980.
    Comprehensive, up-to-date review of all ramifications of antihypertensive therapy during pregnancy.
13. Campbell, D. M., and MacGillivray, I. The effect of a low calorie diet or a thiazide diuretic on the incidence of preeclampsia and on birth weight. *Br. J. Obstet. Gynaecol.* 82:572, 1975.
    Prolonged use of thiazide diuretics during pregnancy leads to reduced infant birth weight.
14. Redman, C. W. G., et al. Fetal outcome in trial of anti-hypertensive treatment in pregnancy. *Lancet* 2:753, 1976.
    Often-quoted paper defending use of methyldopa during pregnancy. For a critical analysis of this paper see Hypertension in Pregnancy by Gant and Worley [2], pp. 99–101.
15. Curet, L. B., and Olson, R. W. Evaluation of a program of bed rest in the treatment of chronic hypertension in pregnancy. *Obstet. Gynecol.* 53:336, 1979.
    Seventy-two hypertensive pregnant women were managed by modified bed rest, avoidance of diuretics, and medication (oral hydralazine) only if diastolic pressure exceeded 110 mm Hg.
16. Arias, F., and Zamora, J. Antihypertensive treatment and pregnancy outcome in patients with chronic hypertension. *Obstet. Gynecol.* 53:489, 1979.

Twenty-nine untreated women were compared with 29 women who were treated with either methyldopa or hydralazine plus a thiazide. Diuretic therapy appeared to have adverse effects.

Pregnancy-Induced Hypertension

Hypertension that is unique to pregnancy is best termed *pregnancy-induced hypertension (PIH)*. PIH is synonymous with preeclampsia-eclampsia (eclampsia being an extension of the preeclamptic process). The old term *toxemia* is being replaced by the more appropriate PIH. Although the cause is unknown, there are many theories, although none of these theories encompasses the entire disease entity. Socioeconomic factors, nutritional deficiencies, and slow, disseminated intravascular coagulation have been postulated as etiologic agents but may be only associated factors. Recent immunologic explanations are intriguing but not proved. It is likely that the final answer will be multifactoral.

Observations that any theory must explain include the following: PIH is principally a disease of primigravid women; it is unique to humans; it has an association with a large amount of trophoblast; there is a coordination with chronic vascular disease; there is a genetic predisposition; a viable fetus is not always present.

Basic physiology demonstrates that hypertension is a consequence of either an increase in cardiac output or an increase in peripheral vascular resistance. Since cardiac output remains at the normal value for pregnancy, PIH is the result of increased peripheral resistance. This vascular resistance is caused by the generalized vasospasm so characteristic of the disease. Early in normal pregnancy, the mother's arteries become more refractory to pressor agents such as angiotensin II (the most potent pressor substance). The cause of this normal vascular refractoriness is not known, but prostaglandins do play a role. Many weeks prior to clinically detectable PIH, there is a loss of refractoriness to infused angiotensin. Angiotensin infusions can actually predict which normotensive patient is destined to acquire PIH in the future. After the loss of vascular refractoriness to angiotensin, but before onset of clinical hypertension, there is a decrease in placental perfusion (as measured by clearance of dehydroisoandrosterone sulfate). It is now appreciated that PIH is a chronic disease process and that hypertension occurs relatively late in its course. By the time that elevated blood pressure is detected, the disease is well established.

The diagnosis of PIH requires the presence of hypertension with proteinuria or edema, or both, after the twentieth week of pregnancy. It is primarily a disease of the first pregnancy—occurring with higher frequency in the young (teenage) and older (>35) primigravida. The diagnosis of PIH in the multigravid woman is often incorrect and should be made only after excluding cardiovascular and renal disease. Hypertension is defined as a recording of greater than 140/90 or any recording that represents an increase of 30 mm Hg systolic or 15 mm Hg diastolic over baseline recordings. Two blood pressure readings taken at least 6 hours apart are required. It is important to realize that a blood pressure of 130/80 may constitute hypertension in the young primigravida with a previous baseline of 90/50. Proteinuria is a more important diagnostic criterion than is edema. Significant proteinuria is defined as 500 mg/dl or more per 24 hours, which correlates well with a 2+ urinary protein. Edema is such a common occurrence that it is often not helpful in diagnosis. Nondependent edema is significant, but as many as 8 of 10 normotensive women demonstrate dependent edema.

Many authorities differentiate between mild and severe pregnancy-induced hypertension. Mild disease consists of minimal to moderate elevations of blood pressure (systolic less than 160, diastolic less than 110), nondependent edema, and less than 2 g of proteinuria in 24 hours. When one or more of the following signs occur, preeclampsia is classified as severe: blood pressure greater than 160/110, proteinuria greater than 5 g in 24 hours (3 + to 4 +), oliguria (less than 400 ml in 24 hours), visual blurring or scotomata, and pulmonary edema or cyanosis.

The diagnosis of PIH usually makes hospitalization mandatory. Management must then be individualized according to the maturity of the fetus and the severity of PIH. If PIH has its onset at 37 or more weeks gestation, little can be gained from procrastination. Even with mild PIH, oxytocin induction is indicated, particularly if the cervix is favorable. Even if the cervix is unfavorable, the pregnancy should not continue past term. Severe PIH, even if associated with a premature fetus, demands intervention. There are also distinct warnings that eclampsia is imminent. These are accelerating hypertension, headache, visual blurring or scotomata, epigastric or right upper quadrant abdominal pain, and tremulousness. These signs require the prompt administration of magnesium sulfate in order to prevent convulsions.

Conservative management is appropriate only when the fetus is premature and the hypertension is not severe. This patient is allowed a regular hospital diet and light ambulation. Vital signs should be checked four times daily while she is awake. Weight is checked daily, and urine protein is checked frequently. Creatinine clearance is obtained weekly and serial sonography is performed every 3 weeks. The mother may be asked to record fetal movements, although nonstress and/or contraction stress tests are usually conducted weekly in those who are managed conservatively. Biochemical monitoring by estriols, human placental lactogen, and pregnancy-specific proteins are of debatable usefulness.

After hospitalization is begun, a spontaneous diuresis can be expected within the first 24 hours. The diuresis is reflected by a decrease in weight and an improvement in blood pressure, in addition to a large urinary output. If the patient becomes normotensive, it must be decided whether or not to continue hospitalization until delivery. It is often cheaper to pay for maternal hospital care than to risk exacerbation of disease, subsequent premature delivery, and the great cost of neonatal intensive care. For the woman who is unwilling or unable to accept hospitalization, home bed rest with daily blood pressure monitoring is second best. Whenever severe preeclampsia occurs, management is straightforward: prevention of convulsions with magnesium sulfate, control of hypertension with intermittent hydralazine, and delivery.

Magnesium sulfate ($MgSO_4$) is a safe and efficient agent to prevent convulsions. Maintenance $MgSO_4$ can be administered by either intramuscular (IM) or intravenous routes. The initial IM dose is 10 g, followed by 5 g IM every 4 hours. Each 5 g of $MgSO_4$ consists of 10 ml of a 50% solution that is given in the upper outer quadrant of the buttock through a 3-inch 20-gauge needle. One ml of 2% xylocaine can be added to each dose for analgesia. The intravenous method consists of 10 g $MgSO_4$ added to 1000 ml of 5% dextrose in water and administered at the rate of 1 g per hour. If signs of impending convulsion persist, the intravenous dose may be increased to 2 g per hour. The intravenous method demands the use of continuous infusion pumps, the availability of personnel for infusion monitoring, the documentation of adequate renal function, and preferably the capability of making serum magnesium determinations on an emergency basis.

Maintenance of $MgSO_4$ should never be continued unless the following criteria are met: patellar reflex is present, respirations are normal, and urine output is at least 100 ml every 4 hours. Before any treatment, the normal serum magnesium level is 1.5 to 2 mEq/l, while the therapeutic maintenance range is 4 to 7 mEq/l. The earliest sign of magnesium toxicity is loss of the patellar reflex; this occurs at 7 to 10 mEq/l. Respiratory depression begins at 10 to 15 mEq/l and cardiac arrest at 30 mEq/l. Calcium gluconate is the antidote to magnesium sulfate. The dose is 1 g (10 ml of a 10% solution) given slowly over 3 minutes. Mechanical respiratory support is also necessary in these cases.

Antihypertensive medication is reserved for patients with diastolic pressures of 110 or greater, and hydralazine is the drug of choice. It is given by intermittent intravenous bolus (5 to 20 mg) or by continuous infusion (180 mg in 500 cc D_5W) when diastolic pressure enters the 90 to 100 range. Because of vasospasm, the patient with PIH has a contracted blood volume. This knowledge is important in management since volume contraction mandates against either volume expansion or depletion. Injudicious fluid therapy may lead to overload and pulmonary edema. In contrast, salt-restriction or the use of diuretics may cause decreased placental perfusion. As a consequence of the diminished blood volume, the patient with PIH cannot withstand the same degree of blood loss at delivery as can a normal woman. A sudden reduction of blood pressure at delivery is usually the result of a profound blood loss.

Severe pregnancy-induced hypertension and its sequel, eclampsia, are largely preventable. The key to prevention is astute management. Patient education, close monitoring, and attention to subtle detail will reduce the morbidity and mortality and expense associated with this disease.

Text
1. Pritchard, J. A., and MacDonald, P. C. Hypertensive Disorders in Pregnancy. In *Williams Obstetrics* (16th ed.). New York: Appleton-Century-Crofts, 1980.
   A most complete review of the place of eclampsia within the syndrome of pregnancy-induced hypertension; 107 references are included.

Review
2. Gant, N. F., and Worley, R. J. *Hypertension in Pregnancy*. New York: Appleton-Century-Crofts, 1980.
   In addition to their original work, the authors give critical analyses of many papers on this topic. This book is an excellent review of basic science, as well as a source of practical advice on management.
3. Soutter, W. P. The haemodynamic pathophysiology of pre-eclampsia. *S. Afr. Med. J.* 58:351, 1980.
   The author reviews the hemodynamic characteristics of pregnancy-induced hypertension. The overall role of therapeutic management is discussed.

Etiology
4. Beer, A. E. Possible immunologic bases of preeclampsia/eclampsia. *Semin. Perinatol.* 2:39, 1978.
   Fascinating evidence and speculation about a possible cause of PIH.
5. Page, E. W. On the pathogenesis of pre-eclampsia and eclampsia. *J. Obstet. Gynaecol. Br. Commonw.* 79:883, 1972.
   A most complete work regarding the pathogenesis of preeclampsia and

*eclampsia. This work promotes the theory of McKay regarding dissemi-
nated intravascular coagulation.*

6. Sheehan, H. L. Renal morphology in preeclampsia. *Kidney Int.* 18:241, 1980.
   *This eminent investigator reviewed the renal morphology found in pa-
   tients who have pregnancy-induced hypertension. This is a classic article
   and speaks very well to the immunohistology problem encountered in the
   study of these patients.*

Vascular Perfusion

7. Madden, J. D., et al. The pattern and rates of metabolism of maternal
   plasma dehydroisoandrosterone sulfate in human pregnancy. *Am. J.
   Obstet. Gynecol.* 125:915, 1976.
   *This paper offers basic understanding of the metabolic pathways of de-
   hydroisoandrosterone sulfate clearance from maternal plasma. The relationship of this calculation to uteroplacental perfusion is explained.*

8. Gant, N. F., et al. A clinical test useful for predicting the development of
   acute hypertension in pregnancy. *Am. J. Obstet. Gynecol.* 120:1, 1974.
   A description of the "roll-over" test.

Complications

9. Assali, N. S., and Vaugh, D. L. Blood volume in pre-eclampsia: Fantasy
   and reality. *Am. J. Obstet. Gynecol.* 129:355, 1977.
   *A good review of the hemodynamic physiology of normal pregnancy and
   the altered hemodynamics unique to preeclampsia.*

10. Bern, M. D., Driscoll, S. G., and Leavitt, T., Jr. Thrombocytopenia com-
    plicating preeclampsia. *Obstet. Gynecol.* 57:28S, 1981.
    *A case report with extensive discussion regarding thrombocytopenia com-
    plicating preeclampsia is offered. The suggestion of an immune-mediated
    phenomenon in preeclampsia is outlined.*

11. Naulty, J., Cefalo, R. C., and Lewis, P. E. Fetal toxicity of nitroprusside
    in the pregnant ewe. *Am. J. Obstet. Gynecol.* 139:708, 1981.
    *The authors demonstrate that prolonged use of nitroprusside can be
    associated with tachyphylaxis in the mother and with the development of
    lethal levels of cyanide in the fetus.*

Management

12. Pritchard, J. A. Management of severe pre-eclampsia and eclampsia.
    Semin. Perinatol. 2:83, 1978.
    *Straightforward management protocol by an author of extensive experi-
    ence.*

13. Chesley, L. C. Parenteral magnesium sulfate and the distribution,
    plasma levels, and excretion of magnesium. *Am. J. Obstet. Gynecol.*
    133:1, 1979.
    *The safety of magnesium sulfate therapy is demonstrated by calculating
    the apparent volume of distribution of magnesium.*

14. Berkowitz, R. Anti-hypertensive drugs in the pregnant patient. *Obstet.
    Gynecol. Surv.* 35:91, 1980.
    *Comprehensive, recent review of all ramifications of antihypertensive
    therapy during pregnancy.*

15. Welt, S. I., et al. The effect of prophylactic management and therapeutics
    on hypertensive disease in pregnancy: Preliminary studies. *Obstet.
    Gynecol.* 57:557, 1981.
    *A prospective evaluation of pregnancy complicated by chronic hyperten-
    sion was carried out in 63 women. The incidence of pregnancy-induced*

hypertension in those treated prophylactically with antihypertensives was lower than in those not treated. Treatment of chronic hypertensive patients is important in preventing preeclampsia.

16. Gilstrap, L. C., Cunningham, F. G., and Whalley, P. J. Management of pregnancy-induced hypertension in the nulliparous patient remote from term. *Semin. Perinatol.* 2:73, 1978.
A strong argument for continued hospitalization until delivery. The uncorrected perinatal mortality rate for the 545 women who accepted this management was only 9 per 1000.

17. Rafferty, T. D., and Berkowitz, R. L. Hemodynamics in patients with severe toxemia during labor and delivery. *Am. J. Obstet. Gynecol.* 138:263, 1980.
The hemodynamics of patients with severe preeclampsia and eclampsia are discussed. The use of pulmonary capillary wedge pressures and other indexes of cardiorespiratory function are advocated.

18. Sehgal, N. N., and Hitt, J. R. Plasma volume expansion in the treatment of pre-eclampsia. *Am. J. Obstet. Gynecol.* 138:165, 1980.
The effects of plasma volume expansion with dextran, plasmanate or simple fluid hydration. There was a significant improvement in the status of those receiving plasmanate or dextran.

19. Benedetti, T. J., et al. Hemodynamic observations in severe preeclampsia with a flow-directed pulmonary artery catheter. *Am. J. Obstet. Gynecol.* 136:465, 1980.
Ten patients with severe preeclampsia were studied with pulmonary artery catheters. This modality is said to provide a useful clinical adjunct in patients with severe disease.

20. Nochimson, D. J., and Petrie, R. H. Glucocorticoid therapy for the induction of pulmonary maturity in severely hypertensive gravid women. *Am. J. Obstet. Gynecol.* 133:449, 1979.
Twenty patients with severe preeclampsia were given betamethasone therapy to mature fetal lungs prior to delivery. Pregnancy-induced hypertension was not found to be a contraindication to glucocorticoid therapy for the induction of lung maturity.

21. Nochimson, D. J., and Petrie, R. H. Glucocorticoid therapy for the induction of pulmonary maturity in severely hypertensive gravid women. *Am. J. Obstet. Gynecol.* 133:449, 1979.
This study was done in 20 hypertensive gravid women with severe pregnancy-induced hypertension. They were treated with betamethasone to induce lung maturity and showed that there was no untoward sequellae for the infant. This is the first study indicating that these compounds can be used safely in severely hypertensive patients.

22. Sibai, B. M., et al. Reassessment of intravenous $MgSO_4$ therapy in preeclampsia-eclampsia. *Obstet. Gynecol.* 57:199, 1981.
The authors indicate that the standard dosage of $MgSO_4$ may be insufficient for many patients. They recommend adjusting the intravenous dosage of $MgSO_4$ for each patient.

23. Anderson, W. A., and Harbert, G. M. Conservative management of preeclamptic and eclamptic patients. *Am. J. Obstet. Gynecol.* 129:260, 1977.
The conservative management, both benefits and risks, of pregnancy-induced hypertensive patients are detailed. Infant outcome is also listed.

24. Cruikshank, D. P., et al. Effects of magnesium sulfate treatment on perinatal calcium metabolism. *Am. J. Obstet. Gynecol.* 134:342, 1979.
The authors demonstrate that magnesium sulfate does not have a detrimental effect on either the mothers' or the babies' calcium levels. In addi-

tion, the magnesium levels in the infants did not appear to be correlated to depression.

25. Zuspan, F. P. Problems encountered in the treatment of pregnancy induced hypertension. *Am. J. Obstet. Gynecol.* 131:591, 1978.
   The author outlines the importance of adequate therapy for the pre-eclamptic patient. The various difficulties with severely ill preeclamptics are discussed.

26. Pritchard, J. A. The use of magnesium sulfate in preeclampsia/eclampsia. *J. Reprod. Med.* 23:107, 1979.
   The importance of the magnesium ion as a therapeutic medication for patients with eclampsia is underscored. The various therapeutic regimens used in the past are detailed.

Eclampsia

Eclampsia is the extension of pregnancy-induced hypertension (PIH) to the point of convulsion or coma, or both. Eclampsia may cause significant morbidity and mortality for both the mother and baby. Maternal mortality may be as high as 10%, whereas perinatal deaths range from 8.6%–27.8%. Fortunately it is a largely preventable illness. The following are considered distinct warnings that convulsion is imminent: Acceleration of hypertension, epigastric–right upper quadrant abdominal pain, visual blurring or scotomata, headache, and tremulousness. The presence of any of these signs demands the prompt administration of magnesium sulfate. However, approximately 20% of women who develop eclampsia will have only mildly elevated blood pressures (80–90 mm Hg diastolic), often without proteinuria or edema. For this reason, all patients who meet the blood pressure criteria of PIH in labor should receive magnesium sulfate therapy.

The cause of the eclamptic convulsion is unknown. Both cerebral vasospasm and cerebral edema are incriminated but are unproved as etiologic agents. One-half of convulsions occur before labor, one-quarter during labor, and most of the remainder within 48 hours postpartum. However, there are documented cases of eclampsia reported up to 11 days postpartum. Seizures are grand mal in character, and typically there is no antecedent aura. Tongue-biting, urinary-fecal incontinence, injury from falls, and, occasionally, fractures are observed as are transient apnea and cyanosis.

Care during the actual convulsion consists of gentle constraint, use of a padded tongue blade, maintenance of an airway, and administration of oxygen as soon as the convulsion ceases. A chest x-ray is obtained to exclude aspiration. Blood for blood count, liver profile, and serum electrolytes is drawn, while an indwelling catheter is placed in the bladder for measurement of hourly output. A stage of agitation is common after the postictal patient regains partial consciousness. A quiet room with subdued light and the presence of a family member are helpful.

Management of eclampsia is straightforward. Convulsions are treated, blood pressure controlled, and delivery accomplished as soon as possible after stabilization of the mother. Timing of delivery does not depend upon the maturity of the fetus.

The agent of choice for the treatment of convulsions is magnesium sulfate. The following regimen has proved efficacious: 4 g of 10% $MgSO_4$ given intravenously (IV) over 4 minutes, followed by a continuous maintenance infusion of 1 g $MgSO_4$ per hour in 75 ml of 5% dextrose in water (D5W) if there is no sign of maternal depression. Occasionally, the maintenance dose will have to be increased to 2 g per hour if urinary output is high. Another regimen used frequently is 4 g of $MgSO_4$ given intravenously over 4 minutes, followed immediately with 5 g (50%) given intramuscularly (IM) in each buttock and intramuscular injection of 5 g every 4 hours. This 14-g loading dose can be given safely to any patient who has not already received $MgSO_4$. Another convulsion within 20 minutes of the loading dose does not require additional treatment. A subsequent seizure occurring 20 minutes or more following the initial dose is treated with additional intravenous (10%) $MgSO_4$ (2 g slowly IV if patient weighs less than 55 kg and 4 g if more than 55 kg. For the rare patient who continues to convulse after the second intravenous bolus of magnesium sulfate, intravenous sodium amobarbital (Amytal) or Dilantin titrated as needed may be helpful.

Magnesium sulfate causes a peripheral neuromuscular blockage via interference with acetylcholine release and action. This is clinically important if succinylcholine is used for muscle relaxation since less drug is required for cesarean section or other surgery. The synergism between $MgSO_4$ and succinylcholine can explain cases of prolonged muscle paralysis postoperatively. Vasodilatation and a central cerebral sedative effect are also noted as actions of this agent. Prior to any therapy, the normal serum magnesium is 1.5–2.0 mEq/l. After a loading dose of 4 g given intravenously and maintenance infusion of 1 g $MgSO_4$ per hour, serum magnesium levels range from 2.2 to 4.1 mEq/l. A maintenance infusion of 2 g per hour results in serum magnesium levels of 2.7–5.5 mEq/l. A 10 g intramuscular dose results in levels of 3.5–6.0 mEq/l within 2 hours. The levels return to normal within 6 hours if no further magnesium is given. A maintenance dose of 5 g IM every 4 hours results in a therapeutic range between 4 and 7 mEq/l.

Because magnesium is excreted by the kidneys, renal disease or oliguria require a reduction or cessation of dose. The earliest sign of magnesium toxicity is the loss of the patellar reflex (occurs at 7 to 10 mEq/l). Respirations are depressed at 10 to 15 mEq/l, and cardiac arrest occurs at about 30 mEq/l. A maintenance regimen of $MgSO_4$ (either intramuscular or intravenous) should never be administered unless these criteria are confirmed: patellar reflex present, respirations normal, and urine output at least 100 ml every 4 hours. Intramuscular regimen is 5 g every 4 hours up to 24 hours postpartum, while intravenous maintenance is 1 g per hour up to 24 hours postpartum. Calcium gluconate is the antidote to magnesium sulfate. The dose for respiratory depression is 1 g (10 ml of a 10% calcium gluconate solution) administered intravenously over 3 minutes. Mechanical respiratory support may be necessary if the patient develops respiratory depression.

The blood pressure may be normal immediately following a convulsion, although the hypertension usually resumes. If the patient remains normotensive or if the convulsion occurs more than 48 hours postpartum, causes of convulsions other than eclampsia should be considered. Other causes include epilepsy, cerebrovascular accident, central nervous system tumor, electrolyte disturbance, and hypoglycemia. However, eclampsia can occur more than 48 hours postpartum.

Intravenous hydralazine is the drug of choice to control the hypertension associated with eclampsia. Its use is reserved for blood pressures of 170/110 or greater. Hydralazine is given by means of constant infusion pump by mixing 100 mg of hydralazine in 250 ml of D5W. Blood pressure is taken every 5 minutes initially and every 15 minutes after becoming stable. The goal of therapy is to maintain the diastolic blood pressure between 90 and 100 mm Hg. If diastolic blood pressure drops below 90 mm Hg, the infusion rate should be decreased or the infusion discontinued. Hydralazine also can be given in intravenous bolus amounts of 5 to 20 mg. One may begin with 5 mg and increase (if necessary) in 5-mg increments until the diastolic pressure is 90–100. On rare occasions, hypotensive episodes may occur. For this reason, constant infusion is favored.

Definitive cure of eclampsia is delivery. It is best to wait until the mother is stable on magnesium sulfate therapy. This usually occurs 4 to 8 hours after the last convulsion. Even if the cervix is unfavorable for induction, oxytocin stimulation may be successful. The fetus should be carefully monitored during labor. Many fetuses of eclamptic women have intrauterine growth retardation. They may have little placental reserve and not tolerate labor. Also, the incidence of placental abruption is greatly increased in eclampsia, and this may lead to sudden deterioration of the fetus. Cesarean section is reserved for customary obstetric indications.

The eclamptic patient, like the one with severe PIH, has a contracted blood volume. Hemoconcentration is a constant finding. Puerperal hemorrhage, even of a magnitude tolerated by the normal pregnant patient, can lead to dangerous underperfusion of vital organs. A sudden reduction of blood pressure at the time of delivery or immediately postpartum is usually the consequence of excessive blood loss. Because of their contracted blood volume, all women with eclampsia should be typed and crossmatched for blood.

The patient frequently may inquire about the risk of recurrence of severe PIH or eclampsia. The young primigravida who has experienced this disease has a much more favorable prognosis than the older multigravida with chronic hypertension and superimposed preeclampsia-eclampsia. There is a 1 in 4 chance of recurrence if the patient is normotensive. With chronic hypertension, the recurrence risk rises to 7 in 10.

Reviews
1. Zuspan, F. P. Toxemia of Pregnancy. In J. J. Sciarra and T. W. McElin (Eds.), *Gynecology and Obstetrics*. Hagerstown, Md.: Harper & Row, 1977. Vol. 2.
   A 20-page review of all aspects of pregnancy-induced hypertension with excellent references.
2. Mendlowitz, M. Toxemia of pregnancy and eclampsia. *Obstet. Gynecol. Surv.* 35:327, 1980.
   An in-depth review of the basic science aspects of the preeclampsia/eclampsia syndrome. Seventy references are detailed.

Etiology
3. McKay, D. G. Discussion of Pritchard, J. S., Cunningham, F. G., and Mason, R. A. Does Coagulation Have a Causative Role in Eclampsia? In M. D. Lindheimer, A. I. Katz, and F. P. Zuspan (Eds.), *Hypertension in Pregnancy*. New York: Wiley, 1976.
   An argument for disseminated intravascular coagulation as a cause of eclampsia.
4. Porapakkham, S. An epidemiologic study of eclampsia. *Obstet. Gynecol.* 54:26, 1979.
   The epidemiologic characteristics in 298 cases of eclampsia were studied. Inadequate antenatal care was a major factor in maternal and perinatal mortality.

Coagulation Changes
5. Pritchard, J. A., Cunningham, F. G., and Mason, R. A. Coagulation changes in eclampsia: Their frequency and pathogenesis. *Am. J. Obstet. Gynecol.* 124:855, 1976.
Overt disseminated intravascular coagulation seen in only a minority of women with eclampsia. However, vasospasm causes endothelial damage, which causes platelet adhesiveness and local fibrin deposition with some laboratory changes in the coagulation profile.

Management
6. Pritchard, J. A., and Pritchard, S. A. Standardized treatment of 154 consecutive cases of eclampsia. *Am. J. Obstet. Gynecol.* 123:543, 1975.
A classic presentation of a successful management protocol by an author with extensive experience.
7. Sibai, B. M., et al. The late postpartum eclampsia controversy. *Obstet. Gynecol.* 55:74, 1980.
Purportedly, eclampsia does not occur before the twentieth week and after a few days postpartum. This study deals with women who were diagnosed as eclamptic by exclusion, although the seizures occurred much later than is commonly acceptable for such a diagnosis.
8. Sibai, B.M., et al. Reassessment of intravenous $MgSO_4$ therapy in preeclampsia-eclampsia. *Obstet. Gynecol.* 57:199, 1981.
This article offers evidence that the current methods of management of $MgSO_4$ in the treatment of patients with eclampsia may not be adequate. Many of the patients thought by clinical grounds to be well controlled had low $MgSO_4$ levels.
9. Zuspan, F. P., and Zuspan, K. J. Strategies for controlling eclampsia. *Cont. Ob/Gyn.* 18:135, 1981.
An in-depth review of the therapeutic choices to treat the eclamptic patient is offered by the authors. Also a nice section on the delivery of the eclamptic patient is detailed.

Prognosis
10. Chesley, L. C., Annitto, J. E., and Cosgrove, R. A. The remote prognosis of eclamptic women: Sixth periodic report. *Am. J. Obstet. Gynecol.* 101:886, 1968.
Long-term follow-up of women who have experienced eclampsia demonstrating no adverse long-term effects on maternal health.
11. Bryans, C. I., Jr. Leon Chesley and the long-term prognosis of eclamptic patients. *J. Reprod. Med.* 25:5, 1980.
The author introduces data collected by Chesley and others regarding the prognosis for eclamptic patients. Much of the classic work leading to the conclusions regarding eclampsia are detailed in this paper.
12. Pritchard, J. A., and Stone, S. R. Clinical and laboratory observations on eclampsia. *Am. J. Obstet. Gynecol.* 99:754, 1967.
Sixty-nine consecutive patients with eclampsia were studied during the intrapartum period. All mothers survived and the perinatal salvage rate was 79% for all fetuses. Management and diagnostic techniques are discussed.

INFECTIONS IN PREGNANCY

Data from the Collaborative Perinatal Project have shown that approximately 5% of all pregnancies are complicated by one or more maternal viral infections. Nonspecific infections such as the common cold, flulike syndromes, gastroenteritis, pharyngitis, and tonsillitis are most common. Generally these are mild, but occasionally a viral infection during pregnancy is of considerable consequence because of its potential effects on the developing embryo, fetus, or neonate. The exact incidence of the more serious infections is not known. Neither has the proportion of congenital anomalies (3%–6% of all infants) nor of spontaneous abortion directly attributable to viral infections been established.

Viruses may cause localized or generalized infection of the fetus, inflammation of the placenta, vasculitis, chromosomal aberrations, or delayed viral disease in the infant. The ultimate consequence of intrauterine infections may be: (1) no significant problem, (2) asymptomatic chronic infection, (3) spontaneous abortion or intrauterine death, and (4) fetal malformation. These infections may also be acquired during parturition and the neonatal period. Viral infections during pregnancy produce very similar signs such as those acquired in the neonatal period. Nervous system manifestations are most common and include microcephaly, mental retardation, seizures, chorioretinitis, cataracts, microphthalmia, cerebral calcification, sensorineural deafness, and central auditory imperception. Failure to thrive, low birth weight, prematurity, purpura, hepatosplenomegaly, jaundice, cardiac lesions, chronic rash, and pneumonitis are extraneural findings often associated with congenital infection.

Rubella, cytomegalovirus, and herpes virus are the most significant causes of infection in man. Crude estimates show that infection in the newborn from all agents occurs in 1%–5% of all babies delivered. Fortunately, severe infection is rarely manifest in the neonate. However, subclinical or mild infections may result in low IQ or subtle defects, e.g., hearing loss, which diminish the social and educational potential of the individual.

Approximately 15%–20% of the adult population is susceptible to rubella, an RNA virus that is transmitted person to person. Symptomatic individuals develop a typical mild exanthematous rash associated with postauricular lymphadenopathy and mild transient arthralgia of the small joints. Isolating the virus from the nasopharynx confirms the diagnosis. Susceptible women have no detectable antibodies in the serum, and seroconversion provides evidence of infection. Hemagglutination inhibition (HI) antibodies appear in the serum with onset of the rash, peak in 2 to 3 weeks, then gradually decrease. The serum, however, remains positive. Complement fixation antibody begins to rise several days following the onset of the rash and eventually disappears. Specific rubella IgM antibody occurs with onset of the rash, persists for 6 weeks, and is helpful in establishing a diagnosis in the neonate.

Susceptible individuals should receive rubella vaccine, preferably before puberty. Puerperal women may be vaccinated, but as many as 20% will not respond. Although the risk of congenital infection following vaccination is extremely low, pregnancy should be prevented for 3 months. In spite of the vaccination program, 20% of adult women remain susceptible—twice the incidence in 1964. This program seems to be effective since no epidemics have occurred since 1964, but a high rate of infection may occur in the future.

Approximately half of those women who contract the rubella infection in the first trimester of pregnancy have spontaneous abortions. Infants born with congenital rubella show a high incidence of cataracts and deafness.

Congenitally infected infants shed the virus and pose a threat to susceptible women.

Cytomegalovirus (CMV), a herpes type virus, can be spread person to person by multiple routes, including venereal contacts. The majority of patients are asymptomatic, but occasionally heterophile negative mononucleosis syndrome is seen. Other features include abrupt onset of a spiking fever up to 104° F, abnormal liver function, and constitutional symptoms such as malaise, chills, and myalgia. The virus may be cultured from the urine, nasopharynx, or cervix of 3%–5% of pregnant women. The hemagglutination inhibition test becomes positive following primary infection and remains positive. Complement fixation antibody develops shortly after the onset of the infection and gradually disappears. Specific CMV IgM is the most sensitive indication of primary infection. Although the virus is rather easily cultured and serologic tests are sensitive, primary infection remains difficult to document.

CMV, which occurs in 0.5%–1.5% of births, is the most common congenital infection in the United States and England and may occur following primary or recurrent maternal infection. An additional 3%–5% of neonates may become infected, presumably because of exposure to infected cervical secretions, infected breast milk, or exposure to close oral contact. As many as 10% of these children may exhibit symptoms.

Therapeutic abortion is warranted in the rare situation of primary infection early in pregnancy because of the teratogenic potential of the virus. Following early infection, viral replication with low grade cellular and tissue injury is the rule, but severe infection is rare. The prognosis for those with obvious disease at birth is poor, and central nervous system and perceptual disabilities are common. Infants born with positive IgM specific antibody but having no clinical disease may have sufficient intellectual, behavioral, neurological, or sensory abnormalities to need special education. CMV is one of the major causes of intellectual disability and, therefore, may be an immense public health problem.

Venereal transmission is common for herpes, a DNA virus. The diagnosis is usually based on clinical appearance of the vesicles, which may be associated with or preceded by pruritus, burning, or hyperesthesia of skin. The vesicles form flat, nonindurated ulcers 2 to 5 mm in diameter that have a grayish white base, do not bleed when scraped, are exquisitely tender and painful, and resolve in 2 to 4 weeks unless they become secondarily infected. Recurrent disease follows essentially this same course except that it is less debilitating, there are fewer ulcers, and lesions usually persist only 1 to 2 weeks. Hemagglutination inhibition, complement fixation, and IgM antibodies are identifiable following infections and show two types of herpes virus, although little benefit is gained in distinguishing the types.

Transplacental infection may result in spontaneous abortion or congenital infection, but this is clearly less likely than with CMV or rubella. Infection by the ascending route via the cervix is rare in the absence of ruptured membranes. Passage through an infected birth canal is clearly the most significant cause of infection. Evidence suggests that 40%–80% of neonates are at risk of infection if they deliver through an infected birth canal. Systemic neonatal herpes has 90% mortality and virtually no neonate is left unscathed. Because women may shed herpes and remain asymptomatic, one must take frequent viral cultures. Although not as reliable, cytology (Pap smear) from the cervix may show evidence of infection. One must therefore prevent fetal contact with the virus. The only proved method of doing this is by avoiding vaginal delivery by performing cesarean section prior to 4 hours after ruptured membranes.

Approximately 15% of women in their childbearing age are susceptible to varicella, a herpeslike virus that is spread by direct contact. The macular rash proceeds to crops of lesions, which may be seen at various stages from vesicles to crusting lesions and are most likely to be seen on the trunk than the extremities. The lesions, which are intensely pruritic and often associated with a low-grade fever, may involve the mucous membranes of the mouth, vulva, and vagina.

Approximately 5% of those susceptible women who become infected during the first 16 weeks of gestation will produce children with congenital defects. Neonates usually escape severe infection because antibody of maternal origin is present and alters the course of the disease. However, 30% of those infants whose mothers are infected 4 days or less before delivery have severe disseminated infection, presumably because they have no maternal antibody protection. Infants born to these mothers should receive high titer varicella zoster immune globulin, which provides protection through passive immunity and also alters the course of the disease in severe neonatal infections.

Rubeola, mumps, influenza, smallpox, hepatitis, and vaccinia have all been proved to cause perinatal infection and congenital malformations. However, a consistent pattern of congenital deformities, newborn infections, or increased early abortion has not been documented.

The responsibility of the obstetrician is to determine susceptibility to viral diseases, to determine appropriate therapy, and to counsel pregnant women affected by viral diseases. Viral cultures, cytology, and serology must be used to identify the causative organism. Currently, passive immunization of the mother or infant exposed to a specific infection is the only means of treating or modifying these diseases. Several vaccines are being tested but only rubella currently has proved to be beneficial. Using antimetabolite therapy, such as ido-deoxyuridine, cytosine arabinoside, and adenosine arabinoside, has been advanced theoretically but is yet to be proved in clinical situations.

Text
1. Hanshaw, J. B., and Dudgeon, J. A. Viral Diseases of the Fetus and Newborn. In A. J. Schaffer and M. Marowitz (Eds.), *Major Problems in Clinical Pediatrics*. Philadelphia: Saunders, 1978.
   This is an authoritative reference book that reviews the etiologies, pathophysiology, classic findings, differential diagnoses, and therapies for viruses known to cause fetal or neonatal infection.
2. Sever, J. L., Larsen, J. W., and Grossman, J. H. *Handbook of Perinatal Infections*. Boston: Little, Brown, 1979.
   This text is a reference for perinatal infections and provides answers to practical questions frequently asked.

Reviews
3. Sever, J. L. Viral infections in pregnancy. *Clin. Obstet. Gynecol.* 21:477, 1978.
   This article reviews the common viral infections associated with congenital infections and gives data accumulated in the United States.
4. Grossman, J. H. Perinatal viral infections. *Clin. Perinatol.* 7:257, 1980.
   The common viral infections associated with perinatal mortality and morbidity are reviewed with emphasis on recent changes in diagnosis, management, and therapy.
5. Schoenbaum, S. C. Specific problems in diagnosis, prevention and management of congenital infections. *Clin. Obstet. Gynecol.* 22:321, 1979.
   Common infections, including viral agents, are discussed and emphasis

is placed on the diseases that can be prevented or treated, or both, and on the future of those diseases for which no therapy is currently available.

Rubella

6. Rossi, M., et al. Maternal rubella and hearing impairment in children. *J. Laryngol. Otol.* 94:281, 1980.

   Severe damage to the hearing apparatus is common, but severe lesions of other organs occur. The timing of maternal infection during early pregnancy leads to different manifestations.

7. Polk, B. F., et al. An outbreak of rubella among hospital personnel. *N. Engl. J. Med.* 303:541, 1980.

   Many personnel are susceptible, and vaccine probably should be given to those at high risk of infection. Care must be taken to insure pregnant women are not exposed to the disease.

8. Krugman, S. Rubella immunization: Present status and future perspectives. *Pediatrics* 65:1174, 1980.

   The success of rubella immunization in preventing nationwide epidemics is reviewed and compared to other successful immunization programs. This method of therapy will likely be used for other viral infections of significance.

9. Gladstone, J. L., and Millan, S. J. Rubella exposure in an obstetric clinic. *Obstet. Gynecol.* 57:182, 1981.

   Recommendations to prevent future rubella exposures in high risk hospital personnel are presented in this article. There was poor compliance with attempts to immunize susceptible persons.

CMV

10. Griffiths, P. D., et al. A prospective study of primary cytomegalovirus infection in pregnant women. *Br. J. Obstet. Gynaecol.* 87:308, 1980.

    This study shows the incidence of CMV in an English population and the incidence of congenital or neonatal defects. It also established that CMV occurs more frequently than rubella, except during epidemics of rubella.

11. Griffiths, P. D., et al. Persistence of high titer antibodies to the early antigens of cytomegalovirus in pregnant women. *Arch. Virol.* 64:303, 1980.

    Methods to determine recurrent infection using levels of various serum antibody detections are discussed. Recurrent infections are known to cause neonatal disease, and determining their recurrence is potentially important.

12. Stagno, S., et al. Comparative study of diagnostic procedures for congenital cytomegalovirus infection. *Pediatrics* 62:251, 1980.

    The reliability and accuracy of diagnostic techniques for viral infections are discussed. A new technique using electron microscopy is described for identification of CMV from fresh urine specimens.

Herpes Simplex and Varicella

13. Grossman, J. H. III, Wallen, W. C., and Sever, J. L. Management of genital herpes simplex virus infection during pregnancy. *Obstet. Gynecol.* 58:1, 1981.

    The clinical course and outcome of 58 pregnancies complicated by genital herpes is presented. The authors' experience with management regarding the appropriate precautions for these women and their infants is outlined.

14. Kibrick, S. Herpes simplex infection: What to do with mother, newborn, and nursery personnel. *J.A.M.A.* 243:157, 1980.

    Guidelines for management of various permutations of herpetic infection are discussed. Specifically, several of the antiviral drugs are discussed in relationship to their usefulness in neonatal infections.

15. Sever, J. L. Reducing the risk of congenital herpes. *Cont. Ob/Gyn.* 17:191, 1981.
    This leading authority in the field of virology offers management techniques with regard to those women who, late in pregnancy, have primary herpes genitalis. Cesarean section is indicated if herpes is found during the last two weeks of pregnancy.
16. Antiviral treatment of varicella zoster and herpes simplex. *Lancet* 1:1337, 1980 (Editorial Comments).
    The treatment regimen for these viruses is described. These general principles may be used in determining therapy for other viral agents.
17. Dudgeon, J. A. Mumps and varicella vaccines. *Arch. Dis. Child.* 55:3, 1980.
    New vaccines are available for these organisms and may be beneficial for use in susceptible individuals.
18. Guinan, M. E., et al. The course of untreated recurrent genital herpes simplex infection in 27 women. *N. Engl. J. Med.* 304:759, 1981.
    The clinical course of recurrent herpes genital infections were studied in 27 women. The duration of pain, viral shedding, and total healing are remarkably similar to previous studies. No cervical or vaginal lesions were ever present in recurrent herpes. These findings have implications for the pregnant patient with herpes.

Urinary Tract Infection in Pregnancy

Urinary tract infection (UTI) in pregnancy may be asymptomatic or symptomatic. If symptomatic, it may be confined to the bladder, causing cystitis, or may be manifested as acute pyelonephritis. To detect asymptomatic bacteriuria (ASB), which occurs in 4%–15% of pregnant women, a routine urine culture should be obtained on the first prenatal visit. Patients who have an initial positive urine usually remain positive throughout pregnancy unless they receive treatment, and at least 30% will develop acute pyelonephritis compared to 1% of women with negative cultures. This can be prevented in most cases by adequate treatment, usually with ampicillin, sulfa, or Furadantin. The persistence or recurrence of infection in spite of treatment suggests an underlying urologic disease such as vesicoureteral reflux and is an indication for urologic workup once pregnancy has been terminated. Although there is an indirect relationship to prematurity, the mechanism is that ASB probably predisposes to pyelonephritis, which is related to premature labor.

Of the symptomatic UTI, cystitis presents with frequency of urination, nocturia, and urgency. Hemorrhagic cystitis occasionally occurs. Cystitis must be distinguished from urethral syndrome (frequency-urgency syndrome) and the physiologic frequency occurring during pregnancy. Patients are usually afebrile, and the diagnosis rests on culture.

Acute pyelonephritis is more serious and is commonly caused by *Escherichia coli*; it is less commonly due to *Klebsiella* or *Proteus* species. Ascending infection from the bladder is more likely to occur during gestation, accounting for the increased incidence in pregnancy. The reason for this is uncertain, but the hydronephrosis, high urinary pH, and poor peristalsis in the ureter that exist during pregnancy, are important factors. It most likely presents with flank pain and tenderness, more commonly on the right side, and symptoms of cystitis and fever with chills are usually present. Since bacteremia is common, this is a dangerous illness with a 3% incidence of septic shock and potential maternal mortality as well as induction of premature labor.

Hydronephrosis is an important aspect in the pathophysiology of urinary tract infection in pregnancy. Mechanical obstruction of the ureters against the pelvic brim by the uterus itself is a most important factor in producing hydronephrosis. The ovarian veins, which dilate tremendously during late pregnancy, are also implicated. Additionally, the high progesterone levels present during gestation may cause ureteral atonicity. The right collecting system is dilated in 92% and the left side in 60% of pregnant women. These changes undergo resolution following delivery and are usually completed by the sixteenth week postpartum.

When urinary tract infection fails to respond to appropriate therapy, the presence of urinary calculi should be considered. The presence of a urea-splitting organism, particularly the *Proteus* species, and a persistently alkaline urine, suggests the presence of calculous disease. The symptoms, namely severe colicky pain, may be absent due to the poor tone of the ureter. While most calculi can be treated expectantly, an infected kidney that is obstructed by a ureteral stone may require emergency decompression by passage of a ureteral catheter through a cystoscope. Rarely, operative removal of a ureteral calculus is necessary. Diagnosis of calculi during pregnancy may be difficult in view of reluctance to utilize x-rays. However, an excretory urogram can be limited to a plain film and a 20-minute film, which is usually sufficient to allow one to arrive at a diagnosis. Sonography and a radionuclide scan are useful in detecting hydronephrosis but are not helpful in determining whether an obstructing calculus is present.

Acute pyelonephritis is associated with premature labor and premature delivery, although other urinary infection appears to have little effect on perinatal mortality. There is also no definite evidence that pyelonephritis produces an increased incidence of pregnancy-induced hypertension or anemia of pregnancy as has been suggested in the past. Renal function may deteriorate if there is preexisting chronic kidney disease prior to pregnancy, but in general pregnancy does not have a detrimental effect on the renal system. If renal infection is present during pregnancy, a 50% decrease in concentrating ability of the kidneys may be found. Glomerular filtration rate is usually not affected unless preexisting chronic renal disease is present, in which case the onset of urinary tract infection could result in acute renal failure.

The diagnosis of urinary tract infection is definitively made by culture of the urine. A midstream clean catch urine specimen should be employed and culture should be performed within 1 hour. A dip culture (e.g., Bactericult) medium can be used as an inexpensive screen for bacteriuria. Routine catheterization to obtain specimens should be avoided because there is a significant danger of introducing infection; the use of a catheter during labor is also associated with significant morbidity.

The postpartum incidence of bacteriuria in patients who have not been catheterized is 4.7%. Following routine catheterization for obtaining specimens, the incidence rises to 9%; if the catheter is used at delivery, there may be an incidence of bacteriuria of 23%. Some of these patients can be expected to progress to chronic urinary tract infection and pyelonephritis. The catheter, therefore, should be avoided if at all possible during pregnancy and labor. Suprapubic aspiration of urine is a safe and accurate method of collection but is poorly accepted by both patients and physicians. Bacteriuria is considered significant if greater than 10^5 colonies of a single organism are present. If several organisms are found, contamination is usually suspected. A count of 10^4 to 10^5 is equivocal and should be repeated, whereas those less than 10^4 are not significant. The presence of any bacteria on culture or gram stain after suprapubic aspiration or catheterization is significant.

Pyuria alone is a poor screening test for urinary tract infection and indicates infective or noninfective inflammation of the urinary tract at any point. Abacterial pyuria is commonly caused by vaginal contamination or the use of antibiotics before culture is taken. Persistent abacterial pyuria may be caused by tumors, ureteral stone, analgesic abuse, glomerular disease, and tuberculosis.

Asymptomatic bacteriuria in early pregnancy or simple cystitis should be treated with antibiotics for 1 week. Preferred agents are ampicillin, cephalosporins, Macrodantin, or sulfa drugs. Sulfa drugs should not be used in late pregnancy as they may produce jaundice in the infant. A recurrent infection may require repeated courses or continuous antibiotic therapy throughout pregnancy. Relapsing infection is highly suggestive of an underlying urologic abnormality in the urinary tract. These patients should have a urologic workup postpartum.

Patients with acute pyelonephritis are usually toxic, ill, dehydrated, and may be in premature labor. They require hospitalization and administration of intravenous fluids and correction of electrolyte imbalance. Intravenous administration of antibiotics is required. Ampicillin, aqueous penicillin, or cephalosporins (alone or in combination with aminoglycoside agents) are the antibiotics of choice. If the condition fails to respond, other antibiotics may be required as dictated by the sensitivity results. For *Pseudomonas* infection, carbenicillin is indicated. If the infection fails to respond to the appropriate antibiotic, ureteral obstruction must be assumed and should be dealt with promptly. Termination of pregnancy to control urinary tract infection is rarely indicated. Occasionally, a localized area of pyelonephritis may progress to abscess formation, which may require percutaneous aspiration or operative drainage.

Reviews
1. Whalley, P. J. Bacteriuria of pregnancy. *Am. J. Obstet. Gynecol.* 97:723, 1967.
   In-depth review of bacteriuria in pregnancy.
2. Polk, B. F. Urinary tract infection in pregnancy. *Clin. Obstet. Gynecol.* 22:285, 1979.
   A general review with 33 references is offered on the etiology, diagnosis, and management of urinary tract infection in pregnancy.
3. Sabath, L. D., and Charles, D. Urinary tract infections in the female. *Obstet. Gynecol.* 55:162, 1980.
   An excellent review regarding urinary tract infections in the female. Diagnosis and treatment as well as prevention are emphasized.

Etiology and Pathogenesis
4. Burke, J. P. Urinary catheter care may increase risk of infection. *J.A.M.A.* 246:30, 1981.
   This article supports the view that infection of the urinary tract is a hospital acquired infection most frequently related to urinary catheterization. Particularly in pregnancy, at labor and delivery, avoidance of catheterization is encouraged.
5. Harris, R. E., and Gilstrap III, L. C. Cystitis during pregnancy: A distinct clinical entity. *Obstet. Gynecol.* 57:578, 1981.
   Acute cystitis in pregnancy was studied in 126 patients. Most of the cases occurred during the second trimester and E. coli *was cultured most fre-*

quently. Only 17% of these patients had recurrence if they were properly treated.

6. Williams, G. L., et al. Vesico-ureteric reflux in patients with bacteriuria in pregnancy. *Lancet* 2:1202, 1968.
   Of patients with symptomatic bacteriuria 32% continue to have bacteriuria 4–6 months postpartum. A high percentage have vesico-ureteral reflux and/or renal scarring.

7. Fairley, K. F., Radford, N. J., and Whitworth, J. A. Spontaneous ascent of infection from bladder to kidney in pregnancy. *Med. J. Aust.* 2:1116, 1972.
   Bladder bacteria may ascend spontaneously to the upper tracts during pregnancy. Fairley localization test used.

Asymptomatic Bacteriuria

8. Kincaid-Smith, P. Bacteriuria in Pregnancy. In E. H. Kass (Ed.), *Progress in Pyelonephritis*. Philadelphia: F. A. Davis, 1965.
   Screening for bacteriuria in early pregnancy allows prevention of acute pyelonephritis and diagnosis of underlying urinary tract abnormalities.

Effects on Fetus and Mother

9. Brumfitt, W. The effects of bacteriuria in pregnancy on maternal and fetal health. *Kidney Int.* 8:113, 1975.
   Asymptomatic bacteriuria leads to acute pyelonephritis in 30% of patients if left untreated.

10. Kincaid-Smith, P. *The Kidney: A Clinico-Pathological Study.* Oxford: Blackwell Scientific Publications, 1975.
    Pregnancy may precipitate acute renal failure in patients with underlying bilateral chronic pyelonephritis.

11. Asscher, A. W. Symptomless Bacteriuria. In E. I. Williams and G. D. Chisholm (Eds.), *Scientific Foundations of Urology.* London: William Heinemann Medical Books, 1976.
    A higher incidence of preeclamptic toxemia, prematurity, and fetal loss is unlikely.

Acute Pyelonephritis in Pregnancy

12. Cunningham, F. G., Morris, G. B., and Mickal, A. Acute pyelonephritis of pregnancy: A clinical review. *Obstet. Gynecol.* 42:112, 1973.
    If it occurs in the third trimester, it can be a serious hazard to maternal well-being. Septicemia occurs in 3% of cases.

13. Kincaid-Smith, P. Renal and Urinary Tract Disorders During Pregnancy. In H. J. Harrison, R. F. Gittes, A. D. Perlmutter, T. A. Stamey, and P. C. Walsh (Eds.), *Campbell's Urology.* Philadelphia: Saunders, 1975.
    An increase in white blood cell count in the urine during pregnancy is a sensitive index of impending acute pyelonephritis.

Hydronephrosis in Pregnancy

14. Derrick, F. C., Rosenblum, R. R., and Lynch, K. M., Jr. Pathological association of right ureter and right ovarian vein. *J. Urol.* 97:633, 1967.
    Observed great enlargement of ovarian veins in pregnancy. Aberrant crossing leads to ureteral compression; 95% of pyelonephritis in pregnancy occurs on the right side.

15. Roberts, J. A. Hydronephrosis of pregnancy. *Urology* 8:1, 1976.
    Obstruction is the main cause of hydronephrosis in pregnancy.

Urinary Calculi in Pregnancy

16. Coe, F. L., Parks, J. H., and Lindheimer, M. D. Nephrolithiasis during pregnancy. *N. Engl. J. Med.* 298:324, 1978.
   Women with urinary calculi have an increased incidence of urinary tract infection during pregnancy, but outcome of pregnancy is not affected in any other way.

17. Jones, W. A., Correa, R. J., and Ansell, J. S. Urolithiasis associated with pregnancy. *J. Urol.* 122:335, 1979.
   There were 20 cases of calculi in 34,081 deliveries over a 12-year period.

Diagnosis

18. Kass, E. H. Bacteriuria and pyelonephritis of pregnancy. *Arch. Intern. Med.* 105:194, 1960.
   Article discusses 10^5 organisms per ml of a single organism in two consecutive clean-catch specimens; correlates well with clinical hazard.

19. Bergstrom, H. Radioisotope renography in pregnancy. *Acta Obstet. Gynecol. Scand.* 54:65, 1975.
   Renography confirms high incidence of dilatation on the right side. Abnormal renogram is therefore not diagnostic of pathological obstruction.

20. Swartz, H. H., and Reichling, B. A. Hazards of radiation exposure for pregnant women. *J.A.M.A.* 239:1907, 1978.
   Undesirable to expose pregnant women to radiation, especially in the first trimester, but risk to the fetus is low enough not to contraindicate medically indicated studies.

21. Mocarski, V. Asymptomatic bacteriuria—a "silent" problem of pregnant women. *Medical Clinical News* 5:238, 1980.
   The problem of asymptomatic bacteriuria as far as diagnosis is concerned is discussed. The various techniques for varying cultures is also listed.

22. Lapides, J. Mechanisms of urinary tract infection. *Urology* 14:217, 1979.
   The mechanism of urinary tract infection is determined. An excellent review is offered regarding various abnormalities of the urinary tract as an etiology.

Complications

23. Naeye, R. L. Causes of the excessive rates of perinatal mortality and prematurity in pregnancies complicated by maternal urinary-tract infections. *N. Engl. J. Med.* 300:819, 1979.
   Perinatal mortality was high in those patients who had urinary tract infections during pregnancy, particularly within 15 days of delivery. Urinary tract infection was coexistent most often with hydramnios, amnionitis, and abruptio placentae.

Treatment

24. Harris, R. E. The significance of eradication of bacteriuria during pregnancy. *Obstet. Gynecol.* 53:71, 1979.
   The incidence of acute antepartum pyelonephritis during a 20-year period decreased from 4% to 0.8% in one institution. Eradication of asymptomatic bacteriuria and follow-up of patients with cystitis who were treated explained the reduction in prevalence.

Venereal Diseases in Pregnancy

Venereal diseases are usually asymptomatic and of those women who develop signs, few will seek medical advice because their symptoms are mild and transient. Furthermore, in pregnancy the clinical course of venereal disease may be even milder. The common venereal diseases that may be contracted in pregnancy include trichomoniasis, gonorrhea, condyloma acuminata, herpes genitalis, and syphilis. Other less common processes will also be mentioned.

The causal agent of trichomoniasis is *Trichomonas vaginalis*. It is transmitted by sexual intercourse, and women usually have more symptoms than men. The subjective symptoms include profuse, frothy, and foul-smelling vaginal discharge accompanied by vulvar itching, dyspareunia, and dysuria. Diagnostically, the wet smear or the more sensitive *Trichomonas* culture medium is utilized. The most effective therapeutic agent is metronidazole (Flagyl), which may be administered orally in doses of either 250 mg three times a day for 7 days or 2 g orally in one dose. Metronidazole may be safely administered in the second and third trimester of pregnancy. Local measures such as povidone iodine sitz baths and sulfur creams are advocated in the first trimester. Treatment of the sexual partner is strongly recommended, especially in recurrent cases.

Gonorrhea is the most common reportable venereal disease in the United States. There were one million cases of gonorrhea reported in 1979. The incidence of gonorrhea in the pregnant population is 2%–5% and 90% of them are asymptomatic. *Neisseria gonorrhea* is almost always spread by genital or oral contact. The gonococcus is most commonly found in the endocervix. From the cervix the gonococcus may extend to the endometrium, oviducts, and pelvic periotoneum. During pregnancy the infection rarely ascends to the upper genital tract, although it can be spread to other organs such as joints, skin, and so on by hematogenous pathways. In uncomplicated cases the gonorrhea usually involves a transient dysuria, mild vaginal discharge, and/or pharyngeal infection symptoms. In complicated cases the gonorrhea may present as gonococcal pyogenic arthritis accompanied by chills and fever.

The definitive diagnosis of gonorrhea is made by culture on modified Thayer-Martin medium in a 5%–10% carbon dioxide atmosphere. Gram stains, even if positive, may be inaccurate. Endocervical cultures yield the best results, although anorectal and pharyngeal cultures should not be forgotten. In every case, both sexual partners should be examined and treated. Finally, a diagnostic serologic test for concomitant syphilis is strongly recommended.

As in the nonpregnant woman, there are several recommended treatments for uncomplicated asymptomatic or symptomatic ambulatory patients with gonorrhea. The treatment of choice is aqueous procaine penicillin-G, 2.4 million units intramuscularly into each buttock, together with 1 g of probenecid orally just before the injection. This treatment will also cure incubating syphilis. Alternately, one may choose to give 3.5 g ampicillin orally, and for pregnant patients who are allergic to penicillin, erythromycin, cefazolin, or spectinomycin may be used. Tetracycline of course should never be used in a pregnant patient. In hospitalized patients, aqueous crystalline penicillin-G, 20 million units, is given intravenously each day until the patient is afebrile and has clinically improved. The regimen is then followed by 500 mg of oral ampicillin taken four times a day to complete a 10-day treatment. Appropriate cultures should be obtained 7 to 14 days after completion of treatment.

Women with known recent exposure to gonorrhea should receive the same treatment as their sexual partner known to have gonorrhea.

Condyloma acuminata (venereal warts) represent a viral venereal disease spread by sexual contact. They are most commonly found in the genital area during the years of maximal sexual activity. The Pap smear is not useful diagnostically because there are no specific cytologic findings. The initial lesion is usually a rough, "cauliflowerlike," warty papilloma on the perineal area. In pregnancy the condyloma acuminata may grow more rapidly and hinder vaginal delivery. The pregnant patient with condyloma acuminata presents special problems because the usual treatment, topical podophyllin, should be avoided throughout pregnancy due to its toxic properties. Thus, during pregnancy destructive methods of therapy (electrocautery or cryosurgery) combined with betadine douches and other hygienic regimens are used. In case of recurrent and persistent condyloma, an autogenous vaccine has been used successfully.

Syphilis is primarily a sexually transmitted disease and approximately 30% of the 25,000 annual cases occur in women. Additionally, there are 350 cases of congenital syphilis reported every year. During pregnancy transplacental infection of the fetus may occur, resulting in either an asymptomatic newborn who later shows the stigmata of congenital syphilis or in an intrauterine death. Syphilis is a chronic infectious process caused by the spirochete *Treponema pallidum*. Due to its small size it can only be identified on dark-field microscopy. After a 10–90 day incubation period, the patient develops an indurated, nontender ulcer known as a chancre. This primary lesion, accompanied by painless regional lymphadenopathy, usually appears on the external genitalia, in the vagina, or on the cervix. The chancre is followed by a bacteremic or a secondary stage if the disease is not treated.

The clinical manifestations of secondary syphilis include skin rash, lesions on the palms and soles, mucous patches on mucosal surfaces, and wartlike growths in the genital area (condyloma lata). In the absence of therapy the clinical manifestations of tertiary syphilis ensue some years after the initial infection and include gummatous involvement of various organs as well as abnormalities in the cardiovascular and central nervous systems.

The effect of syphilis on the fetus depends on the timing of contraction of the disease during pregnancy and the effectiveness of treatment. Recently it has been shown that the placenta is permeable to the treponema throughout pregnancy. However, clinical observation has shown that if a pregnant patient contracts syphilis during the first 16–18 weeks of gestation, it is less likely that the fetus will be affected. Nevertheless, untreated syphilis in pregnancy may result in early spontaneous abortion, premature labor, stillbirth, neonatal death, or congenital syphilis.

The diagnosis of syphilis is best established by serologic testing, or if primary or secondary lesions are present, by dark-field examination at a time when the serologic tests may be nonreactive. Nonspecific (VDRL) and reagin testing (RPR) are screening serologic tests and should be performed on the first prenatal visit as well as during the third trimester. These tests are insensitive in very early or in latent disease and may be positive in patients without syphilis. Therefore, confirmation of the diagnosis requires a treponema-specific test, detecting specific antibodies to the *Treponema pallidum* (Fluorescent Treponemal Antibody Absorption test [FTA-ABS] and Treponema Pallidum Immobilization test [TPI]). Congenital syphilis can also be confirmed by either a dark-field examination in the presence of lesions or by determining the IgM-FTA-ABS titer, which represents infant IgM antibodies produced as a result of active syphilitic infection.

The treatment of incubating syphilis and syphilis of less than 1 year's duration includes benzathine penicillin-G, 2.4 million units total, half in each buttock, intramuscularly. For syphilis of more than 1 year's duration or of unknown duration, the treatment of choice is benzathine penicillin-G, 2.4 million units intramuscularly weekly for 3 successive weeks, a total of 7.2 million units. Erythromycin, which is recommended for syphilitic pregnant patients allergic to penicillin, crosses the placenta poorly and the levels that are achieved in the fetus are not satisfactory. Finally, it should be noted that the treatment of syphilis with long-acting penicillin is not always effective due to the low serum levels of antibiotics in pregnancy as compared to those in the nonpregnant patient; thus, the administration of a long course of short-acting penicillin for the treatment of syphilis in pregnancy would appear to be more efficacious.

Chancroid, caused by *Hemophilus ducreyi*, is an acute, autoinoculable and painful infection of the external genitalia and regional lymph nodes. It can also be transmitted sexually. The diagnosis is made by either culturing material from the ulcers or bubo in a blood-containing media or by biopsing the described lesions. Possible concomitant syphilis or gonorrhea should be ruled out. Treatment with sulfonamides is quite effective.

Granuloma inguinale, caused by *Calymmatobacterium granulomatis* (also called *Donovania granulomatis*), is a disease of low incidence and infectivity spread by sexual intercourse. The initial lesion is a raised, painless papule that progresses to forming central ulcerations with local, deep destruction of the tissues and formation of rectovaginal fistulas and pseudobuboes. The diagnosis is made by demonstrating the characteristic Donovan bodies in material aspirated from lymph nodes. Culture of *C. granulomatis* is also helpful. Biopsy of the lesions is helpful in making the differential diagnosis from malignancy. Tetracycline and erythromycin are effective in the treatment of early lesions, although only the latter can be used in pregnancy. Surgery may be required for correction of advanced tissue destruction.

Lymphogranuloma venereum, caused by *Chlamydia trachomatis,* is a disease that is usually transmitted through sexual intercourse and primarily affects the lymphatics and the lymph nodes (inguinal buboes). Common applications of the disease include rectovaginal fistulas, perirectal abscesses, and polypoid growths of the colon with occasional malignant degeneration. The definitive diagnosis of lymphogranuloma venereum is made by a complement fixation test. Biopsy of the lesions, biochemical tests, and the Frei intradermal test (not specific) can also be used diagnostically. The recommended treatment is sulfonamides for 3 weeks. Surgical management is sometimes indicated for elephantiasis, rectal strictures, and so on.

Molluscum contagiosum is a sexually transmitted viral (pox virus group) cutaneous disease in the genital area. The diagnosis is based on the microscopic examination of the lesion. Freezing and electrodesiccating the lesions are utilized as effective methods of treatment.

Herpes genitalis is discussed in another chapter.

General

1. Dunlop, E. M. C. Sexually transmitted diseases. *Clin. Obstet. Gynecol.* 4:451, 1977.
   The author describes the most common venereal diseases that may be contracted in pregnancy, as well as how each one of them affects the perinatal outcome.
2. Rein, M. F., and Chapel, T. A. Trichomoniasis, candidiasis, and minor venereal diseases. *Clin. Obstet. Gynecol.* 18:73, 1975.
   This review article discusses both the highly prevalent infections, which

have recently been recognized as sexually transmitted, and the less common but more classic venereal diseases.

3. Mumford, D. M., Smith, P. B., and Goldfarb, J. L. Prevalence of venereal disease in indigent pregnant adolescents. *J. Reprod. Med.* 19:83, 1977.
   In this study the authors show that venereal disease in pregnant teenagers of all socioeconomic levels is probably significant, and routine culturing of all pregnant adolescents is strongly recommended.

4. Schneider, G. T. Sexually transmissible vaginal infection in pregnancy: 1. Common infections. 2. Less common infections. *Postgrad. Med.* 65:177, 185, 1979.
   The author describes the common as well as the uncommon sexually transmissible vaginal infections and how each one of them affects the perinatal outcome.

5. Genadry, R. R., Thompson, B. H., and Niebyl, J. R. Gonococcal salpingitis in pregnancy. *Am. J. Obstet. Gynecol.* 126:512, 1976.
   The authors report a case of acute gonococcal salpingitis coexisting with a 14-week intrauterine pregnancy that subsequently was carried to term with good results.

6. Edwards, L. E., et al. Gonorrhea in pregnancy. *Am. J. Obstet. Gynecol.* 132:637, 1978.
   The results of this study show that infection with the gonococcal organism in pregnancy carries a significant risk to both mother and newborn infant, particularly in instances in which the disease is manifested in the intrapartum period.

7. Harter, C. A., and Benirschke, K. Fetal syphilis in the first trimester. *Am. J. Obstet. Gynecol.* 124:705, 1976.
   The authors show evidence of first trimester fetal syphilis in 2 of their 5 cases (40%) despite the widespread belief that the spirochetes of syphilis are unable to cross the placenta in early pregnancy.

Diagnosis and Management

8. Ryan, G. M., Jr. Ambulatory Management of Venereal Disease. In G. M. Ryan, Jr. (Ed.), *Ambulatory Care in Obstetrics and Gynecology.* New York: Grune & Stratton, 1980.
   The author describes the ambulatory management of gonorrhea and syphilis in both pregnant and nonpregnant patients.

9. Sexually transmitted diseases (STD). *ACOG. Tech. Bull.* No. 50; June, 1978.
   An outline of the current treatment of gonorrhea and syphilis as recommended by the American College of Obstetricians and Gynecologists.

10. Nicholas, J., and Fiumara, N. D. Treatment of primary and secondary syphilis. *J.A.M.A.* 243:2500, 1980.
    This study demonstrated that patients infected with primary syphilis become seronegative within 1 year, whereas in those patients infected with secondary syphilis, the blood test becomes nonreactive within two years.

11. Jones, J. E., Jr., and Harris, R. E. Diagnostic evaluation of syphilis during pregnancy. *Obstet. Gynecol.* 54:611, 1979.
    In this study the authors present data indicating that serologic examination of the cerebrospinal fluid should be included in the evaluation of all pregnant patients with positive VDRL and FTA-ABS tests.

12. McCormack, W. M. Management of sexually transmissible infections during pregnancy. *Clin. Obstet. Gynecol.* 18:57, 1975.
    The author describes the management of sexually transmissible infections that appear to complicate pregnancy.

13. Hart, G. The diagnosis of syphilis. *Med. J. Aust.* 2:722, 1975.

In this paper the author briefly outlines those clinical, microscopic, and serological aspects of the diagnosis of syphilis with which all clinicians should be familiar.

14. Holmes, K. K. The chlamydia epidemic. *J.A.M.A.* 245:1718, 1981.
    This article contains an interview with the most knowledgeable person regarding chlamydia and how it affects pregnant and nonpregnant women. This is a must reading for those interested in the chlamydia epidemic in the country.

Cardiac Disease in Pregnancy

The physiologic changes of pregnancy affect the cardiovascular system profoundly. The normal heart adapts readily to the increased work load, but this may not be the case in a patient with cardiac disease. Heart disease is present in 0.5%–2% of pregnant women and with a mortality of about 1%, it represents the principle nonobstetric cause of maternal death.

The cardiovascular alterations in pregnancy are dependent to a large degree on an increase in plasma volume that commences in the first trimester and by 34–36 weeks is up to 50% above nonpregnant levels (20%–100%); this increase slows near term. Red cell mass also increases; this increase is linear to 20%–25% above nonpregnant levels. The increased blood volume appears to be related to increased maternal vascular capacity and to the action of estrogen and progesterone on renin and aldosterone function.

In adapting to the increased blood volume there is a gradual increase in heart rate, peaking at term at 15 beats per minute over nonpregnant levels. Stroke volume increases in early pregnancy, later declines, and at term equals nonpregnant levels. Cardiac output increases from the first trimester, peaks by 20–24 weeks at 30%–40% above nonpregnant levels, and declines during the last 8 weeks. The increased cardiac output is distributed to the uterus, kidneys, and breasts particularly. At term, uterine blood flow averages 500 ml/min. Cardiac output is very sensitive to posture, so that changing from the supine to the lateral position increases output by 27%, with corresponding increases in renal and uterine flow. These changes are in part related to pressure effects of the pregnant uterus on the inferior vena cava.

In labor the cardiac output rises to 25% above prelabor values during uterine contractions, and there is also a progressive increase in output between contractions. At delivery there is a further rise in cardiac output (20%–60%). Following delivery major hemodynamic changes occur due to increased venous return, decreased intravascular space, blood loss, and use of oxytocics. In the puerperium, the blood volume declines and by the third postpartum day has decreased by about 16%.

The New York Heart Association classifies pregnant patients with heart disease according to their functional capacity. In class I patients, objective findings are present with no limitation of activity; class II patients have some limitation of physical activity; class III patients are comfortable at rest but have marked limitation of physical activity; and class IV patients are unable to carry on physical activity without discomfort.

Rheumatic fever causes 60%–80% of cardiac disease in pregnancy. Mitral stenosis (65%), mitral regurgitation (24%), and aortic regurgitation (10%) are the most common lesions seen. Congenital heart disease accounts for 20%–40% of heart disease in pregnancy. Patients with a left-to-right shunt usually tolerate pregnancy well, provided reversal of shunt does not occur. Patients with a right-to-left shunt are cyanosed, and there is a high fetal wastage. Myocardial disease specifically related to pregnancy is referred to as peripartal heart disease and appears to be a type of cardiomyopathy. Hypertensive and arteriosclerotic heart disease are not included in this presentation.

As a rule, the cardiac disease is already known; however, on occasion, the diagnosis may only be made during pregnancy. Such patients must then have chest x-ray, ECG, and cardiology consultation.

Patients are seen weekly by the obstetrician and monthly by the cardiologist. Commonly, hospitalization early in pregnancy and near term is necessary. Symptoms of undue fatigue, palpitations, dyspnea, orthopnea, or anginal pain are given particular attention. The patient must stay within her cardiac reserve, which may entail modified or even complete bed rest. The use of diuretics and limited-salt diet and early admission on the findings of any evidence of pulmonary congestion are the basis of preventing congestive heart failure. Anemias, excessive weight gain, anxiety, and infections must be prevented and treated if found. Dental care is of particular importance. In patients under 30, recurrence of rheumatic fever can be prevented by monthly penicillin injections.

Close surveillance of fetal growth and development is essential in the pregnant cardiac patient since there is an increased incidence of prematurity and low birth weight in the neonates, even in patients in classes I and II. There is a high fetal wastage in patients with cyanotic heart disease. If the maternal hematocrit is over 65%, 75% abort or go into premature labor.

Patients with mitral stenosis tend to develop arrhythmias (10%) or congestive cardiac failure (20%–25%) in pregnancy. The treatment is as for nonpregnant patients, including cardioversion, digitalis, and quinidine, which have been shown not to harm the fetus.

Termination is rarely indicated; however, if congestive heart failure is present within the first 12 weeks and if response to therapy is unfavorable, this may be offered. Termination is also indicated in patients with pulmonary arterial hypertension, Marfan's syndrome, and peripartal cardiomyopathy with persistent cardiomegaly. An alternative is to offer cardiac surgery if the lesion is amenable to correction. If the pregnancy is beyond the sixteenth to twentieth week, termination becomes more of a hazard than the pregnancy itself. Fetal mortality with open-heart surgery is reportedly about 33%. If possible, the surgery should be performed during the second trimester because of possible teratogenic effects.

The best position for the laboring cardiac patient is a semisitting one. The lithotomy position should be avoided because of the increased blood return after delivery. Pain relief is vital; tranquilizers and narcotics may be used in small doses in combination, but epidural anesthesia is the method of choice. The second stage should be shortened with forceps when obstetrically safe. If cesarean section is indicated for an obstetric problem, general anesthesia is the method of choice. Both of these anesthetic techniques minimize increases in cardiac output. Intravenous fluids, preferably dextrose and water, should be administered sparingly; not more than 50 ml per hour should be used as a rule. Oxytocin should be mixed in 200 ml administration units rather than the usual 1,000 ml. Antibiotics in the form of penicillin and an aminoglycoside should be given from the onset of labor and for three days after delivery to prevent endocarditis.

Sixty percent of cardiac deaths occur postpartum, usually from congestive heart failure. Close observation is therefore vital throughout the puerperium. Postpartum tubal ligation should be offered in selected cases, but surgery should be postponed until nonpregnant cardiovascular status is regained.

Contraception for the cardiac patient who does not wish to be sterilized is difficult, since estrogen-containing pills predispose to fluid retention, hyperlipidemia, hypertension, and thromboembolism. The intrauterine device may be associated with infection, both pelvic and valvular. The barrier methods are safe, but their lesser effectiveness lessens their value for these patients. Insertion of an intrauterine device with antibiotic cover appears to offer the best alternative.

Conception is generally discouraged in patients with cardiac valvular prostheses, although some in classes I and II may be allowed to proceed with pregnancy. These patients usually require anticoagulants, and heparin, which does not cross the placental barrier, should be employed.

Peripartal heart disease or cardiomyopathy is a syndrome of cardiac failure occurring in late pregnancy without obvious cause and in a previously normal heart. This is a rare condition that may recur in subsequent pregnancies. Management is as for class III and IV cardiac patients. If heart size does not return to normal after delivery, further pregnancy should be firmly discouraged.

Reviews and Series

1. Ueland, K. Cardiovascular diseases complicating pregnancy. *Clin. Obstet. Gynecol.* 21:429, 1978.
   Sterilization is recommended only for those women with severe cardiac disability who have surgically uncorrectable lesions.
2. Etheridge, M. J., and Pepperell, R. J. Heart disease and pregnancy at the Royal Women's Hospital. *Med. J. Aust.* 2:277, 1977.
   Report details 764 pregnancies in 542 cardiac patients with a 1.3% maternal mortality and a perinatal mortality of 48 per 1000.

Cardiovascular Changes in Pregnancy

3. Ueland, K., and Metcalfe, J. Circulatory changes in pregnancy. *Clin. Obstet. Gynecol.* 18:41, 1975.
   If the placenta is regarded as analogous to a modified arteriovenous fistula, this would be in keeping with the "hypercirculatory state" of pregnancy.
4. Kerr, M. G. The mechanical effects of the gravid uterus in late pregnancy. *J. Obstet. Gynaecol. Br. Commonw.* 72:513. 1965.
   X-rays demonstrated complete obstruction of the vena cava when in the supine position in 90% of pregnant women at term.

Diagnosis

5. Burch, G. E. Heart disease and pregnancy. *Am. Heart J.* 93:104, 1977.
   In pregnancy the heart progressively assumes a more horizontal position. Allowance must be made for this in the interpretation of the chest x-ray and of the ECG.
6. Harvey, W. P. Alterations of the cardiac physical examination in normal pregnancy. *Clin. Obstet. Gynecol.* 18:51, 1975.
   A short, early systolic, grade 1 to 3 murmur is heard in most pregnant women, and the second sound is usually loud and split.

Management

7. Selzer, A. Risks of pregnancy in women with cardiac disease. *J.A.M.A.* 238:892, 1977.
   In order to offer optimal evaluation and counseling, the time to consider heart disease and pregnancy is prior to pregnancy.
8. Shanl, W. L., and Hall, J. G. Multiple congenital anomalies associated with oral anticoagulants. *Am. J. Obstet. Gynecol.* 127:191, 1977.
   Fetal death from hemorrhage has also been reported with oral anticoagulants.
9. Eilen, B., et al. Aortic valve replacement in the third trimester of pregnancy: Case report and review of the literature. *Obstet. Gynecol.* 57:119, 1981.
   A case report outlining the failure of cardiac valve replacement during pregnancy is offered. The literature is reviewed and recommendations made for the management of such surgery.

10. Gladstone, G. R., Hardof, A., and Gersony, W. M. Propranolol administration during pregnancy: Effects on the fetus. *J. Pediatr.* 86:962, 1975.
May initiate premature labor and has produced bradycardia, hypoglycemia, and respiratory depression in the neonate.

11. Schenker, J. G., and Polishuk, W. Z. Pregnancy following mitral valvotomy. A survey of 182 patients. *Obstet. Gynecol.* 32:214, 1968.
Mitral valvotomy is palliative, not curative.

12. Taguchi, K. Pregnancy in patients with a prosthetic heart valve. *Surg. Gynecol. Obstet.* 145:206, 1977.
Complications associated with prostheses include valve regurgitation or obstruction, thromboembolism, cardiac failure, hemolytic anemia, and arrhythmias.

13. Manning, P. R., Mestman, J. H., and Lau, F. Y. K. Management of the pregnant patient with mitral stenosis. *Clin. Obstet. Gynecol.* 18:99, 1975.
Patients with mild or even suspected pulmonary congestion should be hospitalized for bed rest and reassurance.

Less Common Cardiac Lesions

14. Demakis, J. G., and Rahimtoola, S. H. Peripartum cardiomyopathy. *Circulation* 44:964, 1971.
Most patients are older, black, multiparous, and of low socioeconomic status. The syndrome is more common in women who have had toxemia or twins.

15. Davidson, N. McD., and Parry, E. H. O. The etiology of peripartum cardiac failure. *Am. Heart J.* 97:535, 1979.
The etiology is unknown. The mortality rate is around 30% within a few years of onset, in spite of intensive treatment.

16. Gleicher, N., et al. Eisenmenger's syndrome and pregnancy. *Obstet. Gynecol. Surv.* 34:721, 1979.
Reviews the literature. Maternal mortality ranged from 27%–66%.

17. Airas, F., and Pineda, J. Aortic stenosis and pregnancy. *J. Reprod. Med.* 20:229, 1978.
Twenty-three patients reported in the literature; maternal mortality was 17% and perinatal mortality 31%.

18. Deal, K., and Wooley, C. F. Coarctation of the aorta and pregnancy. *Ann. Intern. Med.* 78:706, 1973.
Pregnancy increased the susceptibility to aortic dissection; this increased susceptibility is also found in patients with Marfan's syndrome.

Diabetes Mellitus in Pregnancy

Diabetes mellitus is a condition of relative or absolute insulin deficiency that, during pregnancy, presents serious dangers for the mother and the fetus. Usually for the diabetic gravida there are progressively increasing insulin requirements, as well as increased risks of infection, ketoacidosis, hydramnios, hypertension, and worsening of preexisting proliferative retinopathy. With maternal hyperglycemia, there is rapid transplacental passage of glucose, which results in fetal hyperglycemia and secondary hyperinsulinemia. These metabolic disturbances frequently result in accelerated fetal growth (macrosomia), chemical alteration of fetal hemoglobin (hemoglobin A_{1c}, which may decrease the oxygen-carrying capacity of fetal blood), and a delay in the maturation of fetal lung surfactant. When present during the first trimester, hyperglycemia (as well as ketoacidosis) possibly may be responsible for the severalfold increase in congenital anomalies seen in infants of diabetic mothers. During the neonatal period, these infants are at risk for severe hypoglycemia, hyperbilirubinemia, hypocalcemia, respiratory distress syndrome, the morbidity associated with nonlethal congenital anomalies, and the trauma associated with ill-advised vaginal delivery of the large fetus.

The most frightening problem for obstetricians is the specter of sudden, unexplained stillbirth, a complication that becomes more likely as term approaches. Routine (but now outmoded) premature delivery of infants of all diabetic gravidas, while generally alleviating the stillbirth problem, resulted rather in death or serious morbidity from prematurity for many infants that probably were and would have remained quite healthy in utero. The past few years have witnessed the use of fetal surveillance techniques that allow the obstetrician to identify the majority of fetuses who are not in danger. The remaining small minority in danger of stillbirth are then subjected to further tests of fetal well-being. This minority, as well as the majority considered healthy but near term, are then subjected to analysis of amniotic fluid surfactant. The use of these tests allows an individualized approach to the timing of delivery and has been associated with a marked improvement in the perinatal mortality rate among infants of diabetic gravidas.

Probably the most important element in achieving this improvement has been the aggressive approach to the control of maternal glucose. Studies have demonstrated that, in nondiabetic pregnant women, serum glucose levels are generally in the range of 60–80 mg/dl before meals and rarely reach 100 mg/dl, even postprandially. In addition, studies from Sweden have shown that when the average serum glucose level, as measured several times daily the last few weeks of pregnancy, is less than 100 mg/dl, the perinatal mortality rate approaches that seen in nondiabetic gravidas. On the basis of such studies, many obstetricians consider it desirable to maintain serum glucose concentrations at less than 100 mg/dl at all times.

Such rigid control may be associated with at least occasional episodes of hypoglycemia. Although these episodes (which, curiously, are sometimes not heralded by the expected premonitory autonomic symptoms) are undesirable from the maternal point of view, they do not seem to place the fetus in particular jeopardy. Indeed, some fetuses have survived without apparent damage the treatment of maternal psychiatric disease by insulin shock therapy.

Most women who exhibit glucose intolerance during pregnancy cannot be shown to have this metabolic problem before or within several years after gestation, although they have a high likelihood of developing diabetes during the subsequent two decades. The pregnancy itself is associated with diabetogenic factors, mostly hormonal, particularly as gestation advances.

Although it is well known that certain historical factors such as previous macrosomia or a strong family history of diabetes increase the likelihood of finding gestational diabetes, a sizable fraction of gravidas with this condition will not be identified unless all pregnancies are appropriately screened. Such screening may take the form of determining serum glucose 2 hours following a 50 or 100 g oral glucose load, or following a standard meal containing at least 100 g of carbohydrate. A positive screening test is generally documented by a 3-hour glucose tolerance test using a 100 g glucose load. The values used for a positive test (in mg/dl)—greater than 105 fasting: 190 at 1 hour; 165 at 2 hours; and 145 at 3 hours—are those originally proposed by O'Sullivan and Mahan and represent values more than two standard deviations higher than the mean for nondiabetic gravidas.

The condition of a gestational (class A) diabetic can usually be controlled by an American Diabetic Association diet containing generally the same caloric level advised for nondiabetic gravidas, 2,000 to 2,400 calories. Such a diet avoids refined sugars but provides generous amounts of carbohydrates at frequent times and in complex form. The islet cell stress is thus minimized and the serum glucose levels, whether fasting or postprandial, are generally in the range for nondiabetic gravidas. If control is not maintained by diet alone, or if the woman was on insulin prior to pregnancy, this drug must be used during pregnancy as well. Oral hypoglycemic agents do not provide adequate control, may be teratogenic, and can result in severe and protracted neonatal hypoglycemia. The insulin dosage, whether being initiated during gestation for decompensated class A diabetes or being modified for the previously insulin-dependent woman, is generally provided in at least two injections daily—before the morning and evening meals—since a single injection rarely allows the degree of control required during pregnancy.

Usually, a combination of intermediate-acting (NPH) and short-acting (regular) insulins is given at both times. As a first approximation, two-thirds of the total is given in the morning (two-thirds as NPH, one-third as regular) and one-third is given in the evening (one-half as NPH, one-half as regular). Weekly patterning of plasma glucose levels is made at 0700, 1100, 1600, and 2100 hours by the patients. The 0700 value is considered to reflect the evening NPH dosage; the 1100 value the morning regular dosage; the 1600 value the morning NPH dosage; and the 2100 value the evening regular dosage. Values from 65 to 95 are most desirable. Increments or decrements only as great as −4 to +4 units (and usually less) are made, depending on the deviations in glucose measurements from the desired range (65–95 mg/dl).

If the glucose values are considerably out of this range, repeated glucose measurements and adjustments in insulin dosages are prescribed, as often as daily, until control has been achieved. Such management is usually feasible on an outpatient basis and thereby avoids the expense, family disruption, and unsatisfactory degree of control usually associated with frequent hospital admission. Prolonged hospitalization, although associated with some of the best perinatal outcome statistics yet reported, is generally too devastating economically for most patients, even if supported by excellent insurance.

Useful antepartum fetal surveillance tests include ultrasound examinations and periodic monitoring of the fetal heart rate with such tests as the contraction stress test (CST) or nonstress test (NST), or both. The initial ultrasound examination, usually obtained by the middle of the second trimester, is primarily to corroborate the clinical assessments of gestational age and to establish baseline measurements for later evaluations of fetal growth. Class A, B, and C diabetics, especially when under poor metabolic control, frequently manifest accelerated fetal growth leading, in some cases, to frank macrosomia. On the other hand, class D, F, and R diabetics generally have underlying vascular disease that may place their fetuses at risk for placental nutritional insufficiency and consequent growth retardation. Ultrasound is also useful at times in defining some of the major congenital anomalies.

The use of weekly CSTs (or, in some centers, weekly or more frequent NSTs) has permitted continued gestation when these test results are negative. This has allowed many such pregnancies to deliver closer to term, thus increasing the chances that the condition of the uterine cervix will be sufficiently favorable to attempt a vaginal delivery. For a class A patient whose condition is otherwise uncomplicated and who on diet maintains acceptable metabolic control, these tests of fetal well-being may be unnecessary, unless insulin has been required during a prior pregnancy, she has previously given birth to an unexplained stillbirth, or the current pregnancy continues past 40 weeks gestation.

The use of maternal serum or urinary estriol determinations to assess fetal health is still practiced in some centers. However, these biochemical tests are becoming less popular in the management of the diabetic pregnancy because of the requirement of daily performance and reporting of values.

Although the lecithin/spingomyelin (L/S) ratio has been reported to reliably reflect fetal pulmonary maturation, there have been challenges to this conclusion in diabetic gravidas. On the other hand, the risk of neonatal respiratory distress syndrome appears to be essentially zero if phosphatidylglycerol is demonstrated in the amniotic fluid prior to delivery. This phospholipid test, which also seems reliable in the presence of blood or meconium, is therefore recommended prior to intervention in diabetic pregnancies.

The management of labor and delivery in the insulin-requiring patient obviously depends upon the planned route of delivery. Although cesarean section is necessary in less than half the patients managed as described, the preemptive use of this operation for obvious macrosomia is prudent. If cesarean section is planned, it is best performed early in the morning following the patient's usual evening insulin dose and evening meal and bedtime snack. For the patient under good control, the fasting glucose level (which should be checked) can be expected to be normal; thus the operation usually can be carried out without insulin or without glucose-containing intravenous fluids. The laboring patient must be maintained in lateral recumbency, and the fetus and uterine activity must be continuously monitored electronically. During labor, glucose and insulin infusions, as described by Linzey, combined with hourly checks of blood glucose by fingersticks and on-site reflectance meter measurements, provide a method by which excellent intrapartum metabolic control can be achieved.

The anesthesiologist and the neonatologist should be consulted early in the hospitalization and should be present for delivery. Infant resuscitation, if necessary, should be vigorous, and glucose measurements should be made on cord blood and frequently in the infant during the first few hours of life. A careful search for trauma and congenital anomalies must be made.

Finally, the intense plan of care described herein requires the efforts of many members of the complications clinic team to keep the patient educated, motivated, and encouraged. Continually caring for many diabetic gravidas maintains the proficiencies of these team members in dealing with their complex clinical and sociologic problems and keeps the economics of such care reasonable. Thus, insulin-requiring pregnant diabetics should be considered for referral to a tertiary center able to offer such care.

Diagnosis

1. O'Sullivan, J. B., and Mahan, C. M. Criteria for the oral glucose tolerance test in pregnancy. *Diabetes* 13:278, 1964.
   This study reports the results of standard glucose tolerance tests on a large number of ostensibly normal pregnant women. The values reported are the criteria used by most authorities today for glucose intolerance.

2. O'Sullivan, J. B., et al. Screening criteria for high risk gestational diabetic patients. *Am. J. Obstet. Gynecol.* 116:895, 1973.
   Although historic criteria for suspecting gestational diabetes are helpful, large numbers of patients with it will be missed unless all pregnant women are screened by a provocative test. A glucose level over 130 mg/dl after a 50 g oral glucose load was taken as a positive screening test.

3. Miller, E., et al. Elevated maternal hemoglobin A_{1c} in early pregnancy

and major congenital anomalies in infants of diabetic mothers. *N. Engl. J. Med.* 304:1331, 1981.

One hundred sixteen insulin dependent diabetic women were studied in the first trimester and subsequently during the pregnancy with maternal hemoglobin A_{1c}. The authors conclude that poorly controlled diabetes mellitus early in pregnancy is associated with an increased risk of major malformations and that hemoglobin A_{1c} values can help detect these alterations.

General

4. Sanders, H. J. Diabetes. Rapid advances, lingering mysteries. *Chem. Engin.* 57:30, 1981.
   An excellent summary article on what is known about diabetes mellitus is presented. The chemistry of insulin and new methods that are available to diagnose and treat this disorder are offered.
5. Spellacy, W. N. Insulin, Glucagon, and Growth Hormone in Pregnancy. In F. Fuchs and A. Klopper (Eds.), *Endocrinology of Pregnancy.* Hagerstown, Md.: Harper & Row, 1977. Vol. 2.
   With an identical intravenous glucose stimulus, there is a progressive and marked increase in insulin output and plasma insulin concentration as pregnancy advances. If the ability of the pancreatic beta cells to respond to these demands is exceeded, then the clinical expression is gestational diabetes.
6. Haukkamaa, J., Nilsson, C. G., and Luukkainen, T. Screening, management, and outcome of pregnancy in diabetic mothers. *Obstet. Gynecol.* 55:596, 1980.
   During a 3½-year period, 94 new diabetics were diagnosed by intensive screening. Their management by strict control of maternal glucose was reflected in excellent perinatal mortality rates.
7. Lemons, J. A., Vargas, P., and Delaney, J. J. Infant of the diabetic mother: Review of 225 cases. *Obstet. Gynecol.* 57:187, 1981.
   The maternal and neonatal data on 225 infants of diabetic mothers are presented. There were improved survival rates as well as decreasing morbidity rates for the infants of diabetic mothers.

Management

8. Hawarth, J. C., and Dilling, L. A. Relationships between maternal glucose intolerance and neonatal blood glucose. *J. Pediatr.* 89:810, 1976.
   Maternal hyperglycemia during a glucose tolerance test is a predictor of subsequent neonatal hypoglycemia. This study is one basis for the clinical practice of maintaining "tight" glucose control, even during labor.
9. Karlsson, K., and Kjellmer, I. The outcome of diabetic pregnancies in relation to the mother's blood sugar level. *Am. J. Obstet. Gynecol.* 112:213, 1972.
   The authors obtained mean blood glucose values from 167 insulin-dependent gravidas. If this mean value exceeded 150 mg/dl, the perinatal mortality rate was 24%, 15% if the average value was 100–150 mg/dl, and only 4% in those with values less than 100 mg/dl.
10. Widness, J. A., et al. Glycohemoglobin (Hb A_{1c}): A predictor of birth weight in infants of diabetic mothers. *J. Pediatr.* 92:8, 1978.
    This glycohemoglobin is thought to be a predictor of long-term control of diabetes. These investigators, in a study measuring Hb A_{1c} in cord blood, showed a good correlation with birth weight.
11. Bustos, R., et al. Significance of phosphatidylglycerol in amniotic fluid in complicated pregnancies. *Am. J. Obstet. Gynecol.* 133:899, 1979.

The presence of phosphatidylglycerol virtually assures mature fetal lungs, even in diabetic patients. This method is also valid in the presence of meconium or blood.

12. Huddleston, J. F. Stress and Nonstress Testing. In J. J. Sciarra and R. Depp (Eds.), *Gynecology and Obstetrics.* Hagerstown, Md.: Harper & Row, 1980. Vol. 3.
A rationale for CST use rather than NST in the management of those at highest risk for fetal death is presented. This rationale is based on basic considerations of uteroplacental pathophysiology, interpretations of the clinical literature, and as yet unpublished data from the CST/NST Collaborative Study.

13. Schade, D. S., and Eaton, R. P. Insulin delivery—today's systems, tomorrow's prospects. *Drug Ther.* 24:37, 1981.
This article discusses insulin resistance and inadequate insulin receptor function. Present modalities of insulin administration and future alternative methods are reviewed.

14. Gabbe, S. G., et al. Management and outcome of class A diabetes mellitus. *Am. J. Obstet. Gynecol.* 127:465, 1977.
A monumental study of 261 gestational diabetics managed as outpatients with frequent determinations of fasting blood glucose. Unless complications occurred, term delivery was expected and antepartum fetal monitoring was not begun until 40 weeks. There were no stillbirths or deaths due to trauma or iatrogenic prematurity.

15. Gabbe, S. G., et al. Management and outcome of pregnancy in diabetes mellitus, classes B to R. *Am. J. Obstet. Gynecol.* 129:723, 1977.
In this study, 271 insulin-requiring pregnant diabetics were aggressively managed by hospitalization from 34 weeks onward, with intensive testing and delivery at or near term. The perinatal mortality rate was an impressive 4% and the deaths were primarily due to congenital anomalies.

16. Schneider, J. M., et al. Ambulatory care of the pregnant diabetic. *Obstet. Gynecol.* 56:144, 1980.
With careful surveillance of 108 diabetic pregnancies on an outpatient basis, a 3% perinatal mortality rate was found with an average of only one hospitalization for each patient.

17. Linzey, E. M. Controlling diabetes with continuous insulin infusion. *Contemp. Ob/Gyn* 12:43, 1978.
A useful method is presented to control maternal (and fetal) blood glucose levels during labor. The hourly assessment of blood glucose, by fingerstick and measurement with a glucose oxidase strip and reflectance meter, is useful.

18. Buchwald, H., et al. Treatment of a type II diabetic by a totally implantable insulin infusion device. *Lancet* 1:1233, 1981.
The feasibility of treating a diabetic patient by a continuous intravenous infusion from an implantable pump was tested. An acceptable degree of glucose control was achieved in this patient. Its implications for future treatment are discussed.

Thyroid Disease in Pregnancy

The thyroid gland is altered by the metabolic and hormonal changes of pregnancy. Likewise, the reproductive outcome may be affected by diseases of this organ. Since all forms of thyroid disease are three to four times more common in women than in men, disorders of this gland are not uncommon during pregnancy.

Results of diagnostic tests for thyroid disorders are markedly changed by pregnancy. Increased estrogen stimulates production of thyroxine binding globulin (TBG) and is responsible for the rise in serum thyroxine (T_4) from nonpregnant levels of 4–6 µg/dl to 10–12 µg/dl from 12 weeks gestation until 6 weeks postpartum. Likewise, elevated TBG causes the T_3 resin uptake percentage to be reduced, since there is an increased number of unsaturated binding sites and thus less T_3 available for attachment to the resin. Although total T_4 increases during pregnancy, the free or metabolically active T_4 remains unchanged during this time. Therefore, during pregnancy an elevated T_4 level with a decreased T_3 resin uptake is a normal finding and reflects euthyroidism in the mother.

Thyroid-stimulating hormone (TSH) and the basal metabolic rate (BMR) are increased by the fourth month of pregnancy; however, the former returns to normal by term whereas the latter continues to rise until the gestation is ended. During pregnancy, the radioiodine uptake assessment of thyroid function is contraindicated because the fetal thyroid will concentrate the radioiodine isotope ^{131}I at a rate twenty to thirty times that of the mother, resulting in hypothyroidism in the fetus. Moreover, although the amount of radiation the mother receives is insignificant, there have been frequent reports of microcephaly and malignancies during childhood in children born of pregnancies complicated by the maternal administration of [131]I. Plasma inorganic iodine is also decreased during pregnancy due to the rise in renal clearance of this element. To compensate, the thyroid gland increases in size to produce sufficient T_4, resulting in the normal hypertrophy or "goiter of pregnancy." Other tests such as the protein-bound iodine and butanol-extractable iodine are no longer used for thyroid assessment because of inaccuracies in the results.

Maternal hypothyroidism is relatively uncommon in the pregnant patient. Although there is no indication that fertility per se is affected, menstrual irregularities, oligo-ovulation, and difficulty maintaining a pregnancy once it is achieved are hallmarks of this disorder. While it is well known that T_4 crosses the placenta poorly, T_3 does cross and is necessary for fetal thyroid gland development prior to the twelfth week of gestation. The most common cause of hypothyroidism is iatrogenic, following either surgery or ^{131}I therapy. Idiopathic hypothyroidism has a much more protracted onset and is usually related to Hashimoto's disease. Diagnosis is usually made on the basis of symptoms, physical signs, and laboratory assessment. Typical complaints of fatigue, obesity, coarse skin, thinning of the hair (particularly the eyebrows), myxedematous (facial or tibial) changes, macroglossia, and a subnormal body temperature are signs of this disorder. Paresthesias and delayed deep tendon reflexes are early symptoms in about 75% of patients with hypothyroidism. Postpartum amenorrhea and galactorrhea may be presenting complaints of hypothyroidism after pregnancy has occurred.

Laboratory diagnosis of hypothyroidism rests on a reduction in the amount of T_4 that is produced; levels in the normal nonpregnant range of 4 to 8 µg/dl should be viewed with suspicion if they occur during gestation. Similarly, the hypothyroid patient demonstrates a reduction in T_3 resin uptake to levels lower than the normal pregnant patient.

Once the diagnosis of hypothyroidism has been made, therapy should be instituted immediately with full replacement doses (3 grains of desiccated thyroid) of natural or synthetic agents. Proponents of synthetic compounds stress the purity of these drugs and the ability of added T_3 to cross the placenta. Care must be taken in the older patient to gradually increase the dose of thyroid, since cardiovascular insults can occur if the thyroid deficiency is corrected too rapidly.

Maternal hyperthyroidism is not uncommon, ranging from 0.05%–0.2% during pregnancy. Hyperthyroidism during pregnancy is associated with an increase in the neonatal wastage rate and low birth weight infants. There is no evidence that the pregnancy per se makes the disease process more difficult to control, although there is a propensity for relapse during the postpartum period. The two major types of hyperthyroidism are toxic diffuse goiter (Grave's disease) and toxic nodular goiter (Plummer's disease). The latter is uncommon during pregnancy and may place the patient at risk for thyroid carcinoma. Grave's disease occurs frequently in conjunction with pregnancy and is usually diagnosed by the classic symptoms of weight loss, ocular signs, pretibial myxedema, a resting pulse rate above 100 (fails to slow during a Valsalva maneuver), muscular wasting, and nervousness. The serum T_4 is above normal pregnancy values (>12–13 µg/dl). Similarly, the T_3 resin uptake in the normal nonpregnant range is indicative of thyrotoxicosis during pregnancy.

Treatment is principally medical with surgery infrequently advocated and radioiodine therapy contraindicated. Principally, the thiourea compounds such as propylthiouracil (PTU) are utilized; they inhibit the synthesis of thyroid hormone by blocking iodinization in the tyrosine molecule in the gland itself. Most patients are begun on 100–150 mg PTU every 8 hours and note some relief after 7 days, while euthyroidism may be approached in 3–5 weeks. Upon regression of symptoms and a fall in serum T_4, the dose of PTU should be decreased as much as possible (while still maintaining a maternal euthyroid state) to prevent the occurrence of fetal goiter, since the drug does cross the placenta. PTU, as well as other medications in this class such as methimazole (Tapazole), is complicated by nausea, skin rash, pruritus, and fever in 2%–8% of patients. Only rarely does the development of agranulocytosis dictate withdrawal of the drug, although white cell counts should be performed bimonthly during therapy. In acute cases, propranolol (Inderal) can be used as a short-term measure, particularly during thyroid storm or in preparing the patient for surgery. It is not useful for long-term management due to such neonatal side-effects as hypoglycemia, bradycardia, and hypothermia.

Neonatal thyroid function figures slightly in excess of those found in the mother are evident in the fetus, with free T_4, T_3, and TSH levels increased compared with maternal serum values. Levels in the infant continue to increase until term but decrease by the fifth day postdelivery to normal adult nonpregnant levels. These events are good evidence that the fetal thyroid gland as well as the hypothalamic-pituitary axis in the fetus function independently of the mother.

Neonatal hypothyroidism, resulting from a lack of sufficient thyroid hormone in the fetus, causes generalized developmental retardation, a related effect caused by T_4 content on cerebral protein synthesis. The etiology of the athyreotic cretin is unknown but appears to be related to an inherited disorder allowing maternal antibodies to cross the placenta and affect the developing fetal thyroid. Unfortunately, even if the diagnosis is made at birth, replacement of thyroid hormones cannot change the retarded mental development in children with this condition. Another hypothyroid disorder of infants is goitrous cretinism. In these patients, the thyroid enlargement is not present at birth but develops later from a defect in T_4 synthesis; this is inherited as an autosomal recessive gene. Finally, a number of substances ingested by the mother may adversely affect fetal thyroid function and cause goiter development.

Patients who have taken PTU may give birth to infants with a small goiter, although there is no evidence that PTU or other drugs has a detrimental long-term effect as far as growth and development are concerned. In contrast, iodine ingestion by the mother has been associated with large neonatal goiters at birth. One of the most important problems caused by these large goiters is respiratory distress due to laryngeal pressure. In most infants with goiters, a low serum T_4 and a normal T_3 resin uptake is diagnostic of hypothyroidism. Indeed, a serum $T_4 < 9.5$ µg/dl should increase suspicion of this disorder. X-rays may also be helpful in the diagnosis of cretinism since the lack of thyroid hormone causes a slow rate of skeletal growth; epiphyseal dysgenesis and lack of ossification are thus signs of fetal/neonatal hypothyroidism.

The treatment of neonatal hypothyroidism is adequate thyroid replacement. The athyreotic cretin cannot be helped by this therapy, but those affected by maternal drug ingestion and other causes can be easily treated and the mental retardation avoided.

Neonatal thyrotoxicosis is even more common in the newborn as compared with the mother. Although some infants will receive the 7S immunoglobin (long-acting thyroid stimulator [LATS]) from the mother via placental transfer, diagnosis is usually made on the basis of the total clinical picture (maternal symptoms of the disease in conjunction with goiter, tachycardia, increased T_4, and hyperirritability in the infant). Occasionally serum T_4 and the goiter may be absent, and the positive assay for LATS is thus helpful in some infants. Cardiac decompensation, hepatosplenomegaly, and jaundice also have been seen in these infants. If the hyperthyroidism is mild, usually no treatment is needed. If treatment is necessary, Lugol's solution (1 drop three times a day) or PTU (10 mg every 8 hours) is utilized. Propranolol is reserved for infants with severe cardiac decompensation with thyrotoxicosis. The infants are usually treated for 3–6 weeks and after that period of time require no further treatment.

In summary, maternal and neonatal hypothyroidism are quite rare, although the appearance of goiter due to maternal ingestion of many drugs is becoming more of a problem. On the other hand, maternal hyperthyroidism or Graves' disease, because of its unique increase in incidence among women, is becoming common as is neonatal hyperthyroidism. Characteristic physical and laboratory findings had to prompt recognition of both maternal and neonatal disorders. Immediate therapy in the mother is necessary for both hyperthyroidism and hypothyroidism in order to protect the infant. Recognition of the problem in the infant is critical if the goiter is large and poses immediate problems, as well as for the long-term prevention of mental retardation due to insufficient thyroid.

Thyroid Physiology in Pregnancy

1. Innerfield, R., and Hollander, C. S. Thyroidal complications of pregnancy. *Med. Clin. North Am.* 61:67, 1977.
   A comprehensive review of basic and clinical considerations regarding thyroid gland function during pregnancy. The effects of hypothyroid and hyperthyroid states on the neonate and fetus are discussed. A fine list of references (113) accompanies this article.
2. Schachter, Y., and Roges, T. E. Hyperthyroidism and hypothyroidism. *The Female Patient* 6:47, 1981.
   Interpretations of thyroid laboratory tests are highlighted by the article. The physiodynamics of thyroid hormones are nicely illustrated in this article.
3. Levy, R. P., et al. The myth of goiter in pregnancy. *Am. J. Obstet. Gynecol.* 137:701, 1980.

In a randomized prospective study, the thyroid glands of pregnant and nonpregnant women were palpated. No difference was found. The authors thus conclude that goiter in pregnancy should be considered a pathologic condition.

Hypothyroidism

4. Montgomery, D. A. D. Hypothyroidism in pregnancy. *Br. J. Obstet. Gynaecol.* 85:225, 1978.
   The effects of maternal hypothyroidism on the mother and infant is discussed. The replacement of thyroid was found to be unnecessary.
5. Potter, J. D. Hypothyroidism and reproductive failure. *Surg. Gynecol. Obstet.* 150:251, 1980.
   The effect of hypothyroidism on reproduction in the female is discussed. The author finds the thyroid gland to be significantly related to reproductive failure and offers 75 references.
6. Blignault, E. J. Advanced pregnancy in a severely myxoedematous patient. A case report and review of the literature. *S. Afr. Med. J.* 57:1050, 1980.
   Pregnancy in a myxedematous patient is described, and a review of the literature is offered. This is a relatively rare disorder, but correct diagnosis is very important because of maternal and neonatal complications.
7. Montoro, M., et al. Successful outcome of pregnancy in women with hypothyroidism. *Am. Intern. Med.* 94:31, 1981.
   The influence of hypothyroidism on fertility, gestation, and the offspring are discussed in this article, which includes the study of 9 hypothyroid women during 11 pregnancies. The literature is also reviewed and 21 references are offered.

Hyperthyroidism

8. Burrow, G. N. Hyperthyroidism during pregnancy. *N. Engl. J. Med.* 298:150, 1978.
   Hyperthyroid disease in pregnancy is thoroughly discussed, as is management of maternal hyperthyroidism.
9. Serup, J., and Petersen, S. Hyperthyroidism during pregnancy treated with propylthiouracil. *Acta Obstet. Gynecol. Scand.* 56:463, 1977.
   Hyperthyroidism in pregnancy, both management and diagnosis, is emphasized. Complications of therapeutic modalities are underscored.
10. Mestman, J. H. Management of thyroid diseases in pregnancy. *Clin. Perinatol.* 7:371, 1980.
    This article contains a thorough discussion of the management of each thyroid disorder during pregnancy. It also has an excellent discussion and diagrammatic representation of various thyroid tests available.
11. Sugrue, D., and Drury, M. I. Hyperthyroidism complicating pregnancy: Results of treatment by antithyroid drugs in 77 pregnancies. *Br. J. Obstet. Gynaecol.* 87:970, 1980.
    The treatment of hyperthyroidism in 77 pregnancies is detailed. Medical therapy in the minimal effective dose is recommended over surgery.
12. Curet, L. B. Hyperthyroidism and pregnancy. *Wis. Med. J.* 78:33, 1979.
    A very succinct discussion of the management of both mother and infant during hyperthyroidism is presented.

Fetal/Neonatal Effects

13. Maxwell, K. D., et al. Fetal tachycardia associated with intrauterine fetal thyrotoxicosis. *Obstet. Gynecol.* 55:18S, 1980.
    Fetal tachycardia in the appropriate clinical setting is the hallmark of fetal thyrotoxicosis. In utero diagnosis is detailed.

14. Rodesch, F., et al. Adverse effect of amniofetography on fetal thyroid function. *Am. J. Obstet. Gynecol.* 126:723, 1976.
    The effect of amniofetography on fetal thyroid is thought to be transient impairment of thyroid function. The dye used in amniography is very important.
15. Weiner, S., et al. Antenatal diagnosis and treatment of a fetal goiter. *J. Reprod. Med.* 24:39, 1980.
    Antenatal diagnosis of fetal goiter was documented with sonography. Intraamniotic treatment with thyroxine was successful.
16. Serup, J. Fetal and neonatal hypothyroidism due to antithyroid-drug therapy. *Lancet* 1:10, 1978.
    Fetal and neonatal hypothyroidism due to maternal treatment for hyperthyroidism is noted. Methods for prevention are detailed.
17. Ingbar, S. H., and Woeber, K. A. The Thyroid Gland. In R. H. Williams (Ed.), *Textbook of Endocrinology.* Philadelphia: Saunders, 1968.
    A thorough discussion of considerations involved in diagnosis, management, and prevention of fetal/neonatal disorders related to thyroid disease is presented.
18. Cheron, R. G., et al. Neonatal thyroid function after propylthiouracil therapy for maternal Graves' disease. *N. Engl. J. Med.* 304:525, 1981.
    Eleven women with hyperthyroidism were treated with PTU and 7 of them received a thyroid hormone supplementation (liotrix). The authors emphasized that it is essential to use the smallest possible dose of PTU to treat hyperthyroidism in pregnancy and that careful evaluation of the neonate after delivery is imperative.
19. Fisher, D. A., and Klein, A. H. Thyroid development and disorders of thyroid function in the newborn. *N. Engl. J. Med.* 304:702, 1981.
    An excellent review article on the thyroid function of the developing fetus and newborn infant; 97 references are included.

Hemoglobinopathies in Pregnancy

Hemoglobinopathies are biochemical disorders that function at a molecular level and affect either the production rate or the structural integrity of the normal hemoglobin molecule. There are over 150 abnormal hemoglobins reported, although the most common ones, sickle hemoglobin and C-hemoglobin, are related to the structural changes. Thalassemia, on the other hand, is caused by the abnormally low production of hemoglobin, and heterozygotes of this disorder are quite common. Homozygous sickle cell anemia (HbS-S), hemoglobin SC disease (HbS-C), and hemoglobin S-thalassemia (HbS-Thal) are the most clinically significant and comprise what is known as sickle cell disease (SCD). Since sickle hemoglobin and thalassemia are genetically inherited disorders, the only preventive measure is genetic counselling. The incidence of SCD ranges between 1 in 400 and 1 in 600 patients.

Mild hemoglobinopathies such as heterozygous thalassemia or sickle cell trait (HbSA-S) are more common (1 in 12 to 1 in 150) and pregnancies usually proceed as routine, uncomplicated gestations. In contrast, patients with SCD are at significant risk both for maternal difficulties and perinatal morbidity and mortality. There is an increased incidence of vaso-occlusive crises caused by hydrophobic bonding of sickle hemoglobin in patients with SCD. This condition is aggravated by infections, high altitudes, hypoxia, and acidosis.

Statistics through 1970 revealed a high maternal morbidity and mortality as well as a perinatal wastage rate of up to 50%. Most of these statistics were obtained when conservative therapy such as alkalinization of the serum, vasodilators, anticoagulants, and symptomatic relief of pain were used. Since 1970, intensive medical therapy as well as the use of transfusions has been more successful in yielding good maternal/fetal outcome. There has also been a dramatic decrease in the number of premature or low birth weight babies born to mothers with SCD when these intensive treatments were utilized. There is great disagreement, however, as to the proper mode of therapy. Those favoring intensive medical regimens point to the disadvantages of transfusion, which include hepatitis, transfusion reaction, and late iso-sensitization. They prefer to reserve transfusion for reactive situations such as occur in those patients who begin to have difficulties such as vaso-occlusive crises, extremely low hematocrits (< 15), or infection. On the other hand, there are those who favor giving transfusions prophylactically on a regular basis to prevent such symptoms. Both methods appear to show good results for the mother and the neonate. It should be noted, however, that for those who use the reactive approach, as many as 50% of the patients in their series will at some time or another receive transfusions for complications. This is to be compared to the less than 5%–15% complication rate in those who are transfused prophylactically.

Among those who routinely use transfusions, there is great disagreement on several points. First, many authors state that exchange transfusions should be used to remove as many sickle cells as possible. Others simply transfuse patients with packed cells to elevate the hematocrit, while still others perform hypertransfusions to drive the hemoglobin A level up to and in excess of 60%. There is also disagreement as to what time during gestation to start the transfusions. While many patients are begun on the transfusion regimen in the latter part of gestation, when the risk of complication is the greatest, others, underscoring the possibility of preventing growth retardation, begin transfusions when their patients first attend the prenatal clinic. Finally, there is disagreement as to what components to use for transfusion. Most persons using simple or hypertransfusion methodology advocate the use of packed cells. Those using exchange methods usually opt for buffy-coat poor-washed red cells. Since sensitization to the leukocytes is the most common cause of transfusion reaction, the use of buffy-coat poor-washed red cells is probably advisable. There is also some evidence that washing the red cells, while decreasing their survival time, also decreases the risk of hepatitis.

Those who use the conservative management approach feel that one can judge the severity of SCD in their patients by their previous medical course, as well as by the level of hemoglobin F. This does not seem to be true. The patients, particularly those with the hemoglobin S-C variety who have not had crises in the past, can experience severe morbidity and death during pregnancy. Therefore, the history, while being of some predictive value, is certainly not absolute in its ability to dictate a normal outcome. Furthermore, unless the levels of hemoglobin F are over 25%, they probably do not represent hereditary persistence-of-high-fetal-hemoglobin, which is not associated with a risk in pregnancy. Thus, even though hemoglobin F levels may be 15%–20%, this does not seem to protect routine patients with SCD, and they should be treated with intensive methods.

The method of follow-up after transfusion is fairly standardized. Most patients are seen posttransfusion or without transfusion at 1- to 2-week intervals. In most centers, particularly after transfusion, a hemoglobin electrophoresis is obtained at least every 2 weeks to assess a change in hemoglobin A and hemoglobin S levels. The packed cell volume, reticulocyte count, and platelet counts are also obtained. In those who are receiving transfusion therapy, a reduction in the percentage of hemoglobin S to less than 50% and an increase in hemoglobin A to at least 40% is desirable. In most of these instances, the packed cell volume will be between 30%–35% posttransfusion. Most authors agree that retransfusion should be performed if the hemoglobin A level falls below 20% or the hemoglobin S level rises about 80%. Antisickling agents such as urea and thiocyanate are of little use during pregnancy since the effect of these drugs on the infant is unknown.

The management of pregnancy proceeds along the lines of that used for any complicated, high-risk pregnancy. Care for these patients throughout pregnancy should be in a hospital setting where adequate hematologic consultation is present. Fetal health assessment using the nonstress or contraction stress tests, or both, should be performed beginning at 32–34 weeks and repeated weekly. Some centers use serum or urine estriols, although I have not found them to be helpful in most clinical situations. The use of fetal breathing movements, while applicable in research, is of no practical value at this time. As with other high-risk patients, the counting of fetal movements two to three times each day for a period of 30 minutes to an hour may be helpful in assessing fetal health.

Labor is not induced nor are patients operated upon for hematologic indications. Patients with SCD are allowed to go into spontaneous labor at or near term, although induction for obstetric reasons with pitocin is not contraindicated. During labor, conduction anesthesia with epidural anesthesia can be used if care is taken to avoid hypotension. A skilled anesthesiologist is needed to make this determination. Otherwise, light analgesia with meperidine or butorphanol can be utilized. Electronically monitoring the fetal heart rate and assessment of maternal blood gases is advised. Fetal scalp pH, if indicated by abnormal fetal heart rate tracings, may also be used. Oxygen given at 4–6 l/min should be administered, and some authors advocate alkalinizing maternal serum with 30 cc of 10% sodium citrate added to each 1000 cc of intravenous fluid. Anesthesia for delivery can be regional, pudendal, or local. Nitrous oxide or saddle block anesthesia is also acceptable. Balanced anesthesia for cesarean section is most acceptable, although care must be taken postoperatively not to allow atelectasis to develop. Obviously, conduction anesthesia for abdominal delivery in these patients is also acceptable if approved by the anesthesiologist.

Postpartum care is marked by a particularly intensive search for infections. Most patients managed with transfusion therapy do not have prolonged hospital stays unless infections are evident. Cord blood is screened so that the genetic condition of the baby is known and genetic counseling can take place.

Genetic counseling and education is of paramount importance. Each parent in the prenatal clinic should be notified and counseled as to the implication of her particular hemoglobinopathy. The husband or father should also be tested so that some prediction of risk to the infant can be given. Therapeutic abortion for maternal indications is not indicated in most cases unless severe maternal disease and compromise is already present.

In the near future it may be possible for fetal abnormalities to be predicted by simple amniocentesis in those patients who have sickle cell trait or in whom the production of an abnormal offspring with SCD might be possible. At the present time we must rely on fetoscopy and fetal blood sampling, which carries a 5%–10% fetal mortality rate with each procedure for this diagnosis. Education and intrapregnancy care should be coordinated with the hematologist and sickle cell center.

Contraception is a problem in these patients. Patients with SCD have a defective opsonization and thus do not fight infection well. For this reason, many people propose that use of intrauterine devices is contraindicated. Likewise, because of their problem with vaso-occlusive crises, many physicians will not place these patients on oral contraceptives. Although there is no data to support the idea that oral contraceptive use is contraindicated, most physicians do not prescribe them. Depo-Provera, although not marketed as a contraceptive, is an excellent choice for one since progesterone and progesteronelike compounds have been shown to be desickling agents, at least in vitro. Barrier contraceptives are probably the most prescribed. The use of permanent sterilization should be based on the family size expectations of the couple rather than on the presence of the hemoglobinopathy alone, since reproductive outcome for the mother and baby at this time is good.

Hemoglobinopathies in General

1. Oluboyede, O. A. Iron studies in pregnant and nonpregnant women with Haemoglobin SS or SC disease. *Br. J. Obstet. Gynaecol.* 87:989, 1980.
   The administration of iron has been contraindicated in patients with sickle hemoglobinopathies for some time. The author demonstrates that iron studies performed in 22 pregnant and 18 nonpregnant females with these hemoglobinopathies showed an evidence of iron deficiency and suggests that iron probably does need to be given to these patients during pregnancy.
2. Kaplan, B. H., and Hunt, T. *Hematology: Synthesis of Heme and Globin* (2nd ed.). New York: McGraw-Hill, 1977.
   An in-depth discussion of the etiology and pathophysiology of inherited hemoglobin defects. The hemoglobinopathies in general are approached from the hematologic and biochemical aspect.
3. Motulsky, A. G. Frequency of sickling disorders in U.S. blacks. *N. Engl. J. Med.* 288:31, 1973.
   A discussion of the frequency and prevalence of the various sickle hemoglobinopathies present in the United States.
4. Vichinsky, E. P., and Lubin, B. H. Sickle cell anemia and related hemoglobinopathies. *Pediatr. Clin. North Am.* 27:429, 1980.
   A complete anthology of sickle cell disease, including specific laboratory findings, clinical manifestations, various systems involvement, as well as treatment regimens; includes 90 references.
5. Maugh, T. H., II. Sickle cell (II): Many agents near trial. *Science.* 211:468, 1981.
   A full review article of the future treatment agents for sickle hemoglobinopathies is presented. The practicality of such agents is discussed.

Hemoglobinopathies in Pregnancy

6. Morrison, J. C. Hemoglobinopathies and pregnancy. *Clin. Obstet. Gynecol.* 22:819, 1979.
   A review of current and past pregnancy-related statistics as they apply to sickle cell hemoglobinopathies. Various therapeutic modalities are also included.
7. Cohen, A. W., Russell, M. O., and Mennuti, M. T. Sickle-δβ thalassemia: Mild sickling disorder with serious morbidity in pregnancy. *Obstet. Gynecol.* 58:127, 1981.
   Two patients with sickle-δβ thalassemia are reported. This particular disorder is clinically important because it has serious morbidity during pregnancy but is rarely a problem in the nonpregnant state.

Management

8. Milner, P. F., Jones, B. R., and Dobler, J. Outcome of pregnancy in sickle cell anemia and sickle cell-hemoglobin C disease. *Am. J. Obstet. Gynecol.* 138:239, 1980.

   A review of the literature and detailed look at conservative management in 181 pregnancies (98 patients). Good reproductive outcome was obtained without the use of aggressive treatment in the asymptomatic patient with sickle cell disease.

9. Morrison, J. C., et al. Prophylactic transfusions in pregnant patients with sickle hemoglobinopathies: Benefit versus risk. *Obstet. Gynecol.* 56:274, 1980.

   Analysis of 75 patients with severe sickle cell hemoglobinopathies who received prophylactic transfusions. The advantages and disadvantages of the use of partial prophylactic exchange transfusions are outlined.

10. Key, T. C., et al. Automated erythrocytophoresis for sickle cell anemia during pregnancy. *Am. J. Obstet. Gynecol.* 138:731, 1980.

    A new method of performing exchange transfusions in patients with sickle cell disease—utilizing the extracorporeal pump—is outlined.

11. Charache, S., et al. Management of sickle cell disease in pregnant patients. *Obstet. Gynecol.* 55:407, 1980.

    The management of pregnant patients with sickle cell disease without the use of prophylactic transfusions is presented. The perinatal statistics from 74 pregnancies in 42 patients are equal to those in the literature in whom prophylactic transfusion therapy was used.

12. Cunningham, F. G., et al. Prophylactic transfusions of normal red blood cells during pregnancies complicated by sickle cell hemoglobinopathies. *Am. J. Obstet. Gynecol.* 135:995, 1979.

    The management by prophylactic hypertransfusion of 37 pregnant women with severe sickle hemoglobinopathies is presented. There was a significant reduction in maternal mortality and morbidity and perinatal mortality when compared to previous papers detailing therapy without the use of transfusion from this institution.

Genetic Counseling and Education

13. Foster, H. W., Jr. Managing the sickle cell anemia in pregnant patients. *Contemp. Ob/Gyn* 16:21, 1980.

    This article presents a well-balanced view of managing sickle cell patients but emphasizes educating the patient about her disease process and giving the couple genetic counseling.

14. Alter, B. P. Prenatal diagnosis of hemoglobinopathies and other hematologic diseases. *J. Pediatr.* 95:501, 1979.

    The antenatal detection of hemoglobinopathies has been possible for some by the use of fetoscopy. This article details the methodology and management of such patients and mentions newer methods used in prenatal detection.

15. Morrison, J. C., Propst, M. G., and Blake, P. G. Sickle hemoglobin and the gravid patient: A management controversy. *Clin. Perinatol.* 7:273, 1980.

    This article deals with the various controversies within the area of the gravid patient with sickle hemoglobinopathies; it also stresses the emphasis that should be given to the patient both on antenatal counseling and consumer/provider education.

16. Kan, Y. W. Antenatal diagnosis of sickle cell anemia by DNA analysis of amniotic fluid cells. *Lancet* 2:910, 1978.

    A critically important article detailing a new technique for antenatal diagnosis of hemoglobinopathies that does not involve fetoscopy. The new technique eliminates the risk involved for the latter procedure and will obviously be applied to diagnosing many diseases in the future.

Tuberculosis and Pregnancy

Human tuberculosis (TB) results from an infection by a nonmotile, acid-fast, aerobic rod called *Mycobacterium tuberculosis*. The elimination of crowded living conditions, as much as antibiosis, has accounted for a drop in the mortality rate from 200 per 100,000 at the turn of the century to 10 per 100,000 at the present time. At its peak incidence, TB was primarily a disease of young adults and is now a disorder that usually affects males over the age of 50. It is still a problem during pregnancy, however, particularly in the southeastern United States where it is indigenous. Approximately 30 of 40,000 infants are born in the United States to women with TB each year, for a rate of 1%–3% among pregnancies in high-risk areas.

The diagnosis is made on the basis of clinical and laboratory examination. Ziehl-Neelsen staining and the culture characteristic of *M. tuberculosis*—its production of niacin in vitro—distinguishes it from similar bacteria. The chest x-ray most commonly reveals posterior and apical lung field involvement with cavitation. Physical findings include apical rales with pleural effusion, high spiking fever, and weight loss. Other suspicious signs are choroid tubercles in the eyegrounds, skin lesions, lymphadenopathy with "cold" abscess formation, hepatosplenomegaly, and a low sodium content.

It is recommended that diagnosis be initiated with the first-strength purified protein derivative (PPD) tuberculin skin test (5 tuberculin units per Mantoux test). This test exhibits a delayed hypersensitivity reaction by cellular response and is not humoral or antibody-mediated. False-positive reactions are rare, and false-negatives are less than 2% in infected patients. A second-strength PPD (250 tuberculin units) produces frequent false-positive reactions due to cross-reactivity with "atypical" mycobacteria. In addition, the tine test, while useful for mass screening, should not be used for diagnostic evaluation.

The tuberculin skin tests become positive 4–12 weeks after exposure to disease. They may be negative during the early phases of the disease and should be repeated if TB is clinically suspected. Once positive, the tuberculin skin test will remain positive in 96%–97% of patients. The exception to this rule is in the patient with disseminated miliary tuberculosis in whom the negative skin test rate may be 20%–25%. There is no danger in testing with PPD during pregnancy, although the immune response may be diminished. Cultures also are useful if the results are positive, but they may require long incubations and may be negative even with active disease.

The value of a routine prenatal chest film has been questioned and most do not perform this as a portion of their antenatal assessment. The diagnosis therefore usually rests with a careful clinical history, a meticulous physical examination, and a continuing risk assessment for tuberculosis. Many patients, however, may be clinically asymptomatic, with a positive PPD or recent conversion of a skin test being the only sign of infection.

Because the natural course of active tuberculosis is in no way altered by pregnancy in the untreated patient, the indication for therapeutic abortion is nonexistent. Pregnant women with inactive tuberculosis have been found to be at a 5%–10% risk of reactivation during gestation, which is approximately equal to that for nonpregnant patients. Parturients receiving adequate chemotherapy for active disease have the same excellent prognosis as their nonpregnant counterparts. In addition, there is no increased incidence of spontaneous abortion, fetal compromise, or newborn anomalies in patients with active tuberculosis who receive adequate antituberculosis chemotherapy. Congenital tuberculosis in the newborn, on the other hand, may occur by hematogenous spread from the untreated mother but more commonly is due to aspiration or inhalation of tubercle bacilli in the amniotic fluid before or during labor.

Therapy usually includes double or triple antibiotic combination regimens. Presently, isoniazid (INH), rifampin, or ethambutol are most commonly used. There are certain side effects, most being related to hepatic toxicity in the mother and infant. INH therapy may result in vitamin B_6 deficiency, and this vitamin probably should be supplemented in pregnant women who receive this drug. Resistance to one of these drugs occurs in 2%–3% of all untreated patients, but double therapy has reduced this complication considerably. Streptomycin, cycloserine, ethionamide, and other drugs are not used because of their teratogenicity to the fetus. BCG (bacille Calmette-Guerin) is a vaccine utilizing living, attenuated tubercle bacilli to protect individuals in high-risk situations who were not previously infected. This vaccine depends on a humoral or antibody response to the tubercle bacillus. It is especially effective in young children and in epidemic situations, but it should not be given to people who are known to be PPD positive because hypersensitivity reactions will occur. One of the most common uses for BCG in this country is its administration to infants of mothers with active TB.

Indication for therapy includes active, untreated disease; inactive disease not previously treated; and a recent tuberculin skin test conversion (within 1 year). There is no indication for therapy during pregnancy in tuberculin-positive patients with no clinical evidence of disease or knowledge of recent conversion of the skin test and in those with inactive disease who have been previously treated.

Management of infants born to tuberculous mothers is also of importance. In those with inactive disease that has previously been treated and in whom there is no evidence of reactivation, permanent contact between the mother and infant can be established immediately, and the infant need not receive treatment. Similarly, patients with inactive disease, those with active disease but receiving adequate antituberculous therapy, and those with inactive disease not previously treated but who have shown no progression during gestation, may have early infant contact, providing the mother is reliable in diagnostic or therapeutic efforts. For the newly diagnosed patient with active disease, contact may be allowed if the mother has been receiving chemotherapy for a minimum of 3 weeks and the infant receives preventive INH. Those patients with active disease and less than 3 weeks of treatment and those patients who are recalcitrant or unreliable are not permitted early infant contact, and their newborns should receive BCG vaccination. If BCG is not given, the infant should be tested with PPD tuberculin at 3- to 4-month intervals and the mother examined and x-rayed at those times.

In summary, although tuberculosis is now a disease of aged men, there is a 1%–3% incidence of new tuberculosis or reactivation of old TB appearing in pregnant women. Although pregnancy itself has no effect on the course of the disease, the impact on the mother's life as well as on that of the neonate can be devastating if the disease is not adequately treated. Furthermore, medical treatment of this disease is quite effective and should be used preventively.

General Respiratory System

1. Fishburne, J. I. Physiology and disease of the respiratory system in pregnancy. A review. *J. Reprod. Med.* 22:177, 1979.

A detailed physiologic assessment of changes that occur in the respiratory system during pregnancy with 71 references.

2. Schoenbaum, S. C., and Weinstein, L. Respiratory infection in pregnancy. *Clin. Obstet. Gynecol.* 22:293, 1979.
A detailed assessment of all respiratory infections during pregnancy is given.
3. Weinberger, S. E., et al. Pregnancy and the lung. *Am. Rev. Resp. Dis.* 121:559, 1980.
The authors give an extensive review of the effects of pregnancy on the lung. In addition, various disease states affecting the lung are discussed in detail.

Tuberculosis in Pregnancy

4. Sulavik, S. B. Pulmonary Disease. In G. N. Burrow and T. F. Ferris (Eds.), *Medical Complications During Pregnancy.* Philadelphia: Saunders, 1975.
A comprehensive analysis of tuberculosis in pregnancy and its effect on the mother, fetus, and newborn. An excellent section on diagnosis and classification of tuberculosis is presented.
5. Bjerkedal, T., Bahna, S. L., and Lehmann, E. H. Course and outcome of pregnancy in women with pulmonary tuberculosis. *Scand. J. Resp. Dis.* 56:245, 1975.
The reproductive outcome in 542 women with pulmonary tuberculosis was compared to over 100,000 pregnant women without this respiratory disease. Statistics with regard to infant outcome in both groups were comparable.
6. de March, P. Tuberculosis and pregnancy. Five-to-ten year review of 215 patients in their fertile age. *Chest* 68:800, 1975.
The influence of pregnancy as a relapse factor in pulmonary tuberculosis was studied in 215 patients receiving adequate chemotherapy. Pregnancy, delivery, or lactation does add to the risk of relapse.

Treatment

7. Good, J. T., Jr., et al. Tuberculosis in association with pregnancy. *Am. J. Obstet. Gynecol.* 140:492, 1981.
A retrospective analysis of 27 patients with pulmonary tuberculosis during pregnancy was reviewed. Over half the patients had drug resistant disease which was brought under control with multidrug therapy. Isoniazid, para-amniosalicylic acid, ethambutol, and rifampin all appear to be safe for the fetus.
8. Kendig, E. L. The place of BCG vaccine in the management of infants born of tuberculous mothers. *N. Engl. J. Med.* 281:520, 1969.
The use of BCG vaccine in infants of tuberculosis-positive mothers is detailed. Recommendations for follow-up of these patients are given.
9. Snider, D. E., et al. Treatment of tuberculosis during pregnancy. *Am. Rev. Resp. Dis.* 122:65, 1980.
The authors review the world's literature with regard to experience in treatment of tuberculosis; it recommended that there was no danger to the fetus if isoniazid in combination with ethambutol was used. If a third drug is needed, rifampin should be used, but, due to ototoxicity, streptomycin is contraindicated.
10. Schaefer, G. Watch for genital TB: A guide to diagnosis and treatment. *Contemp. Ob/Gyn* 17:167, 1981.
A comprehensive review of genital tuberculosis and its sequellae. Also, new and in-depth treatment regimens are advocated.

Diagnosis

11. Koplan, J. P., and Farer, L. S. Choice of preventive treatment for iso-
niazid-resistant tuberculous infection. *J.A.M.A.* 244:2736, 1980.

    *INH therapy was assessed with particular reference to tuberculous resis-
    tance. Guidelines for selecting cases at risk for isoniazid resistance and
    recommendations for second and third drugs are detailed.*

12. Warkany, J. Antituberculous drugs. *Teratology* 20:133, 1979.

    *All drugs used for antituberculous therapy are reviewed for adverse effect
    on fetal outcome. Isoniazid, rifampin, and ethambutol were the most use-
    ful and least toxic to the fetus.*

13. Hadlock, F. P., Park, S. K., and Wallace, R. J. Routine radiographic
    screening of the chest in pregnant women: Is it indicated? *Obstet. Gyne-
    col.* 54:433, 1979.

    *The routine radiographic screening of pregnant women to detect signs of
    tuberculosis was assessed in 5,422 cases. Only 11 cases of TB pathology
    were found, and in only 3 were the findings not suspected from history or
    physical examination. The conclusion is that the routine chest film for
    pregnant women, at least for TB, is no longer indicated.*

14. Covelli, H. D., and Wilson, R. T. Immunologic and medical considera-
    tions in tuberculin-sensitized pregnant patients. *Am. J. Obstet. Gynecol.*
    132:256, 1978.

    *Immunologic sensitivity to tuberculin bacilli was studied in 172 pregnant
    patients. Specific studies with lymphocytes in these patients account for
    the variable immune status of the pregnant woman. PPD derivatives are
    still judged to be safe for pregnant women.*

15. Falk, V., Ludviksson, K., and Agren, G. Genital tuberculosis in women.
    Analysis of 187 newly diagnosed cases from 47 Swedish hospitals during
    the ten-year period 1968 to 1977. *Am. J. Obstet. Gynecol.* 138:974, 1980.

    *A 10-year experience of all of the cases of genital tuberculosis in Sweden
    was discussed. The chance of a normal pregnancy even after surgery or
    chemotherapy was very low, whereas the chance of ectopic pregnancy was
    high.*

Pregnancy in the Adolescent

The rate of early childbearing in the United States is one of the highest in the world and ranks among the major health problems facing both the medical community and society, despite the availability of contraceptive information, contraceptive methods, and the legalization of abortion. The adolescent and her infant face increased risk, both obstetric and psychological, making teenage pregnancy neither desirable nor advocated.

It is estimated that of the 21 million teenagers in the country, 11 million are sexually active. Although there has been a general increase in contraceptive use among those sexually active, only 40% will employ some means of contraception at their first exposure to sexual intercourse. Approximately 1 million adolescents (aged 11 to 20) will become pregnant each year. Of these, 400,000 will have an abortion and 600,000 will go on to deliver live infants. Of the live births, 260,000 are to women under 15 years of age. The incidence of adolescent pregnancy is not bounded by social class or race, with 198,329 infants born to white women under the age of 19 as compared to 160,597 infants born to black women of the same age group. Eight out of ten pregnancies are conceived premaritally and 25% of these adolescents have more than one child by age 20.

There are many reasons for the high rate of adolescent pregnancy. The change in the age of menarche from just over 14 years to 12.5 years with fertility occurring by age 14, has certainly played a role. Increased sexual activity at younger ages, with 1 in 5 adolescents having had intercourse by age 16 and two-thirds by age 19, has also contributed to the rising pregnancy rate. The psychological factors associated with the motivation for pregnancy in the adolescent are complex. They may include: a desire to establish identity as an "adult"; escape from responsibility; rebellion against authority figures; desire for love or the need to give love. Also, pregnancy may temporarily bolster self-esteem through peer acceptance or serve as a mechanism through which a relationship with a significant man may be established or maintained. Although all of these factors are considered to be important, no data has been collected to date that would suggest a simple solution to the problem.

Teenage women have twice the risk of complications during pregnancy and delivery as women in their twenties. Adolescent pregnancy has been associated with an increased incidence of both obstetric and social complications that lead to high infant and maternal mortality as well as morbidity. Due to the biologic immaturity of the adolescent, the body is often ill prepared to sustain a pregnancy and provide safe delivery for the infant. Research to identify risk factors in the pregnant adolescent have shown an increased risk of anemia, pregnancy-induced hypertension, premature delivery, stillbirth, cephalopelvic disproportion, and operative delivery. The increased risk of pregnancy-induced hypertension is significant, especially if the pregnancy occurs within 24 months of menarche. The increased incidence of cephalopelvic disproportion in women under age 15 is related to the relative skeletal immaturity of the pelvis, leading to a higher incidence of cesarean delivery, an operation known to be associated with greater morbidity in the mother.

Adolescence is normally a period of high nuturitional needs due to the rapid growth and development of the body. The pregnant state imposes additional nutritional demands on the growing body and may rapidly deplete already limited reserves. The increased incidence of poor nutrition among adolescents due to limitations in economic resources, poor eating habits, and lack of knowledge regarding nutrition has been directly related to the increased incidence of delivery of low birth weight infants, themselves susceptible to increased mortality as well as developmental and neurological handicaps. Pregnant adolescents are also more susceptible to experiencing abnormal labor patterns with prolonged or precipitous labors occurring frequently, both associated with severe neonatal sequelae. Pregnant adolescents may also experience an increased incidence of postpartum hemorrhage and infection.

The psychological ramifications of adolescent pregnancy are enormous. Adolescence is in itself a period of maturational crisis in which the role of child must be evolved to the role of adult. The familiar prepubescent body image must be revised to that of a woman accommodating the changes of normal hormonal development. Psychologically inconsistent, uncertain feelings with unpredictable reactions are characteristic of the adolescent and produce confusion and frustration in themselves as well as in those around them. Experimentation is essential for the adolescent and may certainly play a major role in pregnancy. Likewise, pregnancy may also be viewed as a maturational crisis in which the familiar role of single individual is exchanged for the role of mother and provider. The adolescent parent must be prepared to nurture an infant instead of being nurtured. When pregnancy occurs during adolescence, the young person must deal with two maturational crises at the same time and satisfactory resolution is seldom possible. A "syndrome of failure" associated with adolescent pregnancy has been described. It includes failure to: fulfill developmental tasks of adolescence; remain in school; limit family size; establish stable families; be self-supporting; and have healthy children.

The long-term consequences to adolescent parents can be extremely costly to both society and the individuals involved. Extensive study has revealed that both adolescent mothers and fathers have substantially less education than their classmates; and the degree of educational deprivation is related to the age of the parent at the time of the infant's birth. Adolescent parents are also much more likely to hold low-prestige jobs due to their relatively low educational attainment. Adolescents account for 17% of mothers with eight years of education or less. For teenage mothers, reduced occupational attainment also means lower income and greater job dissatisfaction than that experienced by their classmates. These problems, plus the fact that adolescent parents usually exceed their family size preference, contribute to unstable marriages, divorce, and remarriage.

A poorly planned pregnancy occurring during the adolescent years will also adversely affect intrapersonal relations. Social skills as well as intrapersonal relationship skills may not adequately develop, both having long-term social ramifications. Relationships with family members as well as men may be jeopardized, leading to the development of further social or psychological complications.

Delivery of health care to the adolescent presents a complex challenge. No single health care provider can meet the many needs of the adolescent, but a team of health care providers can be invaluable. Her primary medical care will not differ significantly from prenatal care of any other woman, although she may expect more privacy and confidentiality. She is more likely to keep prenatal appointments and comply with medical regimes if a trusting, nonjudgmental relationship has been established. A nutritionist as part of the health care team is necessary to discuss with the adolescent her body needs and food requirements particular to pregnancy, thereby helping to provide the nutritional requirements for her own growth as well as the growth of her unborn baby. The social worker can provide referral information and counseling regarding pregnancy alternatives. Above all, the pregnant adolescent needs the cooperation and understanding of her parents and school authorities so that it may be possible for her to receive early and comprehensive prenatal care.

Consideration and support must also be given to the adolescent father so that he may be included in health care decisions, labor and delivery, and nurturance of the infant when he chooses to do so.

Adolescent pregnancy is not solely a medical problem and all the solutions cannot be found within the scope of medical practice. Prevention of this problem is the goal to be achieved and may be reached ultimately through comprehensive educational programs. Such educational programs need to be directed toward formation of healthy, mature attitudes toward sexuality and childbearing. Courses need to be integrated in the elementary school curriculum before the teen years and continued throughout childhood and adolescence. Basic information about human reproduction and conception, contraception, fetal growth, antenatal developments, and intrapartum and postpartum experiences as well as infant care should be included. Discussion groups held between adolescents and parents within the structure of church or school may prove beneficial to reduce misconceptions regarding sexuality and pregnancy.

Review

1. Perkins, R. P., et al. Intensive care in adolescent pregnancy. *Obstet. Gynecol.* 52:179, 1978.

   In this article 135 pregnant adolescents were compared to 100 pregnant control women in an older age group. No statistically significant differences were found in outcome statistics if excellent prenatal care was carried out.

Characteristics

2. Hutchins, F., Kendall, N., and Rubino, J. Experience with teenage pregnancy. *Obstet. Gynecol.* 54:1, 1979.

   A study to evaluate the characteristics of teenage pregnancy in an urban, nonwhite, socioeconomically depressed population.

3. Chilman, C. Illegitimate Births to Adolescents. *Adolescent Sexuality in a Changing American Society.* Bethesda, Md.: U. S. Department of Health, Education and Welfare, 1979. Pp. 195–246.

   The effects of unwed parenthood on adolescents have not been clearly established in this book.

4. Thompson, R. J., Cappleman, M. W., and Zeitschel, K. A. Neonatal behavior of infants of adolescent mothers. *Dev. Med. Child. Neurol.* 21:474, 1979.

   A study of the Brazelton neonatal assessment scale administered to 30 infants of adolescent mothers.

5. Chilman, C. *Adolescent Sexuality in a Changing American Society.* Bethesda, Md.: U.S. Department of Health, Education, and Welfare, 1978. Pp. 2–246.

   A well-documented report on adolescent sexuality.

6. Ryan, G. M., and Schneider, J. M. Teenage obstetric complications. *Clin. Obstet. Gynecol.* 21:1191, 1978.

   A review of black, single teenagers (222) who delivered at the University of Tennessee Center for Health Sciences; an increased incidence of hypertension and convulsive disorders was indicated.

7. Klein, L. Antecedents of teenage pregnancy. *Clin. Obstet. Gynecol.* 21:1151, 1978.
   Identification of antecedent factors relative to adolescent pregnancy.

Management

8. Worthington, B., Vermeensch, J., and Williams, S. Nutrition in Pregnancy and Lactation. *Nutritional Needs of the Pregnant Adolescent.* St. Louis: Mosby, 1977.
   A comprehensive overview of nutritional habits and needs for the pregnant adolescent.
9. Shen, J. Teenage Pregnancy. *The Clinical Practice of Adolescent Medicine.* New York: Appleton-Century-Crofts, 1979.
   A concise review of antepartum and postpartum management of the adolescent gravida.
10. Mercer, R. T. *Perspectives on Adolescent Health Care.* New York: Lippincott, 1979.
    A book designed to present ideas and issues about adolescent health care. An excellent resource for a variety of providers.
11. Anyan, W. Pregnancy in Adolescence. *Adolescent Medicine in Primary Care.* New York: John Wiley and Sons, 1978.
    A review of the general health care of the adolescent gravida together with the associated problems.

Mortality, Morbidity

12. Dott, A., and Fort, A. Medical and social factors affecting early teenage pregnancy. *Am. J. Obstet. Gynecol.* 125:532, 1976.
    A literature review and summary of the findings concerning the infant mortality rates of children born to mothers under 15 years of age in Louisiana.
13. Baldwin, W., and Cain, V. The children of teenage parents. *Fam. Plann. Perspect.* 12:34, 1980.
    Tests indicate that children born to adolescent mothers suffer from intellectual deficits. This is largely a result of the economic and social impact of early childbearing on the young mothers.

Services

14. Mahoney, E. Sex education in the public schools: A discriminant analysis of characteristic pro- and anti-individuals. *J. Sex. Research* 15:264, 1979.
    Political-religious views of sex education in the public schools are less dominant than the views of the role of women, family, and sexuality.
15. Ryan, G., and Sweeney, P. Attitudes of adolescents toward pregnancy and contraception. *Am. J. Obstet. Gynecol.* 137:358, 1980.
    Interviews with pregnant teenagers revealed that 87% had knowledge of contraception and were happy about being pregnant.
16. Johnson, C., Walters, L., and McKenny, P. Trends in services for pregnant adolescents. *Health Soc. Work* 4:27, 1979.
    A review of services for pregnant adolescents and recommendations for programs.
17. Paul, E., and Pipel, H. Teenagers and pregnancy: The law in 1979. *Fam. Plann. Perspect.* 5:297, 1979.
    Health care providers can render sex-related medical services to mature minors without parental consent.

Pregnancy in the Grand Multipara

A pregnant woman is considered to be a grand multipara (GM) if she has completed six or more gestations greater than 24 weeks. It has become apparent during the past several years that the percentage of grand multiparous pregnancies has markedly decreased. This reduction was brought about by a national policy of family planning as well as liberal performance of abortions and permanent sterilization procedures. Although GM pregnancies are not seen as frequently as in previous reports, it continues to be an obstetric problem in the indigent patient. The actual severity of obstetric and medical complications that are associated with GM is controversial. Despite the gloomy outlook reported prior to 1950, more recent investigations emphasize a favorable overall outcome. There is a universal agreement, however, that certain complications are more frequently encountered in the GM when compared to other parturients.

Advancing age in the grand multipara may be a causative factor in the increased incidence of associated medical illness frequently reported in these patients. Medical illness common in the GM includes cardiac disease, hypertensive vascular disorders, renal problems, diabetes mellitus, and anemia. Moreover, these illnesses may contribute significantly to the somewhat higher occurrence of certain obstetric complications (such as preeclampsia, placental abruption, and fetal anomalies). The pregnant woman with six or more children is at high risk for developing anemia during pregnancy because of iron and folic acid depletion caused by fetal demands during repeated pregnancies. In addition, she may be unable to give sufficient priority to her dietary requirements during pregnancy because she has to care for several children. The incidence of preeclampsia tends to decrease in relation to increasing parity and advanced maternal age, but the incidence increases to 20% among grand multiparas who are older than 40 years. This increase is expected because of the higher incidence of hypertensive vascular and renal disease after the age of 40.

The incidence of placenta previa is about two to four times more frequent in the grand multipara. It is postulated that underlying atrophy of the endometrium, secondary to changes induced by repeated pregnancies, is the principal causative factor. The incidence of premature separation of the placenta is increased by two to nine times in the grand multipara. The increased incidence of preeclampsia and hypertensive vascular disease in the GM may play a role in the development of placental abruption in these pregnancies.

Although the increased incidence of prematurity is not constant in various series, it seems that most of it is secondary to the increased incidence of obstetric complications (such as preeclampsia and placental accidents) leading to premature terminations of pregnancy. The incidence of infants weighing more than 4000 g is reported to be about 20%. The incidence tends to increase with increased maternal weight at time of delivery, and it is also increased in those who gain more than 30 pounds during pregnancy. Some authors have reported an increased frequency of fetal anomalies in GM pregnancies. This is probably a factor of increased maternal age and the associated increase in diabetes mellitus, rather than mere multiparity.

The incidence of transverse lie, face, and brow presentations is reported to be twice as frequent in the GM than in other parturients. Malpresentations increase with maternal age, with a peak in the GM who is older than 40 years.

While the etiology for increased fetal malpresentations remains uncertain, it may be related to recent data that revealed an increased amount of myometrial elastic tissue in the GM. There is universal agreement that the risk for postparturient hemorrhage (PPH) is significantly increased in the GM. It is claimed that alterations in uterine fiber histology (such as collagen deposited between uterine muscle fibers) interfere with normal postpartum homeostasis. However, recent studies revealed no such changes when uterine tissues were examined with reticulum stains. Because the grand multipara is at increased risk for uterine rupture (spontaneous or from oxytocin), some authors believe the use of oxytocin to stimulate labor should be contraindicated in the GM. It is claimed that repeated pregnancies and increased maternal age will result in a fragile uterine wall. It is also thought that increased hyalinization of blood vessels and sparser myometrial fibers are responsible for this increased fragility. However, the etiology for the increase in spontaneous uterine rupture remains unclear. The cautious, incremental use of oxytocin may be indicated in selected cases.

Reproductive outcome in the grand multipara has markedly improved because of recent advances in obstetric practice. However, the GM remains at increased risk for maternal and perinatal mortality because of potential obstetric complications frequently encountered. Early and frequent prenatal visits, plus referral to a tertiary perinatal center when indicated, will help reduce the increased risks inherent in these pregnancies.

Review

1. Israel, S. L., and Blazar, A. S. Obstetric behavior of the grand multipara. *Am. J. Obstet. Gynecol.* 91:326, 1965.
   A review of 5551 grand multiparas, with a list of medical and obstetric complications showing increased incidence of abnormal outcome statistics.
2. Fuchs, K., and Peretz, A. The problem of the grand multipara: A review of 1677 cases. *Obstet. Gynecol.* 18:719, 1961.
   Complications of pregnancy and delivery in 1677 grand multiparous patients were compared to those of other parturients. Maternal and infant mortality in the grand multipara group did not exceed that of other parturients. Premature separation of the placenta was nine times more common in the GM. The authors recommend that the grand multipara be delivered in a hospital capable of handling emergencies.
3. Huey, J. R., Jr., Al-Hadjiev, A., and Paul, R. H. Uterine activity in the multiparous patient. *Am. J. Obstet. Gynecol.* 126:682, 1976.
   The uterine activity in the grand multipara is found to be of the same intensity as in the primiparous woman. This is particularly true in the second stage of labor.

Complications

4. Ziel, H. A. Grand multiparity—its obstetric implications. *Am. J. Obstet. Gynecol.* 84:1427, 1962.
   Grand multiparity was associated with a significant increase in the number of potentially dangerous complications of pregnancy. In addition, there appears to be a significant increase in the incidence of excessively large infants, unusual fetal presentations, and stillbirths among infants born to grand multiparas.
5. Petry, J. A., and Pearson, B. Obstetric complications with grand multiparity. *South. M. J. 48:820, 1955.*
   The average age in a total of 862 grand multiparas was 37 years and the maternal mortality (0.35%) was twice that encountered in all deliveries.

The incidence of hypertensive disease, toxemia, placental accidents, infant mortality, ruptured uteri, and large infants (> 4000 g) was greater in the grand multipara group.

6. Quinlivan, W. L. Incidence of abnormalities in women of gravidity seven or more. *Obstet. Gynecol.* 23:567, 1964.

   Five hundred women of gravidity 7 or more were analyzed and found to have a high incidence of hypertensive cardiovascular disease, preeclamptic toxemia, antenatal anemia, malpresentations of the fetus, and postpartum hemorrhage, when compared to a group of women of all parities.

7. Scharfman, E., and Silverstein, L. The grand multipara: A survey of 403 cases. *Am. J. Obstet. Gynecol.* 84:1442, 1962.

   The records of 403 grand multiparas during the years 1951 to 1960 were reviewed. The following conditions were more common in grand multiparas than other parturients: placenta previa (threefold increase), postpartum hemorrhage (fivefold), and prematurity (twofold). There was no increase in maternal mortality.

8. Aziz, F. A. Pregnancy and labor of grand multiparous Sudanese women. *Int. J. Gynaecol. Obstet.* 18:144, 1980.

   The authors found that while labor was shorter in the grand multiparous patient, it was much more complicated with regards to hemorrhage and morbidity.

9. Chang, A., et al. The obstetric performance of the grand multipara. *Med. J. Aust.* 1:330, 1977.

   The outcome of pregnancy for the grand multipara is outlined. Techniques for prevention of morbidity in these patients are detailed.

Maternal Effects

10. Solomons, B. The dangerous multipara. *Lancet* 2:8, 1934.

    The author introduced the term the dangerous multipara *after noting that the risk of maternal death increases steadily from the fifth to the tenth pregnancy.*

11. Dilts, P. V., and Greene, R. R. Myometrial changes associated with grand multiparity. *Am. J. Obstet. Gynecol.* 89:1049, 1964.

    Histologic examination of uteri from pregnant and immediately postpartum patients was performed. The relative amount of myometrial collagen did not change with increasing maternal parity or age. However, there was a noticeable increase in paravascular elastic tissue with parity.

Twin Pregnancy

Multiple births have been a subject of great interest to scientists, particularly the endocrinologist and geneticist, and a cause of concern to obstetricians and pediatricians. The incidence of twins in Europe and in the United States is between 10–15 per 1000 births. The rate among the Japanese is about 6 per 1000. The rate in the African black is high, varying from 16 per 1000 in Zambia to 47 per 1000 in Nigeria. The dizygotic twinning rate varies from 10–40 per 1000, but the monozygotic rate is about 4 per 1000 and appears to be relatively constant throughout the world. The incidence of dizygotic twinning is influenced remarkably by race. The incidence in blacks is about 14.9 per 1000, while the incidence in whites is 10.6 per 1000. Other factors include maternal age and parity. The number of twins born increases with the age of the mother until age 30 and then diminishes. There is also increased twinning with increased parity, both findings confirmed by recent studies. Hereditary factors can also influence twinning rates but probably apply only to dizygotic twinning. The monozygotic twin set appears to be a chance phenomenon. Women who were themselves dizygotic twins have much higher twinning rates than the general population, but this is not the case with male dizygotic twins. The incidence of multiple pregnancies has been increased by the use of gonadotropins in the treatment of infertility. It has also been suggested that women who are prone to twinning have a higher level of serum gonadotropin than do other women.

There are two recognized types of twinning. One is called monozygotic (identical or uniovular), and the other is dizygotic (fraternal or binovular). In monozygotic twinning, the two embryos result from the division of a single zygote. When there is early separation of the blastomeres there may be either two distinct placentas with chorionic and amniotic sacs separate (dichorionic-diamniotic), or a single placenta with fused chorionic and amniotic sacs (fused dichorionic-diamniotic). With later division there is a single placenta and a single chorionic plate. This can be associated with either two amniotic sacs (monochorionic-diamniotic), or single amniotic sacs (monochorionic-monoamniotic), which is very rare.

In dizygotic twinning, two ova from either the same or different ovaries are fertilized, and the two zygotes pass down either the same or separate fallopian tubes. There are two placentas, each with chorionic and amniotic membranes (dichorionic-diamniotic). There is a separate implantation of the separate placentas, but if the sites of implantation are close there might be fusion of the placentas and membranes. A superfecundation is the fertilization of two ova from more than one act of coitus in the same menstrual cycle. Superfetation is the fertilization of two ova from different menstrual cycles and is very rare. A third type of twinning has been postulated in which the ovum is fertilized by two sperms. Similarly, a mosaic singleton has often been shown to result from the fertilization of one ovum by two sperms.

It is well known that there are some complications of pregnancy that occur more frequently with twins. It was firmly believed that antepartum hemorrhage was more common in twin pregnancy, but several recent studies have shown that there is no greater incidence of bleeding than in singleton pregnancy. Anemia is generally believed to be more common in twin pregnancy than in singleton, because there have been many reports of lower hemoglobin concentrations. However, it must be emphasized that at least part of this is due to the greater hemodilution of a twin pregnancy, and some studies suggest that there is no greater incidence of anemia in twin pregnancy.

Hydramnios is more likely to occur with twin gestation. The incidence is equal in monozygotic and dizygotic twins, but both are greater than in a singleton gestation. Acute hydramnios is more common in monozygotic than in dizygotic twin pregnancy. Preeclampsia occurs about three times more often in twin pregnancy than in singleton. If, however, primigravida pregnancies only are considered, the incidence is five times that of singleton pregnancy. There appears to be no difference between the incidence of preeclampsia in monozygotic and dizygotic twin gestations.

It has long been known that perinatal death is several times more frequent in twins than in single infants. The perinatal mortality rate, as reported by Naeye in 1978, was 139 per 1000 births for twins and 33 per 1000 for singleton births in the United States. In Addis Ababa, the perinatal mortality rate for twins was 338 per 1000 and for singleton infants was 53 per 1000. The greatest risk to the fetus is due to the frequency of complications occurring during pregnancy, particularly premature onset of labor, premature ruptured membranes, amnionitis, congenital malformation, and twin transfusion syndrome.

Twins are commonly not diagnosed before parturition, not because it is difficult to diagnose, but simply because the examiner failed to keep the possibility in mind. Family history often provides a clue. Recent administration of clomiphene or gonadotropins, or a physical examination (especially during the second trimester) revealing a larger uterus than expected, are all hints of a multiple gestation. The differential diagnosis must include an inappropriate menstrual history, hydramnios, hydatidiform mole, uterine myoma, and closely attached adnexal masses. Especially during the third trimester it is hard to palpate the fetal parts, particularly if the woman is obese or hydramnios is present. It is possible to identify the two separate fetal heart beats if the rates are distinct from each other and from that of the mother.

Diagnosis of twins can be made as early as 6–10 weeks of gestation by ultrasonography. The identification of each fetal head should be made in two perpendicular planes so as not to mistake a cross section of the fetal trunk for a second fetal head. Cross section of the fetal head remains round in both the planes, whereas the trunks do not.

To reduce perinatal mortality and morbidity it is important that delivery of the premature infant be prevented, fetal trauma during labor and delivery be eliminated, and expert pediatric care be provided. To fulfill these goals, it is important to identify twins as early as possible. After identification, the patient should be seen during her prenatal care more often than a woman with singleton gestation. Evaluation of maternal diet and prevention of anemia is important, as is prevention of pregnancy-induced and pregnancy-aggravated hypertension. Several authors have proposed that bed rest is beneficial to twin fetuses by increasing uterine perfusion and perhaps by reducing the physical force that might act on the cervix and promote effacement and dilatation. Several studies have shown a reduction in the perinatal mortality rate with bed rest, and that twin fetuses of these patients weighed more than did the fetus of comparable gestational age if the mother remained ambulatory.

The most common complication with a twin pregnancy is premature labor. If not already being used, bed rest should be attempted at that point. Sedation should not be so intense as to depress the fetus, but beta-adrenergic agents have been reported to prevent labor quite effectively in these cases. If labor has been established, a fetal heart monitor should be applied and two units of crossmatched whole blood should be available. All possible combinations of fetal positions (vertex, breech, transverse lie, and so on) may occur with twins. Once labor has been established, if there is any doubt about the relationship of the twins or the adequacy of the maternal pelvis, x-rays may be helpful. In the event of rupture of the membranes without labor or with prolonged labor with or without effective contractions, the problem is often better handled by cesarean section, unless there is little hope of salvaging the infants because of gross immaturity. However, some obstetricians do use oxytocin in dilute IV infusion to initiate or stimulate labor.

Pudendal block along with nitrous oxide and oxygen inhalation will provide appropriate pain relief for spontaneous vaginal delivery. If both twins present as vertex, the risk is low so vaginal delivery is the best choice. However, if one or both of the twins presents in transverse lie or breech, and if the twins are premature, many use cesarean birth as the method of choice. Breech or transverse lie delivered vaginally, added to prematurity, causes a high perinatal death rate. If the twins are mature, vaginal delivery may still be acceptable. In all cases, sound physician judgment of the individual patient is essential for optimum results.

Review

1. MacGillivray, I. Twin pregnancies. *Obstet. Gynecol. Annu.* 7:135, 1978.
   A review of a long experience with multiple gestations. Etiology, diagnosis, and management are detailed.
2. Keith, L., et al. The Northwestern University multi-hospital twin study: I. A description of 588 twin pregnancies and associated pregnancy loss, 1971 to 1975. *Am. J. Obstet. Gynecol.* 138:781, 1980.
   The rate of poor outcome was highest in mothers who were less than 20 years of age and of low parity, and in those who delivered premature infants (particularly the second twin).

Etiology

3. Wald, N. J., et al. Maternal serum alpha-fetoprotein (AFP) in relation to zygosity. *Br. Med. J.* 17:455, 1979.
   Maternal serum AFP concentrations were uniformly elevated in 102 twin pregnancies.
4. Nylander, P. P. S. Causes of high twinning frequencies in Nigeria. *Prog. Clin. Biol. Res.* 24:35, 1978.
   Social class has a very marked influence on twinning in Nigeria (the rates being highest in the lowest social class).
5. Bracken, M. B. Oral contraception and twinning: An epidemiologic study. *Am. J. Obstet. Gynecol.* 133:432, 1979.
   In this report 4428 women were studied. Those conceiving within 2 months of cessation of oral contraceptives had a twofold increase in the rate of twin gestation.

Sonography

6. Leveno, K. L., et al. Sonar cephalometry in twins: A table of biparietal diameters for normal twin fetuses and a comparison with singletons. *Am. J. Obstet. Gynecol.* 135:727, 1979.
   Mean twin biparietal diameters (BPD) were consistently smaller than those of singletons, the difference averaging 3.5 mm between 16 and 40 weeks gestation.
7. Grennert, L, Persson, P. H., and Gennser, G. Intrauterine growth of twins judged by BPD measurements. *Acta. Obstet. Gynecol. Scand.* 78:S28, 1978.
   The mean BPD values of twins were close to those of singletons in the second trimester. From the thirty-second week on, the twins' mean weekly BPD increment decreased compared to that of singletons.
8. Divers, W. A., and Hemsell, D. L. The use of ultrasound in multiple gestations. *Obstet. Gynecol.* 53:500, 1978.
   Ultrasound was noted to be of only limited use in antenatal diagnosis of intrauterine growth retardation with a significant number of false-positive and false-negative results.

Perinatal Outcome

9. Naeye, R. L., et al. Twins: Causes of perinatal death in 12 United States cities and 1 African city. *Am. J. Obstet. Gynecol.* 131:267, 1978.
   Perinatal mortality among twins in over 54,000 pregnancies was 139 per 1000 compared to 33 per 1000 in singleton births.
10. Medearis, A. L., et al. Perinatal deaths in twin pregnancy: A five-year analysis of statewide statistics in Missouri. *Am. J. Obstet. Gynecol.* 134:413, 1979.

Low birth weight appears to be the major factor in the elevated perinatal death rate in twin pregnancy.

11. Bender, H. G., and Werner, C. Functional aspects of placental maturation in twin pregnancies. *Prog. Clin. Biol. Res.* 24:147, 1978.
The frequency of premature births in twin pregnancies is associated with a corresponding frequency of cases of premature placental maturation. This result confirms various statements in the literature that somatic development in the intrauterine period takes place more rapidly when twins are involved.

Management

12. Grennert, L., and Persson, P. H. Effects of extensive population screening on the outcome of twin pregnancies. *Prog. Clin. Biol. Res.* 24:123, 1978.
Early detection and bed rest in the hospital seem to improve the outcome of twin pregnancy.

13. Weekes, A. R. L., Cheridjian, V. E., and Mwanje, D. K. Lumbar epidural analgesia in labour in twin pregnancy. *Obstet. Gynecol. Surv.* 33:250, 1978.
This report shows that the epidural technique of anesthesia is a safe procedure for relief of pain in labor for twin deliveries.

14. Miller, A. P. Successful vaginal delivery of locked monoamniotic twins. *Obstet. Gynecol. Surv.* 33:163, 1978.
Although the complication is rare, hypertonicity of the uterus, monoamniotic twinning or oligohydramnios may contribute to interlocking of the fetal heads if the first fetus presents as a breech.

15. Pettersson, F., Smedby, B., and Lindmark, G. Outcome of twin birth review of 1636 children born in twin birth. *Obstet. Gynecol. Surv.* 32:79, 1977.
The perinatal loss was 6.4%. Full-term twins had five times the perinatal mortality of the full-term singleton. The perinatal mortality for the first and second twins was equal.

16. Kerenyk, T. D., and Chitkara, U. Selective birth in twin pregnancy with discordancy for Down's syndrome. *N. Engl. J. Med.* 304:1525, 1981.
The use of amniocentesis in multiple gestations for genetic purposes have recently seen one twin labeled normal while the other was abnormal. An aggressive method of management involving exsanguination of the affected twin with subsequent delivery of a normal fetus is detailed.

17. Jouppila, P., et al. Twin pregnancy. The role of active management during pregnancy and delivery. *Obstet. Gynecol. Surv.* 31:534, 1976.
The perinatal mortality rate among 335 twin pregnancies was 8.8%, which was attributed to early diagnosis of twins and maternal bed rest. The interval between the first twin and second was not found to have any significant effect on the perinatal mortality of the second infant.

18. Hunter, A., and Cox, D. M. Counseling problems when twins are discovered at genetic amniocentesis. *Clin. Genet.* 16:34, 1979.
In the presence of twins the likelihood of finding an abnormality may be significantly increased. The need for additional counseling after amniocentesis is stressed.

Rh Isoimmunization

Since the discovery of the ABO and Rh systems, over 100 other blood group antigens have been identified. Maternal isoimmunization to approximately one-third of these antigens can stimulate sufficient maternal antibody to result in hemolytic disease of the fetus or newborn (HDN). Hemolytic reactions represent a rare breach in the immunologic truce that exists between a mother and her fetus. For hemolysis to occur, the fetus must possess an antigen that the mother is lacking, and the mother must be exposed to the antigen. The maternal antibody produced must be immunoglobulin G, which is the only immunoglobulin capable of transfer across the placenta.

ABO incompatibility is responsible for two-thirds of all cases of HDN. Affected infants tend to exhibit jaundice in the first 24 hours of neonatal life but rarely require exchange transfusion for anemia or hyperbilirubinemia. The majority of cases occur with a type O mother and type A or, occasionally, type B fetus. Type O mothers make IgG isoantibodies, whereas type A and B make IgM isoantibodies.

Rh incompatibility is the second most common cause of HDN but is more significant because of its severity. The Rh antigens are found only on human red cells; therefore, isoimmunization occurs only by exposure to human Rh-positive erythrocytes. Since Rh typing became widely available and the transfusion of incompatible blood largely avoided, the most common etiology of Rh isoimmunization is pregnancy. In approximately 10% of all pregnancies in Caucasian women, an Rh-negative woman will give birth to an Rh-positive infant. The incidence for blacks and orientals is approximately 5% and 1%, respectively. The probability that an Rh-negative mother will be isoimmunized by a single Rh incompatible pregnancy is approximately 17%. When mother and fetus are ABO incompatible, a protective effect is seen on Rh isoimmunization, because the fetal cells that find their way into the maternal circulation are immediately destroyed by maternal AB isoantibodies.

The degree of fetal anemia is dependent on the amount of antibody transferred by the mother to the fetus. If the rate of red cell destruction exceeds the compensatory capacity of the fetus, anemia results and extramedullary hematopoiesis becomes intense. Portal vein hypertension develops, followed by ascites, hypoproteinemia, and hepatic failure. Ultimately, generalized anasarca (hydrops fetalis) occurs. The fetus commonly is not jaundiced at birth since bilirubin is transferred to the mother. However, the neonate may rapidly develop increased levels of bilirubin following delivery. Once this exceeds the albumin-binding capacity, it escapes to the tissues and is recognized as jaundice. Bilirubin uptake by the heavily myelinated cells of the basal ganglia, hippocampus, and cerebellum results in kernicterus. Surviving infants with kernicterus have cerebral palsy.

Management of Rh isoimmunization begins at the first prenatal visit when the Rh factor and ABO group are determined. An indirect Coomb's test, regardless of Rh type, should be performed to identify those women who may have isoimmunization to one of the irregular antigens or to ABO. Rh antibody determinations should be repeated, even if no antibodies were identified on the first visit. If an antibody is detected at any stage, more frequent determinations are indicated. A positive indirect Coomb's test alerts the physician to the presence of isoimmunization; antigen identification enables the physician to know if the antigen causes erythroblastosis; and in a previously unsensitized woman, the indirect Coomb's titer gives an estimate of the degree of fetal hemolysis one may expect. Serial antibody titers will usually reflect the condition of the fetus, because the onset, duration, and strength of immunization are known. A titer of 1:16 is felt to be safe since no intrauterine deaths have occurred at this level. In subsequent immunized pregnancies, the titers do not accurately reflect the condition of the fetus. If antibodies are present at the beginning of pregnancy, the fetus may be more severely affected than if the same level of antibody developed later in pregnancy. Thus, serial amniotic fluid analysis should be performed if the Rh antibody titer is greater than 1:16 in a first immunized pregnancy and in all subsequent immunized pregnancies.

In managing the immunized obstetric patient, the clinician must weigh two potentially hazardous conditions: intrauterine death and prematurity. Intrauterine death may be avoided by performing spectrophotometric analysis of amniotic fluid for indirect bilirubin. Liley defined a nomogram comparing the optical density of amniotic fluid at 450 nm and gestational age, which can be used to identify those infants at risk and predict fetal outcome. Prematurity can be avoided by determining the lecithin/sphingomyelin (L/S) ratio, which assesses functional lung maturity. In severe cases of HDN, early delivery may be mandatory and certainly is with functional lung maturity. Severe hydrops fetalis, however, retards fetal pulmonary maturity. The timing of delivery therefore depends on the degree of fetal hemolysis, indicated by spectrophotometric analysis of amniotic fluid; fetal lung maturity, as indicated by the L/S ratio; and clinical acumen.

Unfortunately, hemolysis is so severe at times that the fetus begins to deteriorate at a stage of gestation too early to survive outside. In this situation, intrauterine transfusion is indicated to supply the fetus with sufficient Rh-negative blood to survive until it is mature enough to be delivered. In utero transfusion is associated with a 10% risk of fetal death. For those infants 32 weeks and above, survival rates in the neonatal intensive care nursery are greater than those accomplished by in utero fetal transfusion.

Interdepartmental cooperation is extremely important for the successful outcome of the immunized pregnancy. The neonatologist should be present in the delivery room so that appropriate care can be initiated immediately if necessary. Because the newborn may be so anemic as to need immediate transfusion, one should have O negative maternal-compatible blood available. Crossmatching against maternal blood assures that any antibody that may have crossed transplacentally to the fetus will not cause a problem with the transfusion. Treatment of the affected neonate is aimed at preventing death from anemia and brain damage from kernicterus. By following the hematocrit and bilirubin concentration, one knows when to perform an exchange transfusion.

Rh immune globulin harvested from previously isoimmunized patients has proved to be remarkably successful in the prevention of sensitization to the Rh antigen in subsequent pregnancies. When high titer anti–Rh immunoglobulin (Rhogam) is given within 72 hours of delivery, less than 1% of treated individuals develop subsequent Rh isoimmunization. Unusually large amounts of fetal-maternal hemorrhage may occur with abruptio placenta, cesarean section, manual removal of the placenta, traumatic vaginal delivery, and severe maternal hemorrhage. These conditions may require more than the standard dosage of immunoglobulin, and techniques are available to determine how much should be given. The incidence of Rh isoimmunization following abortion is 4%–5% and is a significant risk to Rh-negative women, and ectopic pregnancy is similar to abortion. Because of the potential for fetal-maternal hemorrhage, Rh immune globulin is indicated for protection in both situations. Although controversial, it is probably advisable to give immune globulin to Rh-negative women following amniocentesis and antepartum hemorrhage.

When an Rh (D)–negative woman delivers an Rh (D)–positive infant, she becomes a candidate for Rh (D)–immunoglobulin therapy. However, she must be D negative and Du negative, she must have no anti-D antibodies in her serum, her infant must be D or Du positive, and the direct Coomb's test on the infant's cord blood must be negative. Should the Coomb's be positive, but due to antibody other than D, the Rh D immunoglobulin should be administered.

Because of reduced family size and prophylactic use of Rh immune globulin, Rh isoimmunization is becoming less and less common. Immunization will continue to be a problem because of inadequate treatment, treatment failures, lack of treatment, and disease associated with the rare antigens. With interdisciplinary cooperation, use of antibody titers, amniotic fluid analysis, intrauterine transfusion, and intensive neonatal management, perinatal mortality secondary to Rh isoimmunization has decreased from 45% to 8%.

The control of Rh disease represents a success story in perinatal medicine and is a model of management for all high-risk pregnancies and of perinatal risking. Patients who are at risk of Rh isoimmunization are identified and sent to high-risk centers for intensive clinical management when antibodies are first detected. The discovery and application of immune globulin to Rh isoimmunization may be considered a major milestone in obstetric care and has virtually eliminated this as a killer of the unborn and neonate.

Reviews

1. Queenan, J. T. *Modern Management of the Rh Problem* (2nd ed.). Hagerstown, Md.: Harper & Row, 1977.
   This text is an authoritative reference that reviews the history, the pathophysiology, the maternal management, and the prevention of Rh disease, and the neonatal management of hemolytic disease of the newborn.
2. Queenan, J. T. Update on Rh and other blood group immunizations. *Contemp. Ob/Gyn* 16:31, 1980.
   Careful screening, early diagnosis, and appropriate therapy remain vital to minimize perinatal mortality and morbidity.

Pathophysiology

3. Beal, R. W. Non-rhesus (D) blood group isoimmunization in obstetrics. *Clin. Obstet. Gynecol.* 6:493, 1979.
   As a consequence of pregnancy and blood transfusion, women will continue to become isoimmunized to blood group antigens other than D. Although these irregular antigens comprise only 2% of all immunized pregnancies, they will become more significant as D isoimmunization is prevented.
4. Davey, M. The prevention of rhesus-isoimmunization. *Clin. Obstet. Gynecol.* 6:509, 1979.
   The Rh blood group system is actually made up of at least five antigens capable of causing isoimmunization. The most common and significant antigen is D, and currently it is the only one that can be prevented.
5. Jennings, E. R., and Clauss, B. Maternal-fetal hemorrhage: Its incidence and sensitizing effects. *Am. J. Obstet. Gynecol.* 131:725, 1978.
   Maternal-fetal hemorrhage occurs in approximately 2% of births and may explain why some women are sensitized during a first pregnancy. How-

ever, administration of anti-D immunoglobulin to Rh-negative neonates is not indicated.

Management

6. Rodeck, C. H., et al. Direct intravascular fetal blood transfusion by fetoscopy in severe rhesus isoimmunization. *Lancet* 1:626, 1981.
   Two fetuses with severe anemia due to rhesus incompatability received an early blood transfusion (23, 25 weeks) with blood being given directly into the umbilical vessel. One grossly hydropic fetus survived indicating that this method, while radical, can be used in some patients.

7. Frigoletto, F. D., Jr., et al. Intrauterine fetal transfusion in 365 fetuses during fifteen years. *Am. J. Obstet. Gynecol.* 139:781, 1981.
   This study reviews 365 consecutive cases of fetuses who received intrauterine fetal transfusions from 22–32 weeks. Of these, approximately 45% survived—55% without hydrops—but a much smaller percentage survived if hydrops or ascites were present. Direct ultrasound guidance offers increased success in this procedure.

8. Clewell, W. H., et al. Fetal transfusion with real-time ultrasound guidance. *Obstet. Gynecol.* 57:516, 1981.
   The technique of intrauterine fetal transfusion using sonographic guidance in 43 patients is described. The technique appeared to be superior to fluoroscopic directed transfusion.

9. Berkowitz, R. L. Intrauterine transfusion, 1980: An update. *Clin. Perinatol.* 7:285, 1980.
   The technique, selection of candidates, and long-term sequelae of this life-saving procedure are discussed. A summary of the survival data is presented, and most physicians feel the procedure should be reserved for babies at 32 weeks gestation or less.

10. Hauth, J. C., et al. Plasmapheresis as an adjunct to management of Rh isoimmunization. *Obstet. Gynecol.* 57:132, 1981.
    Plasmapheresis performed twice weekly is directly related to the reduction of maternal plasma anti-D concentration.

Prevention

11. Freda, V. J., Gorman, J. G., and Pollack, W. Rh factor: Prevention of isoimmunization and clinical trials on mothers. *Science* 151:828, 1966.
    Passive immunity can be achieved by injecting an excess of anti-D antibody into a woman who has been exposed to D-positive cells. This concept evolved after noting the difficulty of sensitizing individuals with ABO incompatible cells.

12. Bowman, J. M. Suppression of Rh isoimmunization. A review. *Obstet. Gynecol.* 52:385, 1978.
    To suppress Rh isoimmunization to its lowest possible level (2–4 per 10,000 pregnancies), Rh immunoglobulin must be given to all Rh-negative isoimmunized women who: (1) deliver Rh-positive babies; (2) abort; (3) undergo amniocentesis, except when the husband is Rh negative. The dosage should be at least 300 μg/30 ml of fetal blood.

13. Tovey, G. H. Should anti D immunoglobulin be given antenatally? *Lancet* 2:446, 1980.
    The controversy over antenatal prophylaxis with Rh immunoglobulin during normal pregnancies with none of the traditional risk factors for sensitization is discussed.

14. Sebring, E. S., and Polesky, H. F. Comparison of fetomaternal hemor-

rhage detection methods and Rh immunoglobulin usage. *Am. J. Clin. Pathol.* 72:358, 1979.

One must have an accurate index of the amount of fetomaternal hemorrhage to know how much Rh immunoglobulin to inject. If one does not quantitate the amount of hemorrhage, the single injection may be inadequate and result in treatment failures.

15. Grimes, D. A., Geary, F. H., Jr., and Hatcher, R. A. Rh immunoglobulin utilization after ectopic pregnancy. *Am. J. Obstet. Gynecol.* 140:246, 1981.

    This study involves a retrospective review of 305 patients treated with Rhogam after ectopic pregnancy. In comparing these to control groups, it was obvious that those Rh negative patients with ectopic pregnancies should receive Rhogam prophylaxis.

16. Stewart, F. H., et al. Reduced dose of Rh immunoglobulin following first trimester pregnancy termination. *Obstet. Gynecol.* 51:318, 1978.

    Because of the greatly reduced blood volume in early pregnancy (approximately 4.2 ml at 12 weeks), smaller doses of Rh immunoglobulin than that in the standard dose vial (300 µg) can be given and still provide complete protection.

17. Lloyd, L. K., et al. Intrapartum fetomaternal bleeding in Rh negative women. *Obstet. Gynecol.* 56:285, 1980.

    One must check the adequacy of the Rh immune globulin dose to be sure enough was given.

18. Hill, L. M., et al. Rh sensitization after genetic amniocentesis. *Obstet. Gynecol.* 56:459, 1980.

    Following amniocentesis in Rh-negative unsensitized women, Rh immunoglobulin should be administered since fetal-maternal hemorrhage may occur.

Prolonged Pregnancy

The terms *postdate, postterm,* and *prolonged pregnancy* refer to a pregnancy extending greater than 42 weeks (294 days) gestation. The term *postmaturity* refers to those pregnancies, 42 weeks or longer, in which there is concurrent intrauterine growth retardation defined by physical assessment in the infant. The incidence of pregnancies extending beyond 42 weeks has been reported as 3.5%–10%. Postmaturity occurs in approximately 20% of prolonged pregnancies, an incidence probably not greater at a gestational age of 42 weeks compared with those pregnancies of 38–42 weeks.

In a classic study of over 15,000 deliveries, Browne did much to highlight the dangers of prolonged pregnancy. The perinatal mortality at 41 weeks gestation was 10.5 per 1000. The mortality rate doubled by 43 weeks, tripled at 44 weeks, and more than quadrupled at 45 weeks. He also observed that the primary cesarean section rate in pregnancies extending beyond 41 weeks was five times as high as for the group of patients who delivered between 38 and 41 weeks; he also emphasized the importance of fetal death before or during labor.

Two schools of thought arose in the early 1960s. Several authors regarded postdate pregnancy as a significant risk to the fetus and advocated termination of pregnancy at 42 weeks to minimize the risk. Others disputed the belief that postdate pregnancy represented a significant risk. They emphasized an increased rate of congenital abnormalities as the cause of death and felt that the complications of induced labor and forced delivery, solely on the basis of prolonged pregnancy, outweighed any advantages. It must be remembered that these experiences and attitudes developed prior to utilization of continuous fetal heart rate monitoring, ultrasonography, and estriol determinations for the assessment of fetal well-being. Further, intensive care neonatal units were not well established. With the introduction of biochemical and biophysical tests for fetal well-being, there has been a movement away from the epidemiological approach in obstetrics in which, for example, all postdate patients are delivered at 42 weeks, or all diabetics are delivered at 36 or 37 weeks. In the more specific approach now used the delivery time for each patient is individualized. Not all patients with a prolonged pregnancy are in jeopardy. The babies at risk are those who exhibit intrauterine growth retardation and oligohydramnios in the postdate pregnancy.

The clinician is faced with a difficult task in the management of prolonged pregnancy. Accurately diagnosing the prolonged pregnancy by differentiating the uncomplicated prolonged pregnancy from the prolonged pregnancy affected by intrauterine growth retardation is very difficult. Establishment of gestational age is best accomplished on a prospective basis starting in the first trimester. Dewhurst found that the length of gestation cannot be reliably estimated in 22% of pregnant women; because of this a careful menstrual history should be obtained at the first visit. Any irregular cycles or abnormal bleeding should be noted. As ovulation occurs 14 days before the next period, 1 day should be added to the expected date of confinement for each day over a 28-day cycle; 1 week must be added for a 35-day cycle. Another source of error is oligomenorrhea following the cessation of oral contraceptive use. Indeed, 70% of postterm pregnancies are a function of delayed ovulation. For a reliable menstrual history, the following criteria are necessary: the patient must be certain of her LMP (last menstrual period) date; the LMP must be normal; a regular 28-day cycle must be present; and no oral contraceptives should have been used for 3 months prior to the LMP.

The first movement is perceived between 18–19 weeks gestation. In a prospective study, 9% of patients had prolonged pregnancy when calculated from the LMP, but in over half of these subjects, the onset of quickening corrected the gestational age to less than 42 weeks. During the first trimester, examination of uterine size is useful only if repetitive monthly examinations are performed. In later pregnancy it is unreliable due to variation in amniotic fluid volume, irregular growth of the uterus, vagarity in umbilical position, and multiple gestation. Fetal heart tones may be elicited at 12 weeks gestation using a doptone and at 20 weeks gestation using a DeLee stethoscope.

Examinations should be performed weekly from 18 weeks on to accurately assess the onset of fetal heart tones. A single biparietal diameter (BPD) obtained between 20 and 28 weeks gestation is accurate within 11 days of the expected date of confinement (EDC). Beyond 30 weeks, a single BPD may be inaccurate by as much as 3 weeks. Paired examinations, at 20–26 weeks gestation and a 30–34 weeks gestation, may determine correct gestational age to within 3 days. Radiologic data (fetograms) have a very high error rate and should not be used to date pregnancies.

When the gestational age is accurately known, the patient who is at 42 weeks gestation (with a cervix favorable for induction) should be induced. The two major clinical problems are: the patient with a confirmed gestation of 42 weeks and an unripe cervix, and the patient with an uncertain gestational age who is seen for the first time having the possible diagnosis of a prolonged pregnancy. Special investigatory methods are available for the assessment of these patients. An isolated BPD in a suspected postdate pregnancy is of no value and will not allow the physician to determine whether the fetus is at term, postdate, or is existing in an unfavorable environment. Some authors recommend performing amniocentesis for a creatinine determination. If the result is less than 2.5 mg/dl, they feel it is unlikely that the patient has a prolonged pregnancy. This may be repeated in 7 days. Further studies are required to confirm whether this approach is indeed correct. The lecithin-sphingomyelin (L/S) ratio has been found to be less than 2.0:1 in 6% of postdate pregnancies. This may be due to fluctuations in the sphingomyelin concentrations near term, since none of the infants developed hyaline membrane disease. Conversely, a high L/S ratio in the range of 4.0:1 may occur before 42 weeks gestation. Thus the L/S ratio does not distinguish the 38-week from the 42-week gestation.

The significance and management of meconium is controversial. Temporary hypoxia may cause peripheral vasocontraction and anal sphincter relaxation. Green and Paul showed that the incidence of meconium-stained amniotic fluid was not higher at greater than 42 weeks compared to that from 38–42 weeks gestation. All patients with meconium-stained fluid were delivered within 48 hours. There was no difference between the group of patients with meconium-stained fluid and those with clear fluid in terms of the 5-minute Apgar score, the incidence of cesarean section for fetal distress, or neonatal complications. Active intervention because of meconium, especially in the presence of an unripe cervix, will result in a high incidence of cesarean section (up to 28%). In contrast, other authors have reported a higher incidence of fetal and neonatal complications associated with meconium-stained amniotic fluid; these were older studies, however. The modern management of the baby delivered from a meconium-stained environment is critically important. DeLee suction by the obstetrician as the head appears over the perineum is the mandatory step. Immediate, vigorous, and thorough tracheal visualization and suction by trained personnel has averted many of the deaths due to meconium aspiration syndrome. In the past, infant mortality was fairly common in this group.

Estriol (E_3) excretion plateaus around 40–41 weeks and declines gradually thereafter. Thus, a rising or plateauing E_3 value mitigates against postmaturity, which is invariably associated with progressively falling E_3 values. Since fetal compromise also reveals a similar trend, the value of an E_3 test has been questioned. However, as long as the E_3 levels remain in the normal range for a particular laboratory and do not represent a decrease of more than 50% from any previous value, the pregnancy may be allowed to continue without interference. The disadvantage of this test is that serial values are usually needed to detect a trend. It is advisable to start collecting baseline levels in the patient with an unripe cervix at 41 weeks gestation. The contraction stress test (CST) and nonstress test (NST) have both been successfully used in the evaluation of the fetus at risk for postmaturity. The more recent NST is rapid, simple, and cost-effective. If early results are confirmed, the NST may replace the CST as the primary biophysical test for fetal well-being.

Continuous monitoring of the fetal heart rate during labor is essential. One study has reported an incidence of fetal distress as high as 38% in these patients. Thus, fetal membranes should be ruptured as early as possible in the intrapartum period and an internal electrode applied. If meconium is present, experienced personnel should be present at the delivery to aspirate the nasal pharynx and hypopharynx of the fetus. If, after delivery, meconium is found on repeated oropharyngeal suction, or if there is evidence of fetal depression (Apgar < 7), the vocal cords should be inspected by direct laryngoscopy and tracheal suction performed. In the vigorous infant (Apgar at 1 and 5 minutes > 8), intubation is not required.

Review
1. Hauth, J. C., et al. Post-term pregnancy, Part I. *Obstet. Gynecol.* 56:467, 1980.
   A review of the etiology, outcome, and management of the postterm gestation.
2. Vorherr, H. Placental insufficiency in relation to postterm pregnancy and fetal postmaturity. Evaluation of fetoplacental function; management of the postterm gravida. *Am. J. Obstet. Gynecol.* 123:67, 1975.
   An excellent review of the fetoplacental function in the postterm pregnancy. A management plan for the postterm gravida is presented; 190 references are available.

Diagnosis
3. Yaffe, H., Hay-Am, E., and Sadovsky, E. Thromboplastic activity of amniotic fluid in term and postmature gestations. *Obstet. Gynecol.* 57:490, 1981.
   The authors studied the thromboplastic activity of amniotic fluid in 45 pregnant women who were post dates. It was found that when the test result time was less than 42 seconds, all of the newborns (22 neonates) had clinical evidence of postmaturity.
4. Rawlings, E. E., and Moore, B. A. The accuracy of methods of calculating the expected date of delivery for use in the diagnosis of postmaturity. *Am. J. Obstet. Gynecol.* 106:676, 1970.
   In a prospective study the authors demonstrated that the accuracy of quickening could prevent needless inductions of labor in 60% of apparent postdate pregnancies.
5. Sabbagha, R. E., Barton, F. B., and Barton, B. A. Sonar biparietal diameter: II. Predictive of three fetal growth patterns leading to a closer assessment of gestational age and neonatal weight. *Am. J. Obstet. Gynecol.* 126:485, 1976.
   The value of ultrasonography in the assessment of gestational age is described.
6. Crowley, P. Non-quantitative estimation of amniotic fluid volume in suspected prolonged pregnancy. *J. Perinat. Med.* 8:249, 1980.
   The relationship of amniotic fluid volume to postterm pregnancy is outlined. A nonquantitative method for estimation of amniotic fluid volume is detailed.
7. Homburg, R., Ludomirski, A., and Insler, V. Detection of fetal risk in postmaturity. *Br. J. Obstet. Gynaecol.* 17:243, 1979.
   The various factors related to risk assessment in the postmature fetus are outlined. A management plan is also detailed.

Management
8. Freeman, R. K., et al. Postdate pregnancy: Utilization of contraction stress testing for primary fetal surveillance. *Am. J. Obstet. Gynecol.* 140:128, 1981.
   Six hundred seventy-nine postdate study patients were surveyed with a contraction stress test (CST). Seventy-five percent of these patients entered labor spontaneously and delivery was elected because of an abnormal test in only 5.4%. The data show that the use of CSTs are helpful in this

condition but that only one of 20 patients past 42 weeks will require intervention for fetal indications.

9. Miyazaki, F. S., and Miyazaki, B. A. False reactive nonstress tests in postterm pregnancies. *Am. J. Obstet. Gynecol.* 140:269, 1981.
   One hundred twenty-five prolonged pregnancies were studied with nonstress tests (NST). Because the major mechanism causing distress is cord compression with oligohydramnios, the contraction stress test (CST) was more useful than the NST as a sensitive indicator in these patients.
10. Green, J., and Paul, R. The value of amniocentesis in prolonged pregnancy. *Obstet. Gynecol.* 51:293, 1978.
    The authors discuss the finding of meconium at amniocentesis in postdate pregnancies. They conclude that meconium is not more common in postdate pregnancies compared to those between 38–42 weeks gestation, and that the decision to deliver the infant should not be made solely on the presence of meconium.
11. Clark, M. J. Use of the oxytocin challenge test in the management of postdate pregnancy. *J. Amer. Osteopathic Assoc.* 79:632, 1980.
    The oxytocin challenge test (OCT) as an assessment of placental function appears to be the best test to adequately manage the postterm gestation.
12. Knox, G. E., Huddleston, J. F., and Flowers, C. E., Jr. Management of prolonged pregnancy: Results of a prospective randomized trial. *Am. J. Obstet. Gynecol.* 134:376, 1979.
    Patients were prospectively managed if the pregnancies were suspected of postmaturity by the use of amniocentesis. The detection of meconium in the amniotic fluid did not seem to be helpful in managing these patients.
13. Schneider, J. M., Olson, R. W., and Curet, L. B. Screening for fetal and neonatal risk in the postdate pregnancy. *Am. J. Obstet. Gynecol.* 131:473, 1978.
    One hundred and four patients with postmature pregnancies were managed by protocol with no increase in perinatal mortality. Perinatal morbidity was increased, and the authors recommended that the intrapartum stage be managed very carefully even if antepartum assessment is normal.
14. Rayburn, W. J., and Chang, F. E. Management of the uncomplicated postdate pregnancy. *J. Reprod. Med.* 26:93, 1981.
    The 101 postdate pregnancies were compared to 322 term pregnancies. When managed by protocol there was no difference in perinatal mortality, but the need for cesarean section or forceps manipulation was increased in the postterm group.
15. Stubblefield, P. G., and Berek, J. S. Perinatal mortality in term and postterm infants. *Obstet. Gynecol.* 56:76, 1980.
    The authors compare the death rate in postterm infants with that for term infants. The diagnosis and management of the postterm infant is emphasized.

Complications

16. Griff, Y. M., et al. Developmental effects of prolonged pregnancy and the postmaturity syndrome. *J. Pediatr.* 90:836, 1977.
    Forty postterm infants were compared to 40 normal control infants during the first year of life. The postterm infants had lower Brazelton and motor scores at birth; at four months they scored lower on the Denver Developmental scale; and at eight months their Bayley motor scores were equivalent to those of the control infants but the mental scores were lower. There was also a high incidence of illness as well as feeding and sleep disorders in the postmature infants.
17. Takahashi, K., et al. Uterine contractility and oxytocin sensitivity in

preterm, term, and postterm pregnancy. *Am. J. Obstet. Gynecol.* 136:774, 1980.

The sensitivity of the uterus to oxytocin in postterm pregnancy appears to be, as in the premature gestation, less than in the term pregnancy. Possible mechanisms for this change are outlined.

Anemias in Pregnancy

Anemia is the most common medical complication associated with pregnancy and occurs in about 50% of pregnant women in this country. Fortunately, in most cases the effect on the mother and fetus is mild. During the first 24 weeks of pregnancy there is a "relative" anemia that occurs because of the hormonally related increase in plasma volume compared to red blood cells. It is not of clinical importance in most patients, and after 24–28 weeks, when the production of erythrocytes increases, it should not be as demonstrable. The absolute anemias occur because of decreased erythrocyte production, increased red cell destruction, or accentuated erythrocyte loss. The most common causes of anemia, other than obvious blood loss, are those of decreased erythrocyte production (collectively called hypoproliferative anemias). These processes usually reflect a deficiency of an essential subcellular component such as iron, folic acid, or vitamin B_{12}.

The effect of anemia on gestation is variable. Maternal deterioration is not usually noted unless the hemoglobin (Hb) is less than 4–6 g%, and packed cell volume (PCV) is less than 12%–18%. On the other hand, delayed wound healing and a higher incidence of infection, as well as a prolonged hospital stay, have been demonstrated by some moderately anemic parturients (Hb < 8 g%, PCV < 25%). Moreover, even with mild anemia (Hb < 10–11 g%, PCV < 30%), the fetus may be affected by intrauterine growth retardation, polycythemia, and other complications.

Making the diagnosis of an anemia during pregnancy is rather difficult, because the historic and physical signs of an anemia, such as malaise, anorexia, and pallor, may be present in a normal gestation. Additionally, laboratory parameters are also changed by pregnancy itself. Nevertheless, most of the necessary tests can be performed on an ambulatory basis, thus making hospitalization (except when the anemia is severe or serious hematologic disease is suspected) usually unnecessary. Classically, patients with an Hb less than 10 g% or a PCV of less than 30%, or both, during pregnancy are considered to be anemic. Although these are useful tools in screening for anemia, they do not yield any indication as to the cause of the anemia. Blood smears indicate the size of the cell, as well as the chromicity, and are valuable in separating the various patterns such as iron deficiency anemia from a folic acid deficiency. Unfortunately, most patients have a mixed or combination effect, and the smear is not always helpful. If there is a large amount of cellular debris and odd-shaped cells, the appearance of the red blood cells may help predict the hereditary anemias or the hemolytic processes (sickle cell, G6PD, and so on). The red blood cell indices are not of great value unless changed to the extreme. The mean cellular hemoglobin concentration (MCHC) is most reliable, and if less than 30 g/dl/RBC, almost always represents an absolute anemia. On the other hand, the mean cellular volume and mean cellular hemoglobin, due to the disproportionate increase in plasma volume, are less useful. The reticulocyte count is helpful since it should be greater than 1% during pregnancy. If not, particularly in the face of a hemoglobin less than 10 g%, a hypoproliferative disorder is usually present, indicating a primary toxic effect, hereditary disorder (thalassemia), or the lack of essential nutrients such as iron and folic acid. On the other hand, the parturient with an anemia and a reticulocyte count of greater than 3% usually has accelerated RBC production in response to excessive blood loss. Other assessments may be helpful, particularly in specific anemias, and are detailed under each process.

Iron-deficiency anemia (IDA) can be implicated in up to 75% of all anemias during pregnancy. The need for iron during a normal gestation is over 1000 mg, an amount that exceeds by 300–400 mg the level of iron available even in the best diets. Thus, even if iron stores are normal and the diet is perfect in its nutritional value, a net loss of iron occurs in each gestation. Therefore, there is a rationale for prescribing supplemental iron to each pregnant woman. The iron in prenatal vitamins is not enough for replacement since it is only taken once a day. Because the absorptive pattern of iron is maximized at 8-hour intervals, iron needs to be taken three times per day. In addition, many factors affect iron absorption. Antacids, oxalates, and phosphates will reduce absorption, while ascorbic acid, lactate, sorbital, and various amino acids increase absorption.

The diagnosis of IDA rests on finding a hypochromic, microcytic RBC smear with an MCHC of less than 30 g/dl/RBC. Although pregnancy changes various iron indices, the findings of a serum iron less than 30 μg/dl, iron binding capacity of greater than 400 μg/dl, and a transferin saturation of less than 15% is virtually diagnostic of IDA. The treatment of iron-deficiency anemia should involve the use of 60 mg of elemental iron (300 mg ferrous sulfate) taken three times a day with meals. The new combination products do not offer any advantages. For those who complain of gastrointestinal side effects, ferrous sulfate syrup can be used, although care must be taken not to stain the teeth. Parenteral iron, while useful in selected cases, is not commonly employed due to frequent side effects and because the compound is rapidly excreted. If the iron is that badly needed, blood transfusions are usually more appropriate.

Folic acid deficiency represents 20%–22% of the cases of anemia during pregnancy. Therefore, folic acid–deficiency and iron-deficiency anemia account for approximately 97% of all anemias during the reproductive years. Most vitamin preparations have enough folic acid to be absorbed and will suffice if the diet is adequate. If not, a folic acid supplement (one-half of 1 mg tablet) should be taken three times a day to take advantage of the same absorptive pattern stated for iron. Tests for folate deficiency are not useful because changes are documented rather late in the disease course. However, hypersegmented neutrophils, macrocytic and hyperchromatic changes in the RBC, and low serum folate all indicate deprivation of folate. Because a deficiency of it is difficult to diagnose, folic acid, like iron, is usually substituted in most pregnancies. Treatment with iron and folic acid is therefore perhaps the best means of anemia prevention and treatment in pregnant patients.

Anemias associated with the defective production of erythrocytes are numerous but clinically they are rarely seen. Various toxins (radiation, chloromycetin) may give rise to an aplastic anemia. Antiinflammatory agents (such as aspirin or indomethacin) also may be toxic to the marrow, as are severe acute infections. A mortality rate of up to 75% has been reported in patients with aplastic anemia, but pregnancy itself usually does not affect the disorder adversely. Chronic inflammation as represented by the autoimmune diseases and neoplasia may also result in an anemia. In these patients, the storage of iron in the form of hemosiderin or ferritin is adequate, but the release mechanism of iron to the red cells and iron mobilization from the storage depot is abnormal. The anemias are usually mild, with a hemoglobin ranging from 8–11 g% and a reticulocyte count of usually less than 1%, indicating a hypoproliferative pattern, but the sedimentation rate is elevated above that seen in pregnant patients. Diagnosis of the specific disorder is made by careful history and physical examination and a high index of suspicion.

Blood-loss anemia during pregnancy also must be ruled out. Early in gestation, ectopic pregnancy and abortion, as well as vaginal and cervical lesions, must be ruled out. Late in pregnancy, placenta previa and abruptio placentae are the most common causes of blood loss. In developing countries, parasites and nontropical and tropical sprue may play a significant role in the etiology. In this country, hemorrhoids associated with pregnancy can also give rise to chronic blood loss, as can peptic ulcer disease and intrinsic bowel disease. These anemias are more easily diagnosed because the common causes usually involve external blood loss.

Acquired hemolytic anemias of pregnancy include those in wich red blood cells are destroyed prematurely. Diseases such as eclampsia and microangiopathic anemias are particularly representative of such disorders. They all have common blood smear abnormalities that feature very bizarre shaped cells. Many of the disease processes have very specific smear abnormalities, such as spherocytosis and porphyria. The social, family, and past history may be very helpful in these cases. Inherited disorders that can cause anemia are discussed in another chapter.

In summary, the anemias of pregnancy are extremely common. Most of them usually represent only mild deviations from normal for most parturients, and the mother and fetus are usually not severely affected. Nevertheless, it is critically important that during pregnancy the cause of such anemias be diagnosed and treated. If a deficiency or other type of anemia is allowed to continue, it could adversely affect the woman later in life or in subsequent pregnancies. Moreover, we do not know what subtle effects mild anemias may have on the offspring. In addition, it must be emphasized strongly that each pregnant woman should be given supplemental folic acid and iron in almost every case, since the effect of pregnancy is to deplete iron and folic acid in quantities greater than it can be restored by the normal diet.

General Hematology

1. Beck, W. S. Erythrocyte Disorders. In J. W. Williams, E. Bentler, A. S. Erslev, and R. W. Rundles (Eds.), *Hematology* (2nd ed.). Philadelphia: McGraw-Hill, 1977.
   A detailed presentation of the cause and effects of various erythrocyte disorders resulting in anemia. The biochemical aspects of the erythrocyte at the subcellular level are presented.
2. Nienhuis, A. W., and Benz, E. J., Jr. Regulation of hemoglobin synthesis during the development of the red cell. *N. Engl. J. Med.* 297:1318, 1977.
   (Three parts.) An in-depth analysis of the factors involved in hemoglobin synthesis in all phases of human life. An excellent treatise for those interested in the subcellular aspects of hemoglobin, and it contains over 500 references.
3. Wigton, R. S., et al. Chart reminders in the diagnosis of anemia. *J.A.M.A.* 245:1745, 1981.
   In a chart review study, these authors showed that the use of chart reminders to flag those charts with low admission hemoglobin levels were ignored by providers in approximately 25% of the cases. Other means of stimulating a physician not to overlook abnormal laboratory results are needed.

Anemias and Pregnancy

4. deLeeuw, N. K. W., and Brunton, L. Maternal Hematologic Changes, Iron Metabolism and Anemias in Pregnancy. In J. W. Goodwin, et al. (Eds.), *Perinatal Medicine*. Baltimore: Williams & Wilkins, 1976.
   An excellent review of the pathophysiology and clinical correlations of anemias from all causes during pregnancy. A very good section also on the mechanism of iron absorption and incorporation into red cells.
5. Morrison, J. C. Anemia Associated with Pregnancy. In J. J. Sciarra (Ed.), *Gynecology and Obstetrics*. Hagerstown, Md.: Harper & Row, 1980. Vol. 3.
   An in-depth review of the various causes of anemia and how they relate to pregnancy. A nice section is also included on laboratory determinations.
6. Horowitz, J. J., and Laros, R. K., Jr. Anemia and pregnancy: A review of the pathophysiology, diagnosis, and treatment. *J. Cont. Education Obstet. Gynecol.* 21:9, 1979.
   A categorized approach to classifications of each anemia process during pregnancy and its effect on gestation; includes 93 references.

Iron Deficiency

7. Kaneshige, E. Serum ferritin as an assessment of iron stores and other hematologic parameters during pregnancy. *Obstet. Gynecol.* 57:238, 1981.
   Serum ferritin was found to be a useful index of the status of iron stores. The results suggested that maternal body iron storage is depleted in all women who are not taking supplemental iron during pregnancy.
8. Beisel, W. R. Iron nutrition: Immunity and infection. *Res. Staff Phys.* 54:37, 1981.
   The relationship of iron deficiency anemia to immunity and infection is covered in great detail. The various laboratory findings as they apply to infection and malnutrition are outlined.
9. Dallman, P. R. Inhibition of iron absorption by certain foods. *Am. J. Dis. Child.* 134:453, 1980.
   The most up-to-date comment on how iron absorption may be increased or decreased; it also includes many other factors relative to absorptive mechanisms.
10. Oral iron. *Med. Lett.* 20:45, 1978.
    Many iron preparations and their indications as well as cost-effectiveness in clinical situations are detailed.

Folic Acid Deficiency

11. Pritchard, J. A., Whalley, P. J., and Scott, D. E. The influence of maternal folate and iron deficiency on intrauterine life. *Am. J. Obstet. Gynecol.* 104:388, 1969.
    A detailed look at the influence of maternal folate deficiency (as well as other elemental deficiencies) on fetal development and the reproductive outcome.
12. Fleming, A. F., Martin, J. D., and Stenhouse, N. S. Pregnancy anemia, iron and folate deficiency in Western Australia. *Med. J. Aust.* 2:479, 1974.
    A study concerning the relationship of complications to folic acid deficiency and iron-deficiency anemia in over 400 women. Complications such as infection, uterine hemorrhage, and premature delivery occurred in the group with anemia.

Other Anemias

13. Knispel, J. W., Lynch, V. A., and Viele, B. D. Aplastic anemia in pregnancy: A case report, review of the literature, and a re-evaluation of management. *Obstet. Gynecol. Surv.* 31:523, 1976.
    Management techniques as well as a review of the literature regarding aplastic anemia during pregnancy; includes 36 references.
14. Peterson, C. M. Problems of iron imbalance. *Drug Ther. (Hosp).* 26:61, 1979.
    An excellent listing in tabular form of the causes of acute blood loss anemias, as well as those anemias with drug-related etiologies.
15. Morrison, J. C. Anemias and Hemoglobinopathies. In G. M. Ryan, Jr. (Ed.), *Ambulatory Care in Obstetrics and Gynecology.* New York: Grune & Stratton, 1980.
    A practical and clinical approach toward the ambulatory diagnosis of most problems with anemias in the pregnant woman. Recommendations concerning unusual hematologic problems, which actually comprise a small percent of the anemias during pregnancy, are outlined.

Preterm Labor

Preterm delivery accounts for over 75% of all perinatal morbidity and mortality in the United States. The infant who survives has often undergone a long stay in a neonatal intensive care unit with many complications, the most serious of which is hyaline membrane disease and its attendant morbidity. Survival, however, is not necessarily intact, as a significant percentage of these children manifest overt neurologic abnormalities and more subtle effects such as a lower IQ score. Also, the emotional and financial strain on the parents is often severe.

The term *preterm* refers to a gestational age of less than 37 completed weeks (259 days). The term *premature* has been used to describe babies born weighing less than 2500 grams. This may be due to preterm birth, or they may be low birth weight babies who are more than 37 weeks gestation but small for gestational age. The incidence in the United States is approximately 13% for black women and 6% for white women.

The etiology of preterm labor can be broadly classified into four headings: pregnancy complications, epidemiologic factors, iatrogenic factors, and unknown cause. The epidemiologic factors are simply entities associated with preterm labor, and there is no evidence that they actually are etiologically involved. Of all these factors, a previous preterm delivery and multiple gestation in the current pregnancy correlate most strongly with spontaneous preterm birth. Patients with one previous spontaneous preterm delivery have approximately a 37% chance of again delivering preterm, and those with two or more preterm deliveries have a 70% chance, while those with twins are twelve times more likely to have a preterm birth.

It is often extremely difficult to distinguish between true preterm labor and so-called false labor. Often, the diagnosis of preterm labor can be made only in retrospect as only 25%–50% of patients with regular painful contractions actually proceed to preterm delivery. Thus, if all patients with regular contractions are treated, many of them will receive unnecessary therapy. The diagnosis may be facilitated by observing the characteristics of uterine contractility and cervical change. With false labor there is often no progressive cervical change and the contractions cease spontaneously. Although the frequency, regularity, or pain of the contractions do not distinguish true labor from false labor, it is more significant when the contractions are regular, become greater in intensity, last longer, are closer together, and changes occur in the cervix.

Many low birth weight infants are mature, growth-retarded infants, and the labor in these patients may be mistaken for preterm labor. This is more likely to occur in the low socioeconomic, high-risk patient who, to make matters more confusing, often has unreliable dates. It is unwise to use tocolytic drugs to forcibly maintain these fetuses in an unfavorable intrauterine environment, and the best way to avoid this situation is to do an amniocentesis for maturity studies and not to treat when fetal pulmonary maturity is indicated. Thus, diagnosis of true labor and fetal maturity are the cornerstone of our ability to manage preterm labor.

Because a large percentage of patients in so-called preterm labor will respond to a placebo, it is not surprising that claims for success have been made for many modes of treatment and therapeutic agents. Due to the effect on the central nervous system, agents such as meperidine, morphine, promethazine, and phenobarbital were used in an attempt to relax the myometrium. Not only are these agents ineffective in reducing uterine activity, but they may in fact cause respiratory depression and increasing uterine contractions in the preterm baby. Diazoxide, a benzothiadiazine derivative, will inhibit myometrial contractions in vitro as well as in vivo. The propensity of diazoxide to produce hypotension and decreased uterine blood flow mitigates against its widespread use as a tocolytic agent. Magnesium sulfate also decreases uterine activity by approximately 10%. In one study it was found to be more effective than alcohol for the treatment of preterm labor. It should be noted, however, that most preeclamptic patients labor spontaneously while receiving full therapeutic dosages of the drug.

Alcohol has been widely used in the United States for treating preterm labor. Although some studies have shown the drug to be effective in the treatment of preterm labor, others have failed to confirm this finding. It is not as effective as other tocolytic agents in the treatment of preterm labor. Common side effects are nausea, vomiting, headache, diuresis, restlessness, dizziness, and disorientation. The inebriated patient requires constant supervision and serious side effects such as severe lactic acidosis and aspiration pneumonia have been reported. Alcohol freely crosses the placenta and the infants born within 12 hours after its administration have a significantly lower Apgar score and a higher incidence of respiratory distress syndrome (RDS).

As the prostaglandins play a central role in the initiation of labor, it is not unexpected that drugs that inhibit prostaglandin synthetase would modify the labor process and be of therapeutic value in stopping preterm labor. Indomethacin crosses the placenta without difficulty, and several animal studies have demonstrated untoward cardiovascular effects. Rat experiments have demonstrated that large doses of indomethacin given to the mother within 18 hours of term delivery results in intrauterine narrowing of the fetal ductus arteriosus. Further evaluations are necessary, and at this time the prostaglandin synthetase inhibitors cannot be recommended for treatment of preterm labor.

The adrenergic stimulants produce their effects through two different receptors, which he called alpha-adrenergic and beta-adrenergic; stimulation of the β-receptors produces uterine relaxation. By 1967, there was further subdivision of the β-receptors into β_1 and β_2. The β_1-receptors mediate the increase in rate and force of the heart, lipolysis, and effects on the intestine.

The β_2-receptors are involved in glycogenolysis and relaxation of the smooth muscles of arterioles, the bronchi, and the uterus. There are, however, no "pure" β_1 or β_2 stimulants.

Isoxsuprine was the first β-sympathomimetic drug to be widely used as a tocolytic agent in the treatment of preterm labor. Although it is effective in suppressing uterine activity, its therapeutic usefulness has been somewhat compromised by its significant degree of cardiovascular β_1 effects such as maternal tachycardia and hypotension. Ritodrine, which has greater β_2 selectivity, is the first drug in the United States approved for the treatment of preterm labor. The mechanism of action of the β-sympathomimetic drugs is to stimulate adenyl cyclase, an enzyme located on the internal surface of the plasma membrane of the target cell. This activates the conversion of adenosine triphosphate to cyclic adenosine monophosphate (AMP) that in turn increases protein kinases, which results in phosphorylation of specific membrane proteins. This action decreases free intracellular calcium ions and thus causes relaxation of the smooth muscle of the uterus.

The most common maternal side effects are palpitations, muscle tremor, nervousness, and restlessness. The patient with diabetes will require careful monitoring of plasma glucose and will usually need increased insulin when she is treated with these drugs. Special care is required when corticosteroids for fetal lung maturity are used in combination with the β-sympathomimetic drugs as pulmonay edema is a serious complication and is more likely to occur with a combination of these drugs and fluid overload. Follow-up studies of infants born to mothers treated with ritodrine have revealed no untoward effects. At the present time β-sympathomimetic drugs are the treatment of choice for preterm labor.

Our ritodrine protocol with appropriate administration and dosage information is as follows. A large-bore indwelling catheter kept open by an intravenous infusion is inserted. It is safer to control the dosage of the drug by using an infusion pump and to piggyback the infusion onto the main intravenous line. The initial dose is 100 μg/min, after which the dose is increased by 50 μg/min every 15 minutes until contractions stop (or not more than one in 15 minutes) or unacceptable side effects develop. One must monitor maternal heart rate and blood pressure, uterine activity, and fetal heart rate throughout infusion. Once the maternal pulse reaches 140 beats per minute, the dose is not increased any further as this is the maximum dosage for that patient. If the pulse goes above 140 beats per minute, or side effects are poorly tolerated, the dose is reduced. It is important to note that the maximum dose is approximately 350 μg/min.

If labor is successfully arrested, continue the infusion for at least 6 hours before starting to wean the patient from the drug in a stepwise fashion over the next 2 hours. Begin oral therapy—10 mg every 4 hours for 24 hours—30 minutes before stopping the infusion; if the uterus remains quiescent, 10 to 20 mg every 4–6 hours should be given until further inhibition of labor is not indicated. During infusion of the drug it is important to regulate the amount of intravenous fluids carefully, especially with long-term usage and when steroids are concomitantly used (maximum of 150 ml/hr). The intravenous infusion may be repeated as necessary, if the patient still meets the selection criteria.

Review

1. Lipshitz, J., and Schneider, J. M. Inhibition of Labor. In J. J. Sciarra (Ed.), *Gynecology and Obstetrics.* Hagerstown, Md.: Harper & Row, 1980. Vol. 3.

This is a comprehensive and detailed review of the etiology and management of preterm labor.

2. Bejar, R., et al. Premature labor. II. Bacterial sources of phospholipase. *Obstet. Gynecol.* 57:479, 1981.
   The diagnosis of chorioamnionitis was studied in groups of patients at risk for premature labor. The authors postulate that premature labor may be initiated by microorganisms with phospholipase A_2 activity.

3. Rush, R. W., et al. Contribution of preterm delivery to perinatal mortality. *Br. Med. J.* 2:965, 1976.
   This is a good epidemiological article that describes the incidence of perinatal mortality associated with the different causes of preterm delivery.

4. Curbelo, V., et al. Premature labor. I. Prostaglandin precursors in human placental membranes. *Obstet. Gynecol.* 57:473, 1981.
   The mechanism of premature labor regarding the amount of prostaglandin precursors in the human amnion was studied prospectively. The amnion seems to be a more important storage place of these precursors than is the chorion.

Etiology

5. Dubin, N. H., et al. Plasma prostaglandin in pregnant women with term and preterm deliveries. *Obstet. Gynecol.* 57:203, 1981.
   In patients who are in preterm labor, plasma prostaglandins were lower than the control group who were in labor at term. This study provides evidence that most cases of preterm labor are not characterized by elevated prostaglandin levels.

Treatment

6. Fuchs, F., et al. Effect of alcohol on threatened premature labor. *Am. J. Obstet. Gynecol.* 99:627, 1967.
   This article resulted in the widespread use of alcohol for the treatment of preterm labor.

7. Merkatz, I. R., Peter, J. B., and Barden, T. P. Ritodrine hydrochloride: A betamimetic agent for use in preterm labor. *Obstet. Gynecol.* 56:7, 1980.
   The results of the United States multicenter trials with ritodrine, which led to its approval by the FDA, are presented.

8. Barden, T. P., Peter, J. B., and Merkatz, I. R. Ritodrine hydrochloride: A betamimetic agent for use in preterm labor. I. Pharmacology, clinical history, administration, side effects, and safety. *Obstet. Gynecol.* 56:1, 1980.
   The pharmacology, administration protocol, and clinical usage of ritodrine hydrochloride are reviewed.

9. Karch, F. E. Suppressing premature labor with beta-adrenergic stimulants. *Drug Ther.* 9:118, 1979.
   The author reviews selective β_2 adrenergic drugs for the suppression of premature labor and concludes that they are more effective than alcohol or placebos.

10. Lipshitz, J., et al. Effects of hexoprenaline on the lecithin/spingomyelin ratio and pressure-volume relationships in fetal rabbits. *Am. J. Obstet. Gynecol.* 139:726, 1981.
    In addition to delaying premature labor, hexoprenaline was also shown in this study to release surfactant in the fetal lung.

11. Bergman, G., and Hedner, T. Antepartum administration of terbutaline and the incidence of hyaline membrane disease in preterm infants. *Acta Obstet. Gynecol. Scand.* 57:217, 1978.

The incidence of respiratory distress syndrome decreased in the infants whose mothers were treated with terbutaline. Evidence is given that this drug assists in protecting the infant from hyaline membrane disease.

Complications

12. Schreyer, P., et al. Metabolic effects of intramuscular and oral administration of ritodrine in pregnancy. *Obstet. Gynecol.* 57:730, 1981.
    The metabolic effects on the mother of intramuscular and oral ritodrine were assessed in this study. Although there were significant alterations in the level of glucose and electrolytes, with careful management, tocolytic agents can safely be used.
13. Freysz, H., et al. A long term evaluation of infants who received a beta-mimetic drug while in utero. *J. Perinat. Med.* 5:94, 1977.
    Forty-two children whose mothers were treated with ritodrine were studied for long-term effects of these drugs. When compared to control infants there were no significant harmful effects on the infant.
14. Ayromlooi, J., Tobias, M., and Desiderio, D. Effects of isoxsuprine on maternal and fetal acid-base balance and circulation. *Obstet. Gynecol.* 57:193, 1981.
    The fetal and maternal cardiovascular effects of isoxsuprine were determined in pregnant ewes. Various side effects in the metabolic area as well as acid-base and oxygenation parameters were reviewed as tolerable for the fetus.
15. Brazy, J. E., and Pupkin, M. J. Effects of maternal isoxsuprine administration on preterm infants. *J. Pediatr.* 94:444, 1979.
    The side effects on the fetus when isoxsuprine was administered to the mother were detailed. The authors found untoward outcome in a number of infants, but in almost all instances it could be related to profound hypertension and tachycardia in the mother.
16. Nuwayhid, B., et al. Hemodynamic effects of isoxsuprine and terbutaline in pregnant and nonpregnant sheep. *Am. J. Obstet. Gynecol.* 137:25, 1980.
    The cardiovascular effects of the β-sympathomimetic drugs were compared in pregnant and nonpregnant ewes. While there were some differences in uterine blood flow, there were no profound effects that would adversely affect the fetus.
17. Smythe, A. R. II, and Skakini, J., Jr. Maternal metabolic alterations secondary to terbutaline therapy for premature labor. *Obstet. Gynecol.* 57:566, 1981.
    The metabolic changes in pregnant women treated with terbutaline for premature labor were studied. Hypokalemia, hyperglycemia, and an increase in lactic acid occurred. Electrolyte and glucose levels should be monitored in patients treated with tocolytic agents.

Premature Ruptured Membranes

Premature rupture of the membranes (PROM) can be a major obstetric complication. PROM is the rupture of membranes prior to the onset of true labor and is often difficult to document. It occurs in as many as 15%–20% of all labor patients. If it occurs at or near term, the sequela for the fetus is not nearly so severe, although the mother has an additional risk of both increased morbidity and a cesarean versus vaginal birth. If it occurs before 37 weeks, PROM is associated with an increased perinatal mortality rate directly related to the rate of prematurity. The goal is to choose an appropriate management plan, one that will yield a healthy neonate while having the least maternal complication. Thus, the decision whether to manage the patient aggressively with induction of labor by pitocin or cesarean birth, or both, versus the conservative approach—observation—is a difficult one in many cases.

The first step is to document PROM. In the history, one should note the time of rupture as well as the presence of meconium or associated symptoms that might herald infection. Next, direct visualization of the cervix via a sterile speculum exam should be accomplished. In most cases, PROM can be documented by observing free-flowing amniotic fluid from the cervical os. Unless one is committed to delivery, internal digital examination (bimanual pelvic) of the cervix should not be performed. While the speculum is in place, the fluid from the posterior fornix should be tested for an alkaline pH (amniotic fluid) using nitrazine paper. In addition, if a sample of the fluid is allowed to dry on a slide, arborization or ferning will be observed under the microscope if amniotic fluid is present. Nile blue sulfate staining for identification of fetal cells or biochemical tests such as diamine oxidase activity are not particularly useful. During the speculum exam, the amount of dilatation and effacement of the cervix should be estimated since this may have a predictive value in determining which patients can be managed conservatively. Also, if acute cervicitis or other vaginal lesions are present, this would indicate a poor prognosis for conservative management.

An abdominal examination should be performed to make certain there is only one baby. In addition, one can usually assess whether the fetus is breech, vertex, or transverse in its presentation. One may check for abdominal tenderness or uterine irritability, both of which often precede amnionitis. Determination of gestational age should also be carried out. Ultrasonography, using the biparietal diameter (BPD), will yield a rough idea of gestational age of the infant. Additionally, fetal viability (cardiac activity) and the presentation of the fetus can be documented. Moreover, if an amniocentesis needs to be performed, the ultrasound can be used to locate the placental position and pockets of amniotic fluid. It is critical that amniotic fluid be obtained since a single ultrasound biparietal diameter measurement is only a guide to fetal maturity. If amniotic fluid can be obtained by means of the sterile speculum exam and is free-flowing, it can be used in performing the lecithin/spingomyelin (L/S) ratio; the values are not significantly different from abdominally collected samples. If fluid is not available by means of vaginal collection, ultrasound-directed amniocentesis is necessary.

The laboratory assessment of amnionitis is, at best, very confusing. If amniotic fluid can be obtained by amniocentesis or by intrauterine catheter, the presence of organisms on gram stain or an increased white cell count have been correlated with amnionitis. There is not a direct correlation with a certain number of organisms or white cells, or both, and clinically apparent amnionitis; many cases may be subclinical. Similarly, the culture, while helpful in treatment if amnionitis develops, is not particularly germane to its immediate diagnosis. Maternal and fetal tachycardia as well as maternal hyperpyrexia are excellent predictors but are relatively late signs in the course of amnionitis. Likewise, exudate coming from the cervix, poor progress in labor, and delayed response to pitocin are clinical determinants that occur late in the course of amnionitis. An increased C-reactive protein and a change in maternal leukocytosis with a shift toward the segmented neutrophils are early signs in predicting amnionitis. Although these can be used as guidelines, there is no definitive test to detect amnionitis.

The fact that approximately 12.8% of term pregnancies and 30.2% of preterm pregnancies are complicated by PROM indicates that there is a major obstetric and neonatal problem. The major consequence of PROM is a clearly increased risk of maternal morbidity and an increased threat to the infant because of prematurity. Although there is an increased fetal infection rate with PROM, this does not correlate directly with the length of time the membranes have been ruptured but rather is related to the degree of prematurity. Therefore, it is most important that a fetal maturity assessment be performed so that an accurate method of management may be outlined. In pregnancies in which there is known, or strongly presumed, fetal maturity (> 37 weeks), the management of PROM should be active: pitocin induction. Since more than 80% of patients at or near term will go into labor spontaneously within 12 hours of premature rupture of the membranes, many advocate at least 4 to 8 hours of observation before patients at this gestational age are induced. Others begin induction immediately, although it appears that this course of management will lead to more frequent cesarean births. Maternal morbidity, therefore, is higher in those immediately started on pitocin because of the greatly increased morbidity of cesarean births versus vaginal delivery.

On the other hand, in those preterm pregnancies in which pulmonary immaturity has been demonstrated, the management should be along the lines of observation. Conservative management is maintained and intervention is undertaken only if signs of infection or fetal compromise are noted. If the fetus is preterm and the mother is in early labor with the membranes being ruptured less than 12 hours with no signs of infection, consideration of tocolytic therapy can be made. This would be an infrequent occurrence, since most patients with spontaneous labor and premature ruptured membranes are those in whom subclinical amnionitis is present. In cases of fetuses with immature pulmonary systems and in which the fetus is at high risk for delivery in 24 to 72 hours—such as transverse lie, breech, or when the cervix is 3–4 cm dilated—corticosteroids can be employed to mature the fetal lungs. In cases in which the position is transverse, incomplete, or compound breech presentation, the patient is not sent home without delivery.

On the other hand, if the vertex is presenting or if there is a frank breech, the mother can be sent home after observation in the hospital for amnionitis. The current regimen in these cases is to monitor the patients in the labor area for a few hours to detect fetal compromise, amnionitis, or labor. They are then observed on the antepartum ward for another 10–12 hours to see how much fluid they are losing and for signs of amnionitis. At the end of the first 24 hours, the patients are ambulated to see what effect this will have on the extrusion of fluid or the development of symptoms. If neither occurs, they are usually sent home on the third day, unless there is one of the abnormal fetal presentations mentioned or signs of amnionitis develop.

The management of delivery depends on many factors. If delivery is indicated, the infant is vertex, and there are no signs of fetal compromise, pitocin induction is begun. If, on the other hand, the premature infant is breech presentation or transverse lie, a cesarean delivery is performed. Although there is data that the infant weighing less than 1000 g, even in the vertex position, is compromised by vaginal delivery, most authorities are awaiting more complete data on this subject. The use of prophylactic antibiotics has not found a place in the management of PROM without amnionitis. On the other hand, if the mother has active amnionitis, we begin the patient on aqueous penicillin and an aminoglycoside or other appropriate antibiotic as a therapeutic measure. In these cases, neonatologists understand why one must use antibiotics and do not feel that the infant will be subjected to additional risks; indeed, most of the infants who come from definitely infected mothers have antibiotics continued in the nursery.

The effect of premature ruptured membranes on the incidence of respiratory distress syndrome is currently undecided. There are many observers who feel that after 24 hours of ruptured membranes, the infants are "protected" from development of hyaline membrane disease. There are other studies, however, that show that when adjusted for weight and other factors, this advantage is not present. The documentation of fetal pulmonary maturity just before delivery is the most sensitive method of assessing the difficulty that that fetus may have concerning the development of hyaline membrane disease.

Text

1. Hertz, R. H., and Rosen, M. G. Clinical Management of Premature Rupture of the Membranes. In J. J. Sciarra (Ed.), *Gynecology and Obstetrics.* Hagerstown, Md.: Harper & Row, 1980. Vol. 2.
   A very practical effort toward addressing the problems in diagnosis and management of PROM is presented.

PROM and RDS

2. Berkowitz, R. L., et al. The relationship between premature rupture of the membranes and the respiratory distress syndrome. An update and plan of management. *Am. J. Obstet. Gynecol.* 131:503, 1978.
   Three hundred and forty infants with PROM were studied. Increasing length of time of PROM was correlated with decreased RDS in infants 33 weeks and older.

3. Jones, M. D., Jr., et al. Failure of association of premature rupture of membranes with respiratory-distress syndrome. *N. Engl. J. Med.* 292:1253, 1975.
   Records of 16,458 births were studied with regard to the relationship of PROM with RDS. The data did not support the hypotheses that there is a lower incidence of RDS after PROM.

Diagnosis

4. Stedman, C. M., et al. Management of preterm premature rupture of membranes: Assessing amniotic fluid in the vagina for phosphatidylglycerol. *Am. J. Obstet. Gynecol.* 140:34, 1981.
   Eighty percent of 55 patients with PROM yielded vaginal fluid. Assessment for phosphatidyglycerol is found to be accurate in predicting fetal lung maturity.

5. Garite, T. J., et al. The use of amniocentesis in patients with premature rupture of membranes. *Obstet. Gynecol.* 54:226, 1979.
   A study to assess the use of amniocentesis as a diagnostic tool in PROM in 59 patients is presented. Amniocentesis appeared to be useful in both diagnosis and prognosis.

6. Ledger, W. J. Bacterial infections complicating pregnancy. *Clin. Obstet. Gynecol.* 21:455, 1978.
   The diagnosis of ruptured membranes is very difficult as is the diagnosis of infection. Multiple techniques for the diagnosis and management of PROM are discussed.

Effect on the Mother and Neonate

7. Varner, M. W., and Galask, R. P. Conservative management of premature rupture of the membranes. *Am. J. Obstet. Gynecol.* 140:39, 1981.
   The conservative management of premature ruptured membranes in 116 pregnancies was reviewed. A decrease in RDS with the progressive duration of ruptured membranes was observed but this increasing duration was not associated with increased risk of infection to the mother or fetus.

8. Miller, J. M., Jr., Pupkin, M. J., and Hill, G. B. Bacterial colonization of amniotic fluid from intact fetal membranes. *Am. J. Obstet. Gynecol.* 136:796, 1980.
   This study shows that there is a wide spectrum of bacteria capable of colonizing amniotic fluid even in the presence of intact membranes. The gram stain and culture of amniotic fluid were helpful, but the presence of organisms did not mean active infections.

9. Schreiber, J., and Benedetti, T. Conservative management of preterm premature rupture of the fetal membranes in a low socioeconomic population. *Am. J. Obstet. Gynecol.* 136:92, 1980.
   Ninety pregnancies with PROM in a low socioeconomic group of patients were studied. Amnionitis developed in 27% of these patients but did not increase in those as the duration of PROM increased. RDS, not infection, was the significant cause of neonatal death.

10. Naeye, R. L., and Peters, E. C. Causes and consequences of premature rupture of fetal membranes. *Lancet* 1:129, 1980.
    Retrospective data from over 6,000 premature infants were studied. Amniotic fluid infections were two- to threefold more common in the cases of premature ruptured membranes. Low Apgar scores and neonatal hyperbilirubinemia were more common in these patients, but parental coitus prior to delivery was not related to infant morbidity.

11. Nochimson, D. J., et al. Comparison of conservative and dynamic management of premature rupture of membranes/premature labor syndrome. New approaches to the delivery of infants which may minimize the need for intensive care. *Clin. Perinatol.* 7:17, 1980.
    A large number of patients in a regional center received meticulous obstetric management to avoid intrapartum stress, hypoxia, and delivery trauma. This approach, with the advent of adequate tocolysis and glucocorticoids, gave optimal infant outcome.

Management of Amnionitis

12. Johnson, J. W. C., et al. Premature rupture of the membranes and prolonged latency. *Obstet. Gynecol.* 57:547, 1981.
    This retrospective study of 8320 patients with PROM concluded that in the absence of chorioamnionitis there appeared to be no benefit to delivery prior to 37 weeks for the baby or the mother. Thirty-four excellent up-to-date references are offered.

13. Gibbs, R. S., Castillo, M. S., and Rodgers, P. J. Management of acute chorioamnionitis. *Am. J. Obstet. Gynecol.* 136:709, 1980.
    The management of chorioamnionitis in a large university hospital study is detailed.

14. D'Angelo, L. J., and Sokol, R. J. Time-related peripartum determinants of postpartum morbidity. *Obstet. Gynecol.* 55:319, 1980.
    Time-related peripartal events in 101 high-risk patients are correlated with postpartum morbidity. PROM was a statistically significant correlate of morbidity, but not when considered alone.

15. Ledger, W. J. Premature rupture of membranes and maternal-fetal infection. *Clin. Obstet. Gynecol.* 22:329, 1979.
   A study regarding the complete diagnosis and management of premature ruptured membranes as it applies to maternal and infant infection; 36 references are offered.

16. Evaldson, G., Lagrelius, A., and Winiarski, J. Premature rupture of the membranes. *Acta Obstet. Gynecol. Scand.* 59:385, 1980.
   The significant factors associated with premature ruptured membranes in a controlled, prospective study were found to be previous genital operations, cervical operations, surgical procedures, and lacerations. Those delivering longer than 24 hours after PROM were found to have significantly more puerperal infections than the control group, and maternal fever was an unreliable prognostic indicator.

Fetal Demise

In about 1% of pregnancies, the mother and the obstetrician are jolted by the realization that the fetus has died in utero. The demise may occur either prior to labor (antepartum) or during labor (intrapartum). Antepartum fetal demise may occur any time in the course of pregnancy. Early intrauterine death is suspected when the uterus is small for dates and fetal heart tones are not heard. After midpregnancy, loss of viability is often heralded by loss of subjective fetal activity as well as cardiac activity.

Confirmation of intrauterine death is more easily detectable since the advent of ultrasonography. A sonogram done early in pregnancy may show disruption of the gestational sac or persistent absence of fetal parts. Later in pregnancy there is an absence of fetal cardiac activity and collapse of the fetus if sufficient interval has elapsed since death. Sometimes plain x-ray will show gas in the cardiovascular system, overlapping of skull bones, or sharp angulation of the spine. If amniocentesis is done, the fluid is brown in color and demonstrates a markedly elevated creatine phosphokinase.

Intrapartum fetal death is that which occurs during labor, with absence of fetal heart tones by scalp electrode confirming the diagnosis. Caution is necessary since the maternal ECG can be transmitted through the fetus and any heart activity that is attributed to the fetus may not be synchronous with that of the mother. If there is any question of fetal viability, the presence or absence of fetal heart activity can be quickly determined by real time ultrasonography.

Management is simplified if the uterus is 14 weeks size or less. Suction curettage is indicated at this time, although coagulation studies should be done prior to surgery. When the uterus is greater than 14 weeks gestational size, there are several management options: observation only, intraamniotic hypertonic saline, prostaglandin E_2 vaginal suppositories, intravenous oxytocin, and hysterotomy.

Those who advocate expectant therapy (observation only) realize that 80% of patients will experience spontaneous labor within 2 to 3 weeks after intrauterine fetal demise. When this occurs, the patient solves her dilemma without attendant risks associated with intervention. Unfortunately, intrauterine demise is a great emotional burden and this management is unacceptable to many patients.

Another drawback to "watchful waiting" is the potential for coagulopathy. Disseminated intravascular coagulation is a frequently mentioned complication. The woman at risk is one in whom the gestation is greater than 16 weeks and who has retained a dead fetus 4 or more weeks. At 5 weeks, there is a 25% incidence of significant hypofibrinogenemia; subsequent risk increases with length of fetal retention.

Hypertonic saline injected intraamniotically is an effective abortifacient. However, it is contraindicated in patients with renal or cardiovascular disease, and its use may increase the risk of coagulation defect. Intravenous oxytocin has had the widest use and is a familiar agent to all obstetricians. Unfortunately, the preterm uterus is insensitive to oxytocin and high dosages (up to 1000 milliunits per minute) have been used. Water intoxication from the antidiuretic effect of oxytocin, uterine rupture, and cardiac arrhythmias have been reported with its use.

Vaginal suppositories of prostaglandin (prostin) E_2 have been approved by the Food and Drug Administration for use in the patient with intrauterine fetal demise at less than 28 weeks gestation. They are easy to administer and the side effects (nausea, vomiting, diarrhea, temperature elevation) are transient. Initially, prostin suppositories seemed a panacea, but they are not risk-free. There have been cases reported of uterine rupture, cervical trauma, and myocardial infarction. Even so, prostin E_2 suppositories in the properly selected patient are safe and effective. The present maximum dose is one 20-mg suppository every 3 hours. As more experience accumulates, it is possible that smaller doses or longer dosage intervals will be effective.

The key to all successful intervention is individual selection. For the patient with a gestation of 14 weeks or less, suction curettage is the choice. In the second trimester, prostin vaginal suppositories can be used. After 28 weeks gestation, the choice is between intravenous oxytocin and intraamniotic saline. After 36 weeks gestation, oxytocin is the undisputed choice. Hysterotomy is reserved for the unusual patient in whom all other options have failed.

A special case is the patient who has had a previous cesarean section and in whom the uterus is too large to use suction curettage. Use of prostaglandin, hypertonic saline, and oxytocin poses the threat of uterine rupture. If the previous cesarean section was lower segment with no evidence of endometritis, labor is usually allowed, although an internal pressure cannula should be placed to monitor uterine contractions. If these conditions cannot be met, hysterotomy is indicated.

Prior to any mode of therapy, coagulation studies should be performed. In the rare patient with hypofibrinogenemia, heparin is indicated if there is no bleeding. A 2–3-day course of heparin will increase the fibrinogen to acceptable levels (> 200 mg/100 ml) prior to attempts to empty the uterus. Cryoprecipitate or fresh frozen plasma may also be used.

Management responsibilities do not cease when the baby has been delivered. Further goals are emotional support of the parents and a search for the cause of the intrauterine death. It is now recognized that the parents experience a grief reaction similar to that occurring with the loss of other family members, and there is a definite need for effective bereavement counseling. In addition to the grief, there is frequently an element of inappropriate guilt. All members of the perinatal team should learn the dynamics of the grief/guilt process, avoid intellectualization, and know the answers to practical questions such as the proper written forms to use, hospital disposal versus burial arrangements, and requests for postmortem studies. Women should not be heavily sedated after experiencing a fetal death. If there is no obvious reason as to why the baby died, the parents should be so counseled. Both parents should also be told that the grief process is a normal reaction and they should discuss their feelings with each other. They should be seen frequently in the office after discharge to see how they are coping with their grief. Autopsy reports should be discussed at length with both parents as soon as possible. Parents should be encouraged to see their baby. Photographs should be obtained in case the parents initially refuse to see the baby but later wish they had.

It is imperative that an etiological search be done. Some potential repetitions might be avoided. In all babies who have congenital abnormalities chromosome studies, complete autopsy, total body x-rays, and full body photographs, should be done or taken. Perinatal death is associated with a tenfold increase in chromosome abnormalities when compared to the general population of live-born infants. Many cases of intrauterine fetal demise are a result of fetal-maternal hemorrhage. This is detected by examining maternal blood for fetal erythrocytes.

Intrauterine death remains a sad reality. The obstetrician must apply both science and art to assure safe management of the mother and emotional support of the couple. In subsequent pregnancies the woman who has experienced previous intrauterine loss must be considered a high risk. She will need to be seen more frequently and to be monitored more aggressively.

Review

1. Paul, R. H., Gauthier, R. J., and Quilligan, E. J. Clinical fetal monitoring. The usage and relationship to trends in cesarean delivery and perinatal mortality. *Acta Obstet. Gynecol. Scand.* 59:289, 1980.
   The effect of fetal monitoring on the prevention of intrapartum deaths is discussed. An extensive bibliography is available regarding all aspects of this problem.

Etiology

2. Liban, E., and Salzberger, M. A prospective clinicopathological study of 1108 cases of antenatal fetal death. *Isr. J. Med. Sci.* 12:34, 1976.
   Good review of etiologic factors contributing to antenatal fetal death.
3. Bauld, R., Sutherland, G. R., and Bain, A. D. Chromosome studies in investigation of stillbirths and neonatal deaths. *Arch. Dis. Child.* 49:782, 1974.
   Demonstrates the need for chromosome studies as a routine step in the evaluation of perinatal death.
4. Vandeputte, I., Renaer, M., and Vermylen, C. Counting fetal erythrocytes as a diagnostic aide in perinatal death and morbidity. *Am. J. Obstet. Gynecol.* 114:850, 1972.
   Shows the value of searching for fetal erythrocytes in the maternal blood in any complication of pregnancy that can be associated with fetal bleeding. Also demonstrates the usefulness of this test in investigating vaginal bleeding during the third trimester of pregnancy and when blood is aspirated during amniocentesis.

Diagnosis

5. Stempel, L. E., and Lott, J. A. Diagnosis of fetal death in utero with amniotic fluid creatine kinase. *Am. J. Obstet. Gynecol.* 138:1173, 1980.
   The authors describe a test using amniotic parameters to diagnose fetal death in utero. Various other modalities are also discussed.
6. Platt, L. D., et al. Diagnosis of fetal death in utero by real-time ultrasound. *Obstet. Gynecol.* 55:191, 1980.
   The use of real time ultrasonography in several modes regarding the diagnosis of fetal demise is discussed.

Management

7. Rozenman, D., Kessler, I., and Lancet, M. Third trimester induction of labor with fetal death in utero. *Surg. Gynecol. Obstet.* 151:497, 1980.
   The management of fetal death in utero was compared over a seven-year period, using saline or rupture of the membranes plus oxytocin induction. The authors demonstrated a clear preference for the latter method.
8. Southern, E. M., et al. Vaginal prostaglandin E_2 in the management of fetal intrauterine death. *Br. J. Obstet. Gynaecol.* 85:437, 1978.
   Results in 709 patients actively managed with prostaglandin E_2 vaginal suppositories following diagnosis of missed abortion or intrauterine fetal demise.
9. Gordon, H., and Pite, N. G. J. Induction of labor after intrauterine fetal death. *Obstet. Gynecol.* 45:44, 1975.
   A comparison between oxytocin and intravenous prostaglandin for the induction of labor.
10. Boehm, F. H., et al. Prostaglandin E_2 vaginal suppositories in pregnancy with an anencephalic fetus. *Obstet. Gynecol.* 55:758, 1980.
    Successful intervention in pregnancies complicated by an anencephalic fetus—a heretofore frustrating management problem.

Treatment

11. Scher, J., et al. A comparison between vaginal prostaglandin E_2 suppositories and intrauterine extra-amniotic prostaglandins in the management of fetal death in utero. *Am. J. Obstet. Gynecol.* 137:769, 1980.
    Prostaglandin by suppository and extraovular administration are compared in cases fo fetal demise. An entire review of management is also presented.
12. Lauersen, N. H., Cederqvist, L. L., and Wilson, K. H. Management of intrauterine fetal death with prostaglandin in E_2 vaginal suppositories. *Am. J. Obstet. Gynecol.* 137:753, 1980.
    Article discusses management with vaginal prostaglandin suppositories of a large number of patients whose fetuses suffered intrauterine demise.
13. Wallenburg, H. C., et al. Intramuscular administration of 15(s)-15-methyl prostaglandin F2 alpha for induction of labour in patients with fetal death. *Br. J. Obstet. Gynaecol.* 87:203, 1980.
    The use of a new prostaglandin analog for the induction of labor is presented. Less side effects were noted with this drug while effectiveness was equal to other drugs.
14. Rozenman, D., Kessler, I., and Lancet, M. Third trimester induction of labor with fetal death in utero. *Surg. Gynecol. Obstet.* 151:497, 1980.
    The induction of labor for fetal demise with a near term uterus is discussed. Advantages and disadvantages of various techniques are delineated.

Management Complications

15. Sandler, R. Z., et al. Uterine rupture with the use of vaginal prostaglandin E_2 suppositories. *Am. J. Obstet. Gynecol.* 134:348, 1979
    Case report of uterine rupture after use of vaginal prostin E_2 suppository in a patient with a surgically scarred uterus.
16. Patterson, S. P., White, J. H., and Reaves, E. M. A maternal death associated with prostaglandin E_2. *Obstet. Gynecol.* 54:123, 1979.
    The first reported fatality associated with the use of vaginal prostaglandin E_2 suppositories.

Crisis Counseling

17. Taylor, T. B., and Gideon, M. D. Crisis counseling following the death of a baby. *J. Reprod. Med.* 24:208, 1980.

    Very practical advice about effective crisis counseling. A must for those professionals desiring to provide emotional support for the bereaved parents.

18. Woods, D. L., and Draper, R. R. A clinical assessment of stillborn infants. *S. Afr. Med. J.* 57:441, 1980.

    This article emphasizes the clinical assessment of stillborn infants. These figures are of assistance in predicting recurrence rates.

19. Hildebrand, W. L., and Schreiner, R. L. Helping parents cope with perinatal death. *Am. Fam. Physician* 22:121, 1980.

    An in-depth review of perinatal death and the role of health care providers in assisting parents.

Maternal Drug Addiction

The pregnant drug addict should be managed by a physician with both skill and interest in high-risk obstetrics. Addicted patients are predisposed to an array of medical and obstetrical complications that makes management both demanding and frustrating. For example, heroin addicts require a "fix" every 4–6 hours—a life-style that is hardly conducive to a healthy pregnancy. In addition, addicts usually abuse more than one drug (a pharmacological nightmare), suffer from poor nutrition, and fail to follow directions or keep appointments. It is no longer believed that addicts are less fertile than the general population. There has even been a report of an increased incidence of multiple births in addicts.

There are four major groups of abused drugs: hallucinogens (tetrahydrocannabinol, LSD, phencyclidine), stimulants (amphetamines, cocaine), depressants (barbiturates, diazepam), and narcotics and other analgesics (heroin, methadone, morphine, hydromorphone, propoxyphene). Unfortunately, there are little scientific data available on the newer drugs or combination of drugs. Meaningful data are available only for heroin and methadone, but even then there are many variables. A majority of patients on methadone maintenance yield to illicit drugs one or more times during the pregnancy; and the quality, content, and adulterants vary widely.

Frequently patients will fail to volunteer the fact of their addiction. Even astute physicians may miss the wide mood changes or may attribute signs of early withdrawal to another illness. Physical findings are scant but more concrete: pinpoint pupils that are unresponsive to light, scars, nasal abnormalities, and needle tracks. Needle marks may be hidden in tatoos or between fingers and toes.

The pregnant addict is at risk for many medical complications. The obstetrician must be alert for hepatitis, endocarditis, venereal disease, abscesses, tetanus, anemia, pyelonephritis, phlebitis, and withdrawal.

The fetus is also at risk. Intrauterine growth retardation and low birth weight are common. It is unknown whether this is a consequence of poor nutrition or a direct result of the drug. Serial sonography offers the best estimation of progressive fetal growth. For an unknown reason, there is an increased risk of premature rupture of the membranes and stillbirth. Meconium aspiration is also a real danger for the fetus. As many as one in three addicted women are reported to have meconium in the amniotic fluid.

Amniotic fluid epinephrine and norepinephrine have been shown to increase during maternal withdrawal, and it is assumed that the fetus experiences stress. This stress probably results in the passage of meconium and its subsequent potential for aspiration.

When a pregnant heroin addict is first encountered there must be a decision made regarding therapy. The choices are: continuation of the habit with street drugs, acute detoxification, and use of methadone. The option of acute detoxification is contraindicated because of the danger of fetal withdrawal. Allowing the patient to continue the habit with street supplies is untenable because of the wide fluctuations of dose, the associated likelihood of fetal withdrawal, and the legal jeopardy.

Methadone, the most acceptable alternative, may be used in three ways. First, methadone may be substituted and gradually withdrawn (slow detoxification). Second, it may be maintained at the smallest dose necessary to prevent maternal withdrawal (usually 10–30 mg daily). Finally, it can be used in such high doses (up to 150 mg daily) that it "blocks" the patient from achieving any effect from the concomitant use of illicit drugs.

The most acceptable form of methadone use is the smallest daily regimen sufficient to prevent maternal withdrawal symptoms. The rationale for methadone therapy is simple; the methadone effect is 24 hours versus 4 hours for heroin. The vicious fix-crave-fix cycle can be broken. Theoretically, fetal withdrawal can be prevented by maintaining a steady maternal level of the drugs.

Cases of maternal withdrawal are not uncommon. In early withdrawal the mother experiences thirst, tremors, anxiety, rhinorrhea, sweating, and nausea. Later there is vomiting, diarrhea, abdominal pain, blood pressure changes, fever, and possibly seizures.

Withdrawal is treated by intramuscular methadone (5–20 mg initial dose, depending on the severity of the symptoms). Intramuscular methadone will achieve its effect within 1 hour. With severe withdrawal it is sometimes necessary to use a short-acting narcotic such as morphine or meperidine. It is also customary to use intramuscular methadone (with concomitant short-acting narcotic if necessary) when withdrawal occurs in labor. Once symptoms abate, the laboring patient receives customary analgesia-anesthesia. Addicts are well known for their low threshold to pain of labor.

Pentazocine (Talwin) is a narcotic antagonist and should never be given to an addict. It can exacerbate withdrawal.

Many addicts may not receive prenatal care or may avoid detection until they come to the hospital in labor. Often, they will have a fix at the onset of labor because of the fear that they will not receive enough medication to alleviate their pain during labor.

The labor in all drug addicts should be intensively monitored. Many of the fetuses are growth retarded and will not tolerate the stress of labor.

The intrauterine environment of the fetus is probably improved while on low-dose maintenance methadone. Average birth weights are higher on methadone than heroin, but, unfortunately, newborn withdrawal symptoms are more severe from methadone.

Neonatal withdrawal is manifested by a host of signs and symptoms. If any one phenomenon is characteristic, it is hyperactivity. Hyperactive manifestations are restlessness, shrill cries, tremors, and spontaneous reflex movements. Other signs are vomiting, diarrhea, fever, and intermittent apnea. The nursery should be notified of all mothers who are drug addicts or suspected drug addicts. Onset of withdrawal can occur immediately or up to 4 days after delivery. Withdrawal of the infants occurs later in those whose mothers received methadone. These infants should be observed as inpatients until they are past the time that withdrawal may occur, since withdrawal at home may be fatal to the infant. Even though highly suggestive to the astute clinician, none of the above signs are pathognomonic. A high index of suspicion is always necessary.

Centers with great experience in maternal drug addiction emphasize the importance of a *team* approach. Psychiatrists, psychologists, social workers, and nurses are necessary for professional expertise and the all-important interpersonal relationship with the patient. Ideally, a social worker should be assigned to the women in the hospital; the worker will then follow up the women after discharge. Infants of mothers who are drug addicts are at great risk for neglect or child abuse.

Review

1. Wagner, G., and Keith, L. Drug Addiction in Pregnancy. In J. J. Sciarra, and R. Depp (Eds.) *Gynecology and Obstetrics.* Hagerstown, Md.: Harper & Row, 1977. Vol. 3.
   Excellent review of the drug problem in pregnancy.
2. Finnegan, L. P. In utero opiate dependence and sudden infant death syndrome. *Clin. Perinatol.* 6:163, 1979.
   A very cogent review regarding the long-term outcome of infants exposed to opiate addiction. Sudden infant death syndrome is emphasized.
3. Ostrea, E. M., and Chavez, C. J. Perinatal problems (excluding neonatal withdrawal) in maternal addiction: A study of 830 cases. *J. Pediatr.* 94:292, 1979.
   A wide range of perinatal concerns in cases of maternal opiate addiction is offered from an experience of 830 cases.

Multiple Births

4. Rementeria, J. L., Janakammal, S., and Hollander, M. Multiple births in drug addicted women. *Am. J. Obstet. Gynecol.* 122:958, 1975.
   An interesting observation of an increased incidence of multiple births in addicted women. Authors suggest that narcotics may cause supraovulation.

Fetal Growth Retardation

5. Raye, J. R., Dubin, J. W., and Blechner, J. N. Alterations in fetal metabolism subsequent to maternal morphine administration. *Am. J. Obstet. Gynecol.* 137:505, 1980.
   Fetal growth retardation is associated with maternal narcotic addiction. It is unknown whether maternal malnutrition or drug effect is the cause. This paper shows that morphine alters fetal glucose homeostatis.

Comparison of Heroin and Methadone

6. Zelson, C., Lee, S. J., and Casalino, M. Neonatal narcotic addiction. *N. Engl. J. Med.* 289:1216, 1973.
   A comparison of effects of maternal ingestion of heroin and methadone. Neonatal problems that are associated with methadone use are discussed. Indiscriminate use of methadone during pregnancy is condemned.

Heroin Addiction

7. Pelosi, M. A., et al. Pregnancy complicated by heroin addiction. *Obstet. Gynecol.* 45:512, 1975.
   This paper presents data from 118 pregnancies of heroin-addicted women.

Methadone Maintenance

8. Statzer, D. E., and Wardell, J. N. Heroin addiction during pregnancy. *Am. J. Obstet. Gynecol.* 113:273, 1972.
Report on 150 pregnant addicts who were maintained on the smallest daily dose of methadone that would prevent withdrawal symptoms.
9. Newman, R. G., Bashkow, S., and Calko, D. Results of 313 consecutive live births of infants delivered to patients in the New York City methadone maintenance treatment program. *Am. J. Obstet. Gynecol.* 121:233, 1975.
Report of extensive experience with methadone maintenance during pregnancy.

The Neonate

10. Naeye, R. L., et al. Fetal complications of maternal heroin addiction: Abnormal growth, infections, and episodes of stress. *J. Pediatr.* 83:1055, 1973.
An explanation of the neonatal abnormalities associated with maternal heroin addiction. Sixty percent of mothers or their infants demonstrated evidence of acute infection (e.g., chorioamnionitis, funisitis, or neonatal pneumonia in association with amnionitis).
11. Zelson, C. Infant of the addicted mother. *N. Engl. J. Med.* 288:1393, 1973.
A succinct appraisal of the infant's problems.
12. Zuspan, G. P., et al. Fetal stress from methadone withdrawal. *Am. J. Obstet. Gynecol.* 122:43, 1975.
An argument against detoxification during pregnancy. Maternal withdrawal is associated with an increase in amniotic fluid epinephrine and norepinephrine.
13. Chasnoff, I. J., Hatcher, R., and Burns, W. J. Early growth patterns of methadone-addicted infants. *Am. J. Dis. Child.* 134:1049, 1980.
The authors delineate that the growth of children is less if the mother was exposed to methadone and some evidence of methadone addiction was found in the infant. Several excellent references concerning the effects of addictive drugs on the infant are given.
14. Rajegowda, B. K., Kandall, S. R., and Falciglia, H. Sudden unexpected death in infants of narcotic-dependent mothers. *Early Hum. Dev.* 2:219, 1978.
This article emphasizes that infants are at risk for sudden infant death syndrome as products of narcotic-dependent mothers. Some morphologic etiologies for this finding are hypothesized.

The Mother

15. Samuels, S. I., Maze, A., and Albright, G. Cardiac arrest during cesarean section in a chronic amphetamine abuser. *Anesth. Analg.* (Cleve.) 58:528, 1979.
The implications of anesthesia for drug-dependent women are emphasized in this article. Mechanisms for detection of abnormal response to anesthesia due to drug dependence and thus prevention are outlined.

Stillbirths

16. Rementeria, J. L., and Nunag, N. N. Narcotic withdrawal in pregnancy: Stillbirth incidence with a case report. *Am. J. Obstet. Gynecol.* 116:1152, 1973.
An attempt to explain the relationship between maternal addiction and increased stillbirths and neonatal deaths.

Hyperemesis Gravidarum

Hyperemesis gravidarum should be distinguished from the "morning sickness" that normally occurs in the first trimester of pregnancy. Although a certain degree of nausea and vomiting is to be expected, it is usually a first symptom of pregnancy and is self-limiting, abating by 12–14 weeks gestation. However, if the symptoms persist and become more severe, fluid and electrolyte imbalance may result and if left untreated can be fatal. The patient with hyperemesis quickly develops nutritional deficiencies as well as fluid and electrolyte disturbances, both of which may also threaten the fetal outcome. Hyperemesis gravidarum is a self-limiting disease and does not extend beyond pregnancy, although it may recur in subsequent pregnancies.

The reported incidence of hyperemesis is 3.5 cases per 1000 deliveries. The etiology of hyperemesis is unknown. Theories of etiology include: vitamin B_6 deficiency due to a change in protein metabolism, impaired function of the adrenal cortex, hyperthyroidism and excess of HCG secretion, psychopathologic and emotional factors, alterations in gastrointestinal physiology, hypersensitivity reaction, and poor nutrition.

The primary clinical manifestation of hyperemesis is frequent and sustained vomiting (usually 4–8 weeks duration) resulting in significant weight loss or dehydration. Other signs of starvation that gradually develop include ketonuria, hypokalemic alkalosis, oliguria, hemoconcentration, and constipation. In diagnosing and treating hyperemesis, other disorders must be ruled out. Hydatidiform mole, gastroenteritis, multiple gestation, hepatitis, cholecystitis, peptic ulcer, gastric carcinoma, and intestinal obstruction all may be mimicked by hyperemesis.

The prognosis is excellent in these cases, providing proper treatment is given. The principle underlying treatment of hyperemesis is the prevention of dehydration and starvation in addition to handling any psychologic component that may be present. Treatment includes hospitalization in a quiet room (isolation may be required for some patients) and a complete physical examination, including documentation of a verbal history that may be helpful in detailing any emotional problems. Physical and laboratory determinations such as temperature; pulse; respiration; blood pressure; weight on admission and daily; urine specimen for routine testing of albumin, sugar, acetone, specific gravity, and bacteria; and strict fluid intake and output recording. Laboratory evaluation of electrolytes (potassium, sodium, blood urea nitrogen (BUN), serum creatinine) should be obtained. In most cases intravenous fluid therapy (5% dextrose in Ringer's lactate or normal saline) is necessary. After the electrolyte results are available, addition of glucose, potassium, chlorides, and so on can be undertaken. In most cases gastric rest gained by not allowing oral intake is helpful. Antiemetics or mild sedatives such as intramuscular phenergan (25–50 mg) or phenobarbital (16–32 mg) 1 hour before meals and at bedtime, can also be used. Vitamin B-complex, C and B_6 (100 mg) added to intravenous solutions are useful. Psychiatric consultation may be necessary, and isolation from family and relatives is helpful in some cases.

Fairweather suggests that when the patient begins to respond to intravenous therapy, as indicated by cessation of vomiting, the return of electrolyte balance to normal, and increase in urinary output, she should be started on small sips of water, 1 ounce hourly. As soon as she can tolerate oral food, she should be given small, frequent meals of fairly dry and easily digested high-energy foods in the form of carbohydrates (fruit drinks, tea, milk). Intravenous therapy should be discontinued as soon as possible, and the diet should progress from liquids to a semisolid diet before solids are introduced (boiled eggs, cooked cereals, toast, dry crackers). Similarly, vitamin therapy, antiemetics, and sedatives can be gradually decreased or discontinued, or both.

Moderate activity should be gradually initiated and weights recorded biweekly. The weight chart, more than any other guide, will show the progress of the patient. As the psychologic component may be significant, the patient should be given an opportunity to discuss any problems and possibly be referred for psychiatric consultation. The patient may be safely discharged from the hospital after the nausea and vomiting have ceased and the patient begins to gain weight. Continued intensive outpatient follow-up is necessary.

There is little evidence that the patient with hyperemesis will deliver a small for gestational age or intrauterine growth–retarded baby due to this syndrome. Similarly, no increased risk of deformities or congenital malformations resulting from hyperemesis is clearly documented. Ketonuria, however, should be avoided since fetal abnormalities are increased if this occurs. Complications from persistent vomiting include hemorrhagic retinitis, rupture of the esophagus, aspiration pneumonitis, electrolyte depletion, acid-base disturbance, and dental erosion. Complications of antiemetic therapy include jaundice, irregular jerky movements, and opisthotonos due to the administration of phenothiazines.

Diagnosis
1. Chirino, O., et al. Barogenic rupture of the esophagus associated with hyperemesis gravidarum. *Obstet. Gynecol.* 52:515, 1978.
   Case report of primigravida with a diagnosis of hyperemesis gravidarum.
2. Eastman, N., and Hellman, L. Nausea and Vomiting in Pregnancy. In *Williams Obstetrics* (13th ed.). New York: Appleton-Century-Crofts, 1966.
   A review of diagnosis and treatment of nausea and vomiting in pregnancy.
3. Fairweather, D. I. Nausea and vomiting during pregnancy. *Obstet. Gynecol. Annu.* 7:91, 1978.
   A synopsis of definitions, etiology, pathology, diagnosis, and treatment of hyperemesis gravidarum.
4. Burrows, G. N., and Ferris, T. F. Nausea and Vomiting of Pregnancy and Hyperemesis Gravidarum. In *Medical Complications of Pregnancy.* Philadelphia: Saunders, 1975.
   A comprehensive review of nausea and vomiting and hyperemesis gravidarum.
5. Fairweather, D. I. Nausea and vomiting in pregnancy. *Am. J. Obstet. Gynecol.* 102:135, 1968.
   An excellent comprehensive review of nausea and vomiting in pregnancy.

Etiology
6. Uddenberg, N., Nilsson, A., and Almgren, P. E. Nausea in pregnancy: Psychological and psychosomatic aspects. *J. Psychosom. Res.* 15:269, 1971.
   A report focusing on the psychological aspects of nausea during pregnancy in an unselected sample of 152 women.
7. Ylikonkala, O., Kauppila, A., and Haapalahti, J. Follicle stimulating hormone, thyrotropin, human growth hormone and prolactin in hyperemesis gravidarum. *Br. J. Obstet. Gynaecol.* 83:528, 1976.

A study investigating the functional capacity of the anterior pituitary gland in hyperemesis gravidarum.

8. Katon, W. J., et al. Hyperemesis gravidarum: A biopsychosocial persepctive. *Int. J. Psychiatry Med.* 10:151, 1980.
   Forty-two women with hyperemesis gravidarum were compared to 115 women with normal pregnancies. Those in the hyperemesis group had a higher mean HCG, suggesting a causal relationship to hyperemesis.

Treatment

9. Worthington, B., Venmeersch, J., and Williams, S. *Nutrition in Pregnancy and Lactation.* St. Louis: Mosby, 1977.
   Simple dietary treatment of nausea and vomiting in pregnancy.

10. Milkovich, L., and Berg, B. An evaluation of the teratogenicity of certain antinauseant drugs. *Br. J. Obstet. Gynaecol.* 83:529, 1976.
    In a study of 11,481 gravidas taking antinauseant drugs it was concluded that phenothiazine, prochlorperazine, meclizine, cyclizine, and bendectin, when taken as recommended, were not teratogenic.

11. Enez, S., Schifrin, B., and Dirim, O. Double-blind evaluation of hydroxyzine as an antiemetic in pregnancy. *J. Reprod. Med.* 7:35, 1971.
    In a double-blind study, hydroxyzine hydrochloride 25 mg taken by mouth was effective in controlling nausea and vomiting. There was no significant fetal wastage or anomalies, or both, between the users and the control group.

12. Reinken, L., and Gant, H. Vitamin B_6 nutrition in women with hyperemesis gravidarum during the first trimester of pregnancy. *Clin. Chem. Acta* 55:101, 1974.
    A study demonstrating that women with hyperemesis gravidarum have a biochemical vitamin B_6 deficiency.

13. Henker, F. Psychotherapy as adjunct in treatment of vomiting during pregnancy. *South. Med. J.* 69:1585, 1976.
    A study of 10 pregnant patients with hyperemesis gravidarum revealed that, combined with routine medical measures, hypnotic suggestion and supportive psychotherapy can reduce the need for drugs.

Complications

14. Duckler, L., and Cohen, H. Hyperemesis gravidarum with gastric carcinoma. *Obstet. Gynecol.* 45:348, 1975.
    A multiparous female was first seen with a diagnosis of hyperemesis gravidarum and was found to have gastric carcinoma.

15. Weston, P., and Lindheimer, M. Intermittent intestinal obstruction simulating hyperemesis gravidarum. *Obstet. Gynecol.* 37:106, 1971.
    A case study of a 24-year-old primigravida who was hospitalized three times for hyperemesis gravidarum; she was eventually found to have an intestinal obstruction.

16. Pedersen, N. T., and Permin, H. Hyperparathyroidism and pregnancy. *Acta Obstet. Gynecol. Scand.* 54:281, 1975.
    Report of a case (and a review of the literature) of a gravida admitted with the diagnosis of hyperemesis gravidarum who was found to be suffering from hyperparathyroidism.

General

17. Kauppila, A., Huhtaniemi, I., and Ylikorkala, O. Raised serum human chorionic gonadotrophin concentrations in hyperemesis gravidarum. *Br. Med. J.* 1:1670, 1979.

An extensive review with 26 references of the psychological, social, and biologic factors in hyperemesis gravidarum. The effect of body type and psychological "gain" were emphasized.

Intrauterine Growth Retardation

Intrauterine growth retardation (IUGR) is a term applied when infants have birth weights that are significantly lower than one would expect. These infants may be born prematurely, at term, or postterm. Various adjectives have been used to describe these infants (small for dates, small for gestational age, fetally malnourished, and dysmature). The IUGR baby is generally identified by a birth weight that is at or below the tenth percentile for the expected birth weight at a given gestational age. Using this criterion, 10% of all babies will be so designated. Although there is marked variability of "normal" birth weight at any given gestational age, the above classification identifies a group of infants at increased risk for perinatal morbidity and mortality. In addition, some of these infants appear to have an increased risk of neurologic impairment in infancy and childhood. The IUGR infant is also at increased risk for certain disorders: congenital anomalies, central nervous system depression from in utero hypoxia, meconium aspiration, cold stress, hypoglycemia, hypocalcemia, hyperviscosity syndrome, respiratory distress, and pulmonary hemorrhage.

Given an infant identified as small for gestational age, various etiologic factors may be responsible. Approximately 10% of these infants can be identified as having chromosomal abnormalities, severe congenital anomalies, or congenital infections (rubella, cytomegalovirus, toxoplasmosis, or syphilis). Mothers with conditions such as essential hypertension, chronic renal disease, cyanotic heart disease, and hemoglobinopathies place the fetus at risk for IUGR. In addition, the mother's nutritional status, socioeconomic level, smoking habits, and her use of alcohol (as well as other drugs) may markedly affect fetal growth. Placental abnormalities associated with IUGR include nonspecific villitis, chronic abruption, multiple gestation, and placental tumors. Despite these numerous, recognized etiologic factors, in approximately 50% of IUGR babies there is no clearly identifiable cause.

Since intrauterine fetal weight cannot be measured and gestational age is often not precisely known, the prenatal diagnosis of IUGR presents a formidable obstetric challenge. Some pregnancies at risk for IUGR can be identified by maternal history and complications. Clinical information such as maternal weight gain and the serial measurement of uterine fundal height are good screening techniques. If gestational age can be accurately determined, if normal intrauterine fetal growth patterns are known, and if methods are available to assess fetal growth, an estimate can be made as to whether the growth is normal or altered (increased or decreased). However, since the genetic growth potential of any given fetus is unknown, and a variable range of normal fetal weight exists for a given gestational age, the accurate identification of the fetus with IUGR remains elusive.

Accurate determination of gestational age is critically important. Correlation of normal and clearly recalled menstrual data with pelvic exam prior to 12 weeks and heart tones heard by a standard fetoscope by 20 weeks provides a fairly accurate estimation of gestational age. Ultrasound can enhance and complement these clinical tools. The most accurate ultrasonic method of assessing gestational age is by measuring crown-rump length during the gestational interval between 7 and 14 weeks. The most commonly used ultrasonic technique for gestational-age determination, however, is that of biparietal diameter (BPD) measurements between 16 and 30 weeks.

The definition of normal fetal growth is difficult since the rate of fetal BPD growth varies as gestation progresses. Normally, the BPD grows 2 mm per week between 30 and 36 weeks and approximately 1.3 mm per week thereafter. Several studies have established that serial BPD measurements can identify whether infants are large, appropriate, or small for gestational age and at risk for IUGR. Because the error in each ultrasonic BPD measurement is approximately 2 mm, serial scans should be spaced at 3-week intervals. Serial values can be compared to "normal" growth curves and decreasing or arrested BPD growth thereby ascertained. The accuracy of serial scans in identifying the infant who at birth will have manifestations and complications of IUGR varies from 50%–70%. Efforts to enhance the ability of ultrasound to diagnose IUGR include the calculation of the ratio of head and abdominal circumferences and the determination of total intrauterine volume. In addition, the presence of oligohydramnios and advanced placental maturation are commonly seen with IUGR. Oligohydramnios, when present, predisposes to umbilical cord compression.

Once a fetus has been diagnosed as having decreased growth, obstetric management should be directed at modifying any associated factors that can be changed. Nutrition can be improved, cigarette smoking stopped, and alcohol use abandoned. Bed rest in the left lateral position will increase uterine blood flow and hopefully will thereby improve nutrition of the fetus. Since these fetuses are at risk for uteroplacental respiratory insufficiency, serial nonstress testing or oxytocin stress testing should be done. Serial measurement of biochemical indicators of placental function such as urinary or plasma estriol and human placental lactogen are controversial but are advocated by some. There are no data to support early delivery of these infants in the absence of documented fetal uteroplacental respiratory distress.

During either spontaneous or induced labor, these patients must be electronically monitored and observed carefully for evidence of fetal hypoxia. This may take the form of recurrent, severe variable, or late decelerations. The fetoplacental unit with IUGR does not have normal reserve, and in the presence of recurrent hypoxic decelerations unresponsive to treatment (lateral positioning, nasal or mask oxygen, and correction of hypotension or hypovolemia), delivery must be effected safely and expeditiously, most often by cesarean birth. These neonates must then be carefully evaluated for the presence of congenital anomalies and infections. In addition, cold stress must be avoided, meconium aspiration prevented with suctioning of the oropharynx and endotracheal intubation to clear the trachea, blood glucose measured, and the hyperviscosity syndrome and respiratory distress treated should they occur. For all these reasons, these infants should be delivered in a facility that can provide for intensive monitoring during labor and delivery and for subsequent rigorous care in the neonatal period.

The data concerning the subsequent growth and development of these infants should be viewed in light of the heterogeneity of the group. If infants with chromosomal abnormalities, congenital anomalies, and infections are exluded, the prognosis is generally good for subsequent physical development and neurologic outcome. Prevention and treatment of hypoxia during labor and the aggressive management of neonatal problems will decrease the chances of morbidity and subsequent damage such as these infants might have suffered in the past.

Etiology

1. Altshuler, G., et al. Placental pathology of small for gestational age infants. *Am. J. Obstet. Gynecol.* 121:351, 1975.
   Sixty-three placentas from intrauterine growth–retarded pregnancies were examined, and abnormalities were found in 58. Abnormalities included ischemic lesions in 43% (often associated with hypertension). Approximately 25% of the placentas showed villitis of unknown etiology.
2. Battaglia, F. Intrauterine growth retardation. *Am. J. Obstet. Gynecol.* 106:1103, 1970.
   The distinction between IUGR infants and premature infants is thoroughly discussed, and the different problems that present themselves in the neonatal period are identified. Difficulties associated with diagnosis and evaluation of subsequent development of IUGR infants is discussed.
3. Peacock, W. G., and Hirata, T. Outcome in low birthweight infants (750 to 1,500 grams): A report on 164 cases managed at Children's Hospital, San Francisco, California. *Am. J. Obstet. Gynecol.* 140:165, 1981.
   A series of 164 low birthweight infants were studied and 62% survived. Of the infants followed for four years or longer, 82% were normal. No obstetric factors correlated with the group that had neurologic handicaps.
4. Hill, D. Physical growth and development after intrauterine growth retardation. *J. Reprod. Med.* 21:335, 1978.
   Several studies concerning the outcome of infants with IUGR are reviewed. An outline for a prospective study to answer questions of growth potential and subsequent outcome was presented.

Diagnosis

5. Belizan, J., et al. Diagnosis of intrauterine growth retardation by a simple clinical method: Measurement of uterine height. *Am. J. Obstet. Gynecol.* 131:643, 1978.
   The tenth, fiftieth, and ninetieth percentile values of uterine height were established in a group of 298 healthy pregnant women. Of 44 neonates with low birth weight for gestational age, 38 had uterine heights below the tenth percentile.
6. Campbell, S., and Thoms, A. Ultrasound measurement of the fetal head to abdomen circumference ratio in the assessment of growth retardation. *Br. J. Obstet. Gynaecol.* 84:165, 1977.
   The mean head to abdomen circumference (H/A) ratio was determined in 568 normal pregnancies. The H/A circumference ratio was also determined in 31 small-for-date fetuses within 1 week of delivery. In all cases, fetal weight predicted from the fetal abdomen circumference measurement was below the fifth percentile weight for gestation.
7. Crane, J., and Kopta, M. Prediction of intrauterine growth retardation via ultrasonically measured head/abdominal circumference ratios. *Obstet. Gynecol.* 54:597, 1979.
   Prospective study evaluated the reliability of ultrasonically determined head/abdomen ratios in detecting IUGR in 47 patients. This technique was able to predict all 10 infants who had apparent uteroplacental insufficiency and IUGR.
8. Gohari, P., et al. Prediction of intrauterine growth retardation by determination of total intrauterine volume. *Am. J. Obstet. Gynecol.* 127:255, 1977.
   A graph for normal total intrauterine volume was constructed from studies of 100 normal patients. The description and use of total intrauterine volumes to identify infants with IUGR was described.

9. Gaziano, E. P., Freeman, D. W., and Allen, T. E. Antenatal prediction of women at increased risk for infants with low birth weight. *Am. J. Obstet. Gynecol.* 140:99, 1981.
Prenatal risk factors for IUGR were studied in 165 women. With the use of these risk factors, 73.5% of cases involving IUGR were correctly classified.

10. Sabbagha, R., et al. Sonal biparietal diameter: Predictive of three fetal growth patterns, leading to a closer assessment of gestational age and neonatal weight. *Am. J. Obstet. Gynecol.* 126:145, 1976.
Fetal biparietal diameters can be separated into one of three percentile rankings: large, average, and small. Under normal conditions, fetuses initially placed in any one of these BPD levels will continue to grow within the confines of the same percentile range.

11. Queenan, J., et al. Diagnostic ultrasound for detection of intrauterine growth retardation. *Am. J. Obstet. Gynecol.* 124:865, 1976.
Serial biparietal diameter measurements were used to evaluate patients for IUGR. The shortcomings of serial scanning to make this diagnosis were emphasized.

Management

12. Arias, F. The diagnosis and management of intrauterine growth retardation. *Obstet. Gynecol.* 49:293, 1977.
Pregnancies in 28 women showing a late flattening type of growth pattern by serial ultrasound, the presence of maternal high-risk factors, and detection of the abnormal growth before 35 weeks gestation almost always terminated with birth of an IUGR infant. The use of the oxytocin challenge test to evaluate fetal status was recommended.

13. Crane, J., et al. Abnormal growth pattern: Ultrasonic diagnosis and management. *Obstet. Gynecol.* 50:205, 1977.
Serial ultrasonography was used to evaluate patients for possible growth retardation in the fetus. Fetuses exhibiting "reduced growth potential"–type patterns had little risk for fetal distress. Fetuses suffering from utero-placental insufficiency frequently exhibited a pattern of biparietal growth arrest in the third trimester.

14. Jones, M., and Battaglia, F. Intrauterine growth retardation. *Am. J. Obstet. Gynecol.* 127:540, 1977.
A review of factors associated with IUGR and methods to identify the growth-retarded infant prenatally were presented. Management of the growth-retarded pregnancy was discussed.

15. Lin, C., et al. Oxytocin challenge test and intrauterine growth retardation. *Am. J. Obstet. Gynecol.* 140:282, 1981.
The NST and OCT in 85 fetuses with IUGR were studied. Thirty-five to forty percent had poor results in these tests and adverse fetal prognosis was accurately predicted for 92% of these infants.

FETAL MALPOSITIONS

Breech Presentation

Breech presentation, described as early as the first century A.D., is one of the most controversial subjects in modern obstetrics. It is defined as the entrance of the fetal buttocks or the lower extremities into the maternal pelvic inlet. The incidence of breech presentation varies from 3%–5% and is almost five times higher among infants weighing less than 2500 g than in those at term. In defining the orientation of the breech, the denominator is the fetal sacrum within the maternal pelvis; thus RSA (right sacroanterior) equates with the sacrum of the fetus being positioned on the right side of the maternal pelvis viewing cephalad. Three types of breech presentation, based on fetal attitude, are described. The first and most frequent (65%) is frank breech, in which both thighs of the fetus are flexed on the abdomen and both legs are extended over the chest. Next, with a frequency of 8%, is the complete breech, in which both thighs of the fetus are flexed on the abdomen and both legs are flexed at the knee. Finally, the incomplete or footling breech, in which one or both lower extremities of the fetus are extended below the level of the fetal buttocks, accounts for approximately 27% of all breeches.

In over half the cases, the etiology of breech presentation is not known. During the second and early third trimester of pregnancy, the ratio of the intrauterine volume to the size of the fetus is large; thus prematurity is the most common known causative factor of breech presentation. In addition, breech presentation results from any condition interfering with the accommodation of the fetus in the uterus. The septate uterus, placenta previa, or uterine myomas predispose to breech presentations. Other factors favoring breech presentation are fetopelvic disproportion, multiparity, multiple pregnancy, hydramnios, and hydrocephaly.

Diagnostically, Leopold's maneuvers are utilized to palpate and identify the fetal head in the uterine fundus and the breech in the pelvis. The first maneuver denotes the head as a hard, spherical, and ballotable mass occupying the fundus of the uterus. The rest of the maneuvers demonstrate the various fetal parts in breech presentation. The fetal heart tones are usually best heard above the umbilicus in the breech presentation. Vaginal examination discloses the breech in the pelvis by palpating the fetal anal orifice, which forms a straight line with the ischial tuberosites laterally. Occasionally on pelvic examination, the breech is confused with a presenting face, shoulder, arm, or anencephalic head. The most useful landmark in making the differential diagnosis is the palpation of the sacrum posterior to the anus.

If the membranes have ruptured, the presence of meconium on the examining finger confirms the diagnosis of breech presentation. If there is any doubt, the diagnosis should be made radiologically or, preferably, by ultrasonography. Additionally, ultrasonography can be used to localize the fetal head and to measure the biparietal diameter, thus assisting, in some cases, in the choice of delivery method (vaginal versus abdominal).

The accurate diagnosis of breech presentation, especially in the primigravida in the third trimester of pregnancy, is of paramount importance for several reasons. As term approaches, spontaneous conversion to the vertex position is less likely to occur. Although a final decision as to the method of delivery in term breech should not be made until after the onset of labor, the physician should be alert for any complications arising from the presentation per se (i.e., malformations and prolapse of umbilical cord). On the other hand, if the diagnosis of breech presentation is made prior to 36 weeks gestation, external version has been suggested. Because of its low success rate (spontaneous reversion to a breech usually occurring) and placental complications, external version has limited usefulness at this time. The use of tocolytic agents in the future, however, may increase its application.

In the past 30 years the rate of cesarean section for breech delivery has increased. Many authors recommend cesarean section for women with breech presentations of large infants (>3800 g), premature rupture of membranes, premature infants (<2000 g), footling breech presentations, or for primigravidas. One study involving 1003 singleton breech presentations demonstrated that the route of delivery (vaginal or cesarean section) made no difference in neonatal mortality in infants weighing more than 2500 g at birth. However, cesarean section significantly lowered the neonatal mortality rate of infants with birth weights between 1000 and 2500 g. The most common conditions contributing to the increased perinatal loss during vaginal breech delivery are birth asphyxia resulting from umbilical cord prolapse (over 10% in footling breech presentations) and arrest of the after-coming head at delivery (premature breech delivery). On the other hand, performing total breech extraction in an attempt to prevent umbilical cord accidents and birth asphyxia results in central nervous system injuries (tentorial tears and intracranial hemorrhages).

Kauppila demonstrated that 7% of term breech infants delivered vaginally, regardless of difficulties at the time of delivery or Apgar scores, were injured (cerebral hemorrhage, Erb's paralysis). He also pointed out that among pupils in special schools, 11.9% were born vaginally in breech presentation, a much higher percentage than in those children with problems who had vertex births. The same infants were found to have abnormal EEG findings in 27.3% of the cases. Other birth injuries contributing to the breech perinatal mortality and morbidity are spinal cord damage, cephalhematomas, damage to the brachial plexus, and injury to intraabdominal organs. Despite the above significant perinatal problems resulting from the conservative management of breech delivery, cesarean section is not recommended as the method of choice in all breech presentations.

When the patient is admitted to the hospital, a decision should be made, as early as possible, whether vaginal delivery or cesarean birth is more appropriate. A useful guide in making this decision has been the "breech scoring index" presented by Zatuchni and Andros in 1967. This index is based on points given for cervical dilatation, station, fetal weight, increasing parity, decreasing gestational age, and type of pelvis. The patients with higher scores can be allowed to labor. However, the final decision regarding the management of the breech presentation should be based on careful clinical observation of patient in labor.

X-ray pelvimetry for evaluation of the pelvic capacity, as well as a flat plate and a lateral view of the abdomen to exclude any evidence of hyperextension of the head, are routinely performed. Whenever possible, real-time ultrasonography should be utilized to rule out the possibility of meningomyelocele, anencephaly, or other malformations that might influence the decision regarding cesarean birth. If an adequate gynecoid pelvis, a well-flexed head (frank or even complete breech presentation), and an infant estimated at greater than 2000 g but less than 3500 g with intact membranes are found, labor is allowed to continue, provided there is progressive cervical dilatation and effacement and normal descent of the presenting part. Continuous electronic monitoring of the uterine contractions and fetal heart rate is recommended. If the membranes rupture (they are kept intact as long as possible), prolapsed cord should be ruled out. Any evidence of acute fetal distress or prolapsed cord would necessitate an emergency cesarean section.

A continuous segmental epidural is considered a good choice for obstetric anesthesia. In situations in which regional anesthesia is not available, successful pudendal anesthesia provides good pain relief at the time of delivery, following routine intravenous analgesia. The delivery of the breech is conducted spontaneously until the umbilicus appears; then the obstetrician gently assists the trunk over a liberal mediolateral episiotomy. The Mauriceau-Veit-Smellie maneuver or the application of the Piper forceps are utilized to deliver the after-coming head.

There are some instances (secondary uterine inertia, acute fetal distress, second twin) in which the fetus must be delivered by breech extraction, provided that the pelvis is adequate and the cervix completely dilated. The breech extraction carries increased risk to both the fetus and the mother, and it should be done only when absolutely necessary.

In summary, vaginal breech delivery should be conducted in carefully selected patients who make adequate progress with no signs of fetal compromise. As data have accumulated, the increased rate of cesarean delivery has resulted in a decreased incidence of perinatal mortality and morbidity in infants having breech presentation. Nevertheless, the optimal decision in the management of breech presentation should be individualized and based mainly on clinical grounds.

Etiology and Diagnosis

1. Sweeney, W. J., III, Hawks, G. G., and Caplan, R. M. Breech Presentation. In J. J. Sciarra (Ed.), *Gynecology and Obstetrics*. Hagerstown, Md.: Harper & Row, 1980. Vol. 2.
   Uterine, Pelvic, fetal, and placental factors predisposing to breech presentation are discussed. Subjective and objective diagnostic symptoms and signs in breech presentation are also described.

Management

2. Zatuchni, G. I., and Andros, G. J. Prognostic index for vaginal delivery in breech presentation at term. *Am. J. Obstet. Gynecol.* 98:854, 1967.
   The authors describe the "breech scoring index," with points assigned for factors of increasing parity, cervical dilatation and effacement, station, fetal weight, gestational age, and type of breech presentation.
3. Collea, J. V., et al. The randomized management of term frank breech presentation: Vaginal delivery versus cesarean section. *Am. J. Obstet. Gynecol.* 131:186, 1978.
   The authors demonstrate that carefully selected cases of term breech presentation can be delivered vaginally.
4. Rovinsky, J. J., Miller, J. A., and Kaplan, S. Management of breech presentation at term. *Am. J. Obstet. Gynecol.* 115:497, 1973.
   In a retrospective analysis of 2145 cases of singleton term breech presentations, the authors demonstrate that although indications for cesarean section should be liberalized, routine elective cesarean section for term breech presentation is not justified.
5. O'Leary, J. Vaginal delivery of the term breech. *Obstet. Gynecol.* 53:341, 1979.
   In a prospective study of 150 term, uncomplicated breech deliveries the author demonstrates the value of a well-defined management program utilizing the breech score, x-ray pelvimetry, and the Friedman labor curve.
6. Mann, L. I., and Gallant, J. M. Modern management of the breech delivery. *Am. J. Obstet. Gynecol.* 134:611, 1979.
   The data provided by this study show that all infants in breech presentation do not require cesarean section for safe delivery.

7. DeCrespigny, L. J. C., and Pepperell, R. J. Perinatal mortality and morbidity in breech presentation. *Obstet. Gynecol* 53:141, 1979.
The data provided by this retrospective study shows that elective cesarean section reduces the perinatal loss of premature infants by reducing the incidence of intrauterine hypoxia and preventing birth trauma.

8. Graves, W. K. Breech delivery in twenty years of practice. *Am. J. Obstet. Gynecol.* 137:229, 1980.
This study comprises a review of all breech deliveries in a partnership practice. Results tend to confirm the increased hazard of vaginal delivery to the premature infant in a breech presentation but are equivocal in those infants whose birth weight is greater than 2500 g.

9. Fall, O., and Nilsson, B. A. External cephalic version in breech presentation under tocolysis. *Obstet. Gynecol.* 53:712, 1979.
In a prospective study the authors show that there are no serious complications in association with attempts at external version in breech presentation under tocolysis.

10. Duenhoelter, J. H., et al. A paired controlled study of vaginal and abdominal delivery of the low birth weight breech fetus. *Obstet. Gynecol.* 54:310, 1979.
In a paired, controlled, retrospective study the authors conclude that delivery by cesarean section is preferable for the low birth weight breech fetus.

11. Haberkern, C. M., Smith, D. W., and Jones, K. L. The "breech head" and its relevance. *Am. J. Dis. Child.* 133:154, 1979.
The authors describe an abnormal head shape, the "breech head," as a factor contributing to birth injury during vaginal delivery of the breech infant.

12. Kauppila, O., et al. Management of low birth weight breech delivery: Should cesarean section be routine? *Obstet. Gynecol.* 57:289, 1980.
In a retrospective study of a total of 434 breech deliveries of low birth weight infants, the authors conclude that for infants of less than 32 weeks gestation primary cesarean section is recommended because of the higher incidence of cerebral hemorrhage in those delivered vaginally.

13. Karp, L. E., et al. The premature breech: Trial of labor or cesarean section? *Obstet. Gynecol.* 53:88, 1979.
In a retrospective study of 66 breech deliveries in premature infants, the authors demonstrate that a trial of labor can be safely undertaken in the presence of a premature frank or complete breech presentation.

14. Correy, J. F. Perinatal mortality in vaginal breech delivery in Tasmania. *Aust. N.Z. J. Obstet. Gynaecol.* 20:106, 1980.
In a survey of 742 vaginal breech deliveries and 26,424 cephalic deliveries of infants weighing 1000 gm or more, the author shows that there is a significantly higher intrapartum and neonatal death rate associated with the preterm breech delivery; cesarean section is recommended for this group.

Outcome

15. Kauppila, O. The perinatal mortality in breech delivery and observations of affecting factors. *Acta Obstet. Gynecol. Scand.* [Suppl.] 39:1, 1975.
The author demonstrates that 7% of term breech infants delivered vaginally, regardless of difficulties at the time of delivery of Apgar scores were injured.

Transverse Lie

Determination of fetal lie is one of the cornerstones in obstetric management of the laboring woman. Obstetric lie is defined as the relationship of the long axis of the fetus to that of the mother. If the fetal spine is parallel to the maternal spine, the lie is longitudinal; if they are at right angles, the lie is transverse. At times the axes are somewhere in between and this represents an oblique lie, often called unstable lie, which almost always converts to longitudinal or transverse during labor. Longitudinal lies are noted in over 99% of laboring patients; transverse and other lies are noted in the remainder.

The presenting part is that portion of the fetus either in the birth canal or in closest proximity to it, and it can ordinarily be felt when a vaginal examination is done. When the fetal lie is transverse, the fetal head and breech occupy opposite iliac fossae. The side of the mother to which the acromion points determines the designation of position (i.e., left or right). In transverse lies, the fetal back may be directed anteriorly, posteriorly, superiorly, or inferiorly, and is designated dorsoanterior, dorsoposterior, dorsosuperior (back up), and dorsoinferior (back down).

The rates for the occurrence of transverse lie range from 0.25%–0.95%. Until 32 weeks gestation, the amniotic cavity is large in relation to the fetal mass and there is no crowding of the fetus by the uterine musculature. Therefore, the mobility of the premature fetus is increased, and noncephalic, nonlongitudinal lies are increased up to that point. The incidence is 0.3%–0.5% in laboring women who continue singleton pregnancies to term.

Many factors are associated with transverse lies. A shortened longitudinal axis of the uterus often requires the fetus to accommodate itself in the transverse direction. The most common situations are implantation of the placenta in the dome of the fundus and placenta previa. Although good statistical data are not available for fundal implantation, approximately 10%–15% of transverse lies are associated with placenta previa or low-lying placenta. Relaxed abdominal wall musculature, especially associated with grand multiparity, allows the fetus to fall forward, interfering with descent and engagement of longitudinal lies. Grand multiparity is associated with approximately one-third of transverse lies, and the grand multipara is ten times more likely to have transverse lie than is a nulliparous woman.

Patients admitted in premature labor are more likely to have a transverse lie because of the greater mobility of the preterm fetus. A contracted maternal pelvis prevents fixation of the fetus by preventing the proper engagement of the fetal head and is one of the few conditions in which a longitudinal lie will convert to a transverse lie. Uterine anomalies that widen the bicornual area make the transverse diameter more favorable. Leiomyoma arising in the lower uterine segment, transverse cesarean section scars, and other pelvic masses may predispose to transverse lie by obstructing the lower portion of the uterus. Hydramnios increases the volume of the uterus and allows for more fetal movement. Fetal anomalies or fetal demise may lead to transverse lie because of increased fetal flexibility. One special feature of multiple pregnancies is that the lie of the second twin is often transverse. Multiple causes are often present. Even with these associated findings, however, the etiology remains obscure in the majority of cases.

The diagnosis is most often arrived at by simple observation: the transverse diameter of the uterus is greater than expected and the fundal height is less than is appropriate for the gestational age. Confirmation can usually be made by obstetric palpation (Leopold's maneuvers). The first maneuver yields no fetal pole in the fundus. The second shows that the fetal head overlies one of the iliac fossae and the breech in the other. The third and fourth maneuvers are usually negative, unless the labor is well advanced and the shoulder is impacted or the arm prolapsed. Palpation of the uterus gives the feel of a hard transverse plane if the back is anterior or the nodular small parts if the back is posterior. Auscultation of fetal heart tones is usually easily done but often is higher on the fundus than expected. Fetogram or sonography, or both, give valuable information as to the exact habitus of the fetus.

Management of the mother with a fetus in transverse lie is dependent on the clinical situation. Many authors advocate repositioning the fetus to the vertex position in those women not in labor any time an abnormal presentation is noted. Unfortunately, external version is a technique with which few obstetricians are familiar and the effect (i.e., remaining in vertex presentation) does not often last. Also, at least 33% of those fetuses in transverse lie will convert before labor. Moreover, external version should not be done if other complications such as abnormal bleeding, premature rupture of membranes, or previously scarred uterus are present.

If the external version maneuvers are attempted and are successful, the head should be held in the lower uterine segment for several contractions to allow the lower uterine segment to accommodate and then should be held in place by an abdominal binder. External version should be attempted before contractions start since once labor ensues, the conversion of the transverse lie is not likely to be successful. Due to a high incidence of complications (i.e., cord prolapse), no attempt should be made to fix the presenting part by artificially rupturing membranes.

Modern management of the pregnant woman with a viable fetus in transverse lie is cesarean section. Internal podalic version is rarely indicated except in twin pregnancies when the second twin is in transverse lie. Because neither the vertex- nor breech-positioned fetus occupies the lower uterine segment, a low cervical transverse incision may cause difficulty during extraction of the fetus. A vertical incision, either low-segment or classic, may be more expeditious.

When the fetus has died, vaginal delivery may be permitted if the conceptus is small. The fetus must double up on itself and the head and thorax must pass into the pelvic cavity (conduplicato corporis) before expulsion. If the fetus is dead but too large to pass through the pelvis, one may attempt for delivery internal version or operations that destroy the fetus. Both of these procedures are hazardous to the mother because of the possibility of rupture of the uterus. Almost always cesarean section is preferable to major intrauterine manipulation even for a dead fetus.

A major management problem is neglected transverse lie. This may result from patient delay in coming to the hospital after initiation of labor or from inaccurate diagnosis. The shoulder may become wedged into the pelvic canal and a hand or arm may prolapse into the vagina. At this point, a vaginal delivery is impossible since the head and thorax cannot enter the pelvis at the same time. If not treated, the uterus eventually forms a pathologic retraction ring (Bandl's ring) and then ruptures, usually resulting in maternal and fetal death. In these cases one must be ready to deal with massive hemorrhage, and large quantities of blood must be available. Because of the uterine manipulation, especially during a neglected labor or during management of a fetal demise, sepsis is frequently encountered. The use of antibiotics early in the course of these infections is recommended. Maternal death occurs from complications of neglected labors such as spontaneous or traumatic (ill-advised in utero manipulation) ruptured uterus, and overwhelming sepsis. Even with optimal care, maternal risks are increased because of (1) association with placenta previa, (2) greater incidence in older women, (3) necessity of operative intervention, and (4) likelihood of maternal sepsis.

Risks to the fetus are also increased. The most likely problems are prolapsed cord, which is the same as with any nonstable lie and fetal prematurity. Because delivery requires manipulation of the fetus, the incidence of birth injuries and birth-related hypoxia are markedly increased. Major intrauterine manipulation (i.e., internal podalic version and extraction) is associated with a corrected neonatal mortality as high as 21% and with infant morbidity as high as 33%. Cesarean section reduces the fetal mortality to approximately 6% and morbidity to approximately 19%. Although cesarean section increases chances of a good neonatal outcome, transverse lie continues to place the fetus at increased risk. One must therefore be ready to care for a very ill infant.

Management of transverse lie is best done in a team effort. Because the uterus must be relaxed for optimal nontraumatic manipulation of the fetus during both vaginal delivery and cesarean section, anesthesia must be available. Because of the high incidence of premature, asphyxiated, or birth-injured neonates, pediatric support is mandatory to treat the potentially sick infant.

In summary, transverse lie occurs in approximately 0.5% of all labors. Maternal and fetal risk are increased, and one must be prepared to deal with massive maternal hemorrhage, maternal sepsis, fetal distress, and prematurity. Cesarean section is the management of choice for most transverse lies. The risk to mother and fetus can be reduced by early recognition of the problem and appropriate obstetric management supported by anesthesia and pediatrics personnel in a team approach.

Reviews

1. Hall, S. C., and O'Brien, F. B., Jr. Review of transverse lie at the Methodist Hospital, Brooklyn, 1924–1958. *Am. J. Obstet. Gynecol.* 5:1180, 1961.
   A review of 25 years experience and changing management trends.
2. Cockburn, K. G., and Drake, R. F. Transverse and oblique lie of the fetus. *Aust. N.Z. J. Obstet. Gynaecol.* 8:211, 1968.
   A review of 12 years experience details incidence, etiology, and maternal and fetal complications of transverse and oblique lie.
3. Steverson, C. S. Transverse or oblique presentation of the fetus. *Clin. Obstet. Gynecol.* 5:946, 1962.
   An extensive summary of the literature with emphasis on etiology, diagnosis, and management.
4. Kawathekav, P., et al. Etiology and trends in the management of transverse lie. *Am. J. Obstet. Gynecol.* 1:39, 1973.
   A discussion of etiology and trends of management in India.
5. Cruikshank, D. P., and White, C. A. Obstetrical malpresentations: Twenty years experience. *Am. J. Obstet. Gynecol.* 8:1097, 1973.
   A review of all common malpresentations.

Management

6. Ranney, B. The gentle art of external cephalic version. *Am. J. Obstet. Gynecol.* 2:239, 1973.
   Safety, success, optimum timing, and technique of external cephalic version are discussed.
7. Pelos, M. A., et al. The "intra-abdominal version technique" for delivery

of transverse lie by low segment cesarean section. *Am. J. Obstet. Gynecol.* 8:1009, 1979.

Illustration of a technique to avoid the classic cesarean section and permit the more desirable low-segment cesarean section.

8. Dutta, G. P., and Bhaumik, I. A study of transverse lie. *J. Indian M. A.* 74:48, 1980.

    Three hundred thirty-three patients with transverse lie were reviewed. Correlation with parity, obstructed labor, and maternal complications were increased.

Abnormal Variants of the Vertex Presentation

The face presentation is a malpresentation in which the head is hyperextended with the occiput in contact with the fetal back. The mentum (chin) is the denominator on the presenting part. The incidence of face presentation is 1 in 500–600 deliveries. It is more common in black patients than in Caucasians. The causes of face presentation are multiple, originating from any factor that either promotes extension or restrains flexion of the head. Pelvic disproportion (contracted inlet), prematurity, multiparity (pendulous abdomen), maternal pelvic tumors, anencephaly, tumors of the fetal neck such as thyroid enlargement, and macrosomia are the major obstetric factors predisposing to extended positions of the head.

The diagnosis of face presentation is not usually made until late in labor and sometimes not until delivery. By utilizing Leopold's maneuvers, one may palpate the cephalic prominence on the same side as the back. A groove can also be recognized between the occiput and the fetal back. The fetal heart tones are best heard on the side of the small parts. On vaginal examination, a face presentation may be confused with a frank breech presentation, but in the latter the anus lies on a straight line with the ischial tuberosities. In a face presentation, the fetal mouth and the malar prominences form the corners of a triangle. The palpation of the nose, the orbital ridges, and the frontal sutures with the anterior fontanel may also help in the diagnosis. An x-ray of the abdomen or ultrasonography may be used to demonstrate the hyperextension of the fetal head as well as any abnormalities of the skull. X-ray pelvimetry will sometimes aid in evaluating the pelvic capacity, knowledge of which is a necessary factor in making a decision regarding the management of the face presentation.

Although the fetus follows the cardinal movements in descent, certain features of the mechanism of labor in a face presentation are at variance. The main difference lies in the presenting diameter at the pelvic inlet. As a result of the mentobregmatic diameter of the fetus presenting at the pelvic inlet in face presentation, engagement occurs much later in labor than in the vertex presentation. During internal rotation, the face (mentum) should pass under the symphysis pubis. Unless the fetus is unusually small or macerated, vaginal delivery cannot be accomplished unless spontaneous internal rotation of the mentum to the anterior position occurs. In the clinical course of labor, minimal prolongation of labor in face presentation has been noted as compared to the vertex presentation.

It has been noted that the incidence of fetal distress in face presentation is much higher than in vertex presentation. Severe variable decelerations due to umbilical cord compression against the pelvis by the hyperextended head are common. Due to the presenting face, the application of the fetal scalp electrode is not suggested unless performed under direct visualization. Likewise, scalp pH sampling may not be possible. When ready for delivery, the patient with a fetus having a face presentation should be taken to the delivery room where preparations for either a vaginal or abdominal delivery should be made, with anesthesia and blood available.

When the face presentation is mentum anterior and the pelvis is adequate, vaginal delivery can be accomplished spontaneously or with outlet forceps applied to the face when it is on the pelvic floor. A particular problem in managing the face presentation occurs when the fetus is in the mentum transverse or mentum posterior positions. Fetuses in many of these positions rotate spontaneously to mentum anterior late in the second stage of labor and there is thus no need for cesarean section. Any attempt (other than manual rotation) to convert a transverse or posterior mentum to anterior by operative procedures (Kielland midforceps, and so on) has resulted in increased maternal and neonatal morbidity. On the contrary, cesarean section performed at the appropriate time in these cases has significantly reduced the maternal and neonatal damage.

Brow presentation is an unstable malpresentation produced when the fetal head is deflexed so that the portion of the vertex between the orbital ridge and the anterior fontanel (brow or sinciput) presents at the pelvic inlet. Since the presenting diameter of the fetal head (occipitomental) measures 14 cm, it is obvious that vaginal delivery cannot be accomplished in most cases unless the brow converts to either an occipital or face presentation or the fetus is very small and the pelvis large. The brow presentation occurs once in 1500 deliveries, with a greater predominance among Caucasian, multiparous patients. Because the causes of inadequate flexion of the fetal head that result in a face presentation can also create a brow presentation, the etiology of brow presentation is similar to that of the face presentation. The diagnosis of brow presentation is suspected by physical examination and is confirmed by x-ray study. Both the occiput and mentum can be palpated by abdominal examination. On vaginal examination, the anterior fontanel, frontal suture, supraorbital ridge, and the root of the nose can easily be identified.

In the brow presentation with a normal labor and an adequate pelvis, it is not unusual for a "brow" to convert to either a face or occipital presentation. In this case, the management is conservative while continuous monitoring of the fetus during labor is carried out. In cases in which the brow persists at a high station after the cervix has been completely dilated and the patient has been pushing for almost an hour, an attempt to manually flex the head and rotate the occiput either anterior or posterior may be made.

Occasionally, the brow is arrested at the level of the midpelvis. In this case, after a manual conversion and rotation has been tried failed, Kielland or Barton forceps may be used to accomplish vaginal delivery successfully. For either manual or instrumental conversion and rotation of the brow, adequate relaxation of the pelvic musculature is required. When the brow presentation persists into late second stage, the prognosis is poor for vaginal delivery. Whenever both manual or forceps conversion of the brow fail, cesarean section is mandatory.

Persistent occiput posterior is defined as failure of the occiput to spontaneously rotate to the anterior or transverse position prior to vaginal delivery. This condition is mostly seen with either an android or platypelloid (flat) pelvis. The incidence of persistent occiput posterior is about 5%, with a greater predominance among black patients. The diagnosis is easily made by palpating the small fontanel posteriorly.

Most often (in 90% of cases), fetuses in occiput posterior position undergo spontaneous rotation, resulting in an uncomplicated vaginal delivery. With a persistent occiput posterior position and prolonged second stage of labor, forceps rotation of the occiput may be attempted (rotation by Scanzoni maneuver or Kielland forceps rotation), provided that other prerequisites for forceps application are present. Another possibility for vaginal delivery is the application of the forceps to the head in the posterior occiput position after which delivery, utilizing a large mediolateral episiotomy, is performed. In either case, the delivery is more successfully completed under adequate anesthesia. Before forceps rotation of the occiput is attempted, a less traumatic manual rotation of the occiput should be attempted.

A review of 552 consecutive cases showed that the persistent occiput posterior position does not represent an increased risk factor to the fetus, and unjustified intervention should be avoided. The basic management of persistent occiput posterior position should be similar to that of occiput anterior positions. Furthermore, when the fetus is in the persistent occiput posterior position (compared to occiput anterior) labor is somewhat prolonged, but the perinatal mortality does not differ significantly. On the other hand, episiotomy extension and minor maternal morbidity are significantly increased in the patients with fetuses presenting in the persistent occiput posterior position.

Etiology and Diagnosis

1. Duff, P. Diagnosis and management of face presentation. *Obstet. Gynecol.* 57:105, 1981.

   The author discusses the incidence, diagnosis, and possible causes of face presentation in a series of 19 infants delivered at Walter Reed Army Medical Center. A management protocol is also outlined.

2. Benedetti, T. J., Lowensohn, R. I., and Truscott, A. M. Face presentation at term. *Obstet. Gynecol.* 55:199, 1980.

   This retrospective study was conducted to investigate the possible relationship between intrapartum fetal heart rate (FHR) abnormalities and face presentation in term infants.

3. Ingemarsson, E., Ingemarsson, I., and Westgren, M. Combined decelerations—clinical significance and relation to uterine activity. *Obstet. Gynecol.* 58:35, 1981.

   A combined variable and late deceleration were found to be positively correlated with uterine hyperactivity and occiput posterior position. These decelerations are discussed as a potential indicator of fetal distress.

Management

4. Hellman, L. M., Epperson, J. W. W., and Connally, F. Face and brow presentation. The experience of the Johns Hopkins Hospital, 1896 to 1948. *Am. J. Obstet. Gynecol.* 59:831, 1950.

   In this study, based on 141 face presentations and 45 brow presentations, the authors concluded that the approach to extended position of the fetal head should be conservative, unless pelvic contraction exists in which case cesarean section is indicated.

5. Phillips, R. D., and Freeman, M. The management of the persistent occiput posterior position. *Obstet. Gynecol.* 43:171, 1974.

   In a retrospective study of 552 cases, the authors demonstrated that the persistent occiput posterior position does not represent an increased risk factor to the fetus, and therefore premature intervention should be avoided.

6. Daw, E. Management of the hyperextended fetal head. *Am. J. Obstet. Gynecol.* 124:113, 1976.

   The author describes the management of delivery in face, star-gazing, and flying presentations of the fetus.

7. Ingemarsson, E., et al. Influence of occiput posterior position on the fetal heart rate pattern. *Obstet. Gynecol.* 55:301, 1980.
   In this study the authors show that variable decelerations are significantly more frequent and more pronounced in the infants presenting the occiput posterior position than in the controls.
8. Levy, D. Persistent brow presentation: A new approach to management. *South. Med. J.* 69:191, 1976.
   This report presents (1) a method of selecting patients for whom conversion with vaginal delivery is feasible and (2) the principles employed in the procedure.
9. Ong, H. C., and Chelvam, P. Brow presentation. *Med. J. Malaysia* 29:299, 1975.
   In this paper the authors present their experience with 6 cases of brow presentation, and they show that fetal prognosis is improved by less interference vaginally and by the more frequent use of cesarean section as the mode of delivery.
10. Ong. H. C., and Teo, S. P. Face presentation. *Med. J. Malaysia* 31:42, 1976.
    In this paper the authors review their experience with 16 cases of face presentation, and they conclude with the old maxim, "if a face is making progress, leave it alone."

Umbilical Cord Prolapse

Prolapse of the umbilical cord is an acute obstetric emergency requiring prompt action to avert fetal injury.The fetal risks are substantial, and most contemporary series still report a perinatal mortality ranging from 12%–24%. Proper management is based on prevention, early recognition, and timely intervention. Frank prolapse is said to occur when the membranes are ruptured and the cord extends into, or beyond the cervix, prior to passage of the major portion of the presenting fetal part. Occult prolapse exists when the cord is situated between the presenting part and the lower uterine segment but does not extend through the cervical canal. The overall incidence of frank prolapse of the umbilical cord is approximately 0.4% of all deliveries.

Although the majority of prolapses occur in association with a vertex presentation, the *relative* frequency is much higher in other presentations. In one series the likelihood of cord prolapse with various presentations is as follows: vertex (0.2%), breech (3.6%), compound (10.0%), oblique (14.8%), and transverse (20.0%). More recent studies have suggested that the frequency of cord prolapse in the frank breech habitus approaches the rate with vertex presentation. Complete and footling attitudes, however, show substantially higher frequencies.

Frank prolapse usually occurs because the umbilical cord is situated between the cervical os and the presenting fetal part at the time of amniotomy or spontaneous rupture of the membranes. Occasionally, it is secondary to obstetric manipulations performed after the membranes have ruptured. In addition to the relationship between fetal presentation and cord prolapse, several other predisposing factors, as well as the well-documented association with prematurity, multiple gestation, and polyhydramnios, have been identified. These factors appear to be the increased frequency of malpresentations and the relative disproportion between the size of the fetus and the maternal pelvis. Several other presumed predisposing conditions are also often cited, although proof of a causal relationship has not been established by clinical studies. Among these are "excessively" long cords, low-lying placentas, and cephalopelvic disproportion.

Unfortunately, up to one-third of umbilical cord prolapses are iatrogenic. Usually they are the result of inappropriate amniotomies, those performed with an excessively high fetal station or an undiagnosed malpresentation. Sometimes they are secondary to elevation of the fetal head to facilitate manual or forceps rotations. Occasionally, they are the result of other obstetric manipulations, such as version and extraction. The majority of these iatrogenic events are avoidable.

Frank prolapse of the umbilical cord may be discovered in three ways: looking, listening, and feeling. The prolapsed cord may be visualized by perineal inspection, speculum examination, or sonography. Bradycardia, resulting from compression of the cord, may be detected by auscultation or electronic fetal heart rate (FHR) monitoring. A pulsating cord may be palpated on digital vaginal exam to confirm the diagnosis. Occult prolapse is suggested by a variable FHR deceleration pattern with an onset coincident with fetal descent or rupture of the membranes, or both. However, the diagnosis can only be confirmed by direct palpation of the pulsating cord or by careful ultrasonographic examination.

The treatment of umbilical cord prolapse with a living infant is prompt delivery. In almost all cases, this means cesarean section. However, some authorities believe that with a completely dilated cervix and the presenting part at a satisfactory station, vaginal delivery with forceps or vacuum extraction is acceptable. In either case, delivery should be accomplished without undue delay. While preparations for cesarean section are underway, it is usually beneficial to reduce the pressure on the cord by placing the patient in the Trendelenberg or knee-chest position while elevating the presenting part manually per vaginum in most cases. Any attempts at replacement of the cord are to be discouraged since they are seldom successful.

Although spontaneous prolapse of the umbilical cord can seldom be prevented, the fetal risks can be minimized by early recognition and prompt intervention. Evaluation of the fetal heart rate should be routinely performed after the rupture of membranes, and careful digital examination is advisable if prolapse is suspected. In cases of possible occult prolapse, evaluation should include sonography, when available, and continuous fetal heart rate monitoring. Most iatrogenic prolapses are preventable. If there is any uncertainty regarding the fetal lie or habitus, elective amniotomy should be delayed until the presenting part is confirmed by sonography, digital examination, or radiologic studies. Amniotomy should be deferred when the fetal station is high, unless internal monitoring or immediate delivery is essential. Obstetric manipulations that disengage the presenting part should be avoided if possible. However, when such procedures are elected, suitable facilities for abdominal delivery should be available.

Prolapse of the umbilical cord complicates approximately 0.4% of all deliveries and represents a serious threat to fetal well-being. The basic principles of management include prevention, early recognition, and prompt intervention. Although most cord prolapses are spontaneous, many are iatrogenic and thus preventable. Certain conditions are associated with an increased risk of prolapse and the clinician should be alert to this possibility. The appropriate intervention is timely delivery, usually by cesarean section. With proper obstetric management, the frequency and risks of umbilical cord prolapse may be minimized.

Diagnosis

1. Donnelly, P. B., et al. Sonographic demonstration of occult umbilical cord prolapse. *Am. J. Radiol.* 134:1060, 1980.
   This report demonstrates the usefulness of ultrasonic examination in confirming the difficult clinical diagnosis of occult umbilical cord prolapse.
2. Goodland, R. C., and Lowe, E. A functional umbilical cord occlusion heart rate pattern. *Obstet. Gynecol.* 43:22, 1974.
   A classification of fetal heart rate patterns with regard to umbilical cord occlusion is presented. Functional details as well as management are outlined.
3. Lenke, R., and Osterkamp, T. A prolapsed umbilical cord into the abdominal cavity in a woman with a previous cesarean section. *Am. J. Obstet. Gynecol.* 138:1224, 1980.
   A short report emphasizing that the umbilical cord can be prolapsed in areas other than the vagina. The use of ultrasonography in detecting prolapsed umbilical cord is detailed
4. O'Leary, J. A., Andrinopoulos, G. C., and Giordano, P. C. Variable decelerations and the nonstress test: An indication of cord compromise. *Am. J. Obstet. Gynecol.* 137:704, 1980.
   Thirty-seven women were observed to show persistent mild variable decelerations on the nonstress test. In 35 of the 37 subjects, umbilical cord problems were noted during labor.

Treatment

5. Savage, E. W., Schuyler, G. K., and Wynn, R. M. Prolapse of the umbilical cord. *Obstet. Gynecol.* 36:502, 1970.
   A good review of the literature showed that in the patients who underwent cesarean section after cord prolapse the perinatal mortality rate was 15% as compared to an overall mortality of 38%. The authors urge the "more liberal use of cesarean section" for treatment of umbilical cord prolapse.
6. Chetty, R. M., and Moodley, J. Umbilical cord prolapse. *S. Afr. Med. J.* 57:128, 1980.
   The problems regarding detection and management of umbilical cord prolapse are detailed.
7. Ward, J. M. Umbilical cord prolapse. *Cent. Afr. J. Med.* 25:12, 1979.
   The various causes of umbilical cord prolapse are discussed, and very practical points on management are offered.

Complications

8. Brandeberry, K. R., and Kistner, R. W. Prolapse of the umbilical cord. *Am. J. Obstet. Gynecol.* 61:356, 1951.
   A classic article demonstrating the hazards of vaginal approach to management. Cord prolapse in 117 cases had a perinatal mortality of 35%. Amniotomy was the cause of prolapse in 37% (1% of all amniotomies).
9. Clark, D. O., Copeland, W., and Ullery, J. C. Prolapse of the umbilical cord. *Am. J. Obstet. Gynecol.* 101:84, 1968.
   The "corrected" perinatal mortality was 16.8% overall, but was only 5.8% for those infants delivered abdominally (29% of total).
10. Niswander, K. R., et al. Fetal morbidity following potentially anoxigenic obstetric conditions: III. Prolapse of the umbilical cord. *Am. J. Obstet. Gynecol.* 95:853, 1966.
    In the Collaborative Study of Cerebral Palsy, over 17,000 deliveries at multiple centers were analyzed; 80 cases of frank prolapse were identified.

The overall perinatal mortality was 34%, and one-quarter of these were secondary to amniotomy.

11. Weber, T., and Secher, N. J. Transcutaneous fetal oxygen tension and fetal heart rate pattern preceding fetal death: Case report. *Br. J. Obstet Gynecol.* 87:165, 1980.
    A fetus weighing 830 g at 27 weeks gestation was carefully monitored but was allowed to expire following prolapse of the umbilical cord. The lethal pathophysiologic effects of cord prolapse are clearly documented.

12. DeCrespigny, L. J., and Pepperell, R. J. Perinatal mortality and morbidity in breech presentation. *Obstet. Gynecol.* 53:141, 1979.
    The contribution in breech presentation of umbilical cord prolapse to perinatal mortality and morbidity is emphasized. Techniques for prevention and increasing one's index of suspicion are offered.

Fetal Abnormalities Associated with Hydramnios and Oligohydramnios

Hydramnios, or the less-used term *polyhydramnios,* and oligohydramnios are abnormalities in the amount of amniotic fluid. Hydramnios means an excess of fluid, and oligohydramnios a reduced amount when compared with normal pregnancies at specific stages of gestation. Both conditions are associated with a higher incidence of congenital fetal anomalies and place the pregnant woman and her fetus at high risk during that gestation.

The presence of 1500–2000 cc of amniotic fluid is usually required to make the clinical diagnosis, since near term the normal pregnant amniotic cavity contains approximately 800–1000 cc. Clinically, hydramnios may be diagnosed by: a uterus that seems larger than the gestational age, a difficulty in palpating the fetus and ballottement of the fetus, as well as fetal heart sounds that are distant and difficult to hear with a fetoscope. Confirmation of the diagnosis is made most reliably by ultrasonography.

The incidence of hydramnios ranges from 0.4%–1.5%. Usually the fluid collects gradually over several days or weeks. In these cases most (35%) are idiopathic, while about 25% are associated with maternal diabetes and 20% with congenital malformation. Other causes include erythroblastosis fetalis and multiple gestation, about 10% each. Nearly 2% of cases are classified as acute hydramnios, which is defined as an excessive amount of fluid developing over a period of hours or days. The greatest risk to the mother is discomfort and premature labor. Pregnancy-induced hypertension is also commonly associated with hydramnios, but it is not known to be causal and is usually noted in the acute type of hydramnios. The perinatal death rate is highest in the group of women with congenitally malformed fetuses (90%), emphasizing the poor prognosis when hydramnios is associated with fetal anomalies.

Fetal anomalies associated with hydramnios include fetal central nervous system disorders, with anencephaly being the most common; gastrointestinal tract (GI) disorders, including esophageal, duodenal, and jejunal atresia; cardiovascular anomalies; hydrops fetalis; and fetal renal anomalies. Hydramnios occurs in approximately 60% of women carrying an anencephalic fetus. This relationship may be explained by defective fetal swallowing, increased urine production, or perhaps transudation of fluid through exposed meninges. While esophageal and duodenal atresia are the most common GI tract disorders associated with hydramnios, other abnormalities such as esophageal compression from congenital goiter, diaphragmatic hernia, and duodenal compression from an annular pancreas have also been incriminated. Indeed, 2%–10% of normal-appearing infants delivered of patients with hydramnios will be noted to have an obstruction of the gastrointestinal tract. Appropriate diagnosis and treatment in early neonatal life is imperative. Increased venous pressure in the fetal/placental circulation may explain hydramnios in reported cases of fetal retroperitoneal fibrosis and placental tumors such as chorioangiomas.

Another common cause of hydramnios is erythroblastosis fetalis secondary to Rh isoimmunization. More recently, nonimmunologic causes are being diagnosed more frequently because of a decreasing incidence of Rh disease in the general population. The incidence of nonimmunologic hydrops is increased one hundred times if the fetal heart is malformed. Other fetal disorders may also result in fetal hydrops and subsequent hydramnios. While rarely mentioned, fetal renal abnormalities such as obstructive uropathies, neoplastic renal dysplasia, and fetal polyuria may be associated with hydramnios.

Treatment is poor at best. Therapeutic removal of large amounts of amniotic fluid periodically has been unnecessary in general but may be very helpful in some cases. Bed rest and control of associated maternal factors, if possible (diabetes mellitus, pregnancy-induced hypertension), is also important.

Oligohydramnios is defined as a reduced amount of amniotic fluid, usually below 400 cc. Like hydramnios it may also be associated with fetal anomalies, the most common of which is renal agenesis. Potter's syndrome (complete renal agenesis) is commonly associated with oligohydramnios. It is a rare condition of a fetus occurring in approximately 0.23–0.34 per 1000 deliveries and is usually not diagnosed prior to birth. Usually associated with renal agenesis is fetal pulmonary hypoplasia, believed to be secondary to the oligohydramnios, which causes a condition whereby normal pulmonary development is prevented. The diagnosis should be considered whenever intrauterine growth retardation and severe oligohydramnios are present.

Other fetal abnormalities associated with oligohydramnios include the postmaturity syndrome. This disorder is characterized by a fetus who is meconium-stained and who has significant loss of subcutaneous tissue, wrinkled skin, long fingernails, numerous metabolic disorders, and various forms of dysmaturity or intrauterine growth retardation.

The diagnosis of oligohydramnios can best be confirmed by ultrasonography. Occasionally, the absence of fetal kidneys can be noted on ultrasonographic examination. Since amniotic fluid in the second half of pregnancy is comprised primarily of fetal urine, any disorder causing a decrease in fetal urinary output may result in oligohydramnios. Fetal urine production occurs at a constant rate of about 10 mm per hour at 30 weeks to 27 mm per hour at 40 weeks. Regardless of the etiology, oligohydramnios places the fetus at greatly increased risk. Usually cord accidents lead to fetal demise, although associated placental and fetal abnormalities may contribute to the high stillbirth rate. One must remember, however, that all pregnancies with oligohydramnios do not harbor an abnormal fetus. In addition, diagnosing the specific amount of amniotic fluid is difficult. For this reason, even when specific fetal anomalies are demonstrated, the fetus should be judged as salvageable and the high-risk pregnancy managed accordingly. Usually, delivery is the only therapeutic tool the obstetrician has to use in cases of oligohydramnios.

Review
1. Wallenburg, H. C. S., and Wladimiroff, J. W. The amniotic fluid. II. Polyhydramnios and oligohydramnios. *J. Perinat. Med.* 6:233, 1977.
   A good review article on excessive, as well as insufficient, amounts of

amniotic fluid during pregnancy, with emphasis on clinical and patho-physiological aspects of these two disorders.

2. Niswander, K. R. The obstetrician, fetal asphyxia, and cerebral palsy. *Am. J. Obstet. Gynecol.* 133:358, 1979.
The effects of fetal asphyxia in causing long-term neurologic problems in the infant is delineated. Difficult management decisions facing the obstetrician in modern perinatal care are discussed.

Diagnosis

3. Jeffcoate, T. N. A., and Scott, J. S. Polyhydramnios and oligohydramnios. *Can. Med. Assoc. J.* 80:77, 1959.
This article reports polyhydramnios in 12 out of 13 cases of esophageal atresia.

4. Keirse, M. J. N. C., and Meerman, R. H. Antenatal diagnosis of Potter's syndrome. *Obstet. Gynecol.* 52:645, 1978.
This article presents a case of bilateral renal agenesis that was diagnosed prior to birth and was made on the basis of severe oligohydramnios and unrecognizable fetal kidneys and bladder on ultrasound.

5. Achs, R., Harper, R. G., and Harrick, N. J. Unusual dermatoglyphics associated with major congenital malformations. *N. Engl. J. Med.* 275:1273, 1966.
The authors review the various dermatoglyphics associated with major congenital malformations. The more unusual or rare the markings, the more likely the child is to have a malformation.

6. Sagar, H. J., and Desa, D. J. The relationship between hydramnios and some characteristics of the infant in pregnancies complicated by fetal anencephaly. *J. Obstet. Gynaecol. Br. Commonw.* 80:429, 1973.
The diagnostic hallmarks of anencephaly are detailed. The relationship between hydramnios and various clinical presentations are discussed.

Incidence

7. Queenan, J. T., and Gadow, E. C. Polyhydramnios: Chronic versus acute. *Am. J. Obstet. Gynecol.* 108:349, 1970.
This article reviews a 20-year period at the New York Hospital, Cornell Medical Center, and reports on 358 cases of polyhydramnios for an incidence of 0.41%.

8. Sergovich, F., et al. Chromosome aberrations in 2159 consecutive newborn babies. *N. Engl. J. Med.* 280:851, 1969.
This article reports on 2159 consecutive newborn babies who were studied for chromosomal aberrations. The frequency of major chromosomal rearrangements are detailed.

9. Ash, P., Vennart, J., and Carter, C. O. The incidence of hereditary disease in man. *Lancet* 13:849, 1977.
The incidence of inherited disease is categorized and discussed by the authors. Percentages for many of the abnormalities are listed.

10. Jacoby, H. E., and Charles, D. Clinical conditions associated with hydramnios. *Am. J. Obstet. Gynecol.* 94:910, 1966.
The authors outline all of the clinical conditions associated with hydramnios. Various management schemes are detailed.

Cause

11. Perlman, M., Potashnik, G., and Wise, S. Hydramnios and fetal renal anomalies. *Am. J. Obstet. Gynecol.* 125:966, 1976.
This article reviews 4 cases of hydramnios associated with renal anoma-

lies; 2 patients had obstructive uropathy and 2 had a neoplastic type of re-nal disease.

12. Wladimiroff, J. W., and Campbell, S. Fetal urine production in normal and complicated pregnancy. *Lancet* 1:151, 1974.
    Fetal urine production occurs at a constant rate of about 10 mm/hr at 30 weeks to 27 mm at 40 weeks. Fetal urine production is usually lower in fetuses with intrauterine growth retardation.

13. Knuppel, R. A. Recognizing teratogenic effects of drugs and radiation. *Contemp. Ob/Gyn* 15:171, 1980.
    The entire spectrum of drugs and radiation as a cause of fetal abnormali-ties is reviewed; 59 references are offered.

14. Hutchinson, D. L., et al. The role of the fetus in the water exchange of the amniotic fluid of normal and hydramniotic patients. *J. Clin. Invest.* 38:971, 1959.
    This classic study details the role of the fetus as the mediator for amniotic fluid. Oligohydramnios and polyhydramnios as they are caused by fetal anomalies are discussed.

Management

15. Etches, P. C., and Lemons, J. A. Nonimmune hydrops fetalis: Reports of 22 cases including three siblings. *Pediatrics* 64:326, 1979.
    This article presents 22 cases of hydrops fetalis not related to Rh disease.

16. Ratten, G. J., Beisher, N. A., and Fortune, D. W. Obstetric complications when the fetus has Potter's syndrome. *Am. J. Obstet. Gynecol.* 115:890, 1973.
    This article discusses the obstetrical complications occurring when the fetus has Potter's syndrome, including a 40% incidence of breech pre-sentation of the infant.

17. Crandall, B. F. Identification and management of some genetic prob-lems. *J. Reprod. Med.* 17:116, 1976.
    A very concise paper dealing with the identification and management of fetal abnormalities.

LABOR AND DELIVERY

The use of medications during the intrapartum period must be carefully assessed because of the effects of the physiologic changes of pregnancy on the mother and the effects of such drugs on the fetus. It is critically important to use antepartal and intrapartum risk assessment to detect maternal and fetal complications before the introduction of other variables such as analgesia and anesthesia medications. Although there is a move toward making the birth process more family-oriented and natural, certain medical prerequisites must be fulfilled. Even for the patient at no risk, intravenous fluids should be administered so that dehydration during labor will be prevented, at the same time assuring an adequate circulating volume. In addition, should any catastrophic event occur, the intravenous line can be lifesaving. Finally, if medication is desired during labor, a precise dosage and convenient route for administration of such drugs is available.

Almost every drug used for analgesia in the mother during labor crosses the placenta and may affect the infant. This is because most analgesic agents are small in molecular weight (less than 1000), are lipid-soluble, and have a high pKa, thus allowing for easy transit across the placenta. The most common type of analgesics administered during pregnancy are the narcotic agents, principally meperidine. While most institutions have discouraged the use of twilight sleep (meperidine combined with a amnesic scopolamine), many times inordinate amounts of meperidine are used during labor for sedation. In most cases, 75–100 mg of meperidine, given in 25-mg increments every 2–4 hours, is sufficient for pain relief during labor and has little effect on the baby other than decreasing the beat-to-beat variability. At these dosage levels, if a depressed fetus is seen, it is invariably not due to the analgesic. Additionally, meperidine can be given just prior to parturition and should not be withheld because the patient is going to deliver within the next 1 or 2 hours.

Morphine, on the other hand, is very rarely used because of the fetal depression associated with excessive doses. Although 5 mg of morphine is equianalgesic with 25 mg of meperidine, does not need to be repeated as often, and is no more depressant, because of adverse publicity, most people currently use meperidine. Other analgesic agents such as butorphanol (Stadol), alphaprodine (Nisentil), or nalbuphine (Nubain) can be used during labor. The advantage of these drugs is that they do not have any metabolites to affect the infant. They are depressant to the fetus as well as to the mother, however, and do not have an antagonist. Nevertheless, if used carefully, they can afford significant pain relief during labor. It also should be mentioned here that the narcotic antagonist naloxone (Narcan) should be used for specific cases of documented maternal and/or fetal respiratory depression due to narcotic overdose. It should not be combined with the analgesic agent because it has respiratory depressant effects on the infant in its own right, and it will reduce the amount of analgesia in the mother.

Sedatives and hypnotics are now used infrequently in labor and delivery suites. Barbiturate usage, at least during the active intrapartum phase, is almost entirely limited to the induction of general anesthesia for cesarean section. Although phenothiazines and similar derivatives have been used for a number of years as adjuncts to narcotic analgesia, they are not synergistic but additive and have the disadvantage of not having any specific antagonist. The drugs do, however, provide good sedation and some analgesia so that less meperidine is used for analgesia. In addition, they are also touted as being able to reduce the incidence of nausea. Most observers feel, however, that the nausea occurring during the intrapartum period is due to supine hypotension and can be corrected by positional changes, not by hypnotic agents. Further, the sedatives have certain side effects, e.g., hypotensive reactions (prochlorperazine [Compazine], chlorpromazine [Thorazine], and triflupromazine [Vesprin]). Promethazine (Phenergan) is also associated (as is the narcotic Nisentil) with platelet abnormalities in both mother and baby. Pentazocine (Talwin) has been demonstrated to correlate with dissociative behavior in certain patients during labor. Diazepam (Valium), on the other hand, has been used in labor and delivery and has been troublesome because of hypothermia in the newborn infant. In summary, the tranquilizing agents are widely used but probably not very effective.

Inhalation analgesia, on the other hand, is rarely used in this country, except for nitrous oxide, which is used primarily just before delivery. In other countries, trichloroethylene (Trilene) and methoxyflurane (Penthrane) are used in administered inhalers. Several maternal deaths due to overdoses in patients who were not closely monitored during labor have led to its decreasing popularity in this country.

Regional anesthesia is more utilized today than ever before in obstetrics. The use of the caudal and more recently the segmental epidural blocks has gained popularity in this country. Epidural analgesia using the amide derivative drugs (lidocaine, bupivacaine) may block only the uterine innervation during labor and has the advantage of also being able to render satisfactory anesthesia for delivery. Complications include inadvertent entry into the spinal canal and hypotension. Paresthesias, particularly a complication of the ester-based local anesthetics (2-chloroprocaine), have been demonstrated after epidural anesthesia. In addition, many obstetricians feel that the use of conduction anesthesia prolongs labor and leads to an increased incidence of fetal transverse position and subsequent midforceps rotation. Despite this, the adverse effects on the mother and fetus are far outweighed by the benefits of this technique.

Psychoprophylaxis (prepared childbirth) has also gained wide attention in this country as a method of analgesia in labor. This method of coping with pain during labor has been shown to be an extremely effective method and, if successful, is very rewarding for the parturient and her support person. If unsuccessful, small doses of analgesic agents can be administered and her active participation in the birth process can still be maintained. An approach of a tailored psychoprophylaxis for each patient is necessary rather than a rigid protocol of analgesia versus no analgesia. In women who "lose control" while attempting psychoprophylaxis, hyperventilation with resultant hypocarbia and epinephrine release has occasionally resulted in hypoxia. Regardless, psychoprophylaxis joins conduction anesthesia as being the most common method of analgesia during labor.

Anesthesia for vaginal delivery still includes the low spinal or saddle block anesthesia. This method provides good relaxation, allows for forceps delivery if necessary, and is extremely safe. Like all methods of conduction anesthesia, hypotension is the principal problem that one must prevent. Another very common method of anesthesia used at the time of delivery and a favorite of those using psychoprophylaxis for labor and delivery is the use of local agents such as lidocaine or carbocaine. These agents deaden the episiotomy site and allow for easy episiotomy repair. Pudendal anesthesia is also frequently used but has a high degree of partial effects even in the best hands.

Fortunately, the use of general anesthesia for vaginal delivery is losing the popularity it once enjoyed in the United States. If general anesthesia is to be employed (other than simple nitrous oxide and oxygen), the patient should be intubated to prevent aspiration. In no case should general anesthesia be given without the patient being intubated, since the obstetric patient is one of the most likely candidates for aspiration pneumonitis.

Anesthetizing for cesarean section likewide can be accomplished by the use of general or regional anesthesia. The regional anesthesia techniques include the epidural or the hypobaric or isobaric spinal. The difference between the modes of spinal anesthesias is that a saddle block utilizes a weighted anesthetic solution so that the block will remain low in the spinal canal. For cesarean section, as with the epidural block, anesthesia up to the T10 dermatome is the objective. With both techniques, hypotension is the principal danger, but this can be avoided by maintaining adequate fluid loads and by wedging (tilting) the patient to prevent the supine hypotensive syndrome.

In another approach, the use of balanced endotracheal anesthesia combined with rapid induction in which intravenous barbiturates and a muscle relaxant are utilized are equally efficacious for anesthesia in abdominal deliveries. If the patient's case is uncomplicated, the team gathered for the event—the anesthesiologists, pediatrician, and obstetrician—may allow the patient her choice as to anesthesia. In complicated cases, the obstetric anesthesiologist in consultation with the perinatologist and neonatologist should decide the best manner of anesthesia for delivery.

The use of new agents (such as the endorphines) is experimental at this time but holds great promise for the future. Other analgesic/anesthesia agents include hypnosis and acupuncture. The value of these techniques, while having been demonstrated to be effective in some studies during labor and delivery, has not been generally accepted by the medical community.

Texts
1. Bromage, P. R. *Epidural Analgesia.* Philadelphia: Saunders, 1978.
   A descriptive text of all methods of pain relief and how they affect the mother, fetus, and newborn.
2. Bonica, J. J. *Principles and Practice of Obstetric Analgesia and Anesthesia.* Philadelphia: Davis, 1972.
   This classic obstetric anesthesia text deals in depth with the pregnant woman and her offspring. This text and its references deal best with the basic science aspect of anesthesia.

Review
3. Endler, G. C. Conduction anesthesia in obstetrics and its effects upon fetus and newborn. *J. Reprod. Med.* 24:83, 1980.
   A review of conduction anesthesia is offered. The effects upon the fetus and newborn are detailed and 42 references are listed.

Parenteral Analgesia
4. Kuhnert, B. R., et al. Meperidine and normeperidine levels following meperidine administration during labor: I. Mother. II. Fetus and neonate. *Am. J. Obstet. Gynecol.* 133:904, 909, 1979.
   The pharmacokinetics of meperidine and its metabolites are delineated in 23 pregnant patients and their offspring, all of whom were intensively studied.
5. Dilts, P. V., Jr. Analgesia for labor and delivery. *The Female Patient* 5:62, 1980.
   The analgesic effects of meperidine are compared to other analgesic

agents, particularly morphine. Guidelines for analgesic usage are presented.

6. James, F. M. A guide to anesthesia for labor and vaginal delivery. *Resid. Staff Physician* 26:89, 1980.

   A comprehensive article that details all methods of analgesia for pain relief during labor and vaginal delivery. A convenient chart to use as a guide with respect to the various methods of analgesia, with advantages and disadvantages, is presented.

7. Myers, R. E., and Myers, S. E. Use of sedative, analgesic, and anesthetic drugs during labor and delivery: Bane or boon? *Am. J. Obstet. Gynecol.* 133:83, 1979.

   A very complete study of all drugs that have been used in the mother for pain relief and their effect on the fetus. Using a very even-handed approach, it lists the positive and negative points related to the use of these drugs during labor and delivery. There are 210 references.

8. Lewis, J. R. Evaluation of new analgesics. Butorphanol and nalbuphine. *J.A.M.A.* 243:1465, 1980.

   Two new, strong analgesic agents and their use in clinical medicine are presented. While generally as effective as morphine and meperidine, they have not been thoroughly tested in obstetrics.

9. Dilts, P. V., Jr. How substances cross the placenta—clinical implications. *Contemp. Ob/Gyn.* 17:89, 1981.

   This excellent article demonstrates a combined approach as to how drugs actually get across the placenta with particular reference to analgesic/anesthetic agents. The chemistry as well as the modes of placental transfer are discussed.

Regional Analgesia/Anesthesia

10. Jouppila, R., et al. Segmental epidural analgesia in labour: Related to the progress of labour, fetal malposition and instrumental delivery. *Acta Obstet. Gynecol. Scand.* 58:135, 1979.

    The effect of segmental epidural anesthesia with bupivacaine on the duration of labor and frequency of malposition at delivery was tested in 100 parturients. There was no difference in the normal progress and outcome of labor with the use of epidural anesthesia.

11. Ralston, D. H., and Shnider, S. M. The fetal and neonatal effects of regional anesthesia in obstetrics. *Anesthesiology* 48:34, 1978.

    The authors have given us a complete overview of the controversies surrounding local anesthetics. An in-depth analysis of their action at the molecular level and a detailed comprehensive viewpoint as to their side effects are presented along with 187 references.

12. DeJong, R. H. The chloroprocaine controversy. *Am. J. Obstet. Gynecol.* 140:237, 1981.

    Chloroprocaine has been widely used for conduction anesthesia. Neurologic complications, however, have recently been reported and the author suggests further testing to make certain the catheter is not in the subarachnoid space prior to final injection.

13. Richard, R. M. Paracervical block—anesthetic hazard to the fetus. *Contemp. Ob/Gyn* 17:97, 1981.

    This round table discussion by several eminent authorities in the field emphasizes the use and abuse of the paracervical block. Although this is not used as widely as in the past, the specific treatment regimes when problems arise with the use of this method are detailed.

General Anesthesia

14. James, F. M., et al. A comparison of general anesthesia and lumbar epidural analgesia for elective cesarean section. *Anesth. Analg.* (Cleve.) 56:228, 1977.
   A comparison of general anesthesia versus epidural anesthesia for cesarean section is detailed in 35 patients. Both techniques yielded good outcome for the baby.
15. Pederson, H., and Finster, M. Anesthetic risk in the pregnant surgical patient. *Anesthesiology* 51:439, 1979.
   Anesthetic risk in the pregnant surgical patient was assessed both retrospectively and prospectively. Step-by-step management techniques to prevent complications is emphasized.

Effects on the Newborn

16. Effect of medication during labor and delivery on infant outcome. AAP Committee on Drugs, in collaboration with the ACOG Committee on Obstetrics: Maternal and Fetal Medicine. May, 1978.
   The American Academy of Pediatrics and American College of Obstetrics and Gynecology prepared a joint statement concerning drugs in pregnancy. This periodical delineates knowns and unknowns about the effects of medication on the infant and makes worthwhile recommendations.

New Techniques

17. Oyama, T., et al. B-endorphin in obstetric analgesia. *Am. J. Obstet. Gynecol.* 137:613, 1980.
   The role of B-endorphin given intrathecally was assessed in 14 obstetric patients. It gave excellent analgesia during labor and is not reansferred across the placenta; there were no fetal effects. A relationship to acupuncture or psychoprophylaxis, or both, and endogenous endorphins is suggested.

Forceps and Vacuum Extraction

The American College of Obstetricians and Gynecologists has defined three categories of forceps operations: outlet forcep, midforcep, and high forcep. The high forceps operation, defined as application of forceps any time prior to full engagement of the fetal head, has been abandoned because of its association with significant fetal and maternal morbidity. Outlet forceps delivery is the application of forceps when the fetal scalp is visible at the introitus without having to separate the labia, the skull has reached the pelvic floor, and the sagittal suture is in the anteroposterior diameter of the pelvis. The midforceps operation is the use of forceps when the fetal head is engaged, but conditions for outlet forceps have not been met. Any forceps delivery other than high forceps requiring artificial rotation, regardless of the station from which extraction is begun, is designated officially as midforceps. Many physicians object to this rigid criterion for the midforceps operation, inasmuch as they believe that the rotation from a left occiput anterior (LOA) position, with the fetal head on the pelvic floor, to the occiput anterior (OA) position prior to delivery, should be listed as an outlet forceps delivery.

There are three types of forceps. The first is the classic model used for low forceps delivery, another group is used for special situations, and a third type is the traction forcep. The routine low forceps delivery is usually accomplished by either the Simpson, Elliott, or Tucker-McLean types, with the last two (overlapping shanks) being utilized primarily for the unmolded head, and the Simpson forceps utilized for the molded head because of the wider shank separation. The specialized forceps, especially the Barton and Kielland types are used for midforceps deliveries. The Barton forceps is used primarily for the infant in the persistent occiput transverse position in a flat pelvis to allow the operator to first pull the fetal head down to the floor of the perineum in the transverse position, and then to rotate the head to the OA position. The Kielland forceps are most often used for persistent occiput transverse position when the head is not on the floor of the perineum as well as for rotation from the occiput posterior position to the occiput anterior position.

When the infant is in the occiput posterior position the operator may wish to rotate the fetal head to the occiput anterior position, using a Scanzoni rotation with two separate applications of the Simpson forceps. For the aftercoming head of a breech, Piper forceps are most often utilized because of their unique shape. Traction forceps are rarely used today in delivering a living fetus because the amount of traction and pressure that one can exert with these types of forceps is significant. When nontraction forceps are used pressures reaching 27–34 pounds have been demonstrated and are considered normal. Pressures exceeding these levels are to be avoided.

Prerequisites for applying forceps include a trained, skillful operator, an engaged fetal head, rupture of the membranes, a fully dilated cervix, a thorough knowledge of fetal position and type of maternal pelvis, as well as a clear indication for their use. Forceps have been incriminated in many fetal injury cases, yet the literature reports conflicting results with their use; most of the trauma being related to the type of forceps that were used, the fetal status prior to the delivery process, as well as the skill of the operator. A large study by the Collaborative Perinatal Project of uncomplicated pregnancies, involving approximately 30,000 babies, followed with periodic exams for up to 4 years, has failed to reveal any conclusive evidence that outlet forceps operation increased the hazard of neonatal death or produced subsequent neurologic impairment of the infants.

While most physicians believe that low or outlet forceps are safe, controversy does exist when the midforceps delivery is discussed. The problem exists because some midforceps operations are easy while others are difficult, and persistence in attempts to effect vaginal delivery may lead to unfavorable results. A situation in which the fetal head is significantly molded, with little or no descent over several hours of second stage labor despite effective pushing and adequate uterine activity, and in which the examiner has difficulty in placing his hand between the pelvic side wall and the fetal skull, is a good example of when a midforceps delivery should *not* be performed. On the other hand, a patient in whom the fetal head is engaged but does not qualify as being at an outlet forcep stage, and in whom adequate pelvic room is perceived, fetal macrosomia is not suspected, and adequate anesthesia is available, a midforceps delivery can probably be attempted without trauma, thereby possibly averting an unnecessary cesarean section.

While any forceps delivery can significantly damage the maternal pelvic tissue, these injuries are usually associated with the more difficult forceps deliveries. Although opinion on the use of the midforceps operation is not unanimous in this country, I believe strongly that midforceps delivery, especially the rotation to occiput anterior from the occiput transverse or posterior position, is an important tool for the obstetrician and should be taught properly in residency programs. Certainly in those situations in which there is fetal distress and performing a cesarean section would prolong significantly the duration of distress, forceps delivery can be lifesaving.

While many physicians attempted to utilize the vacuum principle for vaginal delivery, it wasn't until 1956 that this technique, using the current instrument, was developed to affect delivery. Over the last decade the use of the vacuum extractor for delivery of the fetus has become a controversial subject. The reasons cited for not utilizing this instrument include staff inexperience with its use, technical difficulties such as inability to maintain a partial vacuum, leaks in the tubing following sterilization, parental concern about the chignon on the baby's head at birth, and sporadic reports in the literature alleging brain damage after its use.

Despite these objections, however, many obstetricians believe that proper use of the vacuum extractor should be taught in residency programs, and that each physician in obstetrics should be familiar with its use for selected cases. These cases include positional arrests, fetal distress, uterine hypotonicity unresponsive to oxytocin, any situation in which forceps delivery is required yet general or conduction anesthesia is either undesirable or unavailable, as well as some situations in which a physician is not certain of the fetal position or cannot apply forceps safely, or both. The advantage of the vacuum extraction in positional arrests lies in the fact that the fetal head is not disengaged during application, nor does the vacuum extractor occupy space or cause deflexion of the vertex. Traction on the cup, in fact, promotes flexion, rotation, and descent, important factors in effecting vaginal delivery. Excessive traction on the fetal head is avoided since traction above 25 pounds of pressure will detach the cup.

Its being able to be used in fetal distress when the cervix is not yet completely dilated is another advantage. Use of the vacuum extractor in these cases can effect delivery safely and rapidly, thus avoiding a traumatic forceps delivery or a cesarean section. This method of delivery has been noted to be expecially valuable in cases in which there is a prolapsed umbilical cord and significant fetal heart rate deccleration in the second stage of labor. Another use for the vacuum extractor is in the delivery of the second twin when the presenting part is at a station that would preclude forcep deliveries yet signs of fetal distress are noted.

Maternal complications occurring with the use of the vacuum extractor are usually limited to cervical and vaginal trauma, which is secondary to maternal tissue being included in the cup during application or traction, or both. With increased experience this complication is rare. Complications to the fetus include an artificially induced caput (chignon), which usually resolves within several hours and is completely gone within 1 to 2 days. Minor abrasions and signs of bleeding into the skin of the fetal scalp have been noted to occur in approximately 10%–20% of cases and are usually considered of little importance in overall neonatal care. Cephalhematomas may occur, but these are usually associated with more difficult deliveries and are reported in approximately 5% of cases.

The literature contains a number of reports indicating that the use of this instrument is associated with no evidence of neurologic damage to the fetus, while other reports suggest an increased incidence of abnormalities associated with vacuum extraction. In situations related to fetal distress, second twin, and prolonged labor, it is not surprising that studies may indicate a higher fetal morbidity rate. Whether or not this higher rate is associated directly with the use of the vacuum extractor is unclear at this time, however. Retinal hemorrhages are noted nearly as frequently with use of the vacuum extractor as with a spontaneous delivery. While fetal intracranial hemorrhages have been described, most of these cases have been associated with inappropriate use of the extractor for particularly long periods of time.

In summary, the vacuum extractor, like the forceps, should have a place in each obstetrician's training. When used properly, vacuum extraction is considered safe for both mother and baby; furthermore, its use provides a very effective means of instrumental delivery when the use of forceps is either contraindicated and/or when delivery must be effected quickly. Hopefully, more exposure to this instrument during resident training will increase its safe use in this country.

Review

1. Laufe, L. *Obstetric Forceps.* New York: Harper & Row, 1968.
   Each type of obstetric forcep is discussed in relation to its structure and appropriate use.
2. Chamberlain, G. Forceps and vacuum extraction. *Clin. Obstet. Gynaecol.* 7:511, 1980.
   A scholarly review of the indication and use of forceps and vacuum extraction. The complications of both methods are detailed.
3. Douglas, R. G., and Stromme, W. B. *Operative Obstetrics* (3rd ed.). New York: Appleton-Century-Crofts, 1976.
   A good overall review of the subject of forceps for the beginner.

Midforceps

4. Chiswick, M. L., and James, D. K. Keilland forceps: Association with neonatal morbidity and mortality. *Br. Med. J.* 1:7, 1979.
   These authors described a high neonatal morbidity and mortality associated with forceps rotation.

Midforceps, For and Against

5. James, D. K., and Chiswick, M. L. Kielland's forceps: Role of antenatal factors in prediction use. *Br. Med. J.* 1:10, 1979.
   A retrospective study of the factors singificantly associated with the use of Kielland's forceps. Long and dystonic labors and cephalopelvic disproportion were found to be the most common factors. The relationship of epidural anesthesia is also discussed.
6. Danforth, D. N., and Ellis, A. H. Midforceps delivery—a vanishing art. *Am. J. Obstet. Gynecol.* 86:29, 1963.
   A thorough discussion of the techniques of midforceps deliveries is detailed. The philosophy regarding their use is also discussed.
7. Cook, W. A. R. Evaluation of the midforceps operation. *Am. J. Obstet. Gynecol.* 99:327, 1976.
   The evaluation of midforceps operations from a maternal as well as fetal standpoint are detailed. Historic perspectives are given.
8. Ingardia, C. J., and Cetrulo, C. L. Forceps—use and abuse. *Clin. Perinatol.* 8:63, 1981.
   Low forceps operations do not appear to significantly increase infant morbidity, but midforceps deliveries are a subject of controversy. Suggestions are made for reducing the need for midforceps deliveries and for the more liberal use of cesarean section whenever an easy forceps delivery is not expected.

Vacuum Extraction

9. Schenker, J. G., and Serr, D. M. Comparative study of delivery by vacuum extractor and forceps. *Am. J. Obstet. Gynecol.* 98:32, 1967.

Three hundred cases of vacuum extraction were compared with 300 forceps deliveries in order to evaluate safety of mother and child. The conclusion was that the vacuum extractor was an efficient instrument with special indications but could not be accepted as a general replacement for forceps.

10. Plauche, W. C. Vacuum extraction. Use in a community hospital setting. *Obstet. Gynecol.* 52:289, 1978.
    A good review article listing indications and outcome. Significant trauma to the fetal scalp occurred in 18.7% of infants.

Vacuum Versus Forceps

11. Chalmers, J. A. The vacuum extractor in difficult delivery. *J. Obstet. Gynaecol. Br. Commonw.* 72:889, 1965.
    The indication for vacuum extraction of the fetus when forceps delivery or cesarean section may be inappropriate are detailed. The techniques are also discussed.

12. Kappy, K. A. Vacuum extractor. *Clin. Perinatol.* 8:79, 1981.
    A review article on a difficult subject. The technique, advantages, indications, contraindications, and complications of vacuum extraction are discussed.

13. Greis, J. B., Bieniarz, J., and Scommegna, A. Comparison of maternal and fetal effects of vacuum extraction with forceps or cesarean deliveries. *Obstet. Gynecol.* 57:571, 1981.
    The results of 90 vacuum extraction deliveries were compared to forceps or cesarean section births. Where vacuum extraction was used, infants had less significant problems as did the parturients when compared to the other two groups.

Safety of Forceps

14. Niswander, K. R., and Gordon, M. Safety of the low-forceps operation. *Am. J. Obstet. Gynecol.* 117:619, 1973.
    This study reveals that the prophylactic forcep operation does not increase the hazard of neonatal death or subsequent neurologic impairment of the infant.

15. Holmes, J. M. A safe method of Kielland forceps delivery. *J. Obstet. Gynaecol. Br. Commonw.* 65:310, 1958.
    The author demonstrates the prerequisites for the safe application of midforceps. Although the technique is not as frequently used today, a clear understanding of the requisites when its use is required is necessary.

Review of Complications

16. Plauche, W. C. Fetal cranial injuries related to delivery with the Malmstrom vacuum extractor. *Obstet. Gynecol.* 53:750, 1979.
    A review article regarding the propensity of the vacuum extractor to cause fetal cranial injuries, with an attempt to evaluate early and late neurologic damage between vacuum extractor deliveries and spontaneous vaginal deliveries.

17. Levin, S., et al. Diagnostic and prognostic value of retinal hemorrhages in the neonate. *Obstet. Gynecol.* 55:309, 1980.
    Various damage to the fetus, particularly retinal hemorrhage, is discussed in relation to the use of the vacuum extractor.

Cesarean Section

Cesarean section is the delivery of an infant through an incision in the abdominal and uterine wall. While there are several references to abdominal delivery prior to 1900, few were successful—the maternal death rate averaged over 85%. In this century, better surgical techniques, antibiotics, aseptic techniques, and blood banks have decreased the risk of this procedure considerably. Indications for performing a cesarean section include dystocia, abnormal fetal presentation, fetal distress, hemorrhage, and a multiplicity of other maternal and fetal indications. Approximately half of the primary cesarean sections are performed for cephalopelvic disproportion, with breech presentation (15%), fetal distress (7.6%), and dystocia (29%), being other common indications.

Nearly 25% of *all* cesarean sections are repeat procedures performed because the patient had been delivered of her infant by the abdominal route in a previous pregnancy. This course is followed to avoid the possible consequences of rupture of the uterine scar in labor. The dictum "once a cesarean section, always a cesarean section," however, has become a controversial subject since several studies demonstrate that 50% of fetuses can be delivered vaginally following a previous cesarean section without noticeable maternal, fetal, or neonatal morbidity.

Types of cesarean section include the classic, the low-transverse cervical, the low-vertical cervical, and the extraperitoneal. While the classic incision is made in the fundus of the uterus, the low-cervical incision is performed after the parietal peritoneum has been incised and the bladder reflected downward. This incision is made vertically or transversely in the lower, less muscular segment of the uterine wall, allowing the physician to remove the infant through an area in the uterus that is less likely to rupture during a subsequent pregnancy, more likely to heal without significant complications, and usually yields less bleeding during the operation.

The extraperitoneal cesarean section has recently regained popularity because significant maternal abdominal infections can occur with a transperitoneal approach, especially in the already infected amniotic cavity, and may result in loss of fertility. No definite conclusions have been reached by obstetricians in this country concerning this subject; some studies, however, indicate a decreased incidence of peritoneal infection and serious postoperative complications with its use in selected cases. The type of uterine incision made depends largely on the presentation of the fetus, the location of the placenta, the presence of uterine pathology or other conditions relating to the individual patient.

Hysterectomy performed at the time of cesarean section, called the cesarean hysterectomy, is performed generally for patients who require sterilization or who have coincidental uterine pathology. This procedure has been noted to significantly decrease infectious complications in patients who have severe amnionitis at the time of cesarean section. Although it is a more difficult operation, the cesarean hysterectomy has been shown to be safe in experienced hands and may play a significant role in the overall management of the obstetric patient.

Anesthesia given for cesarean section is generally divided into two categories, balanced general technique or regional blocks, the latter utilizing either the spinal or epidural route. Some procedures have been performed using local anesthesia as well as hypnosis and acupuncture. It is important that the type of anesthesia be selected by an experienced anesthesiologist who understands the physiologic changes of pregnancy and is sensitive to fetal considerations.

While some cesarean sections have to be performed prior to fetal maturity, if performed electively, it is imperative that the physician confirm fetal lung maturity prior to the operation. Some studies have indicated that approximately 10%–20% of all babies in newborn nurseries with hyaline membrane disease are products of elective induction or cesarean section. Reasonable assurance of fetal maturity can be accomplished by any combination of the following methods of assessing gestational age: reliable date of last menstrual period, history of pregnancy landmarks such as fetal heart tones at 20 weeks, quickening, early uterine examinations, ultrasound scanning (best performed between 16 and 30 weeks), or amniocentesis to confirm lung maturity via a series of lung phospholipid studies.

Cesarean section rates have increased in the past 10–15 years from approximately 5% in the middle 1960s to approximately 15% in 1980. While this threefold increase in the cesarean birth rate during the last 15 years has been a source of concern to both physician and general public, there is evidence that this increase has contributed to a lowering of the perinatal mortality rate. One study from California showed that while the cesarean section rate rose from 5% to 15%, the perinatal mortality rate declined from 27.1 per 1000 live births to 16.5 per 1000.

The antithesis for this increased fetal/neonatal benefit appears to be elevated maternal morbidity/mortality rates when cesarean section is compared to vaginal delivery. Maternal mortality associated with cesarean births fortunately has become quite rare, occurring at rates between 20 and 70 for every 100,000 operations. Although the risk of maternal demise is small, it is still higher than that for vaginal delivery. In 1974, a survey of 1527 hospitals showed that the maternal death rate from cesarean section was 80 per 100,000 cesarean deliveries, compared to 27 deaths per 100,000 of all deliveries. Postoperative febrile morbidity, from 10%–50%, depending on whether the cesarean section was done electively or during labor with ruptured membranes, is also increased over that found for vaginal delivery (1%–10%). This increase in maternal morbidity, along with prolongation of hospital stay, increased expense, a loss of initial parental interaction with the newborn, and the potential need for a repeat cesarean section is of concern to both the physician and the public. Each case must be managed individually.

The effect of fetal monitoring on the incidence of cesarean section as well as its effect on maternal morbidity is also a controversial subject. While some studies incriminate fetal monitoring as the reason for the overall increase in cesarean section rates in the past 10 to 15 years, there is also data to support that fetal monitoring alone has not been responsible for this increase. Changes in the management of breech presentation, a reluctance to perform difficult forceps deliveries, and a more aggressive approach to the high-risk obstetric patient, combined with the increased safety of the operation, have all contributed significantly to the increased cesarean section rate. Some studies have actually shown a reduction in the incidence of cesarean sections performed for fetal distress when fetal monitoring has been used liberally. The most recent data indicates that internal fetal monitoring is only one variable contributing to maternal morbidity, and that length of labor, the number of examinations, and the overall status of the patient are equally as important.

Because of the high infection rate following cesarean section, studies have been performed regarding the use of prophylactic antibiotics. In carefully controlled studies it seems that prophylactic antibiotics, especially in the high-risk patient, can reduce the postoperative infection morbidity by approximately 50%. The factors placing a patient at high risk for developing infection include ruptured membranes, multiple examinations, obesity, anemia, difficult operative procedures, placental abnormalities, internal fetal monitoring, and general anesthesia. Because of these convincing data, many obstetricians now treat patients demonstrating any of these high-risk factors with antibiotics, usually beginning treatment with clamping of the umbilical cord so as to diminish administration of antibiotics to the fetus, although others would begin the drugs in the postoperative period.

Risks to the fetus from cesarean section include neonatal depression from general anesthesia, reduced uterine blood flow secondary to either regional anesthesia or the mother's supine position prior to and during surgery, incisional trauma to the fetus while entering the uterus, fetal blood loss while traversing an underlying placenta, injury to the fetus during extraction procedures, as well as a slightly increased incidence of respiratory distress when compared to infants of control patients who were delivered vaginally. Nevertheless, when mothers are appropriately selected, the fetus delivered abdominally today fares much better than his counterpart who was delivered vaginally with the same maternal/fetal indication.

Indications

1. Haddad, H., and Lundy, L. E. Changing indications for cesarean section. A 38-year experience at a community hospital. *Obstet. Gynecol.* 51:133, 1978.

   In a review of a 38-year experience with cesarean section at a community hospital, there was a marked increase in the cesarean section rate after 1972. This was due primarily to an increase in the primary cesarean section rate for cephalopelvic disproportion and labor abnormalities, fetal distress, and the breech presentation.

2. Evrard, J. R., Gold, E. M., and Cahill, T. F. Cesarean section: A contemporary assessment. *J. Reprod. Med.* 24:147, 1980.

   This 1-year retrospective study of cesarean sections noted a total cesarean section rate of 18.5% and a primary rate of 13.4%. The four leading indications for primary cesarean sections were: dystocia, 38.8%; breech presentation, 14.9%; malposition, 11.9%; fetal distress, 11.3%.

3. Bottoms, S. F., Rosen, M. G., and Sokol, R. J. The increase in the cesarean birth rate. *N. Engl. J. Med.* 302:559, 1980.

   This article describes the underlying factors in the change of indications for operative delivery and discusses areas in which cesarean section rates may be altered by changes in obstetrical practice.

4. Monheit, A. G., and Resnik, R. Cesarean section: Current trends and perspectives. *Clin. Perinatol.* 8:101, 1981.

   The authors anticipate that prior cesarean section will not continue to be an indication for the abdominal delivery of subsequent births. Indications for cesarean section are discussed, and the benefits and risks of this procedure are evaluated.

5. Burkman, R. T. Why the increase in c-section. *The Female Patient* 6:55, 1981.

   Improved fetal outcome is the most important impetus for the marked increase in cesarean section. A management plan for making a rational decision for cesarean section is introduced.

6. Rosen, M. G., et al. NIH consensus development statement on cesarean childbirth. *Obstet. Gynecol.* 57:537, 1981.

   A two-year report concerning a consensus development statement on cesarean section by NIH is summarized in this article. It is a must reading for all those interested in the increase in the rate of cesarean sections in our society.

7. Amirikia, H., Zarewych, B., and Evans, T. N. Cesarean section: A 15-year review of changing incidence, indications, and risks. *Am. J. Obstet. Gynecol.* 140:81, 1981.

    A 15-year review of 9718 cesarean sections was performed. Perinatal mortality decreased from 40% to 29% and there were 10 maternal deaths. The indications for cesarean section are detailed.

Once a Section—Always a Section?

8. Saldana, L. R., Schulman, H., and Reuss, L. Management of pregnancy after cesarean section. *Am. J. Obstet. Gynecol.* 135:555, 1979.

    This article reviewed the management of 226 patients with a previous low-transverse cesarean section and reported a 38.5% incidence of vaginal delivery in 145 patients who underwent a trial of labor. There were no uterine ruptures on vaginal exploration after delivery or at the time of repeat cesarean section during labor.

9. O'Sullivan, M. J., et al. Vaginal delivery after cesarean section. *Clin. Perinatol.* 8:131, 1981.

    Patients who have previously had a cesarean section should be allowed to deliver their infants vaginally in subsequent births provided that they are carefully selected, their labors are closely managed, and they are examined for intrauterine defects following delivery. The benefits of a diminished cesarean section rate include decreased maternal morbidity and hospital costs.

10. Shy, K. K., LoGerfo, J. P., and Karp, L. E. Evaluation of elective repeat cesarean section as a standard of care: An application of decision analysis. *Am. J. Obstet. Gynecol.* 139:123, 1981.

    Statistical evaluation data in a hypothetical case study using 10,000 pregnant women in regard to their ability to deliver vaginally after prior cesarean section were studied. Using probability data from the literature, the trial of labor resulted in 37 fewer perinatal deaths and 0.7 fewer maternal deaths than elective repeat cesarean section. In addition, direct costs were reduced.

Cesarean Hysterectomy

11. Haynes, D. M., and Martin, B. J. Cesarean hysterectomy: A twenty-five year review. *Am. J. Obstet. Gynecol.* 134:393, 1979.

    This 25-year review of 149 cesarean hysterectomies suggests that cesarean hysterectomy should remain a part of the obstetrician's repertoire, but that it may not be advisable for strictly elective indications.

Timing

12. Frigoletto, F. D., et al. Avoiding iatrogenic prematurity with elective repeat cesarean section without the routine use of amniocentesis. *Am. J. Obstet. Gynecol.* 137:521, 1980.

    During a 3-year period, there were 1497 repeat cesarean sections performed at one institution. A protocol utilizing menstrual history, early bimanual pelvic examinations, and midpregnancy ultrasonography, as well as selected amniocentesis for confirmation of pulmonary maturity yielded an incidence of potentially preventable respiratory distress in 0.27%.

13. Hayashi, R. H., Berry, J. L., and Castillo, M. S. Use of ultrasound biparietal diameter in timing of repeat cesarean section. *Obstet. Gynecol.* 57:325, 1981.

Patients with repeat cesarean section were delivered without amniotic fluid studies if the biparietal diameter on ultrasound was 9.3 cm or greater at 38 weeks. None of these infants developed respiratory distress.

Effect of Fetal Monitoring on Cesarean Section

14. Haverkamp, A. D., et al. A controlled trial of the differential effects of intrapartum fetal monitoring. *Am. J. Obstet. Gynecol.* 134:399, 1979.
    This prospective study indicates that in a group undergoing electronic fetal monitoring there will be an increased incidence of cesarean section when compared to a group of patients undergoing fetal heart rate auscultation.

15. Boehm, F. H., Davidson, K. K., and Barrett, J. M. The effect of electronic fetal monitoring on the incidence of cesarean section. *Am. J. Obstet. Gynecol.* 140:295, 1981.
    The effect of electronic fetal monitoring on the infant at cesarean section was studied. From the analysis of this data the abdominal delivery for breech presentations and high-risk maternal conditions contributed more to the increase of cesarean section rate than did electronic fetal monitoring.

16. Williams, R. L., and Hawes, W. E. Cesarean section, fetal monitoring, and perinatal mortality in California. *Am. J. Public Health* 69:864, 1979.
    The authors show that fetal monitoring increased while cesarean section rates increased. Also perinatal mortality rates concomitantly were reduced.

Complications

17. Frigoletto, F. D., Ryan, K. J., and Phillippe, M. Maternal mortality rate associated with cesarean section: An appraisal. *Am. J. Obstet. Gynecol.* 136:969, 1980.
    This paper presents a large, consecutive experience from a Level III facility where no maternal deaths secondary to cesarean section occurred.

18. Rubin, G. L., et al. Maternal death after cesarean section in Georgia. *Am. J. Obstet. Gynecol.* 139:681, 1981.
    The cause of death after cesarean section was studied. Pulmonary embolism and cardiorespiratory arrests during general anesthesia were the leading causes of death.

19. Gilstrap, L. C., and Cunningham, F. G. The bacterial pathogenesis of infection following cesarean section. *Obstet. Gynecol.* 53:545, 1979.
    The various microorganisms most likely to cause infection after cesarean section are listed. A discussion regarding therapy as well as prevention are outlined.

20. Gall, S. A. The efficacy of prophylactic antibiotics in cesarean section. *Am. J. Obstet. Gynecol.* 134:506, 1979.
    The use of prophylactic antibiotics was found to be helpful in preventing infections in patients undergoing cesarean section. The incidence of severe complications due to infection, however, was the same in both groups.

Failure to Progress in Labor

The phrase "failure to progress in labor (dystocia)" should be limited to failure to progress in the active phase of labor. Active labor occurs when the cervix reaches 3 cm dilatation and dilates progressively at a rate of approximately 1.5 cm/hour for multigravidas and 1.2 cm/hour for primigravidas. By definition, when there has been no progress in cervical dilatation or descent of the presenting part, failure to progress has occurred. This condition has a multifactorial etiology and immediately resorting to cesarean section is incorrect, since at least 50% of patients will continue on to a normal vaginal delivery when the underlying cause has been identified and correct treatment instituted.

The number and route of any previous deliveries, length of the labors, as well as weight of the infants, should be obtained. Information needed related to the present pregnancy includes the gestational age of the baby, time when labor commenced, status of the membranes, and drugs administered intrapartum. Pulse and blood pressure should be assessed since tachycardia may indicate dehydration, which may affect the quality of the uterine activity. The best method to detect dehydration is specific gravity of the urine; a high value indicates dehydration, which may be corrected by the administration of intravenous fluids. An abdominal examination should *always* be performed before a vaginal examination for the following reasons: (1) identification of the position of the fetal back facilitates determination of fetal position on vaginal examination; (2) the lie of the fetus can be assessed before the vaginal examination is done; and (3) uterine activity may be quantitated. Thus, careful abdominal examination may be helpful in the overall evaluation of the patient in labor and forms the basis on which future progress may be measured.

Several fetal causes of failure to progress in labor may be assessed by abdominal examination. Breech, brow, or face position, as well as oblique or transverse lie, may be causes of dystocia in labor. Flexion of the head should be determined by assessing the relative position of the occiput and synciput, as a deflexed head may result in failure to progress. This is determined by running one hand down the back onto the occiput, which should normally be lower than the hand on the opposite side over the synciput.

The vertex should be checked for engagement. If mobile on the abdominal examination, it is termed free-floating; if fixed in the pelvis, it may still not be engaged. The rule of fifths is used. The head is imagined to be divided into five fifths; when three-fifths of the head are below the pelvic inlet, the head is considered engaged and should be at the level of the spines on vaginal examination. This is determined by placing both hands over the fetal head on abdominal examination. If the fingers converge before reaching the symphysis, the head is not engaged (the largest diameter is still above the pelvic inlet). If the fingers continue to diverge until the symphysis is felt, the head is probably engaged in the pelvis. At this stage, the fetal heart rate should be checked for any abnormalities in rate or rhythm.

Inadequate or incoordinate uterine activity is one of the most common causes of failure to progress in labor. Uterine activity may be assessed by placing the tips of the fingers of one hand over the contracting uterus and assessing the frequency, regularity, and intensity of the contractions. Regular contractions (occurring at intervals of 2–3 minutes and lasting approximately 50–60 seconds, with the uterus becoming hard during contractions) make it unlikely that failure to progress in labor is due to an abnormality of uterine contractility. Activity of lesser degrees may signify hypotonic uterine activity; this may be the cause of failure to progress and may require oxytocin augmentation.

Incoordinate uterine action usually associated with a posterior position of the fetal vertex is another condition commonly related to uterine activity that results in failure to progress. There are clues to this condition. The patient experiences extreme discomfort, located mainly in the lower back or rectum. On palpation, the uterus usually does not feel as hard during contractions as in patients experiencing coordinate uterine activity. Another clue is the timing of the pain relative to the onset and disappearance of the contractions. Usually the examiner can palpate the contractions before the patient feels them and can continue to palpate them after she stops feeling them. In incoordinate uterine action, the patient feels the onset of contractions earlier and continues to feel the pain of the contraction for a longer period of time.

The pelvic examination is also important in assessing the progress of labor. Although prolonged labor in the presence of cephalopelvic disproportion (CPD) may result in edema of the vulva, subsequent outlet dystocia is infrequently a problem. A transverse vaginal septum in the upper third of the vagina may be mistaken for the cervix; thus an incorrect diagnosis of failure to progress is seen in both these cases. Both transverse and longitudinal vaginal septae may cause obstruction to descent of the fetal head and may have to be incised during labor, or abdominal delivery may be employed. Vaginal cysts are rarely a problem in labor.

The cervix may also present problems with dystocia. Normally the cervix is directed posteriorly, but as labor progresses, the cervix moves to a central position. Thus, false labor should be suspected when a patient is admitted in labor and the cervix is found to be closed, long, and pointing posteriorly. This also has clinical relevance in the diagnosis and treatment of premature labor. Effacement describes the length of the cervix in the vagina. Confusion between effacement and thickness of the cervix often exists. In the primigravid patient, the cervix usually effaces completely during the latent phase of labor; if not, dystocia may be suspected. During the active phase of labor, the main concern is dilatation of the cervix. The cervix is usually soft and can be stretched somewhat further than it is dilated. Rarely, cervical dystocia occurs due to previous trauma, and a firm fibrous ring that can be felt around the cervix makes it impossible to stretch digitally. Due to the head pushing on this fibrous ring, local caput of the head can be felt through the os of the cervix. Sometimes cervical dystocia occurs due to incoordinate uterine action; the contractions push the head into the cervix without taking up the lower segment of the uterus to effect cervical dilatation. Again, local fetal caput of the vertex, confined to the degree of cervical dilatation, may be found.

In obstructed labor due to CPD, the cervix may become edematous and thicker as labor progresses instead of thinner. This is due to compression of the lower uterine segment between the fetal head and the inlet of the pelvis. In the presence of CPD, the application of the head to the cervix is poor, and in severe instances, "curtaining" occurs. (Curtaining describes what produces the edematous, loose, poorly applied cervix that protrudes in the vagina after prolonged CPD.) Thus, the failure of progressive cervical dilatation and changes in the thickness and application of the cervix may indicate the presence of CPD.

Vaginal examination also confirms that the presenting part is indeed vertex and not a breech, face, brow, or other positional cause of dystocia in labor. It is important not to confuse a shoulder presentation or transverse lie with any of the above, as cesarean section would be required for these two.

If, on abdominal palpation, it is determined on which side the back is lying, determining the direction of the sagittal suture on vaginal examination should identify the position of the baby. This is especially important, since a posterior position is often associated with incoordinate uterine action and failure to progress in labor. An easily palpated anterior fontanel usually indicates deflexion of the head. The easiest method to distinguish the anterior from the posterior fontanel is to run the examining finger from the sagittal suture over the fontanel and beyond. A midline suture (frontal) that extends from the fontanel would indicate that it is the anterior one.

Caput is edema of the subcutaneous tissues that results from pressure of the head upon one of two structures: the bony pelvis due to CPD (in which case the caput extends beyond the cervical dilatation to the bony pelvis), or a cervix that is not dilating (thereby causing local caput, the extent of which corresponds to the cervical dilatation). Molding is the overlapping of skull bones that occurs when the fetal head passes through the pelvis. This is most readily felt at the posterior fontanel where the parietal bones overlap the occipital bone. Molding rarely occurs at the sagittal suture. The amount of overlap of the bones is often a clue to the degree of CPD present.

It is important to determine the station of the head in relation to the ischial spines. A facile maneuver in the management of CPD is the Müller-Hillis maneuver, by which fundal pressure is applied and descent of the presenting part estimated vaginally. If there is no descent with fundal pressure in the presence of the other signs of CPD, further labor should not be allowed and a cesarean section performed. If there is descent, further labor might be allowed and progress reassessed again at a later stage. A careful, clinical pelvic assessment should be performed to rule out any gross abnormalities of the pelvis.

By a logical and stepwise approach to the patient who fails to progress in labor, the causes can usually be related either to the powers, passage, or passenger. Treatment of failure to progress in labor depends on the correct diagnosis of the underlying cause, which is then treated on its own merit. Resorting to cesarean section is not appropriate in all cases in which failure to progress is diagnosed. In summary, it has been shown that failure to progress in the active phase of labor may have varied etiology. A logical approach to the diagnosis and management of this vague condition is presented. When this approach is used, it becomes unnecessary to be familiar with a long list of the causes of failure to progress.

Diagnosis and Treatment

1. Friedman, E. A. *Labor: Clinical Evaluation and Management* (2nd ed.). New York: Appleton-Century-Crofts, 1978.
   This book deals in great detail with normal and abnormal labor patterns. The abnormal patterns are analyzed and defined and their etiology, therapy, and prognosis are discussed. The effects of endogenous and exogenous factors on the course of labor and examples of several labor aberrations are discussed.

2. Crichton, D. A reliable method of establishing the level of the fetal head in obstetrics. *S. Afr. Med. J.* 48:784, 1974.
   Crichton describes the assessment of the fetal station by abdominal palpation of the relationship of the sinciput and occiput above the symphysis pubis. The information is very useful to distinguish true descent from progressive molding.

3. Seitchik, J. Quantitating uterine contractility in clinical context. *Obstet. Gynecol.* 57:453, 1981.
   This retrospective study compared the uterine contractility of patients in normal labor with that of patients in arrested labor. The data suggested that by averaging three successive contractions, one could differentiate normal from hypocontractile labor and thus select patients for oxytocin augmentation.

4. Friedman, E. A. Failure to progress in labor—evaluation and management. *Contemp. Ob/Gyn* 4:41, 1974.

Patients with cephalopelvic disproportion who manifest arrest of dilatation and descent or a prolonged deceleration phase in labor will almost invariably (98.8%) require cesarean section, regardless of what means are used to promote progress in labor.

5. Friedman, E. A. The labor curve. *Clin. Perinatol.* 8:15, 1981.

The labor curve is useful as a means of following labors in progress and for identifying disorders as they arise. A specific problem, once it is identified, requires a specific remedy. Management of prolonged latent phase, protraction disorders, and arrest disorder with or without cephalopelvic disproportion is discussed.

6. Embrey, M. P., Graham, N. B., and McNeill, M. D. Induction of labour with a sustained-release prostaglandin E_2 vaginal pessary. *Br. Med. J.* 281:901, 1980.

The authors demonstrate that the prognosis for the induction or augmentation of labor is usually unfavorable with an unripe cervix. This status of the cervix can be improved by the vaginal administration of prostaglandin E_2 compounds.

Consequences

7. Shane, J. A. Medical-legal ramifications of difficult labor and delivery. *Clin. Perinatol.* 8:3, 1981.

True clinical cases of difficult labor and delivery problems are presented as examples of situations in which claims of negligence may arise. Optimal and well-documented medical care that includes additional consultation when necessary and active participation of the patient when possible can provide the best defense for such suits.

8. Friedman, E. A., Sachtleben, M. R., and Bresky, P. A. Dysfunctional labor: Long-term effects on infant. *Am. J. Obstet. Gynecol.* 127:779, 1977.

The results of developmental studies done at 3 and 4 years of age in a series of 656 children were correlated with labor pattern and type of delivery. There were significant adverse effects among offspring delivered by midforceps or born following labors with prolonged deceleration or secondary arrest of dilatation or descent.

9. Skelly, H. R., Duthie, A. M., and Philpott, R. H. Rupture of the uterus. The preventable factors. *S. Afr. Med. J.* 50:505, 1976.

A review of 50 cases of ruptured uterus reveals that failure to progress during labor, particularly due to CPD, is a major cause of rupture of the uterus.

10. Knutzen, V. K., Tanneberger, U., and Davey, D. A. Complications and outcome of induced labor. *S. Afr. Med. J.* 52:482, 1977.

Inductions of labor in over 1000 patients were reviewed retrospectively. A 20% cesarean section rate was found, and the perinatal loss was not influenced by induction.

General

11. Miller, F. C. Quantitation of uterine activity. *Clin. Perinatol.* 8:27, 1981.

Quantitation of uterine activity provides a means of evaluating the effect of specific events, such as manipulation, medication, and anesthesia, on uterine activity. The development of techniques to measure uterine activity and the current state of the art are outlined.

12. The Cesarean Birth Task Force. NIH consensus development statement on cesarean childbirth. *Obstet. Gynecol.* 57:537, 1981.

The differences between CPD and dystocia or failure to progress are delineated. This category accounted for the single most important area of increase in the number of cesarean sections performed today.

13. Friedman, E. A. Dysfunctional labor. *Surg. Rounds* 7:46–56, 1980.

Patterns of contractibility of the uterus among women undergoing normal labors are often indistinguishable from those with abnormal progress. The challenge, says the author, is the timely recognition of those not progressing normally.

14. Miller, F. Uterine activity, labor management, and perinatal outcome. *Semin. Perinatol.* 2:181, 1978.

The goal of obstetric care is to accomplish delivery in the most atraumatic method possible. Cesarean section is always the best choice in cases of CPD, abnormal labors, and fetal distress.

15. Thom, M. H., Chan, K. K., and Studd, J. W. W. Outcome of normal and dysfunctional labor in different racial groups. *Am. J. Obstet. Gynecol.* 135:495, 1979.

This study investigated the outcome of spontaneous labor in 1643 vertex presentations. They advocate the use of meticulous attention to the dysfunctional labor to reduce prolonged labor as a cause of stillbirths.

Cephalopelvic Disproportion

Normal labor is characterized by progressive effacement and dilatation of the cervix associated with descent of the fetal presenting part. During the cervical changes that begin during the latent phase of labor or before, the cervix undergoes significant biochemical changes in the ground substance structure, reticulum, and water content. The rate of dilatation accelerates rapidly during the active phase and is complete by the end of the first stage. This cervical effacement and dilatation process is dependent on the presence of regular and orderly uterine contractions of adequate intensity and frequency. Descent of the fetal head begins during the last 2 weeks of gestation in about 80% of primigravidas, is maximal during the deceleration phase of labor, and is complete at the end of the second stage. It is dependent on uterine contractions, maternal pelvic capacity, and soft tissue resistance as well as fetal size, presentation, and position, and moldability of the vertex. The ultimate aim of the conduct of normal labor is an uneventful vaginal delivery of a healthy infant.

Most labors will progress in a normal fashion, leading to spontaneous vaginal delivery, but a small percentage will manifest abnormal patterns of progress in the form of protraction or arrest of dilatation, descent, or both. This dystocia represents a potential adverse effect on the fetus and mother. Consequently, it is prudent that all obstetric attendants be able to recognize these abnormal patterns as early as possible so that an orderly systematic plan of management can be undertaken.

Cephalopelvic disproportion (CPD) is defined as the inability of the presenting part of the fetal head to pass through the maternal pelvis. It occurs in about 1%–3% of all primigravidas, in nearly 30% of those who have a protracted active phase of dilatation or descent, and in about half of the parturients with arrest of descent. In fact, CPD is responsible for most abnormal labor patterns if uterine activity, as measured by intrauterine pressure monitoring, is adequate. The components of CPD are categorized into two factors: (1) maternal factors, which include size and shape of bony pelvis as well as soft tissue resistance; and (2) fetal factors, which include size, presentation, position, and moldability of the fetal head. Clinical evaluation of pelvic capacity can be done by digital examination at the patient's first antepartum visit and typing of the pelvis should be carried out according to the Caldwell-Moloy classification (gynecoid, android, anthropoid, or platypelloid). Attention must be directed to the diagonal conjugate, inclination of pelvic side walls, prominence of ischial spines, the shape of the sacrum, and angle of the suprapubic arch. About 85% will have a clinically adequate pelvic capacity, 1% will have a clearly inadequate pelvis, and the remainder will have a "borderline" pelvis. The following factors indicate a possible contracted pelvis: (1) ability to touch sacral promontory with index finger; (2) convergence of side walls; (3) forward inclination of a straight sacrum; (4) sharp ischial spines with small interspinous diameter; (5) narrow subpubic arch; (6) congenital sacral abnormality; (7) history of difficult labor and unexplained intrapartum fetal death; (8) maternal disease, such as rickets or polio, and trauma; and (9) adolescent pregnancy.

Digital pelvimetry should be repeated during the intrapartum period with attention paid to fetal-pelvic relationship; thus the pelvic capacity can be gauged against the dimensions of the presenting fetal part. Moreover, factors relating to presentation, position, and molding and descent of the fetal head during uterine contraction help one assess the possibility of successful vaginal delivery.

The presence of abnormal progress in labor (dystocia) may be the first evidence of pelvic inadequacy. Because about 45% of patients who develop secondary arrest of dilatation or descent, or both, will have CPD, careful evaluation of these patients is mandatory before any attempt is made at labor stimulation. Ultrasound and x-ray pelvimetry of fetal head size are the most accurate measurements to compare pelvic capacity with fetal head volume. There is, however, much controversy regarding the benefits of x-ray pelvimetry versus clinical assessment. Some believe that its benefits may far outweigh the theoretical risk of potential radiation hazards, while others feel the knowledge imparted by these tests is not useful.

Cephalopelvic disproportion, if not identified and managed promptly, will lead to increased maternal, fetal, or neonatal morbidity as well as mortality. Maternal risks include abnormal thinning of lower uterine segment with possible uterine rupture, pressure necrosis of the bladder, pelvic lacerations associated with instrument delivery, postpartum hemorrhage, and increased postpartum uterine infections. Fetal risks include fetal distress (10%), prolapse of cord, intracranial hemorrhage, skull fracture, and long-term neurologic abnormality.

Proper management of CPD involves early recognition during labor, identification of the cause, and prompt institution of therapy. A good initial history and physical examination, with proper index of suspicion in those with predisposing factors, is the most important first step. Attention should be given to the position and presentation of the fetal head detected by combined abdominal and pelvic examination, with special emphasis on the thrust of the fetal head in the birth canal during contractions or by applying fundal pressure (Müller-Hillis maneuver). The development of dystocia in the form of protraction or arrest disorders should be a warning sign of CPD, which may be verified by means of x-ray cephalopelvimetry.

The association of documented CPD with abnormal patterns in the form of arrest of dilatation or descent is an indication for cesarean section without any further trial of labor. The use of oxytocin stimulation of labor or midforceps procedures in the presence of possible CPD or arrest patterns of labor has no place in modern obstetrics practice because of their potential adverse effects on the fetus and the mother. In other cases of borderline CPD with dystocia, or in patients with inadequate labor alone, the use of Pitocin stimulation may be indicated. Once CPD is diagnosed by any other means, however, cesarean section is the treatment of choice.

Etiology

1. Friedman, E. A. Evaluation and management of pelvic dystocia. *Contemp. Ob/Gyn* 7:155, 1976.
   Detection of dystocia can be approached starting in the antepartum period with intrapartum reevaluation, followed by subsequent detection of those specifically developing abnormal labor patterns, and, finally, by using dynamic clinical and x-ray cephalopelvimetry.
2. Mengert, W. F., and Steer, C. M. Pelvic Capacity. In J. J. Sciarra (Ed.), *Gynecology and Obstetrics.* Hagerstown, Md.: Harper & Row, 1980. Vol. 2.
   Five factors combine to produce cephalopelvic disproportion: size and shape of the bony pelvis, force exerted by the uterus, size of the fetal head, moldability of the head, and presentation and position of the fetal head.
3. Rosen, M. G., et al. NIH consensus development statement on cesarean childbirth. The cesarean birth task force. *Obstet. Gynecol.* 57:537, 1981.
   The inaccurate classification of abnormal labor as CPD is frequent. Methods to avoid this problem are discussed.

Diagnosis

4. Barton, J. J., and Garbaciak, J. A. Is x-ray pelvimetry necessary? *Contemp. Ob/Gyn* 13:27, 1979.
   The authors question the continued use of a procedure that they feel yields information of dubious value. A review of the literature and the results of a year-long study led them to the conclusion that x-ray pelvimetry is unsafe and unnecessary.
5. Schifrin, B. S. The case against pelvimetry. *Contemp. Ob/Gyn* 4:77, 1974.
   The author condemns all x-ray pelvimetry because the technique is incapable of predicting outcome precisely when used alone; he offers a trial of Pitocin stimulation as a substitute in patients with arrested labor.
6. Danforth, D. N. Clinical Pelvimetry. In J. J. Sciarra (Ed.), *Gynecology and Obstetrics.* Hagerstown, Md.: Harper & Row, 1980. Vol. 2.
   The pelvic features that are accessible for clinical examination are the width of the forepelvis, the prominence of the ischial spines, the interspinous diameter, the curvature and position of the sacrum both in the midpelvis and at the outlet, the splay of the sidewalls, the width of the subpubic arch, the transverse diameter of the outlet, and, in some cases, the anteroposterior diameter of the pelvic inlet and outlet.
7. Jagani, N., et al. The predictability of labor outcome from a comparison of birth weight and x-ray pelvimetry. *Am. J. Obstet. Gynecol.* 139:507, 1981.
   Clinical estimates of birth weight versus x-ray pelvimetry were studied in 51 women with dysfunctional labor. The data suggests that neither pelvimetry nor the clinical estimate of birth weight provided a predictive tool for delivery outcome.
8. Krebs, H. B., Petres, R. E., and Dunn, L. J. Intrapartum fetal heart rate monitoring. V. Fetal heart rate patterns in the second stage of labor. *Am. J. Obstet. Gynecol.* 140:435, 1981.
   A total of 1755 heart rate tracings were reviewed in the second stage of

labor. Fetal heart rate abnormalities occurred in 91% of the patterns and were mild so that intervention on the basis of fetal distress or cephalopelvic disproportion was unnecessary.

Treatment

9. Miller, F. Uterine activity, labor management, and perinatal outcome. *Semin. Perinatol.* 2:181, 1978.

   The goal of obstetric care is to accomplish delivery in the most atraumatic method possible. Cesarean section is always the best choice in cases of CPD, abnormal labor, and fetal distress.

10. Stewart, K. S., and Philpott, R. H. Fetal response to cephalopelvic disproportion. *Br. J. Obstet. Gynaecol.* 87:641, 1980.

    One hundred eleven primigravidas with relative CPD were allowed to labor. In the group whose fetuses showed excessive molding, fetal heart rate and pH changes were noted.

11. Petrie, R. H. The pharmacology and use of oxytocin. *Clin. Perinatol.* 8:35, 1981.

    Historically, oxytocin has allowed the obstetrician to pharmacologically induce uterine contractions and to reduce rates of maternal and perinatal morbidity and mortality. The surveillance systems that can help to avoid these potential complications are described.

Intrapartum Fetal Distress

For nearly all persons, the most perilous hours during their early lives are those spent traversing the maternal birth canal. Although the risk of intrapartum fetal death is quite low, there is strong evidence that this risk can be nearly obviated by employing the sophisticated electronic fetal monitoring (EFM) devices now available. However, actual intrapartum demise is probably only a small part of the potential damage related to intrapartum events. Sublethal brain injury may be clinically obvious (such as cerebral palsy) or ascertainable only by special testing (such as in some learning disabilities). Of considerable, and currently largely hypothetical, concern is the potentially even larger number of individuals who may have sustained a mild form of intrapartum neurologic injury. Although such individuals might fall within the normal range on all or most neurobehavioral tests, there is no current method to define genetic intellectual potential and thereby estimate mild neurologic damage. The purposes of this essay are to define fetal distress operationally, to explain how EFM can aid in making this diagnosis, and to outline management designed to alleviate the distress before any permanent damage is done.

Until the introduction and popularization of EFM, the most common diagnostic criterion for fetal distress was an average fetal heart rate (FHR) outside the limits of 120–160 beats per minute. We now understand that, in the absence of such alarming FHR patterns as recurrent late or recurrent severe variable decelerations or the absence of FHR variability, the healthy fetus may indeed have a baseline FHR outside these limits and perhaps be responding appropriately to a stress, such as maternal fever.

There is currently some controversy concerning the appropriateness of routinely employing EFM for all patients. Even though the data is inconclusive, the evidence currently favors the position that EFM as a means of intrapartum fetal surveillance is superior to the less sophisticated methods. The choice of its use remains with the physician and the patient. For operational purposes, the following definition may be reasonable: fetal distress is a precarious fetal condition that, if allowed to persist, may lead to fetal damage or to perinatal death. Implicit in this definition is the philosophy that such a diagnosis indeed can be made prior to any associated fetal damage and that reasonable means do exist for the prevention of damage when and if fetal distress occurs. It is unreasonable to define fetal distress in such a way that once the diagnosis becomes definitive there is a high likelihood of damage having already occurred.

Of all potential stresses on the fetus, the most physiologic is that associated with uterine contractions. Since the blood supply to the intervillous space traverses the myometrium, contractions of even mild intensity temporarily interrupt this blood supply. Thus, ordinary contractions, even those normally occurring in the antepartum period, produce recurrent hypoxic stresses on the fetus. The normally oxygenated fetus has mechanisms to cope with such stresses and tolerates them without ill effects. However, the fetus with suboptimal oxygenation reacts to the hypoxic stresses of uterine contractions by rather symmetrical depressions of the FHR, late in the contraction cycles: the pattern of late deceleration. Myers and his associates, working with fetal monkeys, found that this pattern (when occurring repetitively) invariably implies that fetal hypoxemia is present. Recurrent severe variable (cord compression) decelerations (with slow recovery of FHR to baseline) also imply fetal hypoxemia and thus should be considered with the same degree of concern as recurrent late decelerations.

Fetal hypoxemia, however, at least initially, does not necessarily imply fetal damage. Indeed, it is lactic (metabolic) acidosis, the consequence of prolonged, suboptimal oxygenation, that has a high potential for causing fetal damage. Within the fetal cells, energy production is maintained primarily by the aerobic catabolism of glucose. As long as fetal oxygenation is adequate, glucose is fully oxidized to water and carbon dioxide, and large quantities of energy are thereby produced. Whenever the oxygenation is suboptimal, part or all of the glucose is diverted toward the production of lactic acid and the pH drops as a consequence of a reduction in bicarbonate reserves.

The degree of this metabolic acidosis depends, among other things, on the depth and duration of the hypoxia as well as on the preexisting energy and acid-base states. There has been recent interest in the possibility that the hyperglycemic fetus may produce more lactic acid in response to prolonged hypoxia, and thus have potentially more central nervous system (CNS) damage than does the normoglycemic fetus. This idea, which has been reviewed recently by Beard and Rivers, should cause us to question the wisdom of routinely administering intravenous glucose to laboring patients.

Depression of FHR variability regularly occurs whenever fetal acidosis becomes significant. Therefore, the presence of normal variability can be relied upon clinically to indicate that the fetus, at that particular time and despite whatever otherwise ominous signs are present on the FHR monitor, is not seriously acidotic. Reliance upon FHR variability as an indicator of fetal status, however, depends upon an understanding of several factors. First, the assessment of variability can be made only from internal electrodes, which detect fetal electrocardiographic signals. External Doppler signals are inherently "noisy" and do not represent true variability. Second, fetal sleep and maternal administration of drugs may depress FHR variability without implying fetal metabolic acidosis. If CNS-depressant drugs (such as narcotics, barbiturates, benzodiazepines, and perhaps magnesium sulfate) are given to the mother, the fetal CNS may be depressed as well, and FHR variability as a criterion of fetal status temporarily may be lost. Secobarbital given for sedation in cases of false labor seems particularly potent in depressing variability for many hours subsequent to its use.

The finding of recurrent late or recurrent severe variable decelerations (as well as sudden, prolonged decelerations) then suffices for a diagnosis of fetal distress and should prompt attempts to treat this problem of the in utero perinate. Intrauterine resuscitation has two primary goals: improvement of uterine blood flow to the intervillous space and augmentation of the maternal-fetal PO_2 difference. The first and most crucial goal, improvement in uterine blood flow, is promoted by maintaining the patient in the left lateral decubitus position, by correcting any hypotension (increasing the intravenous infusion rate, elevating the legs, or administering ephedrine sulfate intravenously), and by stopping any oxytocin being administered. If there is a variable deceleration component to the distress pattern (including the prolonged deceleration), then other maternal positions, including the knee-chest position with or without digital elevation of the presenting part, should be tried. The latter maneuver may aid in the diagnosis of occult cord prolapse. The use of tocolytic agents to depress uterine contractions may also become part of the standard therapy for fetal distress in the future.

For the second goal in the treatment of fetal distress, augmentation of the maternal-fetal PO_2 difference, administration of oxygen by mask to the mother can increase fetal oxygenation to some extent, but only if uterine blood flow is adequate. Thus, the procedures enumerated to achieve adequate blood flow should supercede the institution of mask oxygenation. Most frequently, these procedures outlined for intrauterine resuscitation will resolve the abnormal FHR patterns, and labor can be safely permitted to continue. Such fetal distress is then termed *transient.* If the late or severe variable, or both, patterns remain after the intrauterine resuscitative efforts, the distress is termed *persistent,* and consideration of expedient delivery is generally made.

The presence of normal FHR variability (with internal FHR monitoring systems) is reassuring and may well allow some procrastination in the management of persistent fetal distress, although such cases should be considered individually. For example, for a multipara at 8 cm of cervical dilatation and station $+2$, procrastination in the presence of normal FHR variability is usually appropriate. On the other hand, a primigravida, 2 cm dilated and at station -4 with persistent distress, should be considered for prompt delivery, regardless of variability on the FHR record. In the latter case, vaginal delivery is generally many hours distant and the likelihood of fetal metabolic deterioration too great to condone a long delay in delivery.

For cases between these extremes of dilatation and station, especially if the FHR variability is or becomes depressed, ascertainment of normal fetal acid-base status by frequent assessment of fetal-scalp blood pH is an alternative, although an engaged presenting part and at least 4 cm of cervical dilatation are required for these assessments. A pH value of below 7.25 is generally regarded as indicating acidosis severe enough to prompt delivery. Whenever delivery for fetal distress is deemed necessary, the route of delivery must be that by which the fetus is least traumatized. If standard conditions, including adequate anesthesia, are met for a low or midforceps application, then such a procedure may be deemed appropriate; otherwise, cesarean section is the procedure of choice. The distressed fetus is even less likely to tolerate well a traumatic midforceps operation than is the nondistressed fetus, since respiratory distress, intracranial hemorrhage, and necrotizing enterocolitis are more likely to occur in the former.

The initial preparations for cesarean section, including alerting of necessary anesthetic, pediatric, and nursing personnel, should begin at the time that the diagnosis of fetal distress is made and as intrauterine resuscitative efforts are being instituted. Although such instances often will ultimately be termed transient fetal distress, mobilizing the forces necessary to expedite delivery is necessary for that unpredictable minority for whom the distress will be persistent. So that misunderstanding will not occur among these personnel, it may be necessary to thoughtfully educate all providers as to why their immediate presence is required. Ideally, any hospital offering obstetric services should have 24-hour, in-house availability of these support personnel.

In summary, we are currently able, with reasonable accuracy, to detect by EFM the fetus with intrapartum hypoxia (fetal distress). If these recurrent late or recurrent severe variable decelerations are unresponsive to efforts at intrauterine resuscitation, metabolic acidosis with its potential for poor perinatal outcome may follow. Unless CNS-depressant drugs have been administered to the mother, such acidosis is suggested by loss of FHR variability and can be confirmed by assessment of fetal scalp pH. If fetal distress is not responsive to ordinary efforts, expedient delivery must be considered before metabolic acidosis supervenes. With early reaction to fetal distress, assuming appropriate team support and avoidance of fetal trauma during delivery, the incidence of severe neonatal depression should be very low. However, it must be considered inappropriate to withhold intervention until neonatal depression is virtually certain. We must never feel it necessary to apologize for the operative delivery of a healthy baby who, in our best judgment, would have been placed in jeopardy by inaction.

Review

1. Beard, R. W., and Rivers, R. P. A. Fetal asphyxia in labor. *Lancet* 2:1117, 1979.
   Perinatal asphyxia, diagnosable by commonly available electronic techniques is frequently the antecedent of perinatal brain damage. Intrapartum administration of glucose may be potentially detrimental to the fetus.
2. Hagberg, B., Hagberg, G., and Olow, I. The changing panorama of cerebral palsy in Sweden 1954–70. *Acta Paediatr. Scand.* 64:187, 1975.
   This review from Sweden concludes that about half of the cerebral palsy cases in that country probably result from perinatal asphyxia.
3. Neutra, R. R., Greenland, S., and Friedman, E. A. The relationship between electronic fetal monitoring and apgar score. *Am. J. Obstet. Gynecol.* 140:440, 1981.
   A retrospective study of 14,350 babies with and without fetal monitoring was reviewed. In a group of high-risk pregnancies, monitored babies had a more favorable five minute apgar versus the group without monitoring. In the normal patient there was no indication of benefit of monitoring in the prediction of fetal distress.

Uteroplacental Physiology

4. Greiss, F. C., Jr. Pressure-flow relationship in the gravid uterine vascular bed. *Am. J. Obstet. Gynecol.* 96:41, 1966.
   In sheep, the uterine artery is normally maximally dilated and will not further dilate to meet additional needs.
5. Parer, J. T. Normal and impaired placental exchange. *Contemp. Ob/Gyn* 7:117, 1976.
   The basics of uteroplacental physiology are presented. The presentation of factors involved in fetal oxygenation are detailed.

6. Ramsey, E. M. Uteroplacental circulation during labor. *Clin. Obstet. Gynecol.* 11:78, 1968.
   In this paper the author demonstrates the adverse influences of normal contractions on uterine and intervillous space blood flow. At the peak of even modest contractions, intervillous space flow is either severely reduced or it ceases.
7. Goodlin, R. C., Quaife, M. A., and Dirksen, J. W. The significance, diagnosis, and treatment of maternal hypovolemia as associated with fetal/maternal illness. *Semin. Perinatol.* 5:163, 1981.
   Hypovolemia will decrease uterine blood flow and can cause fetal distress. The authors advocate the measurement of plasma volume at various times during pregnancy to rule out abnormal conditions.

Effects of Hypoxia on the Fetus

8. Martin, C. B., Jr., et al. Mechanisms of late decelerations in the fetal heart rate of lambs. *Eur. J. Obstet. Gynaecol. Reprod. Biol.* 9:361, 1979.
   This study demonstrates that late decelerations occur by two mechanisms, both triggered by fetal hypoxemia. If the fetal acid-base status is normal, the deceleration is mediated by the vagal system; if acidemic, the mechanism is direct depression of myocardial rhythmicity.
9. Marx, G. F., Mahajan, S., and Miclat, M. N. Correlation of biochemical data with Apgar scores at birth and at one minute. *Br. J. Anaesth.* 49:831, 1977.
   The cord blood pH correlates better with the immediate condition of the neonate than the condition at five minutes of age. Neonatal ventilation during the first minute of life accounted for this difference, the pH being thereby normalized by the rapid loss of carbon dioxide.
10. Myter, R. E. Lactic Acid Accumulation as Cause of Brain Edema and Cerebral Necrosis Resulting from Oxygen Deprivation. In R. Korobkin and C. Guilleminault (Eds.), *Advances in Perinatal Neurology.* New York: Spectrum Publications, 1979.
    In monkeys subjected to hypoxia, those with low blood glucose concentrations sustained far less brain damage than those that had been given food. This difference in brain damage was related to the concentration of lactate in the brain tissues. Routine administration of glucose intravenous fluids to the laboring patient may be deleterious.
11. Myers, R. E., Mueller-Heubach, E., and Adamsons, K. Predictability of the state of fetal oxygenation from the quantitative analysis of the components of late deceleration. *Am. J. Obstet. Gynecol.* 115:1083, 1973.
    In fetal monkeys, recurrent late decelerations invariably imply fetal hypoxemia, and in the absence of hypoxia late decelerations do not occur, even with fetal acidosis.
12. Painter, M. J., Depp, R., and O'Donoghue, P. D. Fetal heart rate patterns and development in the first year of life. *Am. J. Obstet. Gynecol.* 132:271, 1978.
    In follow-up examinations of children who had prolonged and severe abnormal fetal heart rate patterns during labor these patterns were not found to be detrimental. Although not controlled, it is probably the best study in the literature relating fetal distress to long-term outcome of the children.
13. Low, J. A., et al. The prediction of intrapartum fetal metabolic acidosis by fetal heart rate monitoring. *Am. J. Obstet. Gynecol.* 139:299, 1981.
    Two hundred babies with metabolic acidosis at delivery were compared to an equal number with normal acid-base status. In reviewing the fetal heart rate characteristics during the intrapartum period, it was found

that marked decelerations of any variety as well as late decelerations were predictive of fetal hypoxia and thus metabolic acidosis.

Clinical Use of Fetal Monitoring

14. Cohen, W. R., Schifrin, B. S., and Doctor, G. Elevation of the fetal presenting part: A method of intrauterine resuscitation. *Am. J. Obstet. Gynecol.* 123:646, 1975.
    This report demonstrates that by digitally elevating the fetal presenting part, the diagnosis of occult cord prolapse, as well as its immediate treatment, can be accomplished.
15. Hon, E. H., and Quilligan, E. J. Classification of fetal heart rate: II. A revised working classification. *Conn. Med.* 31:779, 1967.
    This widely quoted publication is the source for the everyday terms related to accelerations and decelerations of the fetal heart rate.
16. Huddleston, J. F., Perlis, H. W., and Harris, B. A., Jr. The case for electronic fetal monitoring. *J. Reprod. Med.* 25:47, 1980.
    Routine electronic fetal monitoring is considered by some to be harmful. In this paper an argument is advanced that such monitoring, properly interpreted, is of value in recognizing (at an early time) those distressed fetuses who might benefit by intervention.
17. Parer, J. T. FHR monitoring: Answering the critics. *Contemp. Ob/Gyn* 17:163, 1981.
    A very complete and succinct article enumerating the studies, both pro and con, regarding fetal monitoring in labor and its relationship to fetal distress. A nice section regarding the technologic advances and the problems they have engendered is offered.
18. Kubli, F. W., et al. Observations on heart rate and pH in the human fetus during labor. *Am. J. Obstet. Gynecol.* 104:1190, 1969.
    The pH of fetal scalp blood is related to the presence of periodic patterns. The presence of accelerations or early or mild-to-moderate variable decelerations were generally associated with normal fetal pH. Severe variable decelerations or recurrent late decelerations of any magnitude were frequently associated with acidosis of the fetal scalp blood.
19. Paul, R. H., et al. Clinical fetal monitoring: VII. The evaluation and significance of intrapartum FHR variability. *Am. J. Obstet. Gynecol.* 123:206, 1975.
    The presence of normal variability in the presence of late and severe variable deceleration patterns was shown to be associated with a better fetal acid-base status than if variability was subnormal. Thus normal fetal heart rate variability is an indicator of normal fetal metabolic status even in the presence of ominous deceleration patterns.
20. Goodlin, R. C. Why fetal monitoring. *Semin. Perinatol.* 5:105, 1981.
    The pros and cons of routine fetal monitoring are described. Both definite and elective indications for its application are delineated.
21. Perkins, R. P. Sudden fetal death in labor. The significance of antecedent monitoring characteristics and clinical circumstances. *J. Reprod. Med.* 25:309, 1980.
    The characteristics of fetal monitoring data found just prior to death are discussed and suggestions for appropriate responses to avoid fetal death are offered. The fetal monitor is an invaluable tool for this reason.
22. Low, J. A., et al. The effect of maternal, labor, and fetal factors upon fetal heart rate during the intrapartum period. *Am. J. Obstet. Gynecol.* 139:306, 1981.
    The effect of various maternal, fetal, and labor characteristics on the diagnosis of fetal distress during delivery was studied in 400 patients.

Changes in variability and baseline rates were observed with abnormal labor whereas variable decelerations were observed with premature infants.

Neonatal Resuscitation

It is the responsibility of each obstetrician to be skilled in the technique of neonatal resuscitation since he may perform the task or direct a team of providers in this action. Each physician and nurse who practices obstetrics must anticipate a need for resuscitation, be able to recognize a newborn who may require special measures, and be able to respond with the appropriate resuscitative measures. The presence of any antenatal or intrapartum risk factor may signal an infant who needs resuscitation. Such risk factors include, but are not limited to, maternal illnesses, extremes of reproductive age, multiparity, drug abuse, hypertension, isoimmunization, prolonged rupture of membranes, and antenatal hemorrhage. Obviously, new risks may arise during labor: malpresentation, premature labor, abnormal fetal heart rate problems, abnormal labor, passage of meconium, presence of maternal medication, and others. Even normal labor is a physiologic stress for the fetus. It is therefore imperative that compulsive fetal monitoring (either frequent auscultation at appropriate times or continuous electronic monitoring) be carried out during labor.

Since the need for potential neonatal resuscitation exists with each delivery, each delivery area should be well equipped and staffed with individuals who are skilled in advanced life support for neonates. Basic equipment includes a radiant heat source, oxygen, suction catheters, oral airways, resuscitation bag, face mask, endotracheal tubes, laryngoscope, umbilical catheters, and three-way stop cocks. Equipment should be checked before each delivery. Medications and fluids such as atropine, sodium bicarbonate, calcium, dextrose, epinephrine, albuminosol, Ringer's lactate, and naloxone should be readily available. Each person attending the delivery should be familiar with the types of resuscitation bags and face masks that are available and should be skilled in their use. Masks, tubes, airways, laryngoscope blades, suction catheters, and umbilical catheters should be available in sizes that are appropriate for both the small and large infant. Physicians should have intimate knowledge of both straight and tapered endotracheal tubes and should be able to select the appropriate size.

One can recognize the need for resuscitation by scrutinizing the infant shortly after birth. The time-honored method of systematic evaluation is the Apgar score. At 1 minute and again at 5 minutes after complete birth of the infant, a score of 0, 1, or 2 is assigned to five parameters: heart rate, respirations, muscle tone, reflex irritability, and color. Since maximal depression of the infant usually occurs approximately 60 seconds after complete delivery, the 1-minute score is the best assessment regarding the need for resuscitation. The 5-minute score, although a rough index, is the best predictor of future morbidity and mortality. A score of 2 is given for a heart rate greater than 100, good quality respirations and crying, active muscular motion, a cough or sneeze in reflex to a catheter in the nares or a vigorous cry in response to gentle flicking of the sole, and a completely pink color. A score of 1 is assigned for the following: heart rate below 100, slow or irregular respiratory efforts, some flexion of the extremities, a grimace in response to nasal catheter or a flick of the sole, and a pink body with blue hands and feet. A score of 0 is given for: absent heart rate, absent respiratory efforts, absent muscle tone, absent response to irritable stimulus, and pale or blue color. The most important parameters are heart rate, respirations, and muscle tone.

There is a spectrum of resuscitative maneuvers. In general, successful resuscitation follows a systematic scheme that follows the alphabet ("ABCDE"): (1) maintenance of an airway, (2) support of breathing, (3) support of circulation, (4) administration of appropriate drugs, and (5) continued evaluation. Depending on the severity of the neonate's depression, any or all of those steps may be required. The clinical observations, which the Apgar system requires, provide the clue to the degree of resuscitative attempts one must initiate and when they should be begun. Infants with an Apgar score of 7–10 at 1 minute represent the majority of infants. These newborns cry within several seconds of birth and respond to the gentle stimulus of suctioning and drying. Such infants require only a warm environment and observation.

Infants who score 4–6 are considered moderately distressed. These infants have abnormal respiration (either depressed or absent), but the heart rate is greater than 100. They are usually limp and cyanotic but demonstrate some response to irritable stimuli. Moderately depressed infants require an oxygen-rich environment as well as gentle suctioning and drying. Since even a normal infant may be born without oxygen reserves, it is essential that the compromised infant receive oxygen. The oxygen may be supplied through a face mask and resuscitation bag, and most infants will have prompt favorable response. Only in the presence of meconium should mask resuscitation not be attempted. If the heart rate falls below 100 or if color and respirations do not improve within 1 minute, endotracheal intubation should be promptly performed.

There is universal agreement that the infant who scores 0, 1, or 2 (and most authorities include 3) is severely depressed. These infants demand immediate attention; it is both meaningless and dangerous to procrastinate until 60 seconds after delivery. This newborn should be immediately dried and placed in the Trendelenburg position under a radiant warmer. The nose and pharynx should be cleared by gentle bulb suctioning, and oxygenation should be started with bag and mask ventilation. Utilizing direct visualization with laryngoscope, the trachea should be intubated and the infant ventilated with oxygen. It is frequently necessary to suction the endotracheal tube. If there is persistent bradycardia, external cardiac massage is required. An umbilical catheter should be placed as soon as possible so that drugs and fluids can be administered.

Every obstetrician should be skilled in neonatal endotracheal intubation. In an emergency it is best to perform oral intubation. For those infants who will require prolonged intubation, a change to the nasal route can be performed later. The laryngoscope is held in the resuscitator's left hand. Its blade is introduced into the right side of the infant's mouth and is used to deviate the tongue to the left. The blade should rest between the base of the tongue and the epiglottis but care must be taken not to place extreme pressure on the surrounding tissue. A gentle upward tip of the laryngoscope blade will expose the glottis, which will appear as a dark vertical slit. Beneath the glottis is a transverse slit, the esophagus. The endotracheal tube should be placed into the glottis and advanced approximately 2.5 cm below the glottis in the term infant but less in a preterm infant. After intubation, one should watch for bilateral chest wall movements and should listen for bilateral breath sounds. Inadvertent intubation of either the esophagus or the right main stem bronchus should be corrected immediately. In the event that the heart rate does not return to 100 or more after 1 minute of ventilatory assistance, it is necessary to perform cardiac compression. Both one-hand and two-hand methods are suitable, but it is essential to be expert with one. In the two-hand method, the resuscitator's hands encircle the chest so that the fingers support the back and the two thumbs lie over the midsternum. Depending on the size of the infant, the thumbs are side-by-side or superimposed. In the one-hand method, the infant's back is supported with one hand and the middle and index fingers of the other hand are used to compress the sternum. With either method, the midsternum is compressed one-half to three-quarters of an inch at a rate of 100 compressions per minute. Ventilation should be provided every fifth compression while the sternum is relaxed.

Severely depressed infants, especially those without immediate response, require administration of drugs and fluid. Ideally all drugs should be administered intravenously. The umbilical vein can usually be quickly catheterized with a 3.5 or 5.0F endhole catheter. Direct needle puncture of the umbilical cord, intramuscular injections, and subcutaneous injections should be avoided if at all possible. Severely depressed infants are frequently hypovolemic and fluid replacement is the first line of treatment after respiration is accomplished; 5% albumisol, Ringer's lactate, or O-negative whole blood crossmatched against the mother can be used. Each of these volume expanders is administered at a dose of 15 ml/kg of body weight.

Intravenous bicarbonate is a time-honored method of correcting acidosis. However, there is an association between bicarbonate infusion and intracranial hemorrhage. The present recommendation is that all sodium bicarbonate be diluted $1:1$ with 5% dextrose in water, and that it should be administered at a slow rate. The initial dose is 2 mEq/l/kg. Ideally, pH and blood measurements should be obtained after the initial dose so that subsequent doses can be calculated according to need. If blood gas measurements are not available, dilute sodium bicarbonate can be slowly administered at a rate of 1 mEq/l/kg every 10 minutes during arrest. In general, this drug is not favored by most neonatologists for initial resuscitation, however.

Epinephrine may be required for persistent bradycardia, cardiac asystole, or hypotension. Epinephrine hydrochloride is administered as a $1:10,000$ solution. The initial dose is 0.1 ml/kg, and it may be repeated every 5 minutes. Calcium is available in more than one form, but 10% calcium chloride is optimal since it results in the delivery of ionized calcium. It should be administered slowly at a dose of 0.3 ml/kg. The calcium chloride may be repeated every 10–20 minutes if favorable responses are obtained. Persistent bradycardia is sometimes treated with atropine sulfate in a dose of 0.03 mg/kg. It is recommended that atropine not be repeated more than twice and it is also not a first-line drug.

The asphyxiated newborn is frequently hypoglycemic. Dextrose can be given as a 25% solution at a dose of 2 ml/kg, but most prefer a more dilute solution. After this initial dose, 10% dextrose can be given as a continuous infusion that is not to exceed 4 ml/kg/hour.

A cause other than asphyxia of neonatal respiratory depression is administration of narcotics to the mother during labor. The drug of choice for infant resuscitation in this case is naloxone hydrochloride in a dose of 0.01 mg/kg. This dose may be repeated every 2–3 minutes. Since naloxone does not cause respiratory depression, it can be given upon suspicion of neonatal narcotic overdose. It is important to remember that the narcotic effect may outlast the action of naloxone, so the infant who has responded successfully to naloxone should be watched for subsequent recurrence of respiratory depression.

Special consideration must be given to the infant who is born with particulate meconium-staining of the amniotic fluid. Thorough suctioning is essential if meconium aspiration syndrome is to be avoided. As delivery becomes imminent, a sterile De Lee suction catheter is placed in the mouth of the physician. As soon as the head is delivered, and even before the remainder of the infant is delivered, a thorough suctioning of the nasopharynx (through the nose) and the hypopharynx (through the mouth) is performed. After the umbilical cord is divided, the larynx is inspected if the infant is not crying vigorously and the trachea is suctioned if meconium is present in the region of the vocal cords. The same procedure is performed whether the infant is delivered vaginally or by cesarean section.

There are few areas of medicine that summon a physician's resuscitative skills as frequently as the delivery area. Communication between perinatal and neonatal physicians is mandatory as is direction among the team of health-care providers in the delivery room. Frequent dialogue with expert neonatologists provides a source for keeping current.

Reviews

1. Advanced cardiac life support for neonates. In Standards and Guidelines for Cardiopulmonary Resuscitation and Emergency Cardiac Care. *J.A.M.A.* 244:495, 1980.
   Thorough review of all aspects of neonatal resuscitation.
2. James, L. S. Newborn and Infant Resuscitation. In E. J. Quilligan, and N. Kretchmer (Eds.), *Fetal and Maternal Medicine.* New York: Wiley, 1980.
   Up-to-date and concise review.
3. Korones, S. B. Evaluation and Management of the Infant Immediately After Birth. In *High-Risk Newborn Infants* (2nd ed.). St. Louis: Mosby, 1976.
   Good reading for both physicians and nurses.
4. Pritchard, J. A., and MacDonald, P. C. The Newborn Infant. In *Williams Obstetrics* (16th ed.). New York: Appleton-Century-Crofts, 1980.
   This leading textbook offers a superb presentation of basic facts.
5. Robie, G., and Bowes, W. A., Jr. Immediate Resuscitation of the Newborn Infant. In E. J. Quilligan (Ed.), *Current Therapy in Obstetrics and Gynecology.* Philadelphia: Saunders, 1980.
   Practical, concise, and up-to-date review of management of the depressed newborn.

Meconium Aspiration Syndrome

6. Simmons, M. A. Cooperation can prevent or lower the risk of meconium aspiration. *Contemp. Ob/Gyn* 11:29, 1978.
   Thorough suctioning of the nasopharynx and hypopharynx has resulted in much lower morbidity and mortality from meconium aspiration syndrome. This article reviews the problem and its management.

Techniques

7. Hilger, J. S., Holzman, I. R., and Brown, D. R. Sequential changes in placental blood gases and pH during the hour following delivery. *J. Reprod. Med.* 26:305, 1981.
   The use of an isolated segment of umbilical cord for blood gas assessment was correlated with infant outcome, with and without resuscitation. It was found that the values obtained from the isolated segment of cord

were equal to those obtained from the infant itself in predicting neonatal acidosis.

8. Shaffer, K. Neonatal resuscitation. *Nebr. Med. J.* 65:88, 1980.
   The author describes the technique of neonatal resuscitation and some of the dangers that can be encountered.
9. Shaffer, K. Neonatal resuscitation: Part II. *Nebr. Med. J.* 65:122, 1980.
   The author details the implications of neonatal resuscitation as well as the outcome.
10. Devore, J. S. Resuscitation of the newborn. *Clin. Obstet. Gynecol.* 19:607, 1976.
    A complete review of the indications, techniques, and management problems regarding resuscitation of the newborn.

Complications

11. Volpe, J. J. Neonatal intraventricular hemorrhage. *N. Engl. J. Med.* 304:886, 1981.
    This excellent article outlines the causes and effects of neonatal intraventricular hemorrhage which often confound prolonged neonatal resuscitation. The pathogenesis as well as outcome data and management is presented.
12. Valman, H. B. Resuscitation of the newborn. *Br. Med. J.* 2:1343, 1979.
    The author describes several complications that can follow resuscitation of the newborn. Methods of preventing these problems are described.
13. Sheehan, P., Barry, P. J., and O'Brian, N. G. Resuscitation at birth and subsequent development to six years. *Ir. Med. J.* 70:107, 1977.
    The authors followed a number of infants who had been resuscitated at birth for severe asphyxia. The results showed that the infants who were adequately resuscitated had very little neurological deficits.
14. Gregory, G. A. Resuscitation of the newborn. *Anesthesiology* 43:225, 1975.
    The author describes indications and problems with resuscitation of the newborn. The outcome of a number of patients is described.

Delivery of the Small and Large Infant

In many cases the size of a fetus tends to be erroneously estimated before birth. Typically, the size of a small fetus is overestimated and the size of a large fetus is underestimated. Such errors may lead to unnecessary emergency situations. In this chapter, the small infant will be arbitrarily defined as one weighing less than 2000 grams. The large infant will be understood to weigh over 4000 grams.

Today, survival of infants weighing between 850 and 1000 g is considered probable. Survival of infants weighing less than 1500 g was unusual before the development of modern high-risk perinatal care, and such infants were usually allowed to be delivered without special attention. The first priority in the care of the small infant (850–2000 g) is to prevent delivery, if reasonably possible. This essay will assume, however, that attempts at prevention of premature labor have been made and have been unsuccessful. The small infant may be premature, growth-retarded, or both, and is very fragile. Labor should be conducted close to a nursery capable of providing the intensive care required by metabolically compromised babies. Particularly in the case of the smaller infants in this group (i.e., under 1500 g), maternal transport to a tertiary-care facility for delivery should be implemented.

Electronic fetal monitoring should be employed with all small infants during labor to facilitate the early detection of hypoxia and acidosis, which, if present, may result in hypoperfusion of lungs, gut, and kidneys, as well as in direct damage to the fetal brain. Hypoperfusion of the lungs may also cause diminution of surfactant production in the true preterm infant, with increased likelihood of respiratory distress syndrome. If the infant is small because of growth retardation, it will be especially at risk of hypoxia during labor although the lungs may be mature. Therefore, if vaginal delivery is elected, the obstetrician should be prepared to intervene surgically at any time for recurrent significant (late or severe variable, or both) decelerations of the fetal heart rate (FHR) and/or significant loss of FHR variability. Severe variable decelerations are very commonly seen late in the labor of women with small fetuses. These decelerations may represent not only pressure on the umbilical cord, but also compression of the fetal thorax. They carry an ominous significance, especially if FHR variability is diminished or if there is a slow return of the FHR to the baseline rate. Labor involving these infants should be conducted in an area where cesarean section can be done rapidly and adequacy of nursing and support personnel is assured.

Breech presentation presents a particular problem in the premature or growth-retarded infant as the head of this infant is often much larger in proportion to the rest of the infant than in the term baby. The body and extremities may be delivered before the cervix is dilated sufficiently to permit the passage of the head. The resulting dystocia with umbilical cord compression predisposes to severe anoxia, and subsequent efforts of the obstetrician may cause severe trauma to the infant's neck or brachial plexus. Several recent studies indicate substantially greater perinatal morbidity in the small breech baby delivered vaginally compared with abdominal delivery. Therefore, I believe that the small infant in breech presentation is best delivered by cesarean section.

When the delivery of premature or growth-retarded infants involves twins, slightly different considerations apply. If the first twin presents in the breech position, exactly the same considerations apply as with a singleton, and cesarean section should be done. If the first twin delivers as a "vertex" and the second twin presents in the "breech" position, extraction of the second twin may be performed, but only if an anesthesiologist expert in the administration of a type of anesthesia that produces maximal uterine relaxation, such as halothane, is available. Otherwise, primary cesarean section is recommended for both twins.

Ultrasonic evaluation of both biparietal diameters is advisable to ascertain that the second twin's head is not substantially larger than that of the first. If both twins present by the vertex and the first has been delivered vaginally, vaginal delivery may reasonably be expected for the second twin. The second fetal heart should be closely observed by electronic monitoring; a scalp electrode is preferable. If the slightest fetal distress develops, or if labor is not effectual, cesarean section should be done. Internal podalic version is not recommended. Vaginal delivery of twins should be carried out in a room equipped for immediate cesarean section, with both the scrub nurse and the anesthesiologist present and ready to proceed. If any difficulty is encountered in delivery of the second twin, cesarean section should proceed immediately.

If the small infant presents in the vertex position, I favor vaginal delivery for those weighing from 1000 to 2000 g. For those below 1000 g, cesarean section appears preferable because of the extreme fragility of the fetal head and its blood vessels. If vaginal delivery is to take place, it should be conducted with great care. A generous episiotomy is indicated. Low forceps offer more protection to the fetal head than prolonged pushing against a rigid perineum. Midforceps should not be employed. Delivery of these fragile infants must occur in a facility where all necessary pediatric and obstetric personnel are present.

Anesthesia and analgesia should be used sparingly in the labor for and delivery of small infants. It has previously been felt that these agents cause neonatal depression and subsequent behavioral abnormalities. On the other hand, sedatives may depress fetal brain metabolism and maternal catecholamine secretion, thus increasing uteroplacental blood flow while reducing the fetal oxygen requirement. I feel that epidural anesthesia for labor, with or without pudenal block for the actual delivery, offers the best prognosis for the infant.

If cesarean section is done, it is done to deliver the infant as gently as possible. In most labors involving small babies, the lower uterine segment is poorly developed. Therefore, attempts to perform a low-transverse section often result in a very difficult delivery with excessive trauma to the infant. Accordingly, most cesarean deliveries of small infants should be by a low-vertical incision. In many cases this incision will have to extend into the upper uterine segment.

Infants weighing more than 4000 g are often delivered vaginally. Although childhood malnutrition and rickets (with their stultifying influence upon the developing female pelvis) are rare, there are increases in both fetal and maternal morbidity and mortality in association with the large fetus. Large fetuses are more commonly male and are associated with postdate pregnancies or those gestations complicated by maternal diabetes. The second stage of labor tends to exceed 2 hours, and there is a higher likelihood of shoulder dystocia. Fetal asphyxia is more common if the baby is large.

For all the reasons noted in the preceding paragraph, the large fetus in breech presentation should be delivered by cesarean section. Breech delivery increases the incidence of prolonged labor, intrapartum asphyxia, and mechanical dystocia. The added risk of fetal macrosomia makes vaginal breech delivery unacceptable. The large fetus in vertex presentation tends to descend slowly through the pelvis. This, in turn, tends to suggest the use of midforceps, which are associated with less than favorable neonatal outcome.

The large fetus arrested in midpelvis is much more appropriately delivered by cesarean section. This is particularly true because of the possibility of shoulder dystocia. Shoulder dystocia is most likely to occur in the presence of fetal macrosomia, maternal obesity, and a history of previous infants weighing over 4000 g. Shoulder dystocia is best treated by being avoided. A head in midpelvis after a second stage of 2 hours or more in a primigravida (or 1 hour or more in a multipara) is a danger signal, and cesarean section must be seriously considered.

If shoulder dystocia does occur, the following sequence of maneuvers should take place. An assistant should apply firm suprapubic pressure on the anterior shoulder so as to engage it under the symphysis. Gentle downward traction (so as not to injure the brachial plexus) should now deliver the anterior shoulder. If the anterior shoulder cannot be thus engaged, a large episiotomy or an episioproctotomy should be performed. The posterior shoulder should be pushed toward the infant's chest so that the shoulder rotates under the pubic arch. This will frequently disengage one shoulder. Rotation of the shoulders and not the head is essential, since twisting the head while the shoulders are locked may result in a broken neck or a damaged brachial plexus in the fetus. If the shoulders are still undelivered, introduce a hand posteriorly and apply pressure in the antecubital fossa of the posterior arm. As the elbow flexes, the forearm and hand are drawn across the baby's chest and out of the vaginal opening. This will disengage the posterior shoulder. If it is necessary to deliver the posterior arm, the operator should be prepared for fracture of the humerus or clavicle, or both, on the affected side, which seems to be an acceptable price for the delivery of a living infant without neurologic injury.

Delivery of the large infant is best conducted with moderate doses of systemic analgesia during labor. Supplementation with inhalation of nitrous oxide (40%–50%) with oxygen (50%–60%) is desirable at delivery. It is important that the mother retain sufficient natural expulsive powers so that she may be able to bring the head down to the perineum, and in this way, difficult forceps operations may be avoided. Regional anesthesia may well be associated with inadequate propulsive force and is undersirable for the actual delivery.

The Small Infant

1. Haesslein, H. C., and Goodlin, R. C. Delivery of the tiny newborn. *Am. J. Obstet. Gynecol.* 134:192, 1979.

   Survival and morbidity of tiny newborns can be improved by tocolytic agents, steroids to stimulate lung maturation, prophylactic antibiotics, and vertical low-segment cesarean section. While some of these recommendations are controversial, the article spotlights the problems of the tiny infant.

2. Hobel, C. J., and Oakes, G. K. Special considerations in the management of preterm labor. *Clin. Obstet. Gynecol.* 23:147, 1979.

   A comprehensive review of labor and delivery in the preterm fetus; 68 references are included.

3. Brenner, W. E., Bruce, R. D., and Hendricks, C. H. The characteristics and perils of breech presentation. *Am. J. Obstet. Gynecol.* 118:700, 1974.

   A study of 1016 breech deliveries. Vaginal delivery of the breech is associated with an increased incidence of prolonged labor, intrapartum asphyxia, and shoulder dystocia. More frequent use of cesarean section will lower the perinatal mortality rates.

4. Goldenberg, R. J., Nelson, K. G. The premature breech. *Am. J. Obstet. Gynecol.* 127:240, 1977.

   The perinatal mortality rate was 432 per 1000 live births in a group of premature breech babies delivered vaginally, versus 107 per 1000 and 154 per 1000 in vertex and cesarean section groups, respectively. It is suggested that low birth weight infants in breech presentation would benefit by cesarean section.

5. Gross, T. L., et al. Amniotic fluid phosphatidylglycerol: A potentially useful predictor of intrauterine growth retardation. *Am. J. Obstet. Gynecol.* 140:277, 1981.

   Delivery of the small infant was assessed by the use of phosphatidylglycerol in 82 pregnancies. A high amniotic fluid PG predicted the SGA infant in 64% of the cases, indicating that this might be a helpful adjunct in the diagnosis of the small baby.

6. Galbraith, R. S., Karchmar, E. T., Piercy, W. N., and Low, J. A. The clinical prediction of intrauterine growth retardation. *Am. J. Obstet. Gynecol.* 133:281, 1979.

   Risk factors for intrauterine growth retardation (IUGR) are enumerated. Two-thirds of IUGR infants are not recognized antenatally. Perinatal mortality of IUGR infants ranged from two to four times that of those in a non-IUGR group.

7. Gross, T. J., Sokol, R. J., and Rosen, M. G. Clinical use of the intrapartum monitoring record. *Clin. Obstet. Gynecol.* 22:633, 1979.
A complete review of clinical monitoring with 42 references. The significance of variable fetal heart decelerations is discussed.

8. Ingemarsson, I., Westgren, M., and Svenningsen, N. W. Long-term follow-up of preterm infants in breech presentation delivered by cesarean section: Prospective study. *Am. J. Obstet. Gynecol.* 131:186, 1978.
Forty-two singleton preterm breech infants delivered abdominally are compared with 48 preterm breech infants delivered vaginally. Asphyxia, infant mortality, neurologic abnormalities, and CNS hemorrhage were all higher in those delivered vaginally.

The Large Infant

9. Golditch, I. M., and Kirchman, K. The large fetus: Management and outcome. *Obstet. Gynecol.* 52:26, 1978.
A review of 801 pregnancies with infants weighing more than 4100 g. The perinatal mortality rate was increased, and the second stage of labor was prolonged. Shoulder dystocia, perineal lacerations, fetal injuries, asphyxia, and hypoglycemia were increased.

10. Houchang, D., et al. Macrosomia—maternal, fetal and neonatal implications. *Obstet. Gynecol.* 55:420, 1980.
This retrospective study compared 287 macrosomic infants with a like number of term-size neonates. Male infants, multiparity, obesity, diabetes mellitus, and a prior history of infant macrosomia were positive correlates. Ten percent of the macrosomic infants versus 3% of the control group required admission to the neonatal ICU.

11. Bowes, W. A., and Bowes, C. Current role of the midforceps operation. *Clin. Obstet. Gynecol.* 23:549, 1980.
A review with 21 references. In the past 30 years, the use of oxytocin augmentation of labor, declining morbidity of cesarean section, and the greater skill of obstetricians in performing the abdominal operation rather than having the vaginal route used have established cesarean section as less hazardous than midforceps in dealing with the abnormal second stage of labor.

12. Benedetti, T. J., and Gabbe, S. G. Shoulder dystocia: A complication of fetal macrosomia and prolonged second stage of labor with midpelvic delivery. *Obstet. Gynecol.* 52:526, 1978.
A high risk factor for shoulder dystocia occurs with a prolonged second stage of labor with the fetus in the midpelvis. When the fetus is judged to weigh in excess of 4000 g, delivery by cesarean section appears to be safer for both mother and fetus.

13. Benedetti, T. J. Managing shoulder dystocia. *Contemp. Ob/Gyn* 14:33, 1979.
A comprehensive discussion with illustrations of the management of shoulder dystocia.

14. Resnik, R. Management of shoulder girdle dystocia. *Clin. Obstet. Gynecol.* 23:559, 1980.
A review with 13 references, excellent illustrations, and well-demonstrated management techniques.

PUERPERIUM

Postpartum Hemorrhage

Postpartum hemorrhage (PPH) is a complication of pregnancy and the puerperium that may result in serious maternal morbidity and even mortality. Defined as blood loss greater than 500 cc, the exact incidence is difficult to determine because clinical estimation of blood loss during delivery is inaccurate, by as much as 50% of the actual loss in many cases. When measured correctly, the mean blood loss during delivery and postpartum in one large series was 505 cc, with 39% of patients losing more than this amount. PPH is considered "early" if it occurs during the first 24 hours postpartum, and "late" if it develops after this time.

Frequent causes of early PPH include uterine atony, accounting for 90% of cases; genital tract lacerations (uterine, cervical, vaginal, and perineal), 6%; and retained placental fragments, 3%–4%. The latter accounts for most cases of late PPH. Other infrequent causes include blood dyscrasias and uterine inversion. The risk of PPH is increased if any of the following predisposing factors are present: (1) overdistention of the uterus due to polyhydramnios, multiple pregnancy, or a large fetus; (2) high maternal parity; (3) prolonged difficult labor, especially after oxytocin induction; (4) history of previous PPH; and (5) hypertensive disease of pregnancy. Other correlates include deep general anesthesia, abnormal placentation such as placenta previa or accreta, abruptio placentae, and a succinate placenta, as well as operative delivery using instrumentation or version/extraction.

The cardinal steps in the management of PPH include early recognition, aggressive correction of hypovolemia, and control of the specific bleeding sites. Patients with the predisposing factors mentioned above should be monitored very closely and blood should be available at the time of delivery. Universal therapy in all patients should include prompt blood and volume replacement, maintenance of good urinary output, and serial monitoring of vital signs, hematocrit, and central venous pressure. After the initial steps are completed, the patient should be examined under general anesthesia, with systematic exploration of the genital tract to identify the cause of bleeding.

Classic management of uterine atony consists of mechanical stimulation of uterine contractions by means of firm, but not vigorous, massage of the uterus through the abdomen and bimanual compression of the elevated, anteverted uterus, with simultaneous administration of oxytocic agents in amounts sufficient to provoke and maintain uterine contractility. Other mechanical maneuvers to stop bleeding include digital compression of the uterine arteries in the paracervical area and compression of the descending aorta against the maternal spine.

Oxytocin should be given by continuous intravenous administration in a dosage as high as 20–30 U/500 ml of Ringer's lactate and never as a bolus, in order to avoid the potential side effects of hypotension, myocardial arrhythmias, and cardiac arrest. Simultaneous administration of 0.2 mg of methylergonovine intramuscularly may be used in those patients who are normotensive if the uterus fails to respond to oxytocin. If the above measures fail to control bleeding from uterine atony, other recommended methods of treatment include instillation of heated solutions into the uterus, intrauterine packing, or surgical intervention.

Packing the uterus is a procedure that is rarely used in modern obstetrics and its efficacy remains controversial. Some authors consider uterine packing a valuable procedure for the control of severe bleeding from uterine atony, while others feel it is unphysiologic, ineffective, contributes to further bleeding, predisposes to infection, and may delay definitive treatment by obscuring the amount of blood loss. I believe that uterine packing may be used as a temporary measure in preparation for surgical management and, on occasions, it may be a lifesaving or uterus-preserving procedure. Surgical intervention should be the last resort in the management of bleeding from uterine atony. Surgery may include laparotomy with the options of either ligation of the uterine arteries, bilateral ligation of the hypogastric arteries, or total/subtotal hysterectomy, depending on the condition of the parturient as well as the desire to preserve future fertility. New techniques involving prostaglandin derivatives may make it possible to avoid surgery in severe cases but they remain research tools at present.

Retained fragments of the placenta can be removed digitally after finding the proper cleavage plane by means of manual exploration just after delivery. This can be facilitated by use of placental forceps to grasp placental fragments and a piece of gauze spread out over the gloved fingers to remove small fragments and adherent placental membranes. Occasionally, curettage of the uterus with a large blunt curette may be necessary. The diagnosis of placenta accreta should be suspected in the absence of a cleavage plane and inability to remove placental fragments. Treatment usually requires hysterectomy, although uterine packing has been used successfully in some cases.

Vaginal and cervical lacerations are usually the result of the use of instruments at delivery. The most common sites for cervical lacerations are at the 3 and 9 o'clock positions. Control of bleeding is usually achieved by simple suture repair after isolating and tying larger vessels individually. Deep lacerations should be closed in layers to avoid hematoma formation, and the repair should start above the apex of the laceration. Vaginal packing may be helpful in preventing venous oozing or bleeding from varicosities.

Laceration of the lower uterine segment or rupture of the uterus should be suspected following difficult forceps operations, internal uterine manipulation, use of oxytocin in a multiparous patient, and vaginal delivery after previous cesarean section. Bleeding from uterine rupture is usually internal and the diagnosis can be confirmed by digital exploration of the uterus. Treatment of uterine rupture includes laparotomy with the options of repair of the rent and total or subtotal hysterectomy, depending on type, extent, and site of the laceration, as well as the patient's condition and desire to preserve her uterus.

Acute puerperal inversion of the uterus is a rare cause of PPH, one that is usually associated with excessive fundal pressure, strong traction on the umbilical cord, and uterine atony. Classic symptoms include shock, hemorrhage, and pain. If the diagnosis is made early and general anesthesia is available, manual replacement is possible in most of the cases. Constant, firm, slow Trendelenburg positioning and filling the vagina with warm sterile saline solution may also be helpful in restoring the organ to its correct position.

The incidence of delayed PPH is about 1 per 1000 deliveries, with most cases occurring between the sixth and tenth day after delivery. Frequent causes are subinvolution of the uterus and retained placental fragments. Other causes include endometritis and withdrawal bleeding from estrogens. Many of these patients can be managed conservatively with oxytocic agents, especially if placental inspection and uterine exploration are done routinely at time of delivery. The use of curettage with simultaneous use of oxytocin is necessary in about 65% of the patients but is associated with potential complications such as uterine perforation and increased incidence of Asherman's syndrome.

The potential complications of PPH include postpartum infection, anemia, transfusion hepatitis, Sheehan's syndrome, and Asherman's syndrome, especially if curettage was part of the management. Sheehan's syndrome, or acute pituitary necrosis, occurs in a small number of patients after severe PPH. It is more commonly seen after prolonged shock with secondary ischemic necrosis of the anterior pituitary gland. Prolactin-secreting cells are the first to be affected by anterior pituitary ischemia, and the diagnosis hence should be suspected early in the absence of lactation. Treatment consists of hormonal replacement.

Review

1. Schrinsky, D. C., and Benson, R. C. Rupture of the pregnant uterus: A review. *Obstet. Gynecol. Surv.* 33:217, 1978.
   Immediate surgical intervention is the cornerstone of treatment of uterine rupture. Choice of surgical procedure depends on extent of the rupture, the patient's condition, and her desire for future childbearing.
2. Fox, H. Placenta accreta, 1945–1969. *Obstet. Gynecol. Surv.* 27:474, 1972.
   Basic pathology is deficiency of the decidua with older multigravida, placenta previa and previous cesarean section being associated factors. Mortality rates and treatment modalities are reviewed and compared.
3. Taylor, E. S. (Ed.). Postpartum Hemorrhage. In *Beck's Obstetrical Practice* (9th ed.). Baltimore: Williams & Wilkins, 1969.
   The various factors associated with postpartum hemorrhage are reviewed. Management aspects of postpartum hemorrhage are also detailed.

Normal Postpartum Blood Loss

4. Pritchard, J. A., et al. Blood volume changes in pregnancy and the puerperium. *Am. J. Obstet. Gynecol.* 84:1271, 1972.
   Average blood loss during vaginal delivery averaged 505 ml in 75 women; 61% lost less than 500 ml, 32% lost between 500 and 1000 ml, and 7% lost more than 1000 ml.
5. Newton, M., et al. Blood loss during and immediately after delivery. *Obstet. Gynecol.* 17:9, 1961.
   Blood loss in 100 normal vaginal deliveries was noted, with an average error of 46% when comparing estimates with measurements.
6. Nelson, G. H. Consideration of blood loss at delivery as percentage of estimated blood volume. *Am. J. Obstet. Gynecol.* 138:1117, 1980.
   A method for delineating accurate blood loss at delivery is given, and the definition of postpartum hemorrhage is offered as a loss of blood at delivery of greater than 15% of the total estimated blood volume.

General

7. Kelly, J. V. Postpartum hemorrhage. *Clin. Obstet. Gynecol.* 19:595, 1976.
   The etiology, predisposing factors, and management of postpartum hemorrhage are summarized.

Treatment

8. O'Leary, J. L., and O'Leary, J. A. Uterine artery ligation for control of post-cesarean section hemorrhage. *Obstet. Gynecol.* 43:849, 1974.
   This article reports 94 cases of bilateral uterine artery ligation. Follow-up in all cases revealed no adverse effects.
9. Hestler, J. D. Postpartum hemorrhage and reevaluation of uterine packing. *Obstet. Gynecol.* 45:501, 1975.

This article reports on 153 patients with postpartum hemorrhage. Uterine packing, surgery, and conservative management are compared.

10. Fribourg, S. R. C., et al. Intrauterine lavage for control of uterine atony. *Obstet. Gynecol.* 41:876, 1973.
The use of intrauterine lavage in the management of uterine atony in 4 patients who failed to respond to the usual conservative measures is presented.

11. Pritchard, J. A., and MacDonald, P. C. Abnormalities of the Third Stage of Labor. In *Williams Obstetrics* (16th ed.). New York: Appleton-Century-Crofts, 1980.
The etiology of postpartum hemorrhage is detailed and active management techniques are reviewed.

Inversion of the Uterus

12. Watson, P., Besch, N., and Bowes, W. A. Management of acute and subacute puerperal inversion of the uterus. *Obstet. Gynecol.* 55:12, 1980.
Eighteen cases of puerperal inversion of the uterus were studied. The most common signs were hemorrhage (94%) and shock (39%). Treatment regimens are summarized.

13. Kitchin, E., et al. Puerperal inversion of the uterus. *Am. J. Obstet. Gynecol.* 123:51, 1975.
Eleven cases of puerperal inversion of the uterus were studied. In all cases manual repositioning was achieved without significant difficulty and the postpartum course was uncomplicated.

Secondary PPH

14. Rome, R. M. Secondary postpartum hemorrhage. *Br. J. Obstet. Gynaecol.* 52:289, 1975.
This article reviews 106 patients with late postpartum hemorrhage. Conservative and aggressive approaches are outlined.

15. Vorherr, H. The Pregnant Uterus: Process of Labor, Puerperium, and Lactation. In N. Assali (Ed.), *Biology of Gestation.* New York: Academic Press, 1968.
The author reviews the steps in postpartum involution of the uterus and outlines several causes of late postpartum hemorrhage.

16. Visscher, H. C., and Visscher, R. D. Early and Late Postpartum Hemorrhage. In J. J. Sciarra (Ed.), *Gynecology and Obstetrics.* Hagerstown, Md.: Harper & Row, 1980. Vol. 2.
A most complete reference to the causes of both early and late postpartum hemorrhage. Steps taken to prevent this complication are discussed.

Puerperal Infections

The standard definition of puerperal morbidity is that proposed by the Joint Committee on Maternal Welfare. To fulfill the criteria, two temperature readings over 100.4°F (38°C) on any two of the first 10 postpartum days, exclusive of the first 24 hours, need to be recorded. The incidence of all postpartum infections is estimated to be from 1%–8%. Although the usual cause of postpartum pyrexia is a bacterial infection of the genital tract, the urinary tract, lungs, breasts, surgical wounds, and intravenous lines may also be the site of puerperal infections.

Cesarean section is the most important single factor predisposing to puerperal endometritis, with an incidence of postoperative morbidity as high as 29%–85%. Prolonged rupture of membranes, prolonged labor, difficult vaginal or forceps delivery, and multiple vaginal examinations all predispose to puerperal infection. Retained products of conception, postpartum hemorrhage, and anemia may also be etiologic factors. It is still unclear as to whether internal fetal monitoring increases the incidence of puerperal sepsis or not.

Most deliveries take place in hospitals so the majority of puerperal infections are nosocomial. The organisms found are usually those indigent to the vagina. An ascending infection composed of aerobic and anaerobic organisms occurs under circumstances favorable to spread, such as trauma, foreign body formation (e.g., suture lines), and hemorrhage. The resulting endomyometritis may spread to the tubes, broad ligaments, peritoneal cavity, and pelvic veins causing pelvic abscesses, peritonitis, or septic pelvic thrombophlebitis. These serious complications are far more frequent after abdominal as opposed to vaginal delivery.

The clinical findings usually are those of a gradual onset of fever from 2–8 days after delivery with evidence of lower abdominal and pelvic pain and tenderness. Early and more severe patterns of onset, especially with evidence of septic shock, suggest less common infections, particularly *Streptococcus pyogenes, Escherichia coli,* and *Clostridium welchii.* The more common mixed infections are more insidious and progress more slowly. *Bacteroides fragilis* is the most frequently encountered anaerobic pathogen. *Staphylococcus aureus* is occasionally found, usually in diabetic patients or in association with cervical suture, episiotomy, or other trauma. The infection is clinically similar to that caused by anaerobes.

The diagnosis is overwhelmingly dependent on clinical findings since accurate bacteriology is technically difficult to obtain. Examination of breasts, lungs, limbs, surgical incisions, and intravenous sites must not be neglected. A vaginal discharge or heavy malodorous lochia may be present; tenderness on pelvic examination, and on occasion the presence of adnexal masses, will usually indicate the site of sepsis. A complete blood count, chest x-ray, urine samples, and wound cultures should be obtained. High vaginal or endocervical cultures do not really indicate the pathogen in the uterine cavity and may be misleading. Transabdominal uterine aspiration is unwarranted and might spread the infection. Blood cultures should be taken but are only positive in about 8% of cases.

Therapy should be instituted without awaiting bacteriologic results since anaerobic cultures require several days. No single antibiotic covers all the potential pathogens, and intravenous antibiotics in combination are usually employed, depending on the severity of the infection. Common combinations include penicillin and an aminoglycoside, reserving agents effective against *B. fragilis* (clindamycin, chloramphenicol) for those women remaining febrile 48–72 hours after the initial therapy.

If the patient fails to respond within 2–4 days of full antibiotic therapy, reexamination and further investigation are required, including pelvic ultrasound and lung scan if pelvic abscess or pulmonary embolism are suspected. A trial of heparin therapy for possible septic pelvic thrombophlebitis is justifiable if these findings are negative. Surgery, including drainage of wound or pelvic abscesses, or curettage for retained products of conception may be necessary. Hysterectomy may be required in cases of severe nonresponsive sepsis. Fortunately, this is very uncommon. Fever due to therapy must also be kept in mind, including drug fever and antibiotic-induced colitis.

Because the factors predisposing to puerperal infections are well known, bacteriologic analysis of amniotic fluid prior to delivery in risk situations, such as premature rupture of the membranes, may provide a guide to therapy. Prophylactic antibiotics are widely employed with cesarean section in patients at increased risk, for instance, when emergency surgery follows prolonged labor. However, the present-day emphasis on antibiotic therapy and prophylaxis has resulted in a widespread neglect of traditional aseptic techniques in obstetrics services across the country. Many puerperal infections could be avoided by reinstitution of these fundamental practices.

Reviews

1. Sweet, R. I., and Ledger, W. J. Puerperal infectious morbidity: A two-year review. *Am. J. Obstet. Gynecol.* 117:1093, 1973.
   Since only 56% of patients with clinical endometritis had standard morbidity, it is suggested that the definition be modified.
2. Gibbs, R. S., and Weinstein, A. J. Puerperal infection in the antibiotic era. *Am. J. Obstet. Gynecol.* 124:769, 1976.
   A comprehensive review of the subject.

Predisposing Factors

3. Ledger, W. J. Premature rupture of membranes and maternal-fetal infection. *Clin. Obstet. Gynecol.* 22:329, 1979.
   Although the incidence of infection increases as the duration of rupture increases, only a minority of mothers and infants are at risk of becoming infected.
4. D'Angelo, L. J., and Sokol, R. J. Time-related peripartum determinants of postpartum morbidity. *Obstet. Gynecol.* 55:319, 1980.
   Duration of labor may be the only time-related peripartum event in assessing the risk for infection in patients having cesarean section.
5. Gibbs, R. S., Listwa, H. M., and Read, J. A. The effect of internal fetal monitoring on maternal infection following cesarean section. *Obstet. Gynecol.* 48:653, 1976.
   In this series, monitoring did not increase the risk.

Bacteriology

6. Ogden, E., and Amstey, M. S. Puerperal infection due to group A beta hemolytic streptococcus. *Obstet. Gynecol.* 52:53, 1976.
   Miniepidemics of Semmelweis' "childbed fever" are reported from time to time. Early onset, high fever, uterine tenderness, with gram-positive cocci on gram stain of the lochia, provide the diagnosis.
7. Benn, R. Anaerobic infection in the puerperium. *Med. J. Aust.* 2:590, 1979.
   Nonsporing anaerobic bacteria, particularly the gram-negative rods such as B. fragilis, appear to be the most important organisms implicated in puerperal infections.

Diagnosis

8. Eng, J., Torkildsen, E. M., and Christensen, A. Bacteriuria in the puerperium: An evaluation of methods for collecting urine specimens. *Am. J. Obstet. Gynecol.* 131:739, 1978.
   It is difficult to obtain an uncontaminated midstream urine in the puerperium. The writers of this report employed suprapubic bladder puncture and found a 1% incidence of significant postpartum bacteriuria.
9. Pezzlo, M. T., et al. Improved laboratory efficiency and diagnostic

accuracy with new double-lumen-protected swab for endometrial specimens. *J. Clin. Microbiol.* 9:56, 1979.
Lavage techniques, abdominal puncture, special swabs, have all been used in an effort to identify the true pathogens in endomyometritis.

10. Bobitt, J. R., and Ledger, W. J. Amniotic fluid analysis. Its role in maternal and neonatal infection. *Obstet. Gynecol.* 51:56, 1978.
Patients with amniotic fluid bacterial colony counts over $10^3/ml$ were at high risk for maternal sepsis, with the neonate also at risk.

11. Ledger, W. J., and Kriewall, T. J. The fever index: A quantitative indirect measure of hospital-acquired infections in obstetrics and gynecology. *Am. J. Obstet. Gynecol.* 48:514, 1973.
A useful measure of febrile morbidity, the fever index is the number of degree hours under the temperature curve but above 99°F.

Therapy
12. Moellering, R. C. Special consideration of the use of antimicrobial agents during pregnancy, postpartum, and in the newborn. *Clin. Obstet. Gynecol.* 22:373, 1979.
Alterations in drug pharmacokinetics in pregnancy, related to increased clearance and greater volume of distribution, may require higher dosage levels of antibiotics.

13. DiZerega, G., et al. A comparison of clindamycin-gentamicin and penicillin-gentamicin in the treatment of post-cesarean section endomyometritis. *Am. J. Obstet. Gynecol.* 134:238, 1979.
The drug regimen containing a drug specific for B. fragilis (clindamycin) proved superior to the standard combination.

14. Gibbs, R. S., Jones, P. M., and Wilder, C. J. Antibiotic therapy of endometritis following cesarean section. Treatment successes and failures. *Obstet. Gynecol.* 52:31, 1978.
Failure of therapy is usually due to a resistant organism, an abscess, or septic pelvic thrombophlebitis.

15. Ledger, W. J., and Peterson, E. P. The use of heparin in the management of pelvic thrombophlebitis. *Surg. Gynecol. Obstet.* 131:115, 1970.
A clinical response following the addition of heparin to the antibiotic regimen provides presumptive evidence of the diagnosis. Operative ligation of the veins is rarely necessary.

Prophylaxis
16. Polk, B. F., and Schoenbaum, S. C. Prophylactic antibiotics in obstetrics. *Clin. Obstet. Gynecol.* 22:379, 1979.
Three situations are considered: cesarean section, premature rupture of membranes, and bacterial endocarditis.

17. Green, S. L., Sarubbi, F. A., and Bishop, E. H. Prophylactic antibiotics in high-risk cesarean section. *Obstet. Gynecol.* 51:569, 1978.
The incidence of febrile morbidity was reduced from 63% to 15%, but the period of postoperative hospitalization was similar.

18. Iffy, L., et al. Control of perinatal infection by traditional preventive measures. *Obstet. Gynecol.* 54:403, 1979.
Contrary to current views, these authors maintain that most puerperal infections are exogenous and spread by health care professionals. All types of nosocomial infection could be controlled if all traditional methods of asepsis were employed.

19. Ledger, W. J. Hospital infections: Gynecologic, obstetric, and perinatal infections. *Ann. Intern. Med.* 89:774, 1978.
Extraperitoneal cesarean section or cesarean hysterectomy have been

advocated as preventive operative techniques for patients at high risk of serious post-cesarean morbidity.

Mortality

20. Evrard, J. R., and Gold, E. M. Cesarean section and maternal mortality in Rhode Island. Incidence and risk factors, 1965–1975. *Obstet. Gynecol.* 50:594, 1977.
    Cesarean section carried twenty-six times the mortality of vaginal delivery. Sepsis was the major cause of death.
21. Vaughan, J., MacDonald, D., and Daly, L. Puerperal pyrexia—A prospective study. *Ir. Med. J.* 72:317, 1979.
    Infection was the leading cause of maternal death. Secondary postpartum hemorrhage was a serious indication of genital infection.

Breast Infection

22. Ezrati, J. B., and Gordon, H. Puerperal mastitis: Causes, prevention, and management. *J. Nurse Midwife.* 24:3, 1979.
    Two forms of infection occur: Mammary cellulitis involving the connective tissue, and mammary adenitis affecting the lobes and ducts. Both may progress to abscess formation.
23. Niebyl, J. R., Spence, M. R., and Parmley, T. H. Sporadic (nonepidemic) puerperal mastitis. *J. Reprod. Med.* 20:97, 1978.
    S. aureus can be cultured in 50% of cases; early antibiotic therapy usually prevents abscess formation and breastfeeding need not be discontinued.

Deep Vein Thrombosis and Pulmonary Embolism

Deep vein thrombosis (DVT) is an infrequent but serious complication of pregnancy because of the ultimate risk of pulmonary embolism and potential fatal outcome. The incidence is about 0.5 to 1 per 1000 pregnancies during the antepartum period and increasing fivefold postpartum. If untreated, 16% of patients will have pulmonary embolism, with a 10%–15% mortality. If adequately treated, however, pulmonary embolism occurs in less than 5%, with a mortality rate of less than 1%.

Pregnancy is considered a state of hypercoagulability due to the progressive increase in all plasma coagulation factors, except XI and XIII, with an associated decrease in the fibrinolytic activity because of a decrease in the level of circulating plasminogen activator. Concurrently, there is progressive venous stasis because of venous dilatation and increased capacitance, as well as increased pressure on the pelvic vessels. This combined effect of hypercoagulability and venous stasis appears to be related etiologically to the greater risk of thromboembolism during pregnancy. The risk of thromboembolism is also increased in the presence of these associated predisposing factors: (1) cesarean section; (2) instrumental or traumatic delivery; (3) increased maternal age or parity; (4) suppression of lactation by estrogens; (5) sickle cell disease or anemia; (6) history of previous thrombophlebitis, (7) maternal cardiac disease; (8) prolonged immobilization; (9) maternal obesity; (10) maternal infection or sepsis; and (11) chronic venous insufficiency.

The diagnosis of DVT during the antepartum period is usually made on the basis of clinical signs and symptoms, with the help of nonspecific, noninvasive techniques. Diagnostic x-ray and radioisotope studies have potential harmful effects on the fetus and are not used. Symptoms include swelling, muscle pain, tenderness, and a positive Homans' sign and Löwenberg test. Unfortunately, reliance on these findings alone will result in an incorrect diagnosis (false-positive or false-negative) in 50% of the cases. Moreover, it is important that DVT be differentiated from superficial inflammation of the vein since the treatment and prognosis are radically different.

Investigations using the I-125 fibrinogen test and venography reveal that about half of the patients with postoperative deep venous thrombosis have no clinical signs, while 45% of those with clinical signs have normal venograms. Diagnosis is most reliable in the presence of significant thrombosis with a tense, swollen limb, and with pain and tenderness extended to the thigh. Noninvasive techniques such as the Doppler ultrasonic velocity flow detector and impedance plethysmography can be helpful in major venous obstruction but are unreliable for minor venous thrombosis. In the postpartum period, ascending contrast phlebograph can be used and is the most sensitive and reliable of all tests for detection of DVT. Its disadvantage is that it is invasive and carries a moderate degree of risk, and hence should not be used as a screening procedure. I-125–labeled fibrinogen is of value in diagnosing lower extremity venous thrombosis and is most valuable in the screening of patients with risk factors during the postpartum period.

The diagnosis of pulmonary embolism depends on the clinical history and course, physical findings, appropriate laboratory tests, and specific procedures. However, the signs, symptoms, and laboratory data are often nonspecific, and about 50% of the cases occur without a previous clinical diagnosis of thrombophlebitis having been made. The most common findings are dyspnea, tachypnea, chest pain, cough, hemoptysis, and tachycardia. The finding of an arterial PO_2 of less than 80 mm Hg in room air with a positive lung scan is useful in confirming the diagnosis. Both anteroposterior and lateral scans should be performed to reduce false-negative results. If positive, the scan signifies a lung perfusion defect but does not delineate the cause. Pulmonary arteriography remains the most specific and reliable diagnostic procedure for the definitive diagnosis of pulmonary embolism.

Symptomatic treatment in the form of bed rest, elevation of the affected extremity, application of moist heat, and the wearing of elastic stockings may be helpful in DVT. Anticoagulant therapy with heparin or warfarin, however, is the definitive mode of treatment for DVT, with or without pulmonary embolism. Heparin is the drug of choice in the antepartum period because it does not cross the placenta due to its large molecular size and negative charge. The usual regimen of heparin is a loading dose of 5000 to 20,000 units, followed by continuous maintenance doses of 1000 units per hour. Others use the loading dose only if a pulmonary embolus is suspected. Adjustment of the maintenance dose should be based on a prolonged Lee-White clotting time or partial thromboplastin time twice normal.

Intravenous heparin therapy should be continued for about 7 to 10 days after resolution of all symptoms. Following this regimen, the patient is switched to low-dose heparin injections. Oral sodium warfarin can be used but is difficult to regulate, with frequent prothrombin time assessment necessary for follow-up care. In addition, warfarin, a small molecule that crosses the placenta readily, has within it the inherent risk of producing congenital anomalies if given during the first trimester. If used later in pregnancy, it can cause fetal anticoagulation, leading to fetal or neonatal hemorrhage.

There is controversy over using anticoagulants in the treatment of DVT and in prophylaxis of embolism during the antepartum period. Usually, one treats an acute episode of DVT with continuous intravenous heparin for 7 to 10 days after symptoms abate, followed by prophylactic low-dose heparin of 5000 units every 12 hours either by the subcutaneous route or by intravenous injections through an implanted Teflon intravenous catheter. Heparin may be discontinued at the time of labor and resumed immediately postpartum for 5 to 7 days, but many continue its use even into operative deliveries without undue hemorrhage. Other less-used regimens include the use of heparin in the first trimester, warfarin in midpregnancy, and, finally, heparin in the last month of gestation. Still others argue against the use of anticoagulants beyond the acute episode, except for those patients with recurrence and pulmonary embolization.

Pulmonary embolism is a serious, life-threatening situation that requires immediate aggressive management. Medical management consists of the same intravenous heparin therapy as for DVT, except for a larger loading dose, and intravenous treatment should be given for a minimum of 2 weeks. Supportive therapy in the form of oxygen therapy to keep maternal PaO_2 above 70 mm Hg, bronchodilators, maternal sedation, and immediate management of shock or congestive heart failure is of equal importance. If embolism develops postpartum, anticoagulation should be continued for about 3 to 6 months following initial therapy. Surgical intervention should be reserved for those with massive embolization with recurrent embolism in spite of adequate medical therapy, and in those in whom anticoagulation is contraindicated.

Septic pelvic thrombophlebitis is usually a complication of postpartum, postabortal, and postoperative anaerobic pelvic infections. The clinical picture includes persistent spiking fever, with or without chills, and tachycardia in spite of adequate antibiotic therapy. The pelvic examination may be normal, and the diagnosis is made on the basis of clinical response to a trial of heparin therapy. The treatment of choice is intravenous heparin and antibiotics for a minimum of 7 days.

The use of "minidoses" of heparin prophylaxis has been reported to decrease the incidence of DVT and fatal pulmonary emboli in patients undergoing major surgery. Standard regimens recommend 5000 units be given subcutaneously 2 hours prior to surgery, to be repeated every 8–12 hours postoperatively until the patient is fully ambulatory. This small dose acts by enhancing the action of antithrombin factor III, which inhibits activation of factor X. Unfortunately, little is known concerning its use in pregnancy, but it may be helpful in patients with high-risk factors such as previous thromboembolic disease, massive obesity, and in those who develop DVT early in the antepartum period. However, more data is needed to document its effectiveness during pregnancy.

Reviews

1. Finnerty, J. J., and Mackay, B. R. Antepartum thrombophlebitis and pulmonary embolism. *Obstet. Gynecol.* 19:405, 1962.

   A review of 208 cases of antepartum thrombophlebitis. In 135 untreated cases, the incidence of pulmonary embolism was 24%, with a maternal and fetal mortality of 11% and 12%, respectively. In the treated group of 73 cases, pulmonary embolism occurred in 4%, with no maternal mortality and 16% fetal mortality.

2. Vorherr, H. Puerperium: Maternal Involutional Changes and Management of Puerperal Problems and Complications. In J. J. Sciarra (Ed.), *Gynecology and Obstetrics.* Hagerstown, Md.: Harper & Row, 1979. Vol. 2.

A very comprehensive assessment of the thrombotic puerperal complications. This chapter outlines most of the classic studies that have been performed regarding pulmonary embolism.

Clinical Findings and Diagnosis

3. Howie, P. W. Thromboembolism. *Clin. Obstet. Gynecol.* 4:397, 1977.
   Blood coagulation factors rise sharply during pregnancy, while there is a marked depression of systemic fibrinolytic activity. During the puerperium, fibrinogen rises and the number of platelets, as well as platelet adhesiveness, increases.

4. Laros, R. K., and Alber, L. S. Thromboembolism and pregnancy. *Clin. Obstet. Gynecol.* 22:871, 1979.
   Signs and symptoms of thrombophlebitis and pulmonary embolism are discussed. Diagnostic procedures such as ultrasound, impedance plethysmography, radio-fibrinogen test, venography, lung scans, and pulmonary angiography are explained.

5. Barnes, R. W., Wu, K. L., and Hoak, J. C. Fallibility of clinical diagnosis of venous thrombosis. *J.A.M.A.* 234:605, 1975.
   Doppler ultrasonic velocity detector was used in 527 cases of possible venous thrombosis. The overall accuracy of the Doppler method was 94% versus 37% for the clinical diagnosis. The findings confirm the unreliability of clinical diagnosis of acute venous thrombosis.

6. Jackson, P. Puerperal thromboembolic disease in "high risk" cases. *Br. Med. J.* 1:263, 1973.
   The author outlines various risk factors for pulmonary embolism in high-risk obstetric patients. Various diagnostic techniques are discussed.

Treatment

7. Mueller, M. J., and Lebherz, T. B. Antepartum thrombophlebitis: Morbidity with long-term heparin and a proposed regimen of therapy. *Obstet. Gynecol.* 34:874, 1969.
   In the antepartum period, heparin therapy for 7–14 days is recommended for an initial episode of DVT. Long-term therapy is advised for ascending or recurrent disease, ileofemoral involvement, or pulmonary embolism. Heparin is discontinued at time of labor, to be resumed 48 hours postpartum for at least 6 weeks.

8. Henderson, S. R., Lund, C. J., and Creasman, W. T. Antepartum pulmonary embolism. *Am. J. Obstet. Gynecol.* 112:476, 1972.
   Twenty patients with antepartum pulmonary embolism were treated with intravenous heparin for 7 to 10 days, followed by sodium warfarin until term. There were two maternal deaths and one fetal death.

9. Josey, W. E., and Staggers, S. R. Heparin therapy in septic pelvic thrombophlebitis; a study of 46 cases. *Am. J. Obstet. Gynecol.* 120:228, 1974.
   Subcutaneous or intravenous heparin was used in the treatment of 28 postpartum, 8 postabortal, and 10 postoperative patients with septic pelvic thrombophlebitis.

10. Kashtan, J., Conti, S., and Baisdell, F. W. Heparin therapy for deep venous thrombosis. *Am. J. Surg.* 140:836, 1980.
    Nearly one-half of a series of 156 patients with venous thrombosis were found to have had a previous episode. Treatment with continuous intravenous heparin in high doses resulted in faster and more complete recovery than when low-dose heparin was used.

11. Salzman, E., and Davies, G. Prophylaxis of venous thromboembolism. *Ann. Surg.* 191:207, 1980.
    The authors describe their method of prophylaxis by using heparin in

women at high risk for venous thrombosis. With only a small incidence of side effects, this is a worthwhile treatment regimen.

Maternal Complications

12. Turnbull, D., et al. Antenatal and postnatal thromboembolism. *Practitioner* 206:727, 1971.
    The authors reviewed 230 maternal deaths from thromboembolism in pregnancy. The rate of fatal cases increased with age and by 10-fold after cesarean section. Death from pulmonary embolism was often sudden, and over 50% of deaths occurred without any warning signs or symptoms.

Fetal Complications

13. Shaul, W. L., and Hall, J. G. Multiple congenital anomalies associated with oral anticoagulants. *Am. J. Obstet. Gynecol.* 127:191, 1977.
    This article reports 11 infants with multiple congenital anomalies following maternal exposure to oral anticoagulants during the first trimester. The most consistent feature was a flattened, hypoplastic nose.

Prophylaxis

14. Gallus, A. S., et al. Prevention of venous thrombosis with small, subcutaneous doses of heparin. *J.A.M.A.* 234:605, 1975.
    Subcutaneous low-dose heparin was found to be effective in reducing the incidence of postoperative calf, femoral, and popliteal vein thrombosis after elective surgery. The incidence was reduced from 36% to 16%, with a slight increase in postoperative bleeding and wound hematoma.
15. Kakkar, V. V., Carrigan, T. P., and Fossard, D. P. Prevention of fatal postoperative pulmonary embolism by low doses of heparin. *Lancet* 2:45, 1975.
    The use of low-dose heparin prophylaxis in patients undergoing abdominal surgery decreases the incidence of DVT and fatal pulmonary emboli.
16. Hirsh, J. Venous thromboembolism: Diagnosis, treatment, prevention. *Hosp. Pract.* 10:53, 1975.
    The author details a very in-depth assessment of thromboembolism. The section on prevention would be particularly excellent for any hospitalized patient.

Postpartum Depression

One of the most significant events in a woman's life is childbearing. In terms of physiologic and psychologic changes, it may surpass that of menarche and menopause. The development of a significant psychiatric disorder during this time, therefore, can be tragic, not only because it may represent a significant disorder in the mother, but also due to the impact on the newborn child and its father. Because of the serious nature of severe postpartum depression, it is imperative that any physician administering health care to pregnant women understand this disorder and be able to identify and treat it in an early stage. The incidence of significant postpartum depression is between 1 and 2.4 per 1000 deliveries, with the symptoms usually beginning in the first 6 weeks postpartum but occasionally not occurring until 3 to 6 months after delivery.

One study of 198 cases of serious psychiatric disorders during pregnancy reported that 46% of these patients had a history of preexisting psychiatric problems, 22% of the illnesses began during the pregnancy, and 32% of the patients presented with a psychiatric disorder in the postpartum period. Of the last group, only one-half were detected prior to discharge from the hospital. Of the patients followed for postpartum depression 70% were multiparas.

Generally, there are two types of postpartum depression: mild and severe. The mild type is quite common and, with close questioning, most patients will admit to some form of depression in the postpartum period. Considering the psychologic and physiologic changes during pregnancy, along with the extreme excitement of the labor and delivery process, it is to be expected that women will often experience an emotional letdown postpartum. After returning home from the hospital, she is alone with her new baby and the realities of caring for the infant. The phone calls, visitors, and attention she received in the hospital have diminished and most women describe a feeling of isolation clinically much like mild depression. Most patients handle this letdown without significant or serious depression. Certain women, however, do not cope with this phenomenon and develop what can be called severe postpartum depression, one requiring extensive treatment and follow-up.

While the etiology of postpartum depression is not known, there are three general elements that may play a significant role. While there is no proof that the massive physiologic changes of a pregnancy contribute to a postpartum depression, most authors comment that biologic changes may play a role. Postpartum levels of estrogen, progesterone, human chorionic somatomammotropin, and human chorionic gonadotropin fall rapidly. In addition, the postpartum patient has just finished a significantly stressful period of labor and delivery that may include blood loss, anesthesia, surgery, and often significant discomfort. Finally, there may be an underlying genetic disposition to psychiatric disorder that stress, either physiologic or psychologic, may uncover.

A second theory, or element, is that of an underlying psychiatric disorder that is revealed by the pregnancy. Studies to define the antecedent psychologic status on subsequent development of postpartum depression, however, have been frustrating. One study of 60 pregnant women noted that none of the women with the poorest premorbid personality function developed serious psychiatric illness during the early postpartum period. Another study of 100 patients with severe postpartum psychiatric disorders noted that psychologic conflicts more frequently centered on difficulties with the mothering role concept, along with considerable ambivalence toward one's own mother, as well as communication problems with the husband. Comparing mothers with and without postpartum psychosis, one study noted that women who developed significant postpartum psychiatric problems were more likely to be emotionally tied to their own mothers and often confused with respect to the identity of their infants as well as themselves. Therefore, at the present time there is no evidence to support the fact that one can identify patients at significant risk for postpartum depression by establishing preexisting psychological problems.

A third theory, or element, is that of negative social factors. The newborn infant may represent a significant financial burden for the mother and family and may bring an added emotional problem to an already unstable marriage. A patient who is involved in her own career may find that the added burden of childrearing presents an ever-increasing dilemma.

While biologic, psychologic, and sociologic factors cannot be definitely determined to play a role in the etiology of postpartum depression, they may, singularly or in concert, play a role in its eventual evolution. Postpartum depression knows no socioeconomic boundaries and may produce considerable problems for any postpartum patient.

Pregnancy itself is a significant psychologic experience. Patients often note changes in mood and sleep patterns and may complain of nightmares. Patients often note ambivalence to childbearing and childrearing, and most women, when questioned, will confess to a fear of delivering an abnormal child and of not being a good mother. Without adequate support from family members or the medical community, many of these fears are augmented and exaggerated. Patients who develop severe postpartum depression will usually complain of loss of appetite, headaches, fatigue, anxiety, insomnia, forgetfulness, and suicidal thoughts, as well as thoughts of injuring the child.

While there is no known way to prevent this disorder, it is extremely important for the physician to maintain a high level of suspicion; when indicated, to alert the husband and family; to help the patient with insomnia by administering a mild sedative for sleep; and to see her in the office in 1–2 weeks rather than waiting the usual 6 weeks for the first postpartum visit. The obstetrician can spend more time with the patient, explaining the process of childbearing to her and her husband in hopes of reducing the stress. In patients who still have ambivalent feelings about the infant at the time of labor and delivery, immediate postpartum maternal-infant bonding may be of some help. This process is accomplished through close physical contact between mother and child in the 1-hour period postdelivery.

Because of an approximate 25% recurrence rate in a patient who had severe postpartum depression with a previous pregnancy, treatment with lithium may be initiated in the immediate postpartum period. Medical treatment of postpartum depression revolves around the use of tricyclic antidepressants or potent tranquilizers for anxiety. Equally important, however, is the involvement of the patient with proper psychiatric therapy. Early diagnosis and therapy is of the utmost importance, and prognosis for this condition is usually good. The authors of one study of 21 patients with puerperal psychosis concluded that the prognosis for spontaneous recovery was excellent and recommended that lithium therapy was not necessary to obtain a cure. They did suggest, however, that because of a high recurrence rate of this type of psychosis, lithium salts may be administered for several weeks beginning just after delivery, as a preventive measure in those patients with a previous history of severe postpartum depression.

General Review

1. Youngs, D. D., and Lucas, M. J. Postpartum Depression: Hormonal versus Alternative Perspectives. In D. D. Youngs (Ed.), *Psychosomatic Obstetrics and Gynecology.* New York: Appleton-Century-Crofts, 1980. Chap. 3.
   This chapter, which is an excellent review on the subject of postpartum depression, discusses biological and psychological factors.
2. Hamilton, J. A. Puerperal Psychoses. In J. J. Sciarra and A. B. Gerbie (Eds.), *Gynecology and Obstetrics.* Hagerstown, Md.: Harper & Row, 1978. Vol. 2.
   This chapter on puerperal psychoses is another good review on the subject, with a special emphasis on diagnosis and treatment.
3. Steiner, M. Psychobiology of mental disorders associated with childbearing. An overview. *Acta Psychiatr. Scand.* 60:449, 1979.
   A complete synopsis of the etiology, diagnosis, and treatment of all mental disorders associated with childbearing is given. The interpretation of underlying disorders and factors is also given.

Incidence

4. Hatherley, L. I., Breheny, J. E., Robinson, F. S., and Beischer, N. A. Psychiatric disorders in obstetrics. *Med. J. Aust.* 2:399, 1979.

This article gives the rate of puerperal psychosis as being 2.4 per 1000 and gives an incidence of psychiatric problems throughout pregnancy as being as high as 7.2 cases per 1000.

Types

5. Treadway, C., et al. A psychoendocrine study of pregnancy and puerperium. *Am. J. Psychiatry* 125:1380, 1969.
   This paper reviews the less well-documented changes in the biochemistry of pregnancy as an etiologic factor in postpartum depression.
6. Yalom, I. D., et al. "Postpartum blues" syndrome. *Arch. Gen. Psychiatry* 18:16, 1968.
   Attempts to define the psychological makeup of patients who are at risk for postpartum depression are frustrating.
7. Lederman, E., et al. Maternal psychological and physiologic correlates of fetal-newborn health status. *Am. J. Obstet. Gynecol.* 139:956, 1981.
   The authors studied 32 primigravida women in pregnancy and labor. Anxiety in labor and plasma epinephrine were significantly correlated with fetal heart rate patterns in labor and with maternal/newborn outcome.

Prognosis and Treatment

8. Kadrmas, A., Winokur, G., Crowe, R. Postpartum mania. *Br. J. Psychiatry* 135:551, 1979.
   Twenty-one patients with puerperal psychosis were studied, with the conclusion that the prognosis for spontaneous recovery is excellent and a recommendation that lithium therapy is not absolutely necessary to obtain cure.
9. Sneddon, J., and Kerry, R. J. Puerperal psychosis. *Br. J. Psychiatry* 136:520, 1980.
   The authors describe the psychodynamics of puerperal psychosis that might effect the long-term progress of the patient.
10. Ketai, R. M., and Brandwin, M. A. Childbirth-related psychosis and familial symbiotic conflict. *Am. J. Psychiatry* 136:190, 1979.
    This study discusses the various family relationships that may have an effect on a woman with puerperal psychosis as to her success or failure of treatment. The prognosis for various groups of patients is outlined.

Genetic Counseling

Genetic counseling is becoming more commonplace in modern obstetrics. It is important that each physician administering health care to pregnant women understand the basics of genetic counseling for the prenatal patient. In the general population there is approximately a 2% incidence of serious birth defects. Screening and counseling can be classified into two major areas: genetic (heredity) and environment. The genetic aspect involves the single factor disorders categorized as autosomal dominant, autosomal recessive, and X-linked recessive, as well as polygenetic and chromosomal aberrations. Environmental factors include viruses, radiation exposure, and drugs such as alcohol and tobacco.

Genetic counseling begins with screening procedures designed to identify that individual who is at greater risk of producing an offspring with genetic abnormalities than the population at large. This identification requires a thorough family and reproductive history, as well as the effects of various environmental factors. The basic principle of counseling involves timing, which in some instances demands prepregnancy intervention and in most, intervention between conception and 16 weeks gestation. Counseling is best performed when both parents are involved and when the needs of both parents are identified. This counseling can be defined as that process that opens lines of communication between the health care provider and patient to allow the imparting of accurate and reliable information. This allows the patient and her partner to make a fundamental decision regarding future management of the pregnancy. Its objective is to provide information, assist in decision-making and adjustment to the problem, and ultimately to decrease the incidence of genetic defects.

Adequate genetic counseling requires that the reason for concern be clearly delineated and that the information presented to the parents is accurate and timely. A thorough family history (pedigree) and physical examination, as well as the use of various diagnostic procedures, are necessary to establish an accurate diagnosis. The risks, benefits, and failures of each of the diagnostic procedures, usually amniocentesis and ultrasound, need to be communicated in a truthful and noncoercive environment. There is a need for accurate data dissemination, with clear alternatives discussed with the couple. Confidentiality is of utmost importance, and the attainment of an atmosphere of trust between health care provider and patient is imperative. Accurate follow-up of each couple who receives counseling is mandatory.

The category of patients most frequently requiring counseling during the prenatal period are patients conceiving after the age of 35. While the risk of having a baby with Down's syndrome in the population under age 30 is approximately 1 per 2000 pregnancies, at age 35 this risk increases to 1 per 356 pregnancies and is increased each year thereafter, reaching 1 in 12 pregnancies at age 49. Presumably, this increasing incidence associated with maternal age is directly related to aging of the ova. In spite of this direct relationship, however, only 10% of the 150,000 pregnant women over age 35 in the United States are assessed each year for chromosomal abnormalities. In addition, if a patient has had a previous baby with Down's syndrome, the risk of this occurring in a subsequent pregnancy is approximately 1% regardless of maternal age. Patients who are known balanced translocation carriers are also at risk of passing a chromosomal aberration to the unborn child and require genetic amniocentesis in most cases..

While several X-linked recessive disorders can be diagnosed directly by enzymatic determination, the more common sex-linked recessive diseases such as hemophilia and Duchenne's muscular dystrophy cannot. In these instances, only sex determination can identify the fetus at risk. One-half of the male offspring can be expected to have the disease, while female offspring will either be normal or carriers.

Another common indication for genetic counseling is the patient who is at risk for delivering a child with a neural tube defect. If a woman has delivered one child with a neural tube defect, such as meningomyelocele or anencephaly, the risk of her delivering a second child with the problem is approximately 5%. Two such affected children increases the risk of the same thing in the third pregnancy to 10%. While ultrasound testing can usually rule out anencephaly, amniotic fluid assays for alpha-fetoprotein are recommended to rule out the neural tube defects not detected by ultrasonic evaluation. In the pregnancy involving a neural tube defect, alpha-fetoprotein levels can be expected to be high. Since disorders other than neural tube defects can also give rise to elevated amniotic fluid alpha-fetoprotein levels, amniography is recommended for a more accurate diagnosis, unless obvious defects are noted by ultrasound examination.

Since 1952 there has been an increasing number of diseases, known as inborn errors of metabolism, that have been determined to be secondary to the absence of a metabolic process. Most of these disorders are inherited as autosomal recessive or X-linked traits. Detection of the approximately eighty inborn errors currently amenable to prenatal diagnosis is generally performed by enzyme activity assay of cultured amniotic fluid cells. These disorders are grouped into categories of lipidosis, mucopolysaccharidosis, amino-acid and related disorders, disorders of carbohydrate metabolism, and miscellaneous hereditary disorders such as sickle cell anemia.

Patients should be informed that genetic amniocentesis is associated with approximately a 1% incidence of spontaneous abortion secondary to the procedure. The amniocentesis should be performed with ultrasonic guidance so as to minimize the risks of maternal and fetal injury. Additionally, it is important that the pregnancy be thoroughly screened with ultrasound prior to the procedure so as to rule out unusual anomalies or twins and to adequately ascertain gestational age. In those women who are Rh-negative with Rh-positive partners, it is recommended that they receive 300 μg of anti-Rh immunoglobulin at the conclusion of the procedure to prevent maternal sensitization secondary to the amniocentesis.

With a basic knowledge of genetic screening and counseling, and with appropriate information concerning risk factors, the physician administering health care to the pregnant woman can play a crucial role in the overall management of the patient at genetic risk. A team approach is essential and involves the genetic laboratory, ultrasound department, blood bank, obstetrician, pediatrician, and a nurse-coordinator whose role involves providing information regarding procedures, reinforcing or initiating counseling information, emotional support of the patient, care of the specimens, and follow-up of outcome. Because of the ever-increasing knowledge in this field, it is imperative that each physician keep abreast of the information in the literature concerning genetic counseling and, when appropriate, apply this information to his or her patient population.

Counseling

1. Bergsma, D. *Birth Defects: Atlas and Compendium.* The National Foundation–March of Dimes. Baltimore: Williams & Wilkins, 1973.
   As a desk reference, this atlas serves as a valuable tool in both identification of genetic risks and risk counseling.

2. Jones, O. W. Genetic counseling. General concepts and principles. *Perinatol. Neonatol.* 16:32, 1981.
   This is an excellent review article regarding the risks of various inheritance patterns. An appropriate management scheme for patients on an ambulatory basis is offered.
3. Marion, J. P., et al. Acceptance of amniocentesis by low-income patients in an urban hospital. *Am. J. Obstet. Gynecol.* 138:11, 1980.
   The incidence of performance of amniocentesis for genetic reasons in low-income patients was studied in over 700 patients. Although genetic services were acceptable to these patients, accessibility and publicity are needed to promote the utilization of the procedure.
4. Adams, M. M., et al. Utilization of prenatal genetic diagnosis in women 35 years of age and older in the United States, 1977 to 1978. *Am. J. Obstet. Gynecol.* 139:673, 1981.
   The authors determined the ratio of use of prenatal diagnosis for advanced maternal age in four states. The utilization ratios ranged between 6% and 28%, were higher in urban areas than rural, and in whites rather than blacks. The use was lowest for those over 40 years of age in whom the risk was the highest.

Genetic Diagnosis

5. Henry, G. P., Peakman, D. C., and Robinson, A. Prenatal genetic diagnosis: Nine years' experience. *Obstet. Gynecol. Surv.* 33:569, 1978.
   The article reviewed the historical background of prenatal genetic diagnosis, the techniques of counseling, and the results of the studies performed over a 9-year period. Techniques of amniocentesis and amniotic fluid cell culturing were discussed.
6. Simpson, J. L. What causes chromosomal abnormalities and gene mutations? *Contemp. Ob/Gyn* 17:99, 1981.
   This superb article combines its basic approach to chromosomal abnormalities from a variety of sources. Principally, the practical recommendations for patient counseling are given.
7. Milunsky, A. Current concepts in genetics. Prenatal diagnosis of genetic disorders. *N. Engl. J. Med.* 295:377, 1976.
   This article reviewed the indications for genetic studies, current methods of prenatal diagnosis of genetic disorders, and problems likely to be encountered, and recommended governmental support of prenatal screening programs because of the prohibitive costs.
8. Queenan, J. T. Can we meet the increasing demand for genetic amniocentesis. *Contemp. Ob/Gyn* 16:77, 1980.
   The problems of clinical centers meeting the demands for genetic amniocentesis are discussed by a forum of experts. They recommended careful analysis of the need of genetic amniocentesis versus the cost.
9. Simpson, J. L., et al. Genetic counseling and genetic services in obstetrics and gynecology: Implications for educational goals and clinical practice. *Am. J. Obstet. Gynecol.* 140:70, 1981.
   The educational goal of genetic counseling as it effects the health care provider is outlined in this article. It was found unnecessary to stress specific details of rare disorders but rather important to emphasize those more common states that the obstetrician-gynecologist is likely to encounter.
10. Golbus, M. S. Teratology for the obstetrician: Current status. *Obstet. Gynecol.* 55:269, 1980.
    A historical review of the role of teratology in obstetric practice and a discussion of common drug categories and their possible fetal effects were presented.

Neural Tube Defects

11. Milunksy, A., and Alpert, E. Prenatal diagnosis of neural tube defects. I. Problems and pitfalls: Analysis of 2495 cases using the alpha-fetoprotein assay. *Obstet. Gynecol.* 48:1, 1976.

    A useful evaluation of the interpretation of alpha-fetoprotein levels was presented in this article, which is the first of five related articles on neural tube defects by the senior author.

12. Stirrat, G. M., et al. Clinical dilemmas arising from the antenatal diagnosis of neural tube defects. *Br. J. Obstet. Gynaecol.* 86:161, 1979.

    The authors review the clinical dilemmas facing the practitioner performing antenatal diagnosis. This is a good summary of issues other than simple medical practices in genetics.

Complications and Risks of Amniocentesis

13. National Registry Study Group. Midtrimester amniocentesis for prenatal diagnosis. *J.A.M.A.* 236:1471, 1976.

    This prospective study of the safety and accuracy of amniocentesis compared outcomes in 1040 women who underwent amniocentesis to 992 matched women who did not. The conclusion was that amniocentesis is both a safe and accurate procedure in midtrimester pregnancy.

14. Chandra, P., et al. Experience with sonography as an adjunct to amniocentesis. *Am. J. Obstet. Gynecol.* 133:519, 1979.

    Results from this study indicated a reduction in the number of bloody amniocenteses, an increase in the number of successful initial taps, and an increase in the proportion of amniotic samples providing useful information, all with the use of sonography as an adjunct to amniocentesis. In addition, sonography was seen as a valuable tool in assessing uterine and fetal abnormalities.

15. Henry, G., Wexler, P., and Robinson, A. Rh immunoglobulin after amniocentesis for genetic diagnosis. *Obstet. Gynecol.* 48:557, 1979.

    Administration of Rh immunoglobulin to Rh-negative women following amniocentesis was recommended in an attempt to reduce the possibility of Rh-sensitization secondary to trauma related to the amniocentesis procedure.

16. Crandall, B. F., et al. Follow-up of 2000 second-trimester amniocenteses. *Obstet. Gynecol.* 56:625, 1980.

    The authors studied 2000 consecutive amniocenteses done in the second trimester. The analysis did not show an increase in perinatal complication because of the amniocentesis.

17. Nolan, G. H., et al. The effect of ultrasonography on midtrimester genetic amniocentesis complications. *Am. J. Obstet. Gynecol.* 140:531, 1981.

    Two groups of patients undergoing midtrimester amniocentesis, one without and one with diagnostic ultrasound for placental localization, were compared. The routine use of ultrasound did not help reduce the number of complications.

18. Menutti, M. T., Brummond, W., and Crombleholme, W. Fetal-maternal bleeding associated with genetic amniocentesis. *Obstet. Gynecol.* 55:48, 1980.

    The diagnosis of fetal-maternal bleeding associated with amniocentesis done in the second trimester is detailed. A case can be made for the administration of RhoGAM on the basis of fetal cells found in the maternal bloodstream.

19. Goplerud, C. P., et al. The selective use of Rho(D) immune globulin (RhIG). *ACOG Tech. Bull.* No. 61, March, 1981.

    The indications for the use of RhoGAM are detailed. This is a vital refer-

ence since many of the standard practices are changed by this issue of the ACOG Technical Bulletin.

Antepartum Fetal Assessment

Although it is currently possible to identify prospectively many of the fetuses at risk for uteroplacental insufficiency (and its associated problems: intrauterine growth retardation, intrauterine fetal demise, and intrapartum fetal distress), the fact remains that the majority of those so identified will tolerate the pregnancy well and intervention for this majority would seem inappropriate. It thus becomes most important in pregnancies associated with these high-risk conditions (e.g., insulin-requiring diabetes mellitus and hypertensive diseases) to separate this majority from the minority who are *not* tolerating well their intrauterine environments and should therefore be considered for delivery. Thus, rather than delivering all babies with a given risk factor at some arbitrary, and likely premature, date, it would be preferable to deliver only those who would be better served by a nursery environment than by the potentially hostile confines of the uterus.

Our abilities to make this distinction are improving greatly. Although there have been many tests proposed for fetoplacental assessment, few have survived. This chapter will describe currently available tests, which rely upon antepartum fetal heart rate (FHR) monitoring, and will comment upon the use of estriol determinations to complement these FHR assessments.

From the electronic fetal monitoring (EFM) techniques developed during the 1960s, Ray and others developed the contraction stress test (CST), and later Rochard and others developed the nonstress test (NST). For a more detailed discussion of uteroplacental respiratory physiology, please refer to the essay Intrapartum Fetal Distress, page 174.

The CST is a test that evaluates the status of fetal oxygenation and, by inference, the status of uteroplacental exchange. This test is conducted after obtaining an informed consent, with standard external EFM equipment, and with the patient in the lateral tilt or semi-Fowler's position (to prevent aortocaval compression). The response of the fetus to spontaneous or oxytocin-induced uterine contractions is noted. An adequate stress to the fetus has been defined arbitrarily as three 40–60-second contractions occurring within 10 minutes. Since the uterus, by this definition, is at times contracting at such an adequate rate in late pregnancy, it is important to observe the monitor strip for about 15 minutes before adding any oxytocin. If this drug is used, it must be given "piggy-back" via a freely flowing intravenous line. Because the uterus may be unpredictably sensitive, the initial rate should be only 0.5 milliunits per minute, and this rate should be increased no more often than every 10–15 minutes. With such an adequate stress, the absence of late decelerations (a negative CST) implies normal fetal oxygenation and is the finding in over 80% of tests.

If the test result is negative, it is necessary to repeat the CST only weekly. This infrequency of testing is possible because of the wealth of data suggesting that only about 0.2% of high-risk fetuses will experience fetal death within a week of a negative test, as so defined. However, if the currently popular 10-minute-window concept is used, this so-called false-negative rate is somewhat higher, about 1%. This concept ignores an occasional late deceleration so long as there is a 10-minute segment of tracing with three contractions and no late decelerations.

The positive test manifests recurrent late decelerations and (if hyperstimulation and supine positioning are excluded) implies that the fetal basal oxygenation is suboptimal. Unfortunately, with external monitoring techniques the precise quantitation of contraction stress is impossible, and this may help explain why up to 50% of fetuses with a positive CST may tolerate labor without further evidence of distress (late decelerations). However, since the obstetrician is alerted in such cases to possible problems, these labors are generally conducted under conditions normally used for intrauterine resuscitation (maintenance of lateral position, intravascular hydration, mask oxygenation, and extreme care in the use of oxytocin and conduction anesthesia). Such care in the conduct of the labor with these potentially fragile fetuses may help to explain the large number of good neonatal outcomes after a positive test (false-positive). However, it is clear that a positive CST does not, in and of itself, preclude a trial of carefully conducted labor.

For nearly 20% of patients, a definite negative or positive result cannot be obtained during a given CST. The majority of these equivocal tests are termed suspicious, which implies that at least one late deceleration is present on the record. The designation of unsatisfactory is used if late decelerations cannot be excluded with certainty or (rarely) if adequate uterine response cannot be achieved with an oxytocin rate of 8–10 milliunits/minute. A third equivocal designation is *hyperstimulation,* a term used for those CST tracings in which contractions occurring more frequently than every 2 minutes or lasting more than 90 seconds are associated with late decelerations. With any of these equivocal designations, no reassurance can be gained from the CST, and the test must be repeated within 24 hours, at which time the great majority will be either negative or positive. In the case of the suspicious CST, only about 10%–15% will be positive on the repeat test, but this is about three to four times the frequency of overall positive tests and underscores the importance of early retesting. The 10-minute-window concept excludes the suspicious and hyperstimulation designations.

The NST is an assessment of central nervous system (CNS) alertness and, by inference, the status of fetal acid-base balance. This test is also performed with standard external monitoring equipment and with the patient in the lateral tilt or semi-Fowler's position. In the case of *intrapartum* monitoring with fetal scalp electrodes, the presence of FHR variability reassures the clinician that the metabolic status of the fetus (specifically the fetal CNS) is sufficiently intact that the CNS can exert normal, controlling influences on the FHR. Since FHR variability assessment is generally impossible with Doppler ultrasound external techniques, the extension of this concept to the antepartum period has been that the metabolically normal fetus will accelerate its FHR briefly in response to spontaneous or provoked fetal movements. Such accelerations with fetal movement (reactive NST) thus imply that the fetus, at the time of the test, has not recently endured hypoxia sufficiently severe to cause a metabolic acidosis.

The reactive NST has been variously defined, but probably the most widely used definition at present is two accelerations with fetal movement (AFMs) of 15 beats per minute within a 20-minute period. Generally, two 20-minute observation periods, combined if necessary with gentle prodding of the fetus who is apparently sleeping, are used before the test is termed nonreactive. The nonreactive NST is generally followed by a CST. The reasoning behind this sequence is to establish whether the nonreactive pattern observed is on the basis of fetal hypoxia, which would be manifested by a positive CST.

The reactive CST is generally repeated every 7 days, so long as there is not a great deterioration in the clinical condition of the mother. The risk of fetal death within a week of a reactive NST is about 1%, essentially the same as with the negative CST when the 10-minute-window interpretation is used, but approximately five times the rate if any late decelerations seen on the tracing preclude a designation of negative to the CST.

The NST, however, has numerous apparent advantages over the CST. The time required for the NST is normally only a fraction of that necessary for the CST. With the NST, there is no need for an intravenous line, and the potential complications occurring with oxytocin administration are obviated. Also, although there are contraindications to performing a CST (such as ruptured membranes, placenta previa, classic cesarean-section scar, and concern over precipitating premature labor), there are essentially none to performing a NST. If the capability exists to perform backup CSTs in a hospital facility, then NSTs can be performed in the office or clinic. These considerations explain why the NST can be performed for more patients and for less cost than the CST. Of course, since the CST may be necessary as follow-up for any NST, the consent form for the NST must also explain the CST.

The usual sequence of fetal deterioration is: normal oxygenation, normal pH (negative CST, reactive NST); then subnormal oxygenation, still normal pH (positive CST, still reactive NST); and finally, subnormal oxygenation, subnormal pH (positive CST, nonreactive NST). If this sequence is correct, one would expect the fetus with the nonreactive NST, positive CST to have the greatest chance of fetal death and damage, and there are suggestions that this is the case. Such a fetus is very unlikely to tolerate labor, whereas the fetus with a reactive NST, positive CST may well tolerate this stress. The fetus with a nonreactive NST, positive CST is also more likely to have such undesirable concomitants as growth retardation, intrapartum fetal distress, low Apgar scores, and perinatal death.

Although it might be advantageous to have then *both* the NST and CST performed weekly on every pregnancy at risk for uteroplacental insufficiency, the improvement in outcome (if real) would be only slight. For this and the obvious logistic and economic considerations, primary management of most of these pregnancies with the NST is probably appropriate and is generally utilized at present.

On the other hand, it might be considered reasonable to do both tests (CST following a 10–15 minute observation for reactivity and uterine activity) on certain of the patients at highest risk. This as yet unpublished data from the CST/NST Collaborative Study (Dr. Roger Freeman, Long Beach Hospital, Los Angeles, CA) would suggest that those conditions most likely to manifest a nonreactive NST, positive CST are: insulin-requiring diabetes, severe chronic hypertension, oligohydramnios, and sonar-consistent intrauterine growth retardation. This list is of no surprise to anyone, as these are clearly the conditions at highest risk for perinatal death or damage. Patients with these conditions, who will generally comprise no more than 10% of the high-risk patients needing these tests, are currently managed in our center primarily by both NST and CST performed in sequence on a weekly basis. Once a positive CST is encountered, the question arises as to its meaning. Although the greatest value of these tests is prevention of unnecessary intervention in over 90% of high risk pregnancies, we, by deduction, assume that within the positive CST group exist those few pregnancies that, without intervention, will eventuate in undesirable outcomes.

Generally, when the CST is positive, evidence of fetal pulmonary maturity is sought by amniotic fluid analysis. For most pregnancies, a lecithin/sphingomyelin (L/S) ratio should suffice, but an assessment for phosphatidylglycerol is also prudent in patients with diabetes and rhesus sensitization. If the tests then indicate pulmonary maturity, delivery is sought. Unless there is an abnormal lie or other obstetrical indication for cesarean delivery, vaginal delivery is attempted if the cervix is at least partially favorable for an induction attempt (Bishop score of 4 or 5). Another disclaimer is that those fetuses showing a positive CST associated with a nonreactive FHR pattern rarely tolerate labor. If the L/S ratio denotes pulmonary immaturity, procrastination may be reasonable only if either *daily* NSTs or *daily* urinary or plasma estriol levels remain reassuring. Otherwise, the baby is probably better served by delivery and placement in an intensive-care nursery facility. As demonstrated by Harris and associates, perinatal outcome for such a potentially morbid pregnancy is probably improved by transferring the fetus in utero to a tertiary care facility for delivery.

Fetal surveillance with CSTs or NSTs is generally begun at 32 to 34 gestational weeks, although for the most worrisome situations, these tests may be begun as early in gestation as one would be willing to act upon an abnormal test result. In most perinatal centers this lower limit is currently 26 to 28 weeks.

With these antepartum FHR tests, the clinician is able with remarkable accuracy to identify within the high-risk group those fetuses who are tolerating their environments acceptably and are not at serious risk for stillbirth within 7 days. The reassuring tests are therefore of great comfort to both doctor and patient. However, within the positive-CST group must then exist those infants destined for poor outcome. Although we cannot at present identify with precision those so destined, it is refreshing to note that even in an indigent obstetrical population, only a fraction of 1% of patients will ultimately undergo a cesarean section on the basis of these tests. The percentage for whom this operation is thereby avoided is certainly many times higher.

Reviews

1. Huddleston, J. F. Stress and Nonstress Testing. In J. J. Sciarra and R. Depp (Eds.), *Gynecology and Obstetrics.* Hagerstown, Md.: Harper & Row, 1980. Vol. 2.
   A review of the pathophysiology of uteroplacental exchange and a historical perspective on the development of antepartum FHR tests. Also included is a perspective on the complementary usefulness of the two tests.
2. Huddleston, J. F., and Freeman, R. K. The Use of the Oxytocin Challenge for the Management of Pregnancies at Risk for Uteroplacental Insufficiency. In R. J. Bolognese and R. H. Schwarz (Eds.), *Perinatal Medicine: Management of the High Risk Fetus and Neonate.* Baltimore: Williams & Wilkins, 1977.
   A presentation of the method and interpretation of the CST. A review of the then-reported large series of CSTs, 4920 tests in 2307 pregnancies at high risk, showed a fetal loss (false-negative) rate of only 2.2 per 1000 tests.
3. Aladjem, et al. Antepartum fetal testing: Evaluation and redefinition of criteria for clinical interpretation. *Semin. Perinatol.* 5:145, 1981.
   The authors completely review the spectrum of antepartum fetal testing. A redefinition of fetal health assessment test suggested by this study is offered.

Fetal Movements

4. Sadovsky, E. Fetal movements and fetal health. *Semin. Perinatol.* 5:131, 1981.
   The author describes the experience in grading fetal movements with fetal health. Direct correlation was found, and he recommends clinical use of this tool.

5. Manning, F. A., et al. Fetal breathing movements and the nonstress test in high-risk pregnancies. *Am. J. Obstet. Gynecol.* 135:511, 1979.
   Observations of fetal breathing movements were made in 223 patients. If the NST was reactive, it correlated highly to the number of fetal breathing movements.
6. Rayburn, W. F., and McKean, H. E. Maternal perception of fetal movement and perinatal outcome. *Obstet. Gynecol.* 56:161, 1981.
   Perception of fetal activity by the mother was studied in 306 patients. This method excelled at predicting the risk of subsequent perinatal distress.

Contraction Stress Test (CST)

7. Bruce, S. E., Petrie, R. H., and Yeh, S. Y. The suspicious contraction stress test. *Obstet. Gynecol.* 51:415, 1978.
   Although the suspicious CST is followed by a positive test much more frequently than a negative test is, there is little evidence to suggest that delivery should be hastened unless a truly positive test can be demonstrated.
8. Gabbe, S. G., Freeman, R. K., and Goebelsmann, U. Evaluation of the contraction stress test before 33 weeks' gestation. *Obstet. Gynecol.* 52:649, 1978.
   Although there had earlier been some concern that the CST was perhaps not valid in the very premature fetus, this study strongly supports the opposite point of view.
9. Garite, T J., et al. Oxytocin challenge test: Achieving the desired goals. *Obstet. Gynecol.* 51:614, 1978.
   Although there may be value in extending to many more pregnant women the reassurance offered by these antepartum FHR tests, we first need to make sure that the tests are given to all those with risk factors clearly indicating a need for this type of surveillance.

Nonstress Test (NST)

10. Keegan, K. A., and Paul, R. H. Antepartum fetal heart rate testing: IV. The nonstress test as a primary approach. *Am. J. Obstet. Gynecol.* 136:75, 1980.
    The use of the NST as the primary approach in the antepartum surveillance of high-risk pregnancies. By reducing to two the number of accelerations within a 10-minute period necessary to declare a test reactive, and by allowing reactivity appearing on a follow-up CST to suffice for a reactive designation, the number of NSTs that require full CSTs becomes quite small.
11. Sampson, M. B., Thomason, J. L., and Work, B. A., Jr. Rapid nonstress test evaluation. *Am. J. Obstet. Gynecol.* 140:467, 1981.
    The use of a polaroid transparency is encouraged to detect if the accelerations meet the criteria for a reactive nonstress test. This assists the clinician in being more accurate and may be helpful in quantitating the results of this important test.
12. Phelan, J. P., and Lewis, P. E., Jr. Fetal heart rate decelerations during a nonstress test. *Obstet. Gynecol.* 57:228, 1981.
    In a review of 2000 NSTs, 94 revealed rate decelerations in response to fetal activity. Three intrauterine fetal deaths occurred and 8.5% showed fetal distress. Variable decelerations occurred in 60%, while in 55% abnormal cord position was observed during or after labor.
13. Visser, G. H. A., et al. Nonstressed antepartum heart rate monitoring: Implications of decelerations after spontaneous contractions. *Am. J. Obstet. Gynecol.* 138:429, 1980.

Fetal outcome in 98 patients with spontaneous late decelerations in the antepartum period was studied. Intrauterine death occurred in 14 fetuses within a week, while 71% of the remaining 84 fetuses were acidemic at the time of birth.

14. Phelan, J. P. The nonstress test: A review of 3,000 tests. *Am. J. Obstet. Gynecol.* 139:7, 1981.

    Of 3000 NSTs performed, 85% were reactive, 14% nonreactive, and less than 1% unsatisfactory. The patients in the nonreactive group showed a significantly higher rate of cesarean section, fetal distress, and perinatal mortality when compared to the reactive group.

15. Slomka, C., and Phelan, J. P. Pregnancy outcome in the patient with a nonreactive nonstress test and a positive contraction test. *Am. J. Obstet. Gynecol.* 139:11, 1981.

    Pregnancy outcome in 41 high-risk pregnancies with a nonreactive NST and a positive CST were studied. Of the group who were allowed to labor 60% had late decelerations and one-third required abdominal deliveries. A case for induction of labor can be made, but close attention is required.

General

16. Schifrin, B. S., et al. The role of real-time scanning in antenatal fetal surveillance. *Am. J. Obstet. Gynecol.* 140:525, 1981.

    The value of real-time ultrasound scanning was investigated in 150 high-risk patients after a nonstress test. The results suggest that this method, particularly after a nonreactive NST, is a most effective and economical way of assessing fetal ill health.

17. Bishop, E. H. Pelvic scoring for elective induction. *Obstet. Gynecol.* 24:266, 1964.

    Classic description of the pelvic scoring system for predicting the success of elective induction of labor.

18. Druzin, M. L., et al. Antepartum fetal heart rate testing: VII. The significance of fetal bradycardia. *Am. J. Obstet. Gynecol.* 139:194, 1981.

    Fetal movements associated with a variable deceleration pattern suggest oligohydramnios and are of prognostic significance.

19. Manning, F. A., et al. Fetal biophysical profile scoring: A prospective study in 1,184 high-risk patients. *Am. J. Obstet. Gynecol.* 140:289, 1981.

    A fetal biophysical profile was used in the evaluation of referred high-risk patients and this profile allowed only six perinatal deaths to occur. In addition, 13 fetuses with major congenital anomalies were detected. This method can be used effectively to screen and manage a high-risk population.

20. Hon, E. H., and Quilligan, E. J. Classification of fetal heart rate: II. A revised working classification. *Conn. Med.* 31:779, 1967.

    The authors, on the basis of their pioneering work in the field, presented in this article the periodic FHR patterns as we commonly use them now.

21. Keane, M. W. D., Horger, E. O., III, and Vice, L. Comparative study of stressed and nonstressed antepartum fetal heart rate testing. *Obstet. Gynecol.* 57:320, 1981.

    NSTs and CSTs were performed on 566 patients. The correlation between a reactive NST and a negative CST was almost 100%, whereas the correlation between the nonreactive NST and a positive CST was only 25%. The CST was a better predictor of morbidity but both tests were highly significant predictors of fetal distress.

22. Harris, B. A., Jr., et al. In utero versus neonatal transportation of high-risk perinates: A comparison. *Obstet. Gynecol.* 57:496, 1981.

    In this report, covering a 3-year period, the authors compare those infants transferred to a tertiary center after delivery with those transferred to the center in utero. Within each of eight risk categories (based on gestational age and birth weight), there was a numerical improvement in favor of in utero referral. This improvement reached statistical significance in three of the eight categories. There also were statistical differences, in favor of fetal transfer, in length of hospital stay and in the need for continuous positive airway pressure or endotracheal ventilation.

Assessment of Fetal Maturity

We are commonly faced with the problem of whether to deliver, or permit to be delivered, fetuses prior to 40 weeks gestation. Among the myriad of problems premature infants face, respiratory distress syndrome (RDS) looms as the greatest impediment to survival. In 1903, hyaline membranes in the lungs of 2 infants who had died of respiratory difficulties were described. Subsequent research by K. Pattle demonstrated that the tiny bubbles isolated from pulmonary-edema foam have prolonged stability. M. E. Avery and P. B. Mead then demonstrated that lung extracts from infants dying of RDS have markedly higher surface-tension values than those from term infants dying of other causes. C. J. Hobel reported the isolation of a substance that reduces surface tension in bovine lung tissue. This substance was later characterized as a complex mixture of lipids, proteins, and carbohydrates. Among the lipids, 90%–95% are phospholipids, the rest being mainly cholesterol. Phosphatidylcholine, or lecithin, comprises about 50% of the surface-active component. A second phospholipid, phosphatidylglycerol, comprises 7%–14% of the surfactant complex. A number of minor surface-active components may be demonstrated as well.

Efforts to predict the success of newborns in coping with the extrauterine environment were originally indirect in nature, relying on measurements of gestational age, such as amniotic fluid creatinine, osmolality, and bilirubin levels; percentage of fat-staining cells in amniotic fluid; radiologic assessment of distal femoral epiphyses; and more recently, ultrasonic evaluation of the biparietal diameter. While all these measurements provide evidence for advancing gestational age, none of them is capable of assessing the ability of the lungs to function in an extrauterine environment. Recently, a number of methods have been described that measure the actual or functional presence of surfactant components elaborated into amniotic fluid from the fetal airways. As a whole, these tests have excellent specificity in that very few infants predicted to have mature lungs will suffer RDS. On the other hand, the tests are not very sensitive, and a large percentage of infants delivered with "immature" pulmonary indices will have no apparent respiratory disease after birth. Several of the more widely used tests are summarized below.

The lecithin/sphingomyelin (L/S) ratio was first described by L. Gluck in 1971. This method has become the standard against which most new tests are compared. It is, unfortunately, rather time-consuming and tedious to perform, involving both separations and chromatography. Although a number of shortcuts on the method have been described, it is generally felt that most of the shortcuts, specifically those eliminating precipitation with acetone, produce a much less reliable result. A lecithin to sphingomyelin ratio of 2.0 is the value above which a fetus is assumed to have functionally mature lungs. Reported false-positive rates range from 0%–5%, depending, among other things, on the patient population involved. False-negative rates, on the other hand, range from 20%–100%, with most studies reporting values between 33% and 50%. Some investigators have subdivided the range below 2.0 into groups above and below 1.5, or another arbitrary value, but the outcome data reported are not consistent. Indeed, there were a large number of well babies born with L/S ratios less than 1.0. False-positives tend to occur primarily among diabetic patients, whereas false-negative results are spread over the entire gamut of patients. The presence of meconium and blood alter the results in an irregular fashion. L/S values above 2.5, however, almost invariably indicate a mature fetus, even in the presence of contaminants.

Phosphatidylglycerol (PG) was described in 1976 and has been used clinically as an extension of the L/S ratio. PG, which first appears around 36 weeks gestation, normally comprises 7%–14% of the phospholipids in mature surfactant. The determination of PG is made in a manner similar to that of the L/S ratio, except that the chromatography is bidirectional. The method has the advantage of separating surface-active components from contaminants such as blood and meconium. Gluck and others have asserted that, barring complicating factors such as asphyxia or infection, the presence of PG virtually assures the absence of RDS, even in diabetic patients. Unfortunately, the test is even more time-consuming and exacting to perform than the L/S ratio and cannot serve as an inexpensive or rapid screening procedure.

The foam stability test was first described by Clements in 1972. Presently, there are several variants of this test, and all are based on the fact that a certain amount of surface-active lipid in solution will stabilize the small bubbles of foam, even in the presence of ethanol, an antifoam agent. The tests involve combining amniotic fluid and ethanol in precisely controlled ratios, agitating the resulting mixture, and observing for persistence of a surface foam. The several forms of the test vary primarily in the percentage ethanol in the mixture(s), details of mixing, and interpretation of results. Clinical reports indicate that when positive, the tests are very reliable. When questionable or negative, the tests have little predictive value. Meconium and blood in amniotic fluid samples tend to produce false-positive results. Vernix does not. The greatest difficulty with these tests is standardization. Because ethanol concentrations are critical and because handling of samples and interpretation of bubble patterns introduces considerable variability, reproducibility of results has tended to vary widely from institution to institution, leading to some skepticism with regard to the use of these tests.

Fluorescence polarization index of amniotic fluid is a simple, highly reproducible test that has not been used widely in this country, partly because the apparatus needed to perform the test (FELMA microviscosimeter) is quite expensive and is manufactured in Israel. The test is based on use of a lipid-soluble dye that fluoresces when struck by polarized light. When the dye is mixed with a solution containing lipids, such as amniotic fluid, and exposed to polarized light, analysis of the degree of polarization of the resulting fluorescence gives information concerning the concentration of lipids in the solution. The method is also referred to as microviscosimetry. Studies to date indicate that results of this test correlate very well with those obtained by L/S ratio and may, in fact, show an even better correlation with newborn outcome than does the L/S ratio. Definitive statements concerning the practicality of this method await more extensive evaluation.

In regard to optical density (OD) of amniotic fluid, it has been suggested that optical density at 650 nm as a measure of turbidity might be related to total amniotic-fluid phospholipid content and thus be predictive of fetal lung maturity. Measurement of optical density has the advantages of being very quick and inexpensive. Comparisons between OD 650 values and L/S ratio have, however, been inconsistent, and not all authors are enthusiastic about the method.

Measurements of various other components of the surfactant system have been described. Some of these include lecithin phosphorus, total amniotic-fluid lecithin, the lecithin button test, total phospholipid phosphorus, palmitic acid and palmitic/stearic acid ratio, and phosphatidic acid phosphohydrolase (PAPase). For various reasons, none of these has enjoyed widespread popularity.

Future development of tests of fetal pulmonary maturity is being directed toward solving the problems of speed and ease of performance, so that the results may be more readily available at the places and times they are needed. The problem of false-negatives, or fetuses with negative indices who do well when delivered, has plagued all the tests in current use and is under careful scrutiny as well.

Review

1. Shields, J. R., and Resnik, R. Fetal lung maturation and the antenatal use of glucocorticoids to prevent the respiratory distress syndrome. *Obstet. Gynecol. Surv.* 34:343, 1979.
   Comprehensive review of anatomic and biochemical development of fetal lung, indices of fetal lung maturity, and the risks and benefits of administration of glucocorticoids for acceleration of fetal lung maturity.

2. Gabbe, S. G. Recent advances in the assessment of fetal maturity. *J. Reprod. Med.* 23:227, 1979.
   Review of various methods of evaluating amniotic fluid surfactant activity. Details of practical difficulties with each method as well as reported false-positive and false-negative rates.

3. O'Brien, W. F., and Cefalo, R. C. Clinical applicability of amniotic fluid tests for fetal pulmonic maturity. *Am. J. Obstet. Gynecol.* 136:135, 1980.
   A tabular presentation of 25 reports describing the clinical experience with the most popular methods developed to date for surfactant analysis of amniotic fluid.

4. Anderson, H. F., et al. Gestational age assessment: I. Analysis of individual clinical observations. *Am. J. Obstet. Gynecol.* 139:173, 1981.
   The authors assess the accuracy of last menstrual period, uterine measurements, first audible fetal heart tones, and quickening. Of these, the last normal menstrual period was the most accurate estimator of fetal gestational age.

Anatomic Development

5. Stahlman, M. T., and Gray, M. E. Anatomical development and maturation of the lungs. *Clin. Perinatol.* 5:181, 1978.
   Illustrated review of embryonic and fetal development of the lung.

Biochemical Development

6. Farrel, P. M., and Hamosh, M. The biochemistry of fetal lung development. *Clin. Perinatol.* 5:197, 1978.
   Detailed description of the development of biochemical pathways for the production of surfactant components. Discussion of the effect of pharmacologic and physiologic influences on development of these pathways.

7. Wallace, R. L., and Herrick, C. N. Pulmonary maturity studies in the evaluation of premature labor. *Am. J. Obstet. Gynecol.* 140:512, 1981.
   Amniocentesis was performed prior to treating patients with tocolytic

therapy who were in premature labor. A second amniocentesis was performed after tocolytic therapy was begun and there was a poor correlation of OD_{650} and an L/S ratio of greater than 2:1.

Measurement of Surfactant Components

8. Gluck, L., et al. The interpretation and significance of the lecithin/sphyngomyelin ratio in amniotic fluid. *Am. J. Obstet. Gynecol.* 120:142, 1974.

   A discussion of the significance of the L/S ratio and of the several variations that had been described by 1974, with emphasis on what appear to be critical steps in the analysis.

9. Clements, J. A., et al. Assessment of the risk of respiratory distress syndrome by a rapid test for surfactant in amniotic fluid. *N. Engl. J. Med.* 286:1077, 1972.

   Original description of the foam stability test. Numerous variations of this test have been subsequently described.

10. Statland, B. E., Sher, G., and Freer, D. E. Evaluation of a modified foam stability test. *Am. J. Clin. Pathol.* 69:514, 1978.

    One of the several simplifications of Clement's foam stability test. This one incorporates simpler methodology intended to improve reproducibility.

11. Spellacy, W. N., et al. Assessment of fetal lung maturity: A comparison of the lecithin/sphyngomyelin ratio and the tests of optical density at 400 and 650 nm. *Am. J. Obstet. Gynecol.* 134:528, 1979.

    As with most tests of pulmonary maturity, the results are correlated with those of a simultaneously run L/S ratio, rather than to newborn outcome.

12. Golde, S. H., et al. Evaluation of the FELMA microviscosimeter in predicting fetal lung maturity. *Obstet. Gynecol.* 54:639, 1979.

    This promising methodology has yet to be widely evaluated because of the expense and difficulty involved in obtaining the necessary apparatus. Newborn outcomes are considered in this paper, and it appears that this method is at least as good as, and perhaps better than, the L/S ratio in predicting RDS.

13. Simon, M. V., et al. Prediction of fetal lung maturity by amniotic fluid fluorescence polarization, L:S ratio, and phosphatidylglycerol. *Obstet. Gynecol.* 57:295, 1981.

    The relationship of amniotic fluid polarization was compared to the L/S ratio and phosphatidylglycerol. Each test detected mature infants who would have been incorrectly classified by at least one of the other tests. The authors recommend using the three tests in combination to reduce the number of false predictions of hyaline membrane disease.

14. Whittle, M. J., et al. Changes in the lecithin:sphingomyelin ratio during labor and the associated fetal heart rate patterns. *Obstet. Gynecol.* 57:335, 1981.

    Fifty-five patients in labor were assessed for L/S ratios, which were then compared to the fetal heart rate pattern. Very low L/S ratios were observed in some patients whose infants did not develop RDS and were significantly correlated to the duration of labor and long-term variability. The possibility is that the amniotic fluid during labor is no longer representative of the lung fluid.

15. Mackenna, J., Hodson, C. A., and Brame, R. G. Clinical utility of fetal lung maturity profile. *Obstet. Gynecol.* 57:493, 1981.

    The usefulness of the lung maturity profile (PG) was assessed in 356 patients. The presence of PG, even with an immature L/S ratio, predicts that the newborn will not get hyaline membrane disease.

GYNECOLOGY

GENERAL GYNECOLOGY

Fibroids (myomata, fibromyomata, leiomyomata) are the most common benign tumors of the female genital tract. They usually occur in the uterus but can also be found in the round ligament, the ovary, and rarely in the labia majora. These growths are solid tumors but may undergo degeneration, in turn sometimes producing some softening of the tumors.

Degenerations, which may be either hyaline, cystic, or fatty, are usually due to diminished blood supply when the tumor becomes large. Red degeneration (or necrobiosis) may occur during pregnancy or postpartum, and it has been reported in the menopause. This is due to venous obstruction producing intense congestion and necrosis. Malignant (sarcomatous) change is a rare complication in the menopausal woman.

Uterine fibroids may be either submucous (growing into the cavity), intramural, or subserous (bulging into the peritoneal cavity). The last-named type of fibroid may develop a pedicle and become attached to other structures—usually the omentum—and obtain extra blood supply from these areas. Knowing the anatomic site of the myomata is important in regard to their symptomatology, complications, and management.

Little has been documented regarding their etiology. It has been established that they are more common, grow more extensively, and occur at a younger age in the black population. They are somehow associated with infertility (either as a possible cause or effect) and appear to be related to hormonal influences. They certainly get larger during pregnancy and with estrogen administration. They diminish in size postmenopausally and regrow or recur after surgical removal. They can be extremely large and multiple yet remain benign. They have been reported in girls as young as 11 years old.

Pathologically, fibroids are distinguished by their definitive pseudocapsule and whorled macroscopic appearance on cross section. Because they arise from a single smooth muscle cell, *leiomyomata* should be the correct term for these tumors. Deposits of calcium, following long-standing degeneration, account for the tumor's gritty feel on cutting and the typical stippled appearance on x-ray.

The most frequent presenting feature is menorrhagia (75% of patients). It is the resultant anemia that may bring the patient to the doctor. Infertility, dysmenorrhea (usually of the congestive type), and the presence of an abdominal mass account for most of the other symptoms. Acute episodes, such as retention of urine due to degeneration, are rarely encountered. Metrorrhagia may also be a complaint. Large numbers of patients harbor symptomless fibroids, many being identified only at routine vaginal or general medical examinations. Autopsy shows that 20% of women over the age of 30 have fibroids without symptoms; and 50% of patients with symptoms present before they are 35.

The majority of signs and symptoms are related to the submucous fibroids, which account for the dysmenorrhea, the menorrhagia (resulting from an increased bleeding surface area), metrorrhagia, and intermittent pain. The submucous fibroid can become pedunculated and be delivered through the cervix. The surface of the tumor may become eroded, become septic, and produce marked metrorrhagia, which will bring the patient to the hsopital. They may also induce abortion, due to interference with placentation, or postpartum hemorrhage from incomplete placental separation.

Intramural fibroids cause the least problems, only producing symptoms because of their size. The mechanism whereby they affect infertility has not yet been elucidated. They are most likely the result, rather than the cause of sterility.

Subserous fibroids are also asymptomatic unless they are very large or become pedunculated. The latter group may cause some peritoneal irritation or rarely, if very mobile, undergo torsion. Even extremely large fibroid uteri seldom produce more than slight mechanical or anatomical obstruction of the ureters. Edema of the legs and increased varicosities in the extremities may also be noted with large tumors.

In the postmenopausal woman, sudden enlargement (with or without pain) could indicate either cystic degeneration or sarcomatous degeneration. The latter occurs in less than 0.5% of patients.

Leiomyosarcomas occur postmenopausally—the average age is 55—and with greater frequency in the black population. Incidence is unrelated to parity. The most common presenting symptom is vaginal bleeding. The tumor is nonencapsulated with a bulging, homogenous, grayish-white, soft pultaceous mass in which the whorled appearance has disappeared. This malignancy must not be confused with cellular leiomyomata. The latter are fibroid tumors that have increased cellularity and closely opposed nuclei microscopically. They have a low mitotic count compared to sarcomas, with little or no anaplasia. They have a propensity to enlarge rapidly during pregnancy.

The benign metastasizing leiomyoma is a condition in which uterine myomata are found together with pulmonary nodules of well-differentiated benign smooth muscle. It is probably related to dissemination of intravenous leiomyomata; this refers to the presence of well-differentiated smooth muscle in the lumina of uterine and pelvic veins. Microscopically, wormlike cords of tumor can be seen extending from the myometrium into veins of the broad ligament. There is no inclination toward extravascular invasion. Clinical symptoms are vaginal bleeding and, infrequently, abdominal enlargement.

Leiomyomatosis peritonealis disseminata is a rare pathological entity. Multiple, 1 cm–2 cm, raised white nodules are seen on the peritoneal surface, including the liver and bowel. These are often associated with large uterine leiomyomas. They are grossly indistinguishable from a disseminated malignant tumor but are benign, both microscopically and in their clinical behavior. The condition is rather metaplastic than metastatic in its pathogenesis.

The diagnosis of myomata is usually clinical. Bimanual pelvic examination reveals a characteristically firm to hard, irregularly shaped, enlarged uterus. Abdominal x-rays may show the soft tissue tumor and the presence of calcification, which, if present, will appear as concentric white rings. Ultrasound may also be helpful as it will confirm that the tumors are not extrauterine masses. Intravenous pyelography may show evidence of pressure effects on the ureters and should be included in the workup. Differential diagnosis includes ovarian tumors, chronic tuboovarian abscess, hydrosalpinx, uterine sarcoma, and adenomyosis.

The management of myomata will depend essentially on the patient's age, parity, and symptoms. It will also be influenced by her desire for future pregnancies. As a rule, a total abdominal hysterectomy (vaginal hysterectomy may be performed if feasible) is the procedure of choice in the older patient in whom fertility is not a factor.

The treatment of leiomyosarcoma is total abdominal hysterectomy and bilateral salpingo-oophorectomy. The 5-year survival rate is only 20.7%. Pelvic recurrence is the most common initial indication of treatment failure. Metastases to peritoneum and lung are next in frequency.

In the younger patient, small submucous fibroids may be removed after cervical dilatation by curettage or be removed with polyp-forceps. When the fibroid has become pedunculated and presents through the cervix, the tumor may be twisted off or the pedicle cut at the base. This is followed by an immediate curettage to ensure that there are no small residual fibroid polyps.

Hysterosalpingography may indicate if submucous fibroids are present and establish the patency, or otherwise, of the fallopian tubes. Laparoscopy may be done prior to definitive surgery to determine whether myomectomy or hysterectomy should be done. The final decision will usually depend on the condition of the tubes.

Myomectomy is performed when there is tubal patency, or tuboplasty is possible, when the uterus is not too large (not more than 20 weeks pregnancy size), and the fibroids are not too numerous. The main complication is hemorrhage at operation and postoperative sepsis. Prophylactic antibiotics should be administered with all myomectomies. The disadvantage of only resecting the fibroids is that there is a 10% recurrence rate. With young patients 50% will conceive in the first 2 years after myomectomy if there are no other infertility factors. Pregnancy rates are only 5%–10% in women over 35 years of age.

Asymptomatic myomata when the uterus is less than 10 weeks in size may be treated expectantly. Two or three examinations annually will indicate if they are dormant or getting larger.

Myomectomies should never be performed during pregnancy. The rare acute red degeneration in pregnancy will respond to pain relief and antipyretics. Occasionally, a fibroid may be removed at cesarean section if it interferes with the procedure. Obstructed labor due to fibroids is extremely rare, and management is by cesarean section. The fibroids shrink rapidly postpartum and surgery should be delayed for at least 6 weeks after delivery.

Books

1. Novak, E. R., and Woodruff, J. D. Myoma and Other Benign Tumors of the Uterus. In E. R. Novak and J. D. Woodruff (Eds.), *Novak's Gynecologic and Obstetric Pathology with Clinical and Endocrine Relations* (8th ed.). Philadelphia: Saunders, 1979.
   A concise presentation of pathology in relationship to the clinical problems of myomata.
2. Howkins, J., and Stallworthy, C. J. Chap. 18. In J. Hawkins and J. Stallworthy (Eds.), *Bonney's Gynecological Surgery* (8th ed.). London: Balliere-Tindall, 1974.
   A clear, concise, well-illustrated, step-by-step approach to myomectomy. It remains the standard text for the surgical approach to fibroids.

Etiology

3. Wilson, E. A., et al. Estradiol and progesterone binding in uterine leiomyomata and in normal uterine tissues. *Obstet. Gynecol.* 55:20, 1980.
   There might be a hormonal basis for myomatous growth. Estrogen receptors are significantly greater in fibroids than in normal myometrium.
4. Fujii, S., et al. Progesterone-induced smooth muscle-like cells in the subperitoneal nodules produced by estrogen. *Am. J. Obstet. Gynecol.* 139:164, 1981.
   Hormonal basis of fibroids via action on subcoelomic totipotential mesenchyme.

Diagnosis

5. Weinstein, D., et al. Hysterography before and after myomectomy. *A.J.R.* 129:899, 1977.

The value of preoperative hysterography in confirming the diagnosis and localization of the myomata is stressed.

6. Neuwirth, R. S., and Amin, H. K. Excision of submucous fibroids with hysteroscopic control. *Am. J. Obstet. Gynecol.* 126:95, 1976.
   A new dimension in the diagnosis and management of submucous fibroids.
7. Samuelsson, S., and Ovall, S. J. The value of laparoscopy in the differential diagnosis between uterine fibromyomata and adnexal tumors. *Acta Obstet. Gynecol. Scand.* 49:175, 1970.
   Laparoscopy may be indicated with subserous fibroids.
8. Hassan, N. Ultrasonic appearance of pedunculated uterine fibroids and ovarian cysts. *J. Natl. Med. Assoc.* 66:432, 1974.
   Ultrasound can be useful in diagnosing fibroids.

Problems in Pregnancy

9. Ogunbode, O., et al. Uterine fibroids and obstetrical labor. *Obstet. Gynecol.* 42:71, 1973.
   A case report and a review of the problem.
10. Lim, O. W., Segal, A., and Ziel, H. K. Leiomyomatosis peritonealis disseminata associated with pregnancy. *Obstet. Gynecol.* 55:122, 1980.
    Pregnancy and delivery is described in this rare association.
11. Muram, D., Gillieson, M., and Walters, J. H. Myomas of the uterus in pregnancy: Ultrasonographic follow-up. *Am. J. Obstet. Gynecol.* 138:16, 1980.
    Close proximity between myoma and placental site increases risk, mainly of antepartum bleeding and premature rupture of membranes.

Effects of Leiomyomata

12. Payne, P., et al. Uterine fibromyomata and secondary polycythaemia. *J. Obstet. Gynaecol. Br. Commonw.* 76:845, 1969.
    Fibroids may secrete erythropoietin, resulting in secondary polycythemia. This may account for the absence of anemia in patients with documented menorrhagia.
13. Rubin, A., and Ford, J. A. Uterine fibromyomata in urban blacks. A preliminary survey of the relationship between symptomatology, blood pressure and haemoglobin levels. *S. Afr. Med. J.* 48:2060, 1974.
    An association between fibroids and hypertension has been sought since the two conditions frequently coexist. This relationship is probably only statistical, however, since both disorders are very common in black patients.
14. Gross, T. G., et al. Recurrent premenstrual acute urinary retention due to uterine myomas. *J. Reprod. Med.* 20:340, 1978.
    Pelvic fibroids may produce acute urinary problems.

Management

15. Russell, K. P. Office gynecology: Fibroids—when not to operate. *Postgrad. Med. J.* 60:245, 1976.
    Knowing when not to operate is as important as knowing when to operate.
16. Babaknia, A., et al. Pregnancy success following abdominal myomectomy for infertility. *Fertil. Steril.* 30:644, 1978.
    Myomectomy considerably improves fertility when no other detectable causes beside myomas are found.
17. Ranney, B., and Frederick, I. The occasional need for myomectomy. *Obstet. Gynecol.* 53:437, 1979.
    The types of myomas and the operative approach are detailed.

18. Frankez, T., and Benjamin, F. Rapid enlargement of a uterine fibroid after clomiphene therapy. *J. Obstet. Gynaecol. Br. Commonw.* 80:764, 1973.
    Fibroids may be altered by hormone therapy.

Rare Complications
19. Mattison, D. R., et al. Haemoperitoneum from rupture of a uterine vein overlying a leiomyoma. *Am. J. Obstet. Gynecol.* 136:415, 1980.
    A cause of acute bleeding associated with fibroids.
20. Hsu, Y. K., et al. Leiomyomatosis in pelvic lymph nodes. *Obstet. Gynecol.* 57:91S, 1981.
    Differentiate from benign metastasizing leiomyoma or from metastatic leiomyosarcoma.

Malignant Fibroids (Leiomyosarcomas)
21. Hannigan, E. V., and Gomez, L. G. Uterine leiomyosarcoma. *Am. J. Obstet. Gynecol.* 134:447, 1979.
    An excellent review of prognostic clinical and pathological features.
22. Azizi, F., et al. Remission of uterine leiomyosarcoma treated with vincristine, adriamycin and dimethyl-triazeno-imidazole carboximide. *Am. J. Obstet. Gynecol.* 133:379, 1979.
    Chemotherapy is of value in producing remissions; prognosis is nevertheless poor.

Prolapse

Weakness of the pelvic supporting structures may allow descent of the pelvic organs within the vagina. This process is termed *genital prolapse*. Descent of the anterior vaginal wall with protrusion of the bladder is called a *cystocele*. If the urethra sags as well, this is a *cystourethrocele*. A protrusion of the rectum through the posterior vaginal wall is termed a *rectocele*; it is frequently found in association with a herniation of intestine through the cul-de-sac, termed an *enterocele*. The degree of descent of the uterus varies and is described as first degree if the cervix reaches the introitus, second degree if the cervix protrudes through the introitus, or third degree if the entire uterus protrudes. One or more of the forms of uterovaginal prolapse may exist in the individual patient.

The fixed, unyielding support of the pelvic organs is derived from the pelvic bones, while the major soft tissue support is afforded by the muscular pelvic floor. This latter is formed by the levator muscles (pubococcygeus, ileococcygeus, and ischiococcygeus). The more superficial perineal muscles and the urogenital diaphragm also provide some limited muscular support, although they are much less important than the levators. In addition to the pelvic floor muscles, certain connective tissues, called the endopelvic fascia, play a vital role in pelvic organ support. These include the paired uterosacral ligaments, passing from the cervix to the sacrum; and lateral thickenings (in the base of the broad ligament) called transverse cervical, cardinal, or Mackenrodt ligaments, which suspend the cervix and upper vagina from the pelvic side walls. The anterior and posterior vaginal walls are also supported by the pubocervical and rectovaginal fascia, respectively.

Prolapse is almost always a result of damage to the pelvic supporting structures during childbirth and is often aggravated by lack of estrogen in the menopause. As in any other hernial conditions, obesity, chronic cough, constipation, and occupations involving much standing and lifting may be contributory factors.

The most common presenting symptom in patients with prolapse is urinary stress incontinence, which results from the loss of support of the urethrovesical angle. This complaint is present in about one-third of patients with cystourethrocele. (The subject of stress incontinence is fully discussed on pages 235–239.) Less annoying symptoms of prolapse include a feeling of "bulging in the vagina" or a "dragging feeling." Rarely with marked prolapse digital pressure may be necessary in order to allow micturition or defecation. Residual urine, due to incomplete emptying of a cystocele, may be a source of urinary tract infections. In major degrees of prolapse, the protruding cervix and vagina may ulcerate, with bleeding and discharge.

The diagnosis of prolapse is made on pelvic examination. The anterior and posterior vaginal walls are examined separately for descent with straining, as is the cervix. Stress incontinence is assessed if present. The size and position of the uterus is outlined on bimanual examination; the uterus is usually axial or retroverted with prolapse. It is not uncommon for the cervix to be well supported and for vaginal wall prolapse to result in elongation of the supravaginal cervix. This must be noted at the time of examination. Particular care is taken to assess levator muscle tone and to establish the presence or absence of an enterocele. The presence or absence of any other pathology must also be noted. There are few specific diagnostic procedures necessary in the absence of stress incontinence. If third degree descencus is present, an intravenous pyelogram is required since ureteric obstruction is common in major instances of prolapse.

The medical treatment of prolapse is confined to patients with mild forms, especially young women in the first few months after childbirth. Conservative therapy includes pelvic floor exercises, weight loss, control of cough, and management of constipation. In older women, estrogens may improve the condition of the vaginal mucosa and relieve minor symptoms. All these measures are also useful in preparing patients for surgery.

Vaginal pessaries have a place as a temporary measure after childbirth, during pregnancy, or in patients in whom surgery is contraindicated. This last group includes aged, medically debilitated women in whom the operative risk appears too great, or those who refuse the procedure. Pessaries are usually made of plastic in the form of rings and are placed in a fashion similar to that of the contraceptive diaphragm. Pessaries should be cleaned and reinserted every few months since, if neglected, they may cause vaginal ulceration. A modern pessary should cause less trouble than a dental plate.

Conservative measures are usually insufficient in all but the mildest cases of prolapse. Surgery is usually required as the definitive therapy, but it must be remembered that prolapse is seldom a health hazard and that surgery should not be recommended unless symptoms warrant the operative risk. Urinary and local vaginal infections or ulcerations must be cleared up prior to the operation. In planning the procedure, the patient's attitude toward future pregnancy, the presence or absence of stress incontinence, and the importance of coital activity to the individual patient must be considered in detail.

As the favored procedure for uterine descent is a vaginal hysterectomy with support of the vaginal vault by the transverse cervical and uterosacral ligaments, it is fortunate that most patients are older. If an enterocele is present, the peritoneal sac is excised and closed, while the uterosacral ligaments are approximated in the midline to prevent further herniation. In most cases, this procedure is followed by anterior vaginal wall repair (colporrhaphy), with particular attention to support of the urethrovesical angle if stress incontinence is a feature. Posterior vaginal wall repair and restoration of the perineal body (colpoperineorrhaphy) completes the procedure, if there is a rectocele and a deficient perineum.

For those women still desirous of further pregnancies, surgery may be delayed. If this is not possible, modified repair procedures may be performed, although these are much less likely to be successful. Should these patients become pregnant, delivery should be by cesarean section. Otherwise, the repair is likely to break down at the time of delivery. In those older women in whom intercourse is no longer a factor, a stronger repair is possible as less attention need be given to maintaining a functional vagina.

Postoperative care is chiefly directed at urinary function and at the relief of pain associated with the posterior repair. Hemorrhage and infection are the major postoperative complications. The incidence of the latter is much reduced by perioperative prophylactic antibiotics, especially in premenopausal patients.

Long-term postoperative complications include dyspareunia and vault prolapse. Dyspareunia may respond to vaginal dilatation and estrogen therapy. Vault prolapse is usually due to failure of enterocele repair. Several operative procedures, both by abdominal and vaginal routes, have been employed for this difficult surgical problem. However, no completely satisfactory method has yet been developed.

Reviews

1. Mills, W. G. The management of genital prolapse. *Br. J. Hosp. Med.* 20:586, 1978.
   It is often difficult to decide which symptoms are attributable to prolapse and whether they are sufficient to warrant surgery.
2. Nichols, D. H. Effects of pelvic relaxation on gynecologic urologic problems. *Clin. Obstet. Gynecol.* 21:759, 1978.
   Important goals of reconstructive surgery include upward relocation of the vesicourethral junction to a point at which it is once again under the influence of intraabdominal pressure, as well as restoration of normal vaginal depth and axis.
3. Porges, R. F. Abnormalities of Pelvic Support. In J. J. Sciarra (Ed.), *Gynecology and Obstetrics* (Revised Ed.). Hagerstown, Md.: Harper & Row, 1980. Vol. 1.
   Excellent summary.

Diagnosis

4. Beecham, C. T. Classification of vaginal relaxation. *Am. J. Obstet. Gynecol.* 136:957, 1980.
   A suggested classification of the various components of vaginal relaxation since no general agreement exists at this time.
5. Baden, W. F., and Walker, T. A. Physical diagnosis in the evaluation of vaginal relaxation. *Clin. Obstet. Gynecol.* 15:1055, 1972.
   Suggests a technique of physical examination for optimal evaluation.

Anatomy

6. Ulfelder, H. The mechanism of pelvic support in women: Deductions from a study of the comparative anatomy and physiology of the structures involved. *Am. J. Obstet. Gynecol.* 72:856, 1956.
   All would have been well had the human female remained a quadruped.

7. Berglas, B., and Rubin, I. C. Study of the supportive structures of the uterus by levator myography. *Surg. Gynecol. Obstet.* 97:677, 1953.
   These workers felt that the levator muscles form a flat plate supporting the vagina and uterus, and that the levator plate responds to changes in intraabdominal pressure.
8. Ball, T. L. Anterior and posterior cystocele: Cystocele revisited; an account of the twilight hours of some antifascialists and fascialists as I knew them. *Clin. Obstet. Gynecol.* 9:1062, 1966.
   Ball questions the existence of the various "fasciae," claiming that often it is the bladder per se that is being sutured during the repair procedure.
9. Week, J. C. Pelvic anatomy from the point of view of a gynecologic surgeon. *Clin. Obstet. Gynecol.* 15:1035, 1972.
   Excellent illustrations.

Medical Therapy
10. Greenhill, J. P. The nonsurgical management of vaginal relaxation. *Clin. Obstet. Gynecol.* 15:1083, 1972.
    Summarizes medical therapy.
11. Kegel, A. H. Early genital relaxation; new technique of diagnosis and nonsurgical treatment. *Obstet. Gynecol.* 8:545, 1956.
    Using Kegel's "perineometer," the patient reads off the pressure achieved each time she exercises her pubococcygeus.

Surgical Procedures
12. Porges, R. F. Changing indications for vaginal hysterectomy. *Am. J. Obstet. Gynecol.* 136:153, 1980.
    Roughly half the cases needed vaginal plastic repair; 67% of these had both anterior and posterior colporrhaphy.
13. Peters, W. A., III, and Thornton, W. N., Jr. Selection of the primary operative procedure for stress urinary incontinence. *Am. J. Obstet. Gynecol.* 137:923, 1980.
    Individualized chiefly on pelvic examination. Anterior vaginal wall descent indicates vaginal operation, no significant descent indicates need for retropubic vesicourethral suspension.
14. Ridley, J. H. Evaluation of the colpocleisis operation: A report of 58 cases. *Am. J. Obstet. Gynecol.* 113:1114, 1972.
    Complete vaginal closure in patients in whom vaginal function is not a factor.
15. Shaw, W. F. The treatment of prolapsus uteri, with special reference to the Manchester operation of colporrhaphy. *Am. J. Obstet. Gynecol.* 26:667, 1933.
    The Fothergill or Manchester procedure, consisting of anterior repair with cervical amputation, has been largely replaced by vaginal hysterectomy with repair.
16. Goodall, J. R., and Power, R. M. H. A modification of the Le Fort operation for increasing its scope. *Am. J. Obstet. Gynecol.* 34:968, 1937.
    Obliterates the central portion of the vagina, leaving lateral channels for drainage. Can be performed under local anesthesia in very debilitated patients, which is seldom required in modern practice.
17. Nichols, D. H. Types of enterocele and principles underlying choice of operation for repair. *Obstet. Gynecol.* 40:257, 1972.
    It is important to distinguish between an enterocele and a sliding hernia at the time of surgery.

Pregnancy

18. Kurzel, R. B., and Nichols, D. H. Genital prolapse during pregnancy. *J. Reprod. Med.* 24:46, 1980.

    Genital prolapse rarely may be due to congenital weakness, as with this patient who was born with severe urogenital defects. (Spina bifida may also be associated with prolapse.)

19. Scott, J. S. Prolapse and Stress Incontinence of Urine. In C. J. Dewhurst (Ed.), *Integrated Obstetrics and Gynaecology for Postgraduates* (2nd ed.). Oxford: Blackwell, 1976. P. 650.

    Details the procedures of Currie, Hunter, and Shirodkar, all of which are designed to enable the woman to retain good reproductive function.

Vaginal Inversion

20. Ranney, B. Enterocele, vaginal prolapse, pelvic hernia: Recognition and treatment. *Am. J. Obstet. Gynecol.* 140:53, 1981.

    Emphasizes the recognition of early cul-de-sac relaxations during abdominal or vaginal hysterectomy.

21. Symmonds, R. E., et al. Posthysterectomy enterocele and vaginal vault prolapse. *Am. J. Obstet. Gynecol.* 140:852, 1981.

    Of 190 patients, 90% were repaired per vaginum. Abdominal-presacral suspension advised only if preservation of vaginal function is desired.

22. Pelosi, M. A., et al. Use of dermal graft in the surgical repair of vaginal vault prolapse. *Obstet. Gynecol.* 55:385, 1980.

    Summarizes the causes and treatment, and details yet another operative approach.

Stress Incontinence

Stress urinary incontinence (SUI) can be defined as an involuntary loss of urine from an intact urethra that occurs without any conscious desire to void and as a result of a rise in intraabdominal pressure. It is by far the most common cause of urinary incontinence in the female. Minor degrees of stress incontinence may occur in at least 50% of nulliparous women. However, only 1% of all patients requiring surgical correction are nulliparous. The mean parity of patients with significant SUI is 5.2. Thus, pregnancy and childbirth play an undoubted role in the causation of SUI in susceptible subjects by damaging the supports of the bladder neck and urethra. SUI is four times as common in whites than in blacks, but the reason for this is uncertain.

The following are the five mechanisms responsible for continence. (1) The bladder neck or internal sphincter consists of smooth muscle derived from the detrusor muscle fibers. Most patients with SUI have incompetence of this sphincter. (2) The distal sphincter mechanism, which is a smooth muscle sphincter and surrounds the middle and lower portion of the urethra, is a relatively weak sphincter in the female. Both smooth muscle sphincters are innervated by alpha-adrenergic receptors. (3) The external sphincter is a striated muscle that surrounds the middle third of the urethra and acts together with the pelvic floor musculature. Reflex contractions of these muscles, occurring with sudden rises of abdominal pressure, tend to prevent stress incontinence. Damage to this sphincter mechanism is therefore important in the pathogenesis of SUI. (4) The resilience and elasticity of the urethral lining epithelium plays a small additional role in continence. This is important in elderly patients with estrogen lack and atrophic changes in the distal urethral epithelium. (5) The upper third of the urethra lies above the pelvic diaphragm and thus is intraabdominal. This assures that any rise in intraabdominal pressure is transmitted to both bladder and the upper urethra simultaneously. Prolapse of the upper urethra below the pelvic floor therefore eliminates this mechanism.

Patients with grade I SUI complain of transient leaking of urine with sudden increases of intraabdominal pressure such as occurs with coughing, sneezing, or exertion during sporting activities. Incontinence does not occur in bed at night. In grade II, the symptoms are more severe, with incontinence occurring with lesser degrees of exertion such as during walking, standing up from a sitting position, or even sitting up in bed. Grade III incontinence is so severe that there is almost continuous leaking while the person is erect, or with virtually any movement while lying down. About 5%–10% of patients also have incidental urinary tract infection that requires control.

The general physical examination should be directed toward the detection of neurologic disease, chronic respiratory conditions, large bowel pathology, and the presence of a pelvic mass. Signs of senile atrophy should be observed and the appearance and size of the urethral meatus noted. The presence and extent of descent of the anterior vaginal wall is noted when the patient coughs or strains. At the same time, cystocele, rectocele, and uterine prolapse are sought. The patient should be examined when the bladder is comfortably full. Stress incontinence can be demonstrated when the patient is coughing. Failing this, the table may be tilted downward 45 degrees. If this technique fails, she can be tested while in the erect position with a receiver between the thighs.

The Bonney test consists of digital elevation of the vagina on either side of the bladder neck, which prevents demonstrable stress incontinence. This is an unreliable test as only the slightest compression of the urethra itself will prevent all forms of incontinence. The Q-tip test is performed by inserting a lubricated Q-tip into the urethra. Anterior rotation of the Q-tip with straining indicates prolapse of the bladder base. Cystoscopy and urethroscopy should be performed to rule out any other pathology in the bladder. An excretory urogram should be done prior to any surgical procedure.

SUI must be distinguished from other forms of incontinence such as true incontinence caused by diverse pathology, e.g., pelvic fracture, radiation, and surgical trauma. Urinary fistulas into the vagina usually produce constant dribbling incontinence, but a small fistula may leak only during stress. Rarely, an ectopic ureteral opening into the female genital tract presents with pseudostress incontinence. Chronic urinary retention may also present with stress as well as overflow incontinence. Urgency incontinence is usually readily distinguishable with careful history-taking, but there is a select group of patients with bladder hyperreflexia whose symptoms and signs are indistinguishable from SUI. This condition must be demonstrated by urodynamic evaluation since surgery in this type of patient is likely to have a disastrous result. "Giggle incontinence" is an inborn abnormality in which a detrusor contraction is initiated by laughter.

The anatomy of the urethra can be demonstrated radiologically by taking lateral x-rays of the pelvis with the patient in the erect position after passing a beaded metal chain into the bladder. The position of the chain demonstrates the bladder base and position of the urethra. Alternatively, contrast can be introduced via a catheter. Observations are made while the patient is resting, while coughing, during Valsalva's maneuver, and while voiding. Normally the bladder base remains above the lower border of the pubis. In stress incontinence, the bladder neck drops lower than this position. The normal posterior urethrovesical angle is not greater than 90 degrees. Since the distal urethra is fixed, descent of the bladder base will result in flattening of this angle and in a funnelled appearance of the bladder neck (type I). With further prolapse, the urethra comes to lie almost horizontally, making a posterior urethrovesical angle of more than 180 degrees (type II). It must be remembered that loss of this angle is not the cause of stress incontinence but only a sign of bladder neck incompetence and prolapse of the bladder base.

It is important to carry out a filling cystometrogram and simultaneous measurement of rectal (intraabdominal) pressure, using carbon dioxide or water, in order to detect patients with bladder hyperreflexia. By measuring both pressures simultaneously, it is possible by subtraction to detect uninhibited bladder contractions. Reflex contraction of 15 cm of water or more, which the patient cannot inhibit, is abnormal. In some cases, the hyperreflexia can only be detected while the patient is erect (postural hyperreflexia). Other stimuli such as coughing or hopping may initiate a detrusor contraction. When a significant bladder contraction occurs immediately after coughing, symptoms closely resemble those of true SUI. Some 16% of all patients who present with SUI have some degree of hyperreflexia.

The urethral pressure profile is done by measuring the pressure along the length of the urethra. The maximum closing pressure and functional length of the urethra are generally reduced in patients with SUI. The urethral pressure profile study is important in detecting patients with severely decompensated urethral musculature, usually as a result of scarring from previous repeated surgery. These patients will have a very low maximum closing pressure.

Conservative therapy can be tried in mild cases of SUI. Pelvic floor exercises and faradic stimulation of the perineal muscles are occasionally successful. Alpha-adrenergic receptor stimulants may be tried to increase tone in the bladder neck and urethral smooth muscle. Elderly patients with atrophic vaginitis may be improved by being given small doses of conjugated estrogen. Incontinence associated with detrusor hyperreflexia requires treatment with anticholinergic agents or a bladder relaxant. Urinary tract infection must be cleared. Surgery should be offered to patients who have significant SUI.

There are numerous operations designed to cure stress incontinence. No single operation is universally successful and controversy exists as to which type of operation is best used for which type and grade of defect. Anterior vaginal repairs are aimed at repairing the defective pelvic floor and buttressing the bladder neck with sutures apposing the pubocervical fascia (Kelly's operation). Retropubic vesicourethral suspension operations produce elongation of the urethra, anterior angulation to reconstitute the posterior vesicourethral angle, and fixation to prevent descent of the bladder neck. Two operations included in this group are the Marshall-Marchetti procedure and the Burch operation. Sling operations are generally used only for those patients with excessively low urethral pressure profiles resulting from scarring. Materials that can be employed include rectus sheath, fascia-lata, or prosthetic material. When there has been loss of urethral length from previously failed operations, a urethra-lengthening procedure (Young-Dees-Leadbetter) may be required. When all else has failed, urinary diversion may be the last resort for intractable incontinence.

Review

1. Hodgkinson, C. P. Stress urinary incontinence in the female. *Surg. Gynecol. Obstet.* 120:595, 1965. *Collective review.*

Etiology and Pathogenesis

2. Turner-Warwick, R., and Brown, A. D. G. A urodynamic evaluation of urinary incontinence in the female and its treatment. *Urol. Clin. North Am.* 6:203, 1979.
   New concepts of continence and incontinence based on urodynamic findings.
3. McGuire, E. Urethral sphincter mechanism. *Urol. Clin. North Am.* 6:39, 1979.
   Physiology of continence. Inferior and posterior displacement of the urethra into the vagina during stress results in transient incontinence.
4. Forney, J. P. The effect of radical hysterectomy on bladder physiology. *Am. J. Obstet. Gynecol.* 138:374, 1980.
   Stress incontinence may occur after radical hysterectomy due to denervation.
5. Malpas, P., Jeffcoate, T. N. A., and Lister, U. M. The displacement of the bladder and urethra during labor. *Br. J. Obstet. Gynaecol.* 56:949, 1949.
   A probable cause of stress incontinence.

Detrusor Hyperreflexia

6. Mayo, M. E. Detrusor hyperreflexia: The effect of posture and pelvic floor activity. *J. Urol.* 119:635, 1978.
   Postural changes occur in 60% of women with detrusor hyperreflexia. Reflex pelvic floor muscle relaxation often occurs simultaneously.
7. Weprin, S. A., and Zuspan, F. P. The standing cystometrogram. *Am. J. Obstet. Gynecol.* 138:369, 1980.
   Diagnosis and management of incontinence due to detrusor hyperreflexia. Of patients with SUI 16% have detrusor hyperreflexia.

Diagnostic Studies

8. Green, T. H. Development of a plan for the diagnosis and treatment of urinary stress incontinence. *Am. J. Obstet. Gynecol.* 83:632, 1962.
   Loss of posterior urethrovesical angle is constantly seen in SUI (type I). Angle of inclination of urethra increases with descent of bladder neck (type II). Type I is treated with vaginal repair; type II requires suprapubic repair.
9. Tanagho, E. A. Simplified cystography in stress urinary incontinence. *Br. J. Urol.* 46:295, 1974.
   Cystographic comparison of normal women and patients with stress incontinence. Findings of failed surgery are described.
10. Fantl, J. A., et al. Bead-chain cystourethrogram: An evaluation. *Obstet. Gynecol.* 58:237, 1981.
    Radiographic observations of stress incontinence do not differ significantly from those of detrusor instability.
11. Robertson, J. R. Urethroscopy—The neglected gynecological procedure. *Clin. Obstet. Gynecol.* 19:315, 1976.
    Air cystoscopy used to observe and detect incompetence of the bladder neck.
12. Ostergard, D. R., and McCarthy, T. A. Diagnostic procedures in female urology. *Am. J. Obstet. Gynecol.* 137:401, 1980.
    Newer diagnostic procedures include urethroscopy, urodynamics, cystometry, urethral closure pressure profiles, uroflowmetry, electromyography of the pelvic floor, and radiologic procedures.

Therapy

13. Marshall, V. F., Marchetti, A. A., and Krantz, K. E. The correction of stress incontinence by simple vesicourethral suspension. *Surg. Gynecol. Obstet.* 88:509, 1949.
    Sutures appose paraurethral tissues and bladder neck to the back of the pubis.
14. Barnett, R. M. The modern Kelly plication. *Obstet. Gynecol.* 34:667, 1969.
    This article discusses the anterior vaginal approach in which plicating sutures are placed at the bladder neck.
15. Stamey, T. A. Endoscopic suspension of the vesical neck for urinary incontinence. *Surg. Gynecol. Obstet.* 136:547, 1973.
    Use of a cystoscope and specially designed needles to insert suspending sutures on either side of the urethrovesical junction.
16. Tanagho, E. A. Colpocystourethropexy: The way we do it. *J. Urol.* 116:751, 1976.
    Discusses the retropubic operation in which the anterior vaginal wall on either side of the bladder neck is sutured to Cooper's ligament.
17. McGuire, E. J., and Lytton, B. Pubovaginal sling procedure for stress urinary incontinence. *J. Urol.* 119:82, 1977.
    Pubovaginal autogenous fascial sling is used for cases with maximum urethral pressure profile less than 10 cm of water.
18. Turner, A. G. An appraisal of maximum faradic stimulation of pelvic muscles in the management of female urinary incontinence. *Ann. R. Coll. Surg. Engl.* 61:441, 1979.
    Sphincter weakness improved in 10 of 15 patients after 12 maximum stimulations under general anesthesia.
19. Fantl, J. A., Hurt, W. G., and Dunn, L. J. Detrusor instability syndrome: The use of bladder retraining drills with and without anticholinergics. *Am. J. Obstet. Gynecol.* 140:885, 1981.
    High rate of success with bladder retraining drills not significantly different when combined with anticholinergics.
20. Richardson, A. C., Edmonds, P. B., and Williams, N. L. Treatment of stress urinary incontinence due to paravaginal fascial defect. *Obstet. Gynecol.* 57:357, 1981.
    Repair of paravaginal break in the pubocervical fascia in 233 procedures yielded satisfactory results in 95% followed 2–8 years.

Dysmenorrhea, Pelvic Pain

Primary dysmenorrhea is painful menstruation in the absence of pelvic disease. Dysmenorrhea is termed *secondary* if it is related to organic pelvic disease such as endometriosis, pelvic inflammatory disease (PID), the presence of an intrauterine device (IUD), adenomyosis, or fibroids. It would appear that from 14%–26% of young women complain of dysmenorrhea, with a peak incidence some 5 years from menarche.

The cause of primary dysmenorrhea is probably multifactorial, since some patients respond to almost any therapy (including placebo), while others do not respond at all. Psychological and social factors, including a "low pain threshold," overanxious parents, faulty sexual education and outlook, have all been implicated in the pathogenesis of the symptom. However, it is now known that in most, if not all, cases, the excessive uterine production of prostaglandin is involved in the etiology of the disorder.

Prostaglandins are derived from arachidonic acid by the action of an enzyme complex termed *prostaglandin-synthetase*. In women with primary dysmenorrhea, excessive amounts of endometrial, menstrual, and circulating prostaglandin or metabolites, or both are found, the effect of which is excessive uterine contraction with uterine ischemia and spasmodic pain. Since ovulation seems essential for primary dysmenorrhea to occur, it is likely that ovarian hormones are involved, with increased late cycle estradiol possibly being the cause of excessive prostaglandin production.

Clinically, primary dysmenorrhea begins with the first ovulatory cycles, is worse just before or at the beginning of menses, and is improved with increased age, regular intercourse, and after pregnancy. Nausea, dizziness, headaches, and diarrhea (prostaglandin effects) are frequently associated symptoms. Physical examination is negative.

The pain of secondary dysmenorrhea often starts well before the period, lasts several days, and occurs in later life. Deep dyspareunia and menorrhagia may be related symptoms. Physical examination frequently reveals the associated organic disease.

Management of patients includes counseling and reassurance of girls and mothers. If simple analgesics are ineffective, the use of prostaglandin-synthetase inhibitor drugs alleviates pain in 60%–100% of cases. Many drugs are available, including mefenamic acid, ibuprofen, and naprosyn. These drugs need be taken for only 1 or 2 days and have few side effects, other than minor gastrointestinal disturbances.

In women who also desire oral contraceptives, the inhibition of ovulation that this kind of contraception provides is also highly effective in therapy; in nonresponders they can be combined with the prostaglandin-synthetase inhibitors. In the few patients resistant to all measures, laparoscopy to exclude pelvic disease is called for. At this time cervical dilatation and curettage should also be done to exclude or treat the rare instances of cervical stenosis or adhesions. Very occasionally, a presacral neurectomy may be required for serious and refractory dysmenorrhea.

Pelvic pain is a prominent complaint in about a third of patients presenting to gynecologic clinics. In many instances, an organic cause of the pain may be apparent, while in others no discernable etiologic factor is present. In both circumstances, psychological and emotional factors are involved to a degree greater than found when most other areas of the body are involved.

The pelvic viscera are innervated by autonomic nerves. The lumbar and lower thoracic sympathetic ganglia and superior, middle, and inferior hypogastric plexuses constitute the sensory pathways. Fibers from the uterus course through the uterosacral ligaments, while the nerves from the ovaries and tubes pass in the infundibulopelvic ligaments to the inferior mesenteric plexuses. Pain caused by a diseased pelvic viscus is often referred to the skin supplied by the same spinal cord segments. Thus gynecologic pain is often referred to the anterior abdominal wall and lower sacrum.

The many possible organic causes of pelvic pain include bowel pathology, such as appendicitis and diverticulitis; or the urinary tract may be the source of pain, as in pyelonephritis or urinary calculi. Disorders of the lumbosacral vertebrae may also cause pain, as in sacroiliac strain or vertebral disc syndromes. The gynecologic events initiating pain include rupture, distention, or ischemia of a viscus, or mechanical inflammatory irritation of the pelvic peritoneum. Common disorders to be found in this category include salpingitis, endometriosis, and accidents to ovarian cysts. Pregnancy complications, in particular ectopic and abortive pregnancies, are important causes. Finally, pelvic cancers may cause pelvic pain, usually as a late finding.

There is a large group of women who complain of pelvic pain in whom no pathology can be detected. This condition has been described under many names, such as "pelvic congestion syndrome," "pelvic sympathetic syndrome," and most recently as "enigmatic pelvic pain." These patients have real pain caused by a functional disorder of the genital or extragenital pelvic organs.

The features of this disorder vary widely, but some findings are common. The patients are usually parous and always premenopausal. Deep dyspareunia and premenstrual worsening of symptoms are often seen. Leukorrhea, menorrhagia, and bladder irritability are common features. Bowel dysfunction is rare, which helps differentiate the problem from colonic spasm.

Psychological studies, while not entirely satisfactory, indicate a high incidence of neuroticism and anxiety in these cases. While they deny emotional and personal problems, they usually admit to feelings of sexual unattractiveness and complain that relationships with their husbands are unrewarding. It must be kept in mind, however, that it is conceivable that these psychological changes may result from, rather than be the cause of, the chronic pain.

The clinical management of a patient with pelvic pain is based on a thorough history and careful physical examination. Further investigations will be indicated by the clinical findings. Workup should include cervical smear, urine culture, and complete blood count. An intravenous pyelogram may be indicated on occasion.

In recent years, the definitive diagnostic procedure in doubtful cases has been laparoscopy. In fact, in a 1-year review of diagnostic laparoscopies in Great Britain during 1977–1978, 10,825 of 20,971 were performed for the diagnosis of pelvic pain.

Therapy is directed at the cause in patients with organic disease. In those women in whom no organic etiology has been found, a sympathetic analysis and understanding of the woman and her environmental problem(s) are called for. She must be reassured that no serious disease is present. Early referral to a psychiatrist is unnecessary and may be counterproductive, although in some circumstances such help can be useful when suggested in a manner calculated not to offend the patient.

Surgery has an occasional place in the treatment of pain that has failed to respond to medical therapy. The usual procedure is a presacral neurectomy, which is the surgical division of the superior hypogastric plexus. This procedure, when performed, is generally part of a wider surgical approach to a patient with endometriosis. It is seldom indicated in patients without organic disease. The operation provides central pain relief only, since ovarian sympathetic denervation should not be attempted in that compromise of the ovarian blood supply is almost inevitable.

The use of hysterectomy in patients without organic disease is controversial and should be avoided since, if the procedure fails, subsequent therapy is more difficult. Nevertheless, it has been curative on occasion and has a place in therapy. Finally, in patients with intractable pelvic pain due to malignancy, neurosurgical procedures such as cordotomy and rhizotomy are occasionally of great benefit.

Dysmenorrhea

1. Editorial. Primary dysmenorrhoea. *Lancet* 1:800, 1980.

Suggests that the terms spasmodic *(primary) and* congestive *(secondary) dysmenorrhea no longer be used.*

2. Smith, R. P., and Powell, J. R. The objective evaluation of dysmenorrhea therapy. *Am. J. Obstet. Gynecol.* 137:314, 1980.
   Microtransducer intrauterine pressure recordings demonstrated a decrease in frequency and strength of contractions following the administration of a fenemate.

3. Ylikorkala, O., Puolakka, J., and Kauppla, A. Serum gonadotrophins, prolactin and ovarian steroids in primary dysmenorrhoea. *Br. J. Obstet. Gynaecol.* 86:648, 1979.
   Postovulatory progesterone is apparently necessary for prostaglandin synthesis.

4. Heinrichs, W. L., and Adamson, G. D. A practical approach to the patient with dysmenorrhea. *J. Reprod. Med.* 25:236, 1980.
   Contains overall schema for the management of patients with pelvic pain.

5. Trobough, G. E. Pelvic pain and the IUD. *J. Reprod. Med.* 20:167, 1978.
   Dysmenorrhea is increased in incidence and severity by most IUDs, but therapy with prostaglandin-synthetase inhibitors is usually successful.

6. Dingfelder, J. R. Primary dysmenorrhea treatment with prostaglandin inhibitors: A review. *Am. J. Obstet. Gynecol.* 140:874, 1981.
   Reviews the literature.

Pelvic Pain

7. Jeffcoate, T. N. A. Pelvic pain. *Br. Med. J.* 3:431, 1969.
   Differential diagnosis discussed.

8. Christ, J. C., and Lotze, E. C. The residual ovary syndrome. *Obstet. Gynecol.* 46:551, 1975.
   In this report 5% of women whose ovaries were retained at a primary surgical procedure require a second extirpative operation, usually because of pain.

9. Henker, F. O. Diagnosis and treatment of nonorganic pelvic pain. *South. Med. J.* 72:1132, 1979.
   Greatest barrier to successful therapy was refusal of patients to accept the psychologic factors in their illness.

10. Renaer, M., et al. Psychological aspects of chronic pelvic pain in women. *Am. J. Obstet. Gynecol.* 134:75, 1979.
    Article discusses results of psychometric testing employing psychological questionnaires such as the Minnesota Multiphasic Personality Inventory.

11. Malinak, L. R. Operative management of pelvic pain. *Clin. Obstet. Gynecol.* 23:191, 1980.
    Presacral neurectomy appears to have little effect on bladder, bowel, or uterine function.

12. Goldstein, D. P., et al. Laparoscopy in the diagnosis and management of pelvic pain in adolescents. *J. Reprod. Med.* 24:251, 1980.
    Of 140 patients in the age group 10 to 19, only 19 had no organic pathology.

Endometriosis

Endometriosis is the condition in which endometrial tissue occurs aberrantly in various locations. It is not a neoplasm, although it can, on rare occasions, be the site for the development of a malignant growth. It occurs in two forms: adenomyosis (sometimes called internal endometriosis), in which endometrial glands and stroma extend diffusely through tissue spaces in the myometrium and are by convention located more than one high power field from normal surface endometrium on microscopic examination; and external endometriosis (usually abbreviated to endometriosis) in which the glands and stroma are located outside the uterus, usually on other pelvic or abdominal organs, although it can occur almost anywhere in the body.

Adenomyosis is thought to represent a downgrowth from the basal endometrium, but it may be due to venous or lymphatic embolization. Because it is composed of basal type endometrium, which is normally insensitive to hormonal stimulus, secretory activity occurs in less than 30% of cases. On gross examination, the lesion is not encapsulated and has a honeycomb appearance. Clinically, the condition is usually found in older, multiparous women. Menorrhagia is the most common symptom, and the large uterus may also cause pelvic discomfort, bladder and bowel pressure, deep dyspareunia, and even a noticeable abdominal mass. It is, however, rare for the uterus to be larger than a 12–14 weeks gestation.

Treatment for symptomatic adenomyosis is hysterectomy. Rarely, in the young woman still desirous of having children, local excision with metroplasty may be attempted.

The etiology of endometriosis is not known, but there are three major theories. The first theory is that of retrograde endometrial spill with local implantation. This would also explain endometriosis in abdominal incisions and on a traumatized cervix or vagina. To explain endometriosis in sites such as the ureter, urethra, or umbilicus, another theory suggests that the coelomic epithelium, which forms the müllerian ducts from which the endometrium arises, can, at any time in adult life, be restimulated by some unknown mechanism and be transformed once again into endometrial tissue. Finally, endometriosis in pelvic lymph nodes or distant sites, such as the lung or limbs, can be explained by the theory of lymphatic or vascular embolization.

Endometriosis may be found in teenagers and after the menopause but occurs most commonly in upper middle-income white women between the ages of 30 and 40 who have delayed marriage and childbearing. The incidence of infertility is approximately 30%–40% in patients with the disease, and the remaining sufferers are usually of low parity.

Half of the patients with endometriosis are asymptomatic. For this reason it must always be considered in infertile women. Other symptoms of endometriosis depend more on the site of involvement and its nerve supply than the size of individual endometriomata or the extent of the involvement. The ovary is the most common site, occurring in approximately 40% of cases. Its involvement leads to menorrhagia, epimenorrhea, and epimenorrhagia. Involvement of the cul-de-sac and uterosacral ligaments, the next most common site, causes a fixed retroversion and is associated with deep dyspareunia. Progressively worsening dysmenorrhea is another common secondary symptom. Painful defecation, due to bowel involvement, or hematuria, due to bladder involvement, are symptoms more rarely encountered. The diagnosis must always be considered in cases of vague, chronic abdominal pain. Rupture of an endometriomatous cyst may cause acute abdominal pain accompanied by all the signs of an "acute abdomen."

If the lesions are small and few, pelvic examination may be completely negative. More extensive pathology produces tender, nodular swellings along the uterosacral ligaments, or a tender, fixed retroverted uterus, and tender, fixed ovarian tumors with surrounding fibrosis. These patients are often incorrectly diagnosed as suffering from pelvic inflammatory disease.

The correct diagnosis of endometriosis depends on a thorough history, careful physical examination, and confirmation by laparoscopy. Early lesions appear as bluish-purple or reddish-brown "powder burn" lesions of the peritoneal surface. There is often an excessive amount of peritoneal fluid containing large amounts of prostaglandin. This has been postulated as the possible cause for the associated infertility—perhaps by affecting tubal transport—in those patients with minimal lesions.

Laparoscopic visualization of a lesion is considered sufficiently diagnostic to allow treatment to begin, even in the absence of a histologic diagnosis. Histologic specimens may not always supply a pathologic diagnosis because there may have been so much pressure or scarring that the endometriomatous tissue, e.g., in the case of a "chocolate" or tarry cyst of the ovary, can no longer be seen.

The best therapeutic regimen for the treatment of endometriosis depends on the age of the patient, the severity of the symptoms, the desire for pregnancy, and the stage of the disease determined by laparoscopic examination. If the patient is asymptomatic, she should be advised of the condition, checked by pelvic examination every 6 months, and advised to undertake pregnancy if she so desires. Although pregnancy may not cure endometriosis, it usually causes considerable involution of the lesions.

Therapy based on the induction of pseudopregnancy with a combination oral contraceptive (or with medroxyprogesterone acetate) given continuously for a period of 6–9 months was based on the observation of what occurred during pregnancy. This therapy is indicated in unmarried patients with maximal symptoms and minimal palpable findings and in patients with recurrent disease after a previous conservative operation.

Short-term hormonal therapy for 6–8 weeks may also be used prior to conservative surgery to make identification and excision of lesions simpler and more complete. The pregnancy rates, after hormonal treatment of endometriosis in appropriate cases, have varied from 20%–90%. Hormonal treatment does not cure endometriosis and is only advised for those infertile patients in whom moderate degrees of surface ovarian endometriosis are demonstrated at laparoscopy.

Improved results, with a higher fertility rate, have been claimed for a new agent, danazol, a synthetic derivative of testosterone. It is thought to act as an antigonadotropin on the hypothalamus and as a direct androgenic and progestogenic suppressor of the endometrium. The dosage of danazol is 800 mg daily for 6 months. It is expensive, and the most commonly described undesirable side effects are menopausal symptoms, weight gain, edema, and mild virilization.

In the majority of patients whose major complaint is infertility, conservative surgery produces the best results. Such surgery involves excision rather than electrocoagulation of visible endometrial implants, removal of ovarian endometriomata, ventral suspension of the uterus together with an appendectomy. In the presence of severe dysmenorrhea, a presacral neurectomy is frequently performed. In older patients in whom pregnancy is not a consideration and relief of pain is the main objective, a total hysterectomy and bilateral salpingo-oophorectomy with excision of any other visible endometriomatous lesions and lysis of adhesions is the treatment of choice. These women may be placed on maintenance estrogen therapy postoperatively since exacerbation of the endometriosis is uncommon.

Rarely, surgery is indicated for obstruction of the rectosigmoid at the level of the cul-de-sac, due to an endometrioma, or for small bowel obstruction of the distal ileum or at the ileocecal junction. In the latter case, obstruction is most likely due to adhesions between loops of bowel with subsequent kinking.

Malignant change is rare, occurring in less than 1% of patients; the lesion is an endometrioid adenocarcinoma. The prognosis for 5-year survival is good, averaging more than 70%. Stromal endometriosis is a rare myometrial tumor composed of endometrial stroma. It often spreads locally, but true malignant change with remote metastases due to sarcomatous transformation is extremely uncommon.

Review

1. Kistner, R. W. Endometriosis and infertility. *Clin. Obstet. Gynecol.* 22:101, 1979.
   It is not known whether the infertility is the cause or effect.
2. Malinak, L. R. Infertility and endometriosis: Operative technique, clinical staging and prognosis. *Clin. Obstet. Gynecol.* 23:925, 1980.
   The author feels that pregnancy rates are higher with primary surgery and recurrence of disease is more common after medical therapy.

Etiology

3. Ridley, J. H. The histogenesis of endometriosis. *Obstet. Gynecol. Surv.* 23:1, 1968.
   None of the theories explains why all women do not get the disease.
4. Scott, R. B., TeLinde, R. W., and Wharton, L. R., Jr. Further studies on experimental endometriosis. *Am. J. Obstet. Gynecol.* 62:1082, 1953.
   Six of ten monkeys with experimentally induced, retrograde menses developed endometriosis.
5. diZerega, G. S., Barber, D. L., and Hodgen, G. D. Endometriosis, role of ovarian steroids in initiation, maintenance, and suppression. *Fertil. Steril.* 33:649, 1980.
   Estrogen is essential for its development and continued activity.

Clinical Presentation

6. Simpson, J. L., et al. Heritable aspects of endometriosis. I. Genetic studies. *Am. J. Obstet. Gynecol.* 137:327, 1980.
   An apparently unaffected patient with an affected first-degree relative has a 7% risk of developing endometriosis. A polygenic/multifactorial form of inheritance seems most likely.
7. Wentz, A. C. Premenstrual spotting: Its association with endometriosis but not luteal phase inadequacy. *Fertil. Steril.* 33:605, 1980.
   A previously unrecognized association.
8. Naples, J. D., Batt, R. E., and Sadigh, H. Spontaneous abortion rate in patients with endometriosis. *Obstet. Gynecol.* 57:509, 1981.
   Significant increase in the four years prior to diagnosis with significant decrease after conservative surgery.
9. Mostoufizadeh, M., and Scully, R. E. Malignant tumors arising in endometriosis. *Clin. Obstet. Gynecol.* 23:951, 1980.
   Rare, but the true incidence is not known. Endometrioid carcinoma, clear cell carcinoma, stromal sarcoma, and mixed mesodermal adenosarcoma have been described.

Diagnosis

10. Cohen, M. R. Laparoscopy and the management of endometriosis. *Obstet. Gynecol.* 23:81, 1979.
    Used for follow-up of therapy as well as for diagnosis and staging.
11. The American Fertility Society. Classification of endometriosis. *Fertil. Steril.* 32:633, 1979.

Endometriosis classified as stage I through IV (mild, moderate, severe, and extreme), depending on the extent of the disease.

Medical Management

12. Biberoglu, K. I., and Behrman, S. J. Dosage aspects of danazol therapy in endometriosis: Short-term and long-term effectiveness. *Am. J. Obstet. Gynecol.* 139:645, 1981.
    Lower doses produced similar results but side effects were still present.
13. Hammond, C. B., and Haney, A. F. Conservative treatment of endometriosis. *Fertil. Steril.* 30:497, 1978.
    It is difficult to adequately compare medical versus conservative surgical therapy because of preselection of cases for surgery.

Surgical Management

14. Buttram, V. C. Surgical treatment of endometriosis in the infertile female: A modified approach. *Fertil. Steril.* 32:635, 1979.
    Conservative technique described in detail.
15. Meyers, W. C., Kelvin, F. M., and Jones, R. S. Diagnosis and surgical treatment of colonic endometriosis. *Arch. Surg.* 114:169, 1979.
    Radiographic findings are nonspecific.
16. Moore, J. G., et al. Urinary tract endometriosis: Enigmas in diagnosis and management. *Am. J. Obstet. Gynecol.* 134:162, 1979.
    If the ureter is involved, danger to renal function is great, and castration is nearly always indicated, in addition to freeing the ureter.

Pediatric Gynecology

Childhood is the time from birth until the onset of puberty. Puberty is the early stage of adolescence, culminating in menstruation. The problems encountered during these periods include congenital abnormalities of the internal and external genitalia, sometimes associated with intersex states, as well as gonadal dysgenesis. Vulvovaginitis is not uncommon, and the onset of menstruation may be premature or be associated with problems of abnormal bleeding. Tumors of the genital tract, although rare, may be highly malignant. Social problems, often associated with childhood abuse or sexual molestation, or both, are all too common. The management of these problems, difficult in itself, is compounded by the physical and emotional immaturity of the patients. In obtaining the history and performing the physical examination, the clinician must exercise great care and sensitivity. Special training and skills are necessary in order to cope with the more difficult conditions encountered. This chapter will outline some of these areas, while others are to be found in those chapters related to puberty and adolescence.

Vulvovaginitis comprises 85%–90% of the genital problems in premenarchal children. Symptoms include burning, pruritus, and discharge. The causes are protean, with allergic and chemical reactions or bacterial infections being the most common. The history must include inquiry for infections in family members, and the examination requires the use of small instruments specifically adapted for pediatric use, employing a vaginoscope if possible. In the absence of such instruments, a nasal speculum may be satisfactory. Vaginal fluid should be examined with wet preparation for monilia, trichomonas, and pinworms, and bacterial culture obtained, including gonococcal culture. When the clinical picture is suggestive of tumor or diethylstilbestrol (DES) exposure, cytology should be included.

Therapy of monilial, trichomonas, and gonococcal infections is as for adults, but with the appropriate dosage alterations. The nonestrogenized vagina may be infected by many other bacterial pathogens including salmonella, shigella, and *Hemophilis vaginalis*. Local therapy with adult nitrofurazone urethral suppositories used intravaginally together with specific instructions to the mother regarding hygiene of the area is generally successful. Every variety of chemical may set up an allergic vulvitis, and careful inquiry into detergents and soaps used may suggest the cause. Synthetic panties and tight clothing may be implicated and should be replaced by loose cotton clothing. In about 5% of cases, a foreign body in the vagina is the cause and can be suspected if the discharge is particularly foul and malodorous. General anesthesia may be required if removal of the object is likely to be difficult.

Almost every tumor of adults has also been reported in children, but the pattern of childhood neoplasms is generally somewhat different. Vulval tumors are usually benign and include hymenal cysts of the newborn, which generally disappear within a few weeks. Condylomata acuminata, viral warts similar to those in the adult, may be found. Vulval teratomas, hemangiomas, and lipomas have also been reported.

Vaginal and cervical tumors in children are very similar and may be considered together. Girls with these tumors commonly seen by the gynecologist are those whose mothers were treated with DES or other estrogens during pregnancy. In these patients, there is a high risk of the development of vaginal adenosis, in which condition islands of glandular tissue lined with columnar-celled epithelium are found in the vagina. A number of other structural abnormalities of the vagina, cervix, and internal genitalia have also been described. The importance of these changes is that an increased incidence of clear-cell adenocarcinoma of the vagina has been found in DES-exposed offspring; close observation of these girls is therefore essential. Fortunately, malignant change is very rare before puberty, so that in the absence of symptoms, regular surveillance with cytology, colposcopy, and pelvic examination may be postponed until menstruation is established.

Mesodermal mixed tumors, botryoid sarcomas, are rare tumors, generally of the vagina in children and of the cervix in adolescents. The initial appearance may be similar to that of a simple polyp, but growth and metastasis are early and rapid. Radical surgery with cytotoxic therapy offers the best chance of cure.

Nonneoplastic ovarian cysts occasionally occur in children or infants. These cysts are generally follicular or corpus luteal. Unless complications occur, conservative management is preferable.

Ovarian neoplasms in children have a malignancy rate of 35% overall. The tumors in some 65% are of germ cell origin (teratoma, dysgerminoma, endodermal sinus tumor, gonadoblastoma, choriocarcinoma) or derived from specialized stroma in 12% (granulosa-theca cell, Sertoli-Leydig cell). The remaining tumors are chiefly epithelial, as in the adult.

The patient is usually first seen clinically with abdominal pain or an abdominal mass. Stromal tumors and germ cell tumors may cause isosexual precocious puberty. Treatment is complicated by the necessity for preserving developmental and reproductive function whenever possible. For this reason, lesions clinically confined to one ovary are generally treated by unilateral adnexal excision. Radiotherapy and chemotherapy are important modalities reserved for advanced disease or as adjuncts to definitive surgical therapy in those lesions with greater malignant potential, such as the papillary serous epithelial tumors.

Congenital anomalies of the genital tract in chromosomally normal females can result from agenesis or abnormalities of tissue fusion and canalization. Since the wolffian and müllerian systems develop in close proximity, anomalies of the urinary tract are commonly associated.

Remnants of the wolffian duct persisting in the broad ligament may form parovarian cysts, or in the vagina, Gartner's duct cysts. If large or causing symptoms, excision or marsupialization is required.

Müllerian agenesis may occur, or fusion failures and arrested development may cause a wide variety of uterine abnormalities. These range from the minor arcuate deformity or a subseptate uterus to a double uterus (didelphys) with one (unicollis) or two (bicollis) cervices. Longitudinal or transverse vaginal septa can be found in association. These malformations seldom cause problems in children provided the uterovaginal canal is open.

The upper two-thirds of the vagina are formed by canalization of müllerian tissue, and the lower one-third forms from the urogenital sinus. Varying degrees of failure of canalization exist, including imperforate hymen, transverse vaginal septum, and absence of the vagina. The clinical result in babies may be the formation of a mucocolpos in response to maternal estrogens. However, there are usually no symptoms until puberty when the onset of cryptomenorrhea will result in cyclic pain, with the accumulation of blood in the patent areas of the genital tract. Surgery is then indicated, ranging from simple hymeneal incision to the construction of an artificial vagina, depending on the anatomic situation. In severe cases, the degree of hematocolpos, hematometra, and hematosalpinx may necessitate hysterectomy.

The sex of an individual may be considered from four aspects: chromosomal (XX or XY), gonadal (ovary or testes), external genital (phenotype), and sex of rearing (psychologic).

Intrauterine development is along female lines whatever the chromosome pattern or even in the absence of a gonad. Male differentiation occurs because the fetal testis secretes müllerian inhibiting factor, which halts the development of uterus, tubes, and upper vagina and stimulates wolffian development. The testis also secretes testosterone, which masculinizes the external genitalia but has no effect on internal genitalia.

Intersexual states occur when there are bisexual gonads or extragonadal genital organs of the opposite sex. Abnormal sexual differentiation due to chromosomal abnormalities includes Turner's (XO) and Klinefelter's (XXY) syndromes. Abnormalities at the gonadal level include true hermaphrodites in whom an ovary and testis or an ovotestis are present.

End organ resistance causes the androgen insensitivity (testicular feminizing) syndrome in chromosomal males with functioning testes who are phenotypically female.

The external genitals of true females may be masculinized by circulating androgens as in the adrenogenital syndrome (congenital adrenal hyperplasia) or as a result of the administration of progestins in early pregnancy.

A newborn with ambiguous genitalia requires early sex assignment for which pediatric consultation is essential. In general, coital function as an adult is the major concern. In the first week of life, salt-losing adrenal hyperplasia may be fatal, so serum electrolytes must be closely monitored in these infants.

Investigations include buccal smears, karyotyping, steroid studies, and radiology of the urogenital sinus. In most instances, laparotomy with gonadal biopsy can be avoided. Management of the various conditions may include surgery to the external genitals in early infancy and construction of the vagina in the late teens. Gonadectomy is indicated before puberty when there is a risk of malignancy. Exogenous steroids may be required to induce feminization. Patients with congenital adrenal hyperplasia are treated with corticosteroids. Education and counseling of the parents is essential.

Vulvovaginitis
1. Huffman, J. W. Premenarchal vulvovaginitis. *Clin. Obstet. Gynecol.* 20:581, 1977.
   The organisms may originate from the respiratory tract since up to 12% of patients have had a preceding upper respiratory infection.
2. Capraro, V. J. Gynecologic examination in children and adolescents. *Pediatr. Clin. North Am.* 19:511, 1972.
   Even if a one-finger vaginal examination is not possible, rectoabdominal examination is usually feasible.
3. Farrell, M. K., et al. Prepubertal gonorrhea: A multidisciplinary approach. *Pediatrics* 67:151, 1981.
   Children should be hospitalized since this greatly facilitates contact identification.
4. Stumpf, P. G. Increasing occurrence of condylomata acuminata in premenarchal children. *Obstet. Gynecol.* 56:262, 1980.
   Papova virus probably acquired from an infected family member.

Tumors
5. Herbst, A., et al. Clear-cell adenocarcinoma of the vagina and cervix in girls: Analysis of 170 registry cases. *Am. J. Obstet. Gynecol.* 119:713, 1974.
   Radical hysterectomy with vaginectomy is the treatment of choice; radiotherapy is also employed if lymph nodes are involved.
6. Stillman, R. J., et al. Ovarian failure in long-term survivors of childhood malignancy. *Am. J. Obstet. Gynecol.* 139:62, 1981.
   In 12% of 182 cases, the only risk factor was location of the ovaries in relation to radiation treatment fields.
7. Breen, J. L., and Maxson, W. S. Ovarian tumors in children and adolescents. *Clin. Obstet. Gynecol.* 20:607, 1977.
   Because the ovary in early life is abdominal and descends into the pelvis only at puberty, most childhood ovarian tumors present as abdominal masses.
8. Schilsky, R. L., et al. Gonadal dysfunction in patients receiving chemotherapy for cancer. *Ann. Intern. Med.* 93:109, 1980.
   Does not appear to cause profound ovarian dysfunction in young girls. Still under evaluation.

Congenital Anomalies of the Genital Tract
9. Beazley, J. M. Congenital anomalies of the female genital tract excluding intersex. *Clin. Obstet. Gynecol.* 20:533, 1977.
   An ectopic ureter is an uncommon source of vague watery discharge. Diagnosis may be difficult.
10. Gurin, J., and Leiter, E. Associated anomalies of müllerian and wolffian duct structures. *South. Med. J.* 74:805, 1981.
   All patients with congenital uterine or vaginal anomalies should have an intravenous pyelogram.

Intersex
11. Jones, H. W., Jr., and Park, I. J. Intersex. *Clin. Obstet. Gynecol.* 20:545, 1977.

For gonadal assignment, a testis must possess seminiferous tubules and an ovary must have oocytes.

12. Money, J., Hampson, J. C., and Hampson, J. L. Hermaphroditism; recommendations concerning assignment of sex, change of sex and psychologic management. *Bull. Johns Hopkins Hosp.* 97:284, 1955.
    Gender role is chiefly dependent upon sex assigned at birth.

13. Bercee, B. B., and Schulman, J. D. Review. Genetics of abnormalities of sexual differentiation and of female reproductive failure. *Obstet. Gynecol. Surv.* 35:1, 1980.
    Y chromosomal material, even in the absence of a demonstrable Y chromosome, is probably an absolute requirement for the presence of testicular tissue or the H-Y antigen, or both.

14. Scully, R. E. Gonadoblastoma. A review of 74 cases. *Cancer* 25:1349, 1970.
    The Y chromosome carries genetic determinants for testicular formation. There is a high incidence of malignancy in dysgenetic gonads associated with a Y chromosome, and the gonad should be removed.

15. Manuel, M., Katayama, K. P., and Jones, H. W., Jr. The age of occurrence of gonadal tumors in intersex patients with a Y chromosome. *Am. J. Obstet. Gynecol.* 124:293, 1976.
    Suggests that gonads be removed before puberty in most patients but may procrastinate until fully feminized in cases of testicular feminization.

Laparoscopy

Inspection of the internal pelvic organs with an illuminated telescope through a small incision in the gas-distended abdominal cavity is termed *laparoscopy (celioscopy, peritoneoscopy).* The major diagnostic application of the procedure is in evaluating female infertility, with particular regard to tubal patency and ovarian evidence of ovulation. The other major diagnostic application lies in the elucidation of the symptom of pelvic pain. The presence of endometriosis, pelvic inflammatory disease, or ectopic pregnancy explains the symptom, or the absence of organic pathology may provide reassurance to both patient and physician. Diagnostic laparoscopy may also be helpful in the staging and follow-up of patients with pelvic cancer.

The most common indication for therapeutic laparoscopy is for tubal sterilization procedures. The fallopian tubes may be fulgurated with electrocautery or closed by clips or bands. Many other surgical procedures have been performed with the laparoscope. These include removal of intraabdominal foreign bodies (particularly perforated intrauterine devices); ovarian biopsy in patients with endocrine disorders, such as suspected ovarian failure; or the fulguration of endometriotic implants. Skilled laparoscopists aspirate ovarian cysts, capture intact ova, ventrosuspend the uterus, lyse tubal adhesions, and perform fimbriolysis and salpingostomy.

Laparoscopy is contraindicated in patients with severe cardiorespiratory disease, diffuse peritonitis, or ileus. Diaphragmatic herniation or osteotomy are also contraindications. It is relatively contraindicated, dependent to a large degree on the operator's skill or experience, in the obese patient and those with abdominal scars from previous surgery.

Peritoneoscopy may be regarded as a minor surgical but a major anesthetic procedure. This is because general anesthesia with endotracheal intubation and muscle relaxation is the usual anesthetic employed. However, regional or local anesthesia is also satisfactory, particularly when the operation is carried out on an outpatient basis.

Celioscopy is carried out with the patient supine, her legs supported by stirrups angled 15 degrees downward, and her buttocks protruding over the edge of the table. This position is essential because manipulative instruments are introduced through the uterine cervix to enhance visualization by the ability to move the pelvic organs during the procedure. Furthermore, these instruments are canalized so that colored dyes (indigo carmine or methylene blue) may be injected for the assessment of tubal patency.

The first step in the procedure is creating the pneumoperitoneum. Gases used are carbon dioxide (CO_2) or nitrous oxide (N_2O) and are introduced through a spring-loaded needle (Veress, Palmer) generally inserted subumbilically. Gas is insufflated at 1 liter/minute and gas pressure should not exceed 20 mm Hg. The usual amount of gas required varies from 2–5 liters. When liver dullness to percussion is lost, the patient is placed in the Trendelenburg position and the needle is withdrawn.

Next is the introduction of the telescope. A 1 cm subumbilical incision through skin and fascia is made. A trocar and valve sleeve are introduced at an angle of 45 degrees toward the pelvis. The trocar is removed, and the telescope is passed through the sheath. The gas insufflator is attached on automatic flow to maintain the pneumoperitoneum. The fiberoptic light source is attached to the telescope and viewing commences. Telescope diameters vary from 4–10 mm, and their objectives are usually angled 180 degrees forward. If a double-channeled operating laparoscope is used, the placement of ancillary instruments through further incisions may be obviated.

Additional instruments, if required, are passed through a second or third incision, generally placed in the iliac fossae through a smaller trocar and cannula. These incisions are made under direct laparoscopic vision. A wide variety of ancillary instruments are available. These include tubal clip or band applicators, ovarian biopsy forceps, apparatus for suction or aspiration, electrocautery instruments capable of coagulation or cutting, forceps, graduated probes, scissors, loops, and needles.

The mortality rate for diagnostic laparoscopy is 11 per 100,000, and the incidence of laparotomy for intraabdominal complications is 8.5 per 1000. Complications may occur due to anesthesia, improper gas insufflation, perforation of viscera or vessels, and complications of operative procedures, including hemorrhage or burns.

Anesthetic complications are related to increases in intraabdominal pressure over 20 mm Hg, particularly when CO_2 is the insufflating gas. Reduced pulmonary excursion and CO_2 absorption result in hypercarbia, causing cardiac arrhythmias and cardiac arrest (1 per 5000 procedures). Careful technique with close cardiac and abdominal pressure monitoring, together with active ventilation, minimizes the incidence of this problem. The alternative use of N_2O, which does not cause hypercarbia and is nonirritant, is not entirely without problems since it is an ignitable gas and is only slowly absorbed. This must be kept in mind, particularly when electrocautery is used.

Preperitoneal and omental emphysema are common minor problems associated with introduction of the gas. An overdistended abdomen may result in hypotension due to decreased venous return; this is easily dealt with by releasing the tension. Gas embolism is a rare complication, more serious with N_2O since CO_2 is rapidly absorbed.

Almost every conceivable viscus or vessel has been injured by the Veress or other cannulas. The majority of these injuries are minor and require no special attention other than close observation. Of course, immediate laparotomy is necessary for major bleeding or visceral injury.

When operative procedures are performed, bleeding is the most common complication encountered. Hemostasis can generally be obtained by electrocoagulation, although laparotomy may be required. The more serious complications are related to electrical burns. These arise from accidentally touching adjacent tissues or to sparking of the current to these structures. Bowel burns are commonly involved and, if recognized and superficial, may be treated conservatively since most resolve. In those cases in which unrecognized bowel burns become progressive, a picture similar to that of pelvic inflammatory disease or appendicitis develops. Laparotomy with bowel resection, together with antibiotic therapy, is then necessary. Hazards of electric burns are lessened by the use of bipolar rather than unipolar electrodes, while regular inspection and testing of equipment with particular regard to insulation is mandatory. Many surgeons avoid these problems by the use of clips or bands rather than electrosurgical techniques when performing tubal sterilization.

Reviews

1. Taylor, P. J., and Cumming, D. C. Laparoscopy in the infertile female. *Curr. Probl. Obstet. Gynecol.* 2:3, 1979.
   The scope of this review extends farther than the title would suggest; includes 152 references.
2. Loffer, F., and Pent, D. Indications, contra-indications and complications of laparoscopy. *Obstet. Gynecol. Surv.* 30:403, 1975.
   Diagnostic laparoscopy requires special training, while operative laparoscopy requires an even greater degree of expertise.

Anesthesia

3. Magno, R., et al. Acid-base balance during laparoscopy. The effect of intraperitoneal insufflation of carbon dioxide and nitrous oxide on acid-base balance during controlled ventilation. *Acta Obstet. Gynecol. Scand.* 58:81, 1979.
   There is a sharp rise in $PaCO_2$ and a fall in pH with CO_2, but no change with N_2O, in acid-base balance.
4. Aribarg, A. Epidural analgesia for laparoscopy. *J. Obstet. Gynaecol. Br. Commonw.* 80:567, 1973.
   Unfortunately, both induction and recovery time are slow; analgesia is excellent, however.
5. Chapin, J. W., Hurlbert, B. J., and Scheer, K. Hemorrhage and cardiac arrest during laparoscopic tubal ligation. *Anesthesiology* 53:342, 1980.
   In their discussion of two cases, the authors refer to Phillips' review of over 100,000 pelvic laparoscopies from the literature, which indicated a 0.65% incidence of hemorrhage and a 0.3% incidence of cardiac arrest.
6. Weeless, C. R., Jr. Outpatient laparoscope sterilization under local anesthesia. *Obstet. Gynecol.* 39:767, 1972.
   Generally suitable for sterilization with the Falope ring of Yoon or the Hulka clip. Nitrous oxide is used since it is nonirritant.
7. Fishburne, J. I. Anesthesia for laparoscopy: Consideration, complications, and techniques. *J. Reprod. Med.* 21:37, 1978.
   Reports a mortality rate from cardiac arrest of 1 per 8000 procedures.

Technique

8. Semm, K., and Mettler, L. Technical progress in pelvic surgery via operative laparoscopy. *Am. J. Obstet. Gynecol.* 138:121, 1980.

Describes a set of instruments for grasping, cutting, sucking, and ligating, as well as an endocoagulation technique said to be safer than that of high-frequency current coagulation.

9. Hasson, H. M. Open laparoscopy. A report of 150 cases. *J. Reprod. Med.* 12:234, 1974.

A special cannula is inserted through a small laparotomy incision; sutures ensure a gas-tight seal. Especially useful in the obese or when adhesions are suspected.

10. Philipsen, T., and Hansen, B. B. Comparative study of hysterosalpingography and laparoscopy in infertile patients. *Acta Obstet. Gynecol. Scand.* 60:149, 1981.

For a conclusive evaluation of the tubal factor, hysterosalpingography should be replaced by laparoscopy according to the findings in this series of 168 patients investigated by both techniques.

11. Cohen, M. R. Culdoscopy vs peritoneoscopy. *Obstet. Gynecol.* 31:310, 1968.

Endoscopy via the cul-de-sac (culdoscopy) has largely been replaced by the abdominal approach.

Applications

12. Mumford, S. D., and Bhiwandiwala, P. P. Tubal ring sterilization: Experience with 10,086 cases. *Obstet. Gynecol.* 57:150, 1981.

Safety and efficacy found comparable to other methods of tubal occlusion.

13. Drake, T. S., and Grunert, G. M. The unsuspected pelvic factor in the infertility investigation. *Fertil. Steril.* 34:27, 1980.

Following a normal outpatient infertility evaluation, 30 of 38 women were found to have adhesions or endometriosis at laparoscopy; half of these women went on to have term pregnancies following therapy.

14. Sulewski, J. M., et al. The treatment of endometriosis at laparoscopy for infertility. *Am. J. Obstet. Gynecol.* 138:128, 1980.

The procedure was used for diagnosis, staging, and therapy of 100 patients with mild to moderate disease; 40 women conceived.

15. Asch, R. H. Laparoscopic recovery of sperm from peritoneal fluid in patients with negative or poor Sims-Huhner test. *Fertil. Steril.* 27:1111, 1976.

Casts doubt on the reliability of the postcoital test and suggests a further application of laparoscopy in the infertility workup.

16. Yuzpe, A. A., and Rioux, J. E. The value of laparoscopic ovarian biopsy. *J. Reprod. Med.* 15:57, 1975.

The major complication, as in fulguration of endometrial implants, is damage to the ureter.

17. Rosenfeld, D. L., and Gascia, C. R. Laparoscopy prior to tubal reanastomosis. *J. Reprod. Med.* 17:247, 1976.

Essential element of workup prior to tubal surgery for infertility.

18. Steptoe, P. C., and Edwards, R. G. Birth after the reimplantation of a human embryo. *Lancet* 2:266, 1978.

Laparoscopic recovery of oocytes is an essential step in the technique of extracorporeal fertilization (test-tube baby).

Complications

19. Cunanan, R. G., Jr., Courey, N. G., and Lippes, J. Complications of laparoscopic tubal sterilization. *Obstet. Gynecol.* 55:501, 1980.

The complication rate was under 1% in 5018 cases; bleeding accounted for one-half of the problems.

20. Peterson, H. B., et al. Deaths associated with laparoscopic sterilization

by unipolar electrocoagulating devices, 1978 and 1979. *Am. J. Obstet. Gynecol.* 139:141, 1981.
Two deaths, both following bowel injury. The authors recommend no longer using unipolar electrocoagulation.
21. Loffer, F. D., and Pent, D. Pregnancy after laparoscopic sterilization. *Obstet. Gynecol.* 55:709, 1980.
Electric methods have lower failure rates than mechanical methods but are less readily reversed; when pregnancy occurs there is a high incidence of ectopic gestation.

Hysterectomy

The uterus may be removed through an incision in the abdominal wall. A total abdominal hysterectomy is the removal of both corpus and cervix. On rare occasions the cervix may be left in situ, which is a subtotal hysterectomy. An alternative method, vaginal hysterectomy, is removal of the uterus through the vagina. At the time of hysterectomy, one or both tubes or ovaries may also be removed. For instance, in postmenopausal patients requiring hysterectomy, it is customary to remove the adnexa, a procedure termed a *bilateral salpingo-oophorectomy*. Hysterectomy in the treatment of cancer is not included in this discussion but is dealt with in the discussion on radical surgery in the oncology section, page 411. Hysterectomy is the most common major operation performed. In 1976, there were 751,000 hysterectomies, and it was estimated that more than half of the female population would have had the procedure by age 65.

Hysterectomy is indicated in selected patients with fibroids, adenomyosis, endometriosis, cervical intraepithelial neoplasia, endometrial hyperplasia, benign ovarian growths, as well as genital prolapse, pelvic inflammatory disease, and obstetric catastrophes. Increasingly, the procedure is also used for patients with contraceptive difficulties and menstrual problems related to pain and bleeding unresponsive to medical therapy.

Preoperative workup to exclude preinvasive or invasive cancer is necessary, including colposcopy, curettage, or cone biopsy if indicated by results of Pap smears or endometrial biopsy. In nonurgent cases, anemia and local infections should be treated prior to surgery. Many surgeons require intravenous pyelogram and barium enema before the operation. Adequate counseling is essential, especially regarding menstrual, reproductive, and sexual function since the procedure carries profound physical and psychological implications.

The vaginal approach is used in 30%–35% of hysterectomies. The usual indication is pelvic relaxation, although the method is suitable for any hysterectomy in skilled hands, provided no contraindications exist. These include the presence of intraabdominal or pelvic pathology, necessitating abdominal exploration; a uterus too large to remove vaginally; or a narrow subpubic angle that would limit access. The vaginal route is associated with an easier convalescence but a higher incidence of febrile morbidity than the abdominal procedure.

Abdominal hysterectomy is performed through a transverse or vertical abdominal incision, with most gynecologists favoring the former. No clear consensus exists regarding the age at which normal ovaries should be removed as prophylaxis against cancer. In view of the adverse effects of castration on menopausal symptoms, osteoporosis, and vascular disease, many gynecologists remove these organs only in perimenopausal or postmenopausal patients. No similar controversy exists regarding the subtotal procedure, which should be reserved only for emergency situations in which operating time is a crucial factor or when technical difficulties render cervical removal hazardous. This is because the retained cervical stump may cause problems later, including vaginal discharge, infections, and cervical cancer. The safety of total hysterectomy is increased by the use of an intrafascial technique, although this is not suitable for patients with cervical precancer; in these women an extrafascial approach is indicated.

In both vaginal or abdominal hysterectomy, it is important to support the vaginal vault (cuff) with the transverse cervical and uterosacral ligaments as prophylaxis against vault prolapse, an uncommon late complication of hysterectomy. Most gynecologists close the cuff routinely, although many leave it open if infection is present in order to provide pelvic drainage.

On occasion there is postoperative bleeding that may be early or late and present as frank bleeding or with pelvic hematoma. Vaginal or abdominal resuturing will be necessary in most instances, although late hemorrhage from the cuff will usually respond to vaginal packing.

Postoperative infections are not uncommon and may be in the urinary tract, abdominal or vaginal incisions, adnexa, or lungs. In severe cases, pelvic abscess, peritonitis, wound dehiscence, septicemia, and septic pelvic thrombophlebitis may occur. Febrile morbidity is most common in premenopausal patients undergoing vaginal hysterectomy. Utilization of prophylactic antibiotics in high-risk patients has markedly lessened the incidence of all these infectious complications, although routine use does remain controversial.

Thromboembolism is a major cause of postoperative mortality. The use of low-dose prophylactic heparin may lessen the incidence, especially in patients at high risk such as the markedly overweight.

Injuries to bladder, ureters, or bowel are very uncommon but, if not recognized and repaired at the time of surgery, may lead to serious infections and urinary or fecal fistulas. Complications common to major abdominal or pelvic surgery, such as anesthesia, blood transfusion, drug reaction, and ileus and intestinal obstruction, must also be considered.

The emotional and psychosexual sequelae of hysterectomy are of great significance. The incidence of depression after the procedure has been estimated as being two to three times more frequent than after other operations. Hormone replacement in premenopausal patients undergoing surgical castration, and adequate preoperative and postoperative counsel and support are important elements of care.

From this review of the complications, though the more serious are uncommon, it is clear that the added risks do not warrant using hysterectomy purely for sterilization. Nevertheless, it remains one of the safest major procedures, with a mortality varying between 0.05% and 0.2%, one-eighth that of cholecystectomy and one-half that of appendectomy. The average patient may expect to be discharged from 5 to 7 days after surgery, and few procedures improve the quality of life more than an indicated hysterectomy in a well-informed patient.

Reviews
1. Joel-Cohen, S. J. The place of the abdominal hysterectomy. *Clin. Obstet. Gynecol.* 5:525, 1978.

The author is well known for his application of time and motion studies to speed up and simplify gynecologic procedures.

2. Feroze, R. M. Vaginal hysterectomy and repair. *Clin. Obstet. Gynecol.* 5:545, 1978.
   The present-day discussion concerns the relative merits of vaginal hysterectomy, in the absence of prolapse, and abdominal hysterectomy.

Series

3. Porges, R. F. Changing indications for vaginal hysterectomy. *Am. J. Obstet. Gynecol.* 136:153, 1980.
   Two hundred fifty-two vaginal hysterectomies were analyzed. Of the 252, 33% had fibroids of up to 14 weeks gestational size. In 32% of cases, all or a portion of the adnexa were also removed.

4. Amirikia, H., and Evans, T. N. Ten-year review of hysterectomies: Trends, indications, and risks. *Am. J. Obstet. Gynecol.* 134:431, 1979.
   In this article 6435 hysterectomies were analyzed. Fibroids, adenomyosis, and endometriosis were the indications in 77%.

5. Stumpf, P. G., Ballard, C. A., and Lowensohn, R. Abdominal hysterectomy for abortion-sterilization. A report of 500 consecutive cases. *Am. J. Obstet. Gynecol.* 136:714, 1980.
   Ballard has also reported 200 cases of vaginal hysterectomy for abortion-sterilization. Although the results of both of these series were excellent, present opinion would favor safer and simpler procedures.

Incidence

6. Bunker, J. P. Public health rounds at the Harvard School of Public Health. *N. Engl. J. Med.* 295:264, 1976.
   The concept of preventive hysterectomy as a cancer prophylaxis is not justified since the operative mortality nearly balances those who would avoid death from cancer.

7. Selwood, T., and Wood, C. Incidence of hysterectomy in Australia. *Med. J. Aust.* 2:201, 1978.
   The incidence is similar to that of the U.S.A. and twice that of England and Wales. The authors discuss the possible reasons for the difference.

Management

8. Sack, R. A. The value of intravenous urography prior to abdominal hysterectomy for gynecologic disease. *Am. J. Obstet. Gynecol.* 134:208, 1979.
   Benefits include the demonstration of unsuspected pathology, defense against malpractice suits, and assistance in the prevention of urinary tract injury.

9. Hamod, K. A. Single-dose and multidose prophylaxis in vaginal hysterectomy: A comparison of sodium cephalothin and metronidazole. *Am. J. Obstet. Gynecol.* 136:976, 1980.
   The antibiotic need not be broad-spectrum, but it should be one that has activity against either anaerobic or aerobic flora.

10. Williams, T. J., Johnson, T. R., and Pratt, J. H. Time interval between cervical conization and hysterectomy. *Am. J. Obstet. Gynecol.* 107:790, 1970.
    Unless hysterectomy is done within 48 hours of conization, 6 weeks should elapse before proceeding, since an increase in morbidity may be expected otherwise.

11. Brown, S. E., Allen, H. H., and Robins, R. N. Use of delayed primary wound closure in preventing wound infections. *Am. J. Obstet. Gynecol.* 127:713, 1977.

The incidence of wound infections was much reduced by the use of delayed primary wound closure in high-risk patients, such as the obese and those with an infectious disease process.

12. Pratt, J. H., and Jefferies, J. A. Retained cervical stump: A 25-year experience. *Obstet. Gynecol.* 48:711, 1976.
The indications for removal of the cervix following a subtotal hysterectomy appears to be similar to the indications for removal when the rest of the uterus is still present.

13. Sloan, D. The emotional and psychosexual aspects of hysterectomy. *Am. J. Obstet. Gynecol.* 131:598, 1978.
Reviews the often conflicting evidence and makes a plea for allowing the patient to play a real role in her own management.

14. Funt, M. I., Benigno, B. B., and Thompson, J. D. Residual adnexa: Asset or liability. *Am. J. Obstet. Gynecol.* 129:251, 1977.
In this study, only 1.4% of 1507 women with adnexal conservation required further surgery and none developed a malignancy.

15. Stuart, G. C. E., Allen, H. H., and Anderson, R. J. Squamous cell carcinoma of the vagina following hysterectomy. *Am. J. Obstet. Gynecol.* 139:311, 1981.
This analysis of 29 cases indicates the importance of follow-up since vaginal cancer may follow hysterectomy for cervical dysplasia or for unrelated diseases.

Complications

16. Beland, G. Early treatment of ureteral injuries found after gynecologic surgery. *J. Urol.* 118:25, 1977.
A convincing argument for early definitive surgery of ureteral operative injuries.

17. Genton, E., and Turpie, A. G. G. Venous thromboembolism associated with gynecologic surgery. *Clin. Obstet. Gynecol.* 23:209, 1980.
Diagnosis, treatment, and prophylaxis of venous thromboembolism.

18. Sinclair, R. II., and Pratt, J. II. Femoral neuropathy after pelvic operation. *Am. J. Obstet. Gynecol.* 112:404, 1972.
Sciatic and femoral neuropathy have been reported following vaginal hysterectomy due to improper positioning of the patient during surgery.

19. Ledger, W. J., Campbell, C., and Willson, J. R. Postoperative adnexal infections. *Obstet. Gynecol.* 31:83, 1968.
Cuff hematoma, cuff abscess, pelvic cellulitis, and adnexal abscess may follow hysterectomy, especially that done by the vaginal route.

20. Ananth, J. Hysterectomy and depression. *Obstet. Gynecol.* 52:724, 1978.
In some instances, a premorbid personality may be the cause of both hysterectomy and depression.

21. Kaltreider, N. B., Wallace, A., and Horowitz, M. J. A field study of the stress response syndrome. Young women after hysterectomy. *J.A.M.A.* 242:1499, 1979.
Of 28 women, 12 had a mild stress response while 5 had serious intrusive and avoidant symptoms 1 year after nonelective hysterectomy for benign disease.

22. Centerwall, B. S. Premenopausal hysterectomy and cardiovascular disease. *Am. J. Obstet. Gynecol.* 139:58, 1981.
A premenopausal simple hysterectomy is associated with a threefold increase in subsequent coronary heart disease.

23. Rosenberg, L., et al. Early menopause and the risk of myocardial infarction. *Am. J. Obstet. Gynecol.* 139:47, 1981.
Surgical castration before age 35 increased the risk 7.2 times.

INFECTIOUS AND VENEREAL DISEASES

Gonorrhea is an inflammation of the urogenital tract caused by a gram-negative, intracellular diplococcus, *Neisseria gonorrhoeae*. The organism is extremely fastidious, requiring aerobic conditions with a 10% carbon dioxide (CO_2) atmosphere, and has a predilection for columnar and transitional epithelium. Transmission is usually sexual, although it may be spread by other means of direct contact such as delivery through an infected birth canal.

Gram-staining, although worth doing, yields a high false-negative rate (60%–70%), and diagnosis is really dependent on successful culture. Best results are obtained by employing selective media such as Modified Thayer-Martin (MTM) or Transgrow (MTM in 10% CO_2). A candle jar provides an acceptable CO_2 atmosphere. Direct plating on fresh media with incubation at optimal temperatures (35°–36°C) will increase successful growth of the organism. The characteristic colonies are oxidase-positive, and the organism ferments glucose with the production of acid. Specific fluorescent antibody-staining of smears can be used as an adjunct in diagnosis, particularly in sites from which culture is often unsuccessful, such as skin lesions, or in cases in which partial therapy has prevented cultural recovery of organisms.

Gonorrhea ranks number one of all the reported communicable diseases. In 1976, over one million cases were reported in the United States, and it is estimated that only 1 of 5 cases is reported, since the majority of patients are treated by private physicians who frequently do not report the infection to a health department. As is true of all venereal diseases, gonorrhea has an increased incidence in social groups with high rates of sexual promiscuity, is frequently associated with other venereal infections, and is most common among teenagers and young adults. The condition is rare in very young, in the very old, and in religious orders practicing celibacy. There is a high rate of concurrent infection in sexual contacts, the site of infection frequently depending on the mode of sexual relationship. It has long been thought that it is the female who is generally asymptomatic, but studies carried out on the consorts of infected females have shown a high asymptomatic carrier state in the male as well.

The incubation period is usually from 3–7 days after exposure. The acute phase may last for weeks and then gradually, without treatment or with partial therapy, pass on into a chronic phase. Such cases may represent up to 60%–80% of the total number of infected females. The endocervix, urethra, and Bartholin and paraurethral glands are the usual sites of infection. Complaints include vaginal discharge, dysuria, menstrual irregularity, and abdominal pain, including right upper quadrant pain (Fitz-Hugh–Curtis syndrome). Abscess formation may occur in Skene's glands and in Bartholin's glands. Upward spread from the endocervix occurs in from 10%–15% of patients (an increased shedding of the organism during menses has been noted). Gonococcal salpingitis is associated with abscess formation in some 10%–15% of patients. Spread of the organism is along the mucosal surfaces and the tube lumen may fill with purulent exudate, with secondary involvement of the ovaries and adjacent peritoneum. Frequently, secondary bacterial invasion has by this time replaced the original gonococcal infection. In up to 15% of cases, abscess rupture may occur, with diffuse peritonitis.

Primary gonococcal infections also occur in other mucosal sites, including the anorectal area and the oropharynx. Extragenital infection is not uncommon; at this time gonococcal arthritis is the most common type of infectious arthritis. The arthritis is most likely to appear and spread during pregnancy, usually during the second and third trimester. The condition may be monoarticular or polyarticular. Skin lesions are commonly present with the arthritis. They begin as small red papules, evolving through vesicular and pustular stages to a lesion with a necrotic center superimposed on a hemorrhagic base. Healing is usually spontaneous. Gonococcal endocarditis and meningitis have also been reported.

Nonsexual transmission of the gonococcus occurs in neonatal infections and as a cause of vulvovaginitis in young girls. During delivery, the infant is exposed to the birth canal flora, including gonococcal organisms if they are present. Gonococcal ophthalmia neonatorum has an incidence below 1% but is being increasingly reported. Gonococcal vaginitis is responsible for under 2.5% of cases of leukorrhea in children and is accompanied by very prominent symptoms. It is very rare for this type of infection to become widespread, although a few cases of peritonitis and of arthritis secondary to gonococcal vaginitis have been described.

In private physicians' offices, routine testing of all sexually active individuals yields a 2.3%–2.8% positive culture, while in a venereal disease clinic this increases to 12%. A single cervical swab gives an 80%–90% positive rate. The gram-stain is much less helpful and false-negative results may be found in 60%–70% of patients tested. The optimal site for culture is the endocervix, but cultures should also be taken from the rectum, pharynx, urethra, and vagina. In approximately 10% of patients anal culture is the only site yielding positive results. The organism is less commonly cultured from purulent fluids, the incidence of positive cultures ranging from 25%–50%. The explanation for this is uncertain. Since exposure to one venereal disease increases the risk of exposure to others, a serum test for syphilis, e.g., the rapid plasma reagin test (RPR), should be taken at the same time; this test does not become positive for several weeks, however, and will therefore have to be repeated within 1 to 3 months after the initial test.

The Center for Disease Control (CDC) regularly updates the recommended treatment schedules for the various types of gonococcal infections. At present, uncomplicated gonococcal infections are best treated by aqueous procaine penicillin G, 4.8 million units injected intramuscularly with 1 g of probenecid by mouth. Ampicillin, 3.5 g, with 1 g of probenecid by mouth or spectinomycin, 2 g in one intramuscular injection, are also effective. Patients allergic to penicillin can be treated with tetracycline hydrochloride, 0.5 g orally four times a day to a total dose of 10 g. Pharyngeal and anal infections may not respond well to treatment.

All patients with incubating syphilis should be cured by the regimens mentioned except spectinomycin. Follow-up is essential. Cultures should be repeated from the infected sites as well as from the anal canal 3–7 days after therapy. All sexual partners should be examined, have cultures done, and be treated. Treatment failures are generally due to reinfection or noncompliance with treatment schedules; however, penicillin-resistant gonococci (beta-lactamase producers) are becoming more common, and posttreatment isolates should be tested for penicillinase production. These organisms are usually sensitive to spectinomycin.

Pregnant women should have endocervical cultures done at their first prenatal visit and a second culture done in the third trimester. The same treatment regimens are suitable for pregnant women, with the exception of tetracycline because of its potential toxic effects for mother and fetus. Patients with acute gonococcal salpingitis frequently require hospitalization; they may then be treated with crystalline penicillin G, 20 million units intravenously per day until improvement occurs, followed by oral ampicillin, 0.5 g orally four times a day to complete 10 days of therapy; or with intravenous tetracycline, 0.25 g intravenously four times a day until improvement occurs, followed by 0.5 g orally four times a day to complete 10 days of therapy. The management of disseminated gonococcal infections, as in the arthritis-dermatitis syndrome, and of gonococcal infections in pediatric patients, are also covered in the Center for Disease Control bulletins but are outside the scope of this review. Gonococcal ophthalmia is generally prevented by treatment of the newborn with ophthalmic ointment or drops containing tetracycline or erythromycin, or by the application of 1% silver nitrate solution.

In pregnant women, infection due to the gonococcus carries a significant risk for both mother and neonate. There is an increased incidence of premature ruptured membranes and chorioamnionitis, as well as a high spontaneous abortion and prematurity rate. In untreated cases there is a high incidence of puerperal morbidity.

Management of gonococcal infection is not considered complete until patient education, localizing of contacts for therapy, and reporting of the infection have been carried out.

Review

1. Spence, M. R. The role of the gonococcus in salpingitis. *J. Reprod. Med.* 19:31, 1977.
   The organism invades the secretory cells of the tubal epithelium, leading to sloughing of both secretory and ciliated cells.
2. Nolan, G. H. Gonococcal infections in the female. *Obstet. Gynecol.* 42:156, 1973.
   Succinct account of the infection in children and in adults in both the genital and extragenital forms.
3. Holmes, K. K., Counts, G., and Beaty, H. Disseminated gonococcal infection. *Ann. Intern. Med.* 74:979, 1971.
   Disseminated disease is more common with asymptomatic gonorrhea than with symptomatic infection.
4. Litt, I., Edberg, S., and Finberg, L. Gonorrhea in children and adolescents: A current review. *J. Pediatr.* 95:595, 1974.
   Venereal and nonvenereal modes of transmission are possible, and the possibility of childhood sexual abuse must be considered.

Epidemiology

5. Handsfield, H. H., et al. Asymptomatic gonorrhea in men, diagnosis, natural course, prevalence and significance. *N. Engl. J. Med.* 290:117, 1974.
   The asymptomatic carrier state occurs in 40%–70% of those males infected. Asymptomatic males, therefore, are a major factor in the current gonorrhea pandemic.
6. Lucas, J. B., et al. Diagnosis and treatment of gonorrhea in the female. *N. Engl. J. Med.* 276:1454, 1967.
   In females, latent cases represent 60%–80% of the total number of infected females.
7. Wiesner, P. J. Penicillin-resistant gonococci: Result of plasmid promiscuity. *South. Med. J.* 70:769, 1977.
   An epidemic of penicillinase-producing gonococci was expected after the Vietnam War but fortunately never materialized, possibly due to vigorous attempts at prevention by local health departments and the CDC.
8. Forslin, L., Falk, V., and Danielsson, D. Changes in the incidence of acute gonococcal and nongonococcal salpingitis. A five-year study from an urban area of central Sweden. *Br. J. Vener. Dis.* 54:247, 1978.

In Sweden, nongonococcal infections, probably due to chlamydia, are now more common than gonococcal.

Genital Gonorrhea

9. Draper, D. L., et al. Scanning electron microscopy of attachment of *Neisseria gonorrhoeae* colony phenotypes to surfaces of human genital epithelia. *Am. J. Obstet. Gynecol.* 138:818, 1980.
Transition cells of squamocolumnar area showed the greatest adherence of gonococci.

10. Thompson, S. E., et al. Auxotypes and antibiotic susceptibility patterns of *Neisseria gonorrhoeae* from disseminated and local infections. *Sex. Transm. Dis.* 5:127, 1978.
Some gonococci have unique nutritional needs (auxotypes) for arginine, hypoxanthine, and uracil, although only a high susceptibility to penicillin and resistance to human serum appear linked to virulence.

11. Hedberg, E., and Spetz, S. L. Acute salpingitis. Views on prognosis and treatment. *Acta Obstet. Gynecol. Scand.* 37:131, 1958.
Gonococci can attach to sperm and be transported to the fallopian tubes by the semen.

12. Sweet, R. L., Draper, D. L., and Hadley, W. K. Etiology of acute salpingitis: Influence of episode number and duration of symptoms. *Obstet. Gynecol.* 58:62, 1981.
The gonococcus may initiate acute salpingitis. Secondary invasion of the upper genital tract by cervical and vaginal organisms may then occur.

13. Eschenbach, D. A., and Holmes, K. K. Acute pelvic inflammatory disease: Current concepts of pathogenesis, etiology, and management. *Clin. Obstet. Gynecol.* 18:35, 1975.
The classic picture of fever, abdominal and adnexal tenderness, pain on cervical excitation, and a purulent discharge are not always present. Urinary frequency, urgency, and dysuria as well as menstrual irregularity are common misdiagnosed symptoms of gonorrhea in women.

14. Monif, G. R., et al. Cul-de-sac isolates from patients with endometritis, salpingitis-peritonitis, and gonococcal endocervicitis. *Am. J. Obstet. Gynecol.* 126:158, 1976.
Secondarily invading organisms are commonly found in patients with salpingitis. It must be kept in mind that vaginal contamination of the culdocentesis sample is very likely so these cultures may be misleading.

Extragenital Gonorrhea

15. Muller-Schoop, J. W., et al. Chlamydia trachomatis as possible cause of peritonitis and perihepatitis in young women. *Br. Med. J.* 1:1022, 1978.
Acute fibrinous perihepatitis (Fitz-Hugh–Curtis syndrome) may complicate gonorrhea, but other organisms, including chlamydia, have also been incriminated.

16. Klein, E. J., et al. Anorectal gonococcal infection. *Ann. Intern. Med.* 86:340, 1977.
Of females with gonorrhea 44% show a positive anorectal culture. This may be due to anal intercourse or autoinoculation from vaginal secretions.

17. Wiesner, P., et al. Clinical spectrum of pharyngeal gonococcal infection. *N. Engl. J. Med.* 288:181, 1973.
It is more likely that the organism is transferred via fellatio than cunnilingus. Treatment may be difficult.

18. Gelfand, S., Massi, A., and Garcia-Kuzbach, A. Spectrum of gonococcal arthritis: Evidence for sequential states and clinical subgroups. *J. Rheumatol.* 2:83, 1975.
Early (septicemic) phase of migratory polyarthritis with fever is followed

by septic phase with inflammation and effusion in one joint. Blood culture is diagnostic in the early phase and joint culture in the later.

Neonatal and Pediatric Gonorrhea

19. Crede, K. S. F. Die berhutung der angoentzundung der neugeborenen. *Arch. Gynaekol.* 17:50, 1881.
    The incidence of asymptomatic gonococcal infection in pregnant patients ranges from 1%–6% so that the prophylactic use of silver nitrate (Crede's classic solution) or antibiotic ointments is routine in the prevention of ophthalmia neonatorum.
20. Burry, V. F. Gonococcal vulvovaginitis and possible peritonitis in prepubertal girls. *Am. J. Dis. Child.* 121:536, 1971.
    The prepubertal, nonestrogenized thin vaginal mucosa is susceptible to invasion by gonococci, with acute vulvovaginitis and marked symptomatology.

Diagnosis

21. Caldwell, J. G., et al. Sensitivity and reproducibility of Thayer-Martin culture medium in diagnosing gonorrhea in women. *Am. J. Obstet. Gynecol.* 109:463, 1971.
    The culture medium contains antibiotics selective for optimal gonococcal growth.
22. Tronca, E., et al. Demonstration of *Neisseria gonorrhea* with fluorescent antibody in patients with disseminated gonococcal infection. *J. Infect. Dis.* 129:583, 1974.
    Article discusses a sophisticated laboratory technique not generally available.

Treatment

23. Gonorrhea: CDC recommended treatment schedules—1979. *Obstet. Gynecol.* 55:255, 1980.
    There have been few major changes in recommended treatment regimens. Unfortunately, an effective gonorrheal vaccine has yet to be developed.
24. Curran, J. W. Management of gonococcal pelvic inflammatory disease. *Sex. Transm. Dis.* 6:174, 1979.
    Results of five published studies were compared and it was concluded that no change in recommended treatment regimens should be made.
25. Weiler, P. G., and Maddox, D. E. Some perspectives on the problem of gonorrhea. *J. Ky. Med. Assoc.* 75:16, 1977.
    Antibiotic prophylaxis has not been widely used for fear of bacterial resistance. Nevertheless, results are good, and the method should be considered in selected patients.
26. Curran, J. W., et al. Gonorrhea in the emergency department: Management, case follow-up, and contact tracing of cases in women. *Am. J. Obstet. Gynecol.* 138:1105, 1980.
    Test-of-cure, follow-up of untreated cases, and contact investigation is essential to adequate management of gonorrhea.

Syphilis

Syphilis is an infectious disease caused by a spirochete, *Treponema pallidum.* The infection is spread by sexual intercourse or by intrauterine transmission (congenital syphilis).

The incubation period averages 21 days, with a primary sore (chancre) appearing at the site of infection; this remains from 1 to 6 weeks. The chancres, which are commonly seen on the genitalia, mouth, and anus, are usually painless. Regional adenopathy is common. Diagnosis is dependent on a positive darkfield examination demonstrating the organism in a direct scraping from the lesion. Serologic tests are often nonreactive at this stage. The differential diagnosis includes neoplasm, chancroid, lymphogranuloma venereum, granuloma inguinale, herpes, and fungal infection.

A secondary stage of infection appears within 6–8 weeks of the primary stage. This stage is characterized by lesions of skin and mucous membranes. The disease is systemic and generalized adenopathy is often present. The skin lesions take many forms and must be differentiated from common skin eruptions, including drug reactions and acute exanthemata. Condylomata on the genitalia and mucous patches on the genitals, mouth, and lips are characteristic. Serology is invariably positive and like the chancre, the lesions are highly infective.

A subclinical latent stage follows that can last for many years and is diagnosed only by the presence of positive serology. During early latency (1–4 years) relapses with mucocutaneous lesions may occur. Thereafter there are no relapses, and the syphilis is noninfectious except in the pregnant woman who may infect her fetus.

Late syphilis includes cardiovascular and neurosyphilis, although any tissue may be involved. Serology is usually reactive.

The clinical spectrum of syphilis acquired in utero includes stillbirth, neonatal death, neonatal illness in the first months of life, and development of the stigmata of congenital syphilis in later life.

Serologic tests are nontreponemal and treponemal. The former detect antibody against a nonspecific antigen and are used for screening purposes. If positive, they may be repeated quantitatively, and the titers may be used as a guide to therapeutic response. The Venereal Disease Research Laboratory (VDRL) test and the rapid plasma reagin (RPR) test are examples. Treponemal tests measure specific antitreponemal antibody and are used to establish the diagnosis. These tests include the fluorescent treponemal antibody-absorption (FTA-ABS) test, and for the diagnosis of congenital infection the FTA-ABS-IgM test for fetal IgM antibodies. The treponemal tests are more expensive and difficult and are not quantitative. They are specific and sensitive and should be used to confirm a doubtful diagnosis, not for screening or for evaluating response to treatment.

False-positive reactions with nontreponemal tests are common. These reactions are termed *acute* (less than 6 months) and may occur with many infections or pregnancy, and *chronic* (over 6 months), found with collagen diseases, drug addiction, aging, and malignancy. These false reactions are rare with the treponemal tests but do occur, and the clinical picture must be considered in deciding whether the patient has syphilis, another disease, or both.

Parenteral penicillin in the form of a single dose of 2.4 million units benzathine penicillin G is the usual treatment of primary, secondary, and latent syphilis in pregnant and nonpregnant patients or contacts. If penicillin is contraindicated, tetracycline in a total dose of 30 g over 10 days or erythromycin in similar dosage provide alternative therapy. Late syphilis is also treated with penicillin in doses up to 10 million units. Congenital syphilis in the neonate may be treated with a single dose of benzathine penicillin G 50,000 units/kg if the spinal fluid is normal. Adverse reactions to therapy include penicillin sensitivity and the Jarisch-Herxheimer reaction. Because serious anaphylaxis usually begins within 30 minutes of treatment, all patients should be kept at least this time period after injection.

Follow-up with quantitative VDRL tests at 1, 3, 6, and 12 months is essential. If serology does not become nonreactive or reach a fixed low titer, reinfection, relapse, or neurosyphilis should be excluded.

Reviews

1. Rudolph, A. H., and Duncan, W. C. Syphilis—diagnosis and treatment. *Clin. Obstet. Gynecol.* 18:163, 1975.
   Syphilis remains one of the most common reportable communicable diseases. It is vital that doctors understand the diagnosis and therapy of this condition, one that is devastating if untreated but highly responsive to adequate medication.
2. Felman, Y. M., and Nikitas, J. A. Syphilis serology today. *Arch. Dermatol.* 116:84, 1980.
   Reviews the various currently used serologic tests, both nontreponemal and treponemal.

Syphilis in Pregnancy

3. Holder, W. R., and Knox, J. M. Syphilis in pregnancy. *Med. Clin. North Am.* 56:1151, 1972.
   Infection acquired during pregnancy results in stillbirth or neonatal death in 50% and in damage to virtually all the infants. Infection prior to pregnancy carries a perinatal mortality of 10%–20% with 10%–40% residual stigmata in the survivors.
4. Hager, W. D. The transplacental transmission of spirochetes in congenital syphilis: A new perspective. *Sex. Transm. Dis.* 5:112, 1978.
   Syphilis can be transmitted transplacentally at any stage of pregnancy. Serology should be obtained in early pregnancy and repeated in the third trimester.
5. Oppenheimer, E., and Hardy, J. Congenital syphilis in the newborn infant: Clinical and pathological observations in recent cases. *Johns Hopkins Med. J.* 129:63, 1971.
   Neonates may appear normal or exhibit rhinitis ("snuffles"), hepatosplenomegaly, lymphadenopathy, chorioretinitis, or skin rashes. In children, stigmata include dental abnormalities ("mulberry molars," peg-shaped incisors), saddle nose, rhagades, periostitis ("saber shins"), and neurosyphilis.
6. Bryan, E. M., and Nicholson, E. Congenital syphilis. A study of physical and biochemical aspects. *Clin. Pediatr.* 20:81, 1981.
   All but one of the affected, and only one of the unaffected, infants had high immunoglobulin M (IgM) levels.
7. Jones, J. D., and Harris, R. E. Diagnostic evaluation of syphilis during pregnancy. *Obstet. Gynecol.* 54:611, 1979.
   The authors recommend routine cerebrospinal fluid FTA-ABS testing on pregnant patients with positive serology to exclude the presence of tertiary syphilis.

Diagnosis

8. Mackey, D. M., et al. Specificity of the FTA-ABS test for syphilis. An evaluation. *J.A.M.A.* 207:1683, 1969.
   This sensitive, specific test for syphilis should not be used to assess therapy since it remains positive after adequate therapy of the disease.
9. McKenna, C. H., et al. The fluorescent treponemal antibody absorption (FTA-ABS) test leading phenomenon in connective tissue diseases. *Mayo Clinic Proc.* 48:545, 1973.

On occasion, positive serology may indicate a disease process much more serious in its implications than syphilis. Systemic lupus erythematosus for instance, can exhibit a false-positive FTA-ABS reaction.

10. Rosen, E., and Richardson, N. A reappraisal of the value of the IgM fluorescent treponemal antibody test for the diagnosis of congenital syphilis. *J. Pediatr.* 87:38, 1975.

   IgG may be passively transferred from the mother, but IgM is not transferred. The presence of IgM is therefore said to indicate fetal involvement. This test is controversial since other workers have reported negative results in one-third of infants with the disease.

11. Catteral, R. D. Systemic disease and the biological false positive reaction. *Br. J. Vener. Dis.* 48:1, 1972.

   If possible, the cause of the false-positive reaction should be identified.

12. Chapel, T. A. The signs and symptoms of secondary syphilis. *Sex. Transm. Dis.* 7:161, 1980.

   Almost a fourth of the patients were not aware that they had mucocutaneous lesions.

Treatment

13. Thompson, S. E., III. Treatment of syphilis in pregnancy. *J. Am. Vener. Dis. Assoc.* 3:159, 1976.

   Penicillin is standard therapy; erythromycin and cephalosporins may be used if penicillin is contraindicated. Tetracyclines should not be used during pregnancy.

14. Center for Disease Control. Syphilis—CDC recommended treatment schedules 1976. *Morbid. Mortal. Weekly Rep.* 25:101, 1976.

   The CDC recommendations for treatment of the spectrum of syphilitic disease.

15. Schroeter, A. L., et al. Therapy for incubating syphilis: Effectiveness of gonorrhea treatment. *J.A.M.A.* 218:711, 1971.

   Standard gonorrhea therapy is successful in clearing incubating syphilis, but it will not clear established infection.

16. Warrell, D. A., et al. Physiologic changes during the Jarisch-Herxheimer reaction in early syphilis. A comparison with louseborne relapsing fever. *Am. J. Med.* 51:176, 1971.

   A systemic response to therapy of syphilis in some patients characterized by flulike symptoms and usually responsive to conservative measures.

17. Rudolph, A. H., and Price, E. V. Penicillin reactions among patients in venereal disease clinics. A national survey. *J.A.M.A.* 223:499, 1973.

   Penicillin reactions occurred irrespective of negative history or of previous penicillin usage.

Vaginitis

Vaginal discharge is the most common gynecologic complaint brought to the physician's attention. It is important to distinguish between leukorrhea and an infected vaginal discharge. Leukorrhea may be either mucinous, due to reactive hypersecretion from cervical polyps or "erosions"; or hyperestrogenic (postovulatory or birth control pill); or due to hyperdesquamation from an exaggerated response of the vaginal mucosa to normal or abnormal hormonal stimulation. The leukorrhea due to this last is classically a nonadherent, abundant, whitish discharge. There may be an associated itch in 30% of patients.

Tense and anxious women may have a marked increase in the normal secretions. It is estimated that 60% of women with excessive or abnormal discharges will have negative bacterial cultures. Reassurance and confirmation of its noninfective origin will be adequate therapy.

Vaginitis in childhood usually follows local trauma. Contamination may occur from soiled linen, towels, or toilets, or from insertion of foreign bodies. Vaginal examination under anesthesia is frequently indicated for adequate exposure and exploration to exclude pathology or for the removal of foreign bodies. Swabs for culture may be taken without the use of a speculum. The most common organisms found are *Escherichia coli*, although on occasion, sexual molestation may result in gonococcal infection.

Nonspecific vaginal discharge in adults may be related to foreign bodies such as forgotten diaphragms, cotton balls, sponges, or tampons. There is also an increased discharge associated with the birth control pill and the intrauterine device (IUD). Tight underwear or nylon may cause chafing, thus producing itching, vulvitis, and vaginitis with excessive discharge. Allergies to clothing, feminine sprays, soaps, and douches may produce profuse leukorrhea. These conditions frequently become secondarily infected due to damage to the epithelium by chemicals or following scratching from the intense pruritus.

Atrophic vaginitis results from loss of natural estrogens. It is seen post radiation and postoophorectomy, and in the menopausal woman. The mucosa is easily fractured, and initially a nonspecific, often blood-stained discharge occurs. Invasion by pathogenic organisms may follow.

In descending order of frequency, the three common organisms causing vaginitis in women of reproductive age are *Trichomonas vaginalis, Candida albicans,* and *Gardnerella vaginalis.* Recently *Chlamydia trachomatis* and *Mycoplasma hominis* have also been incriminated. *Herpes* virus vaginitis is rare; the lesions of this increasingly common sexually transmitted disease are usually encountered on the vulva or cervix (see page 44). Ultimately, diagnosis is dependent on observation or culture of the specific organism.

T. vaginalis is sexually transmitted, usually in the immediate postmenstrual phase. The discharge is characteristically malodorous, frothy, and yellow in color. The infection may produce vulvovaginal erythema and edema. The pH of the discharge is 5.0–5.5. In its most severe form, petechiae with swollen vaginal papillae ("strawberry vagina") may be seen. It must be stressed, though, that many infections have reddened vaginas with malodorous discharges.

Specimens for examination should be taken from the posterior vaginal wall fairly high up. The swab is then placed in a saline tube and rotated several times. The cotton-tipped applicator is then placed on a slide and a cover slip applied. Motile trichomonads will be seen without the use of specific stains. Trichomonads are also seen on routine Papanicolaou smears.

Metronidazole (or analogues), 250 mg taken three times daily for 7 days, or 2 g as a single dose, will cure 90% of cases. It is important that the male partner be treated as well. Metronidazole should not be used in the first trimester of pregnancy. It may be used, however, if symptoms are severe thereafter. If metronidazole is contraindicated, trichomoniasis can be treated with local applications of povidone-iodine at night for a week at a time. If alcohol is taken with it, metronidazole may produce side effects such as nausea and dizziness. If occurring during pregnancy, 15% of *Trichomonas* infections are combined with candidiasis.

C. albicans is the most important of the specific agents causing vaginitis in pregnant women, though the fungus can be present in the vagina as a commensal, exciting neither reaction nor symptoms. In the last two decades there has been a worldwide increase in fungal diseases. This is ascribed to the administration of antibiotics, corticosteroids, cytotoxic agents, and oral contraceptives. The gut is the usual reservoir for the fungus. Diabetes also increases the risk of candidal infection.

The acidity of the pregnant vagina favors the establishment and multiplication of the *Candida*. The rise in candidal vaginitis in pregnancy is reflected by the change in the ratio of *Trichomoniasis* from 7:1 to 15:1 in favor of moniliasis.

Candidiasis occurs in about 6%–28% of all women, but its incidence is doubled in pregnancy. Symptomatic candidiasis occurs in 15%–43% of patients. Complaints include leukorrhea, pruritus, and dyspareunia. Examination usually reveals classic features: a red, edematous vulva and vagina with a thick, creamy discharge that adheres in patches to the vaginal wall. Removal may leave petechiae. Malodor is usually due to associated *G. vaginalis* or trichomoniasis.

Diagnosis is made by microscopy of the discharge mixed with 10% potassium hydroxide. Distinct, translucent spores and hyphae (filaments) are seen after the potassium hydroxide destroys the cellular elements. A saline wet mount may demonstrate spores, filaments, pus cells, and lactobacilli. Confirmatory cultures can be made by plating the discharge on Nickerson's medium.

Nightly insertions of miconazole cream placed high up in the vagina for a week are usually quite efficacious. A repeat course is sometimes necessary. Oral medication with nystatin may be required if repeated infection occurs by way of the bowel.

Vaginitis caused by *G. vaginalis* is often called "nonspecific" vaginitis. It is probably a sexually transmitted disease and occurs when the pH is low in the vagina (hyperestrogenic states). If the leukorrhea is heavy, there is usually a mixed infection. Many patients are asymptomatic, while others have mild pruritus and burning. The discharge is invariably malodorous, grayish, and homogenous. Because it is a surface infection, inflammation is rare. The vaginal pH is 5.0–5.5. A wet mount will show clumps of dark, stippled epithelium ("clue cells") with the Gardnerella rods. There are few pus cells and often no lactobacilli. Gram stain confirms small gram-negative rods. Treatment with antibiotic creams may be adequate, although oral ampicillin and, more recently, metronidazole appear to be more effective.

C. trachomatis are bacterialike organisms that require specialized culture techniques. They are mostly associated with cervicitis and salpingitis. They are usually harbored in the urethra of the male, causing "nonspecific urethritis." Their role in vaginitis is not yet clear. They respond well to tetracyclines.

Two groups of mycoplasmas, *M. hominis* and *Ureaplasma urealyticum* (they have the ability to hydrolyze urea), have been implicated as causal agents of genitourinary diseases. Postpubertal colonization occurs primarily through sexual contact. The vaginal pH is usually high. They may have a role in "nonspecific vaginitis" when no recognized pathogen can be found, although their role in vaginitis has not yet been evaluated.

Atrophic vaginitis is characterized by a pale, thin, diffuse redness. The mucosa is smooth with ecchymoses and petechiae and loss of the normal rugae. The discharge is variable, from blood-stained, thick or watery, to purulent. The pH is only slightly acidic. Cultures reveal mixed, nonspecific bacterial flora. Vaginal cytology demonstrates an abundance of parabasal or basal epithelial cells. Rapid relief of the burning, itching, and dyspareunia is obtained with local estrogen cream. In severe cases with other symptoms of the menopause, oral estrogens may be used as well. Secondary infection, as with any nonspecific infection, may be treated by local sulphonamide preparations.

Among the smaller group of nonspecific bacterial infections, the most frequent isolates are the *Diphtheroid bacilli, E. coli,* and the anaerobes *Bacteroides fragilis, Peptostreptococcus,* and *Bacteroides melaninogenicus.* Unless associated with pelvic inflammatory disease, the anaerobes produce a mild, nonspecific vaginitis with moderate leukorrhea.

Allergic and chemical vulvovaginitis may be treated with local corticosteroid preparations. Estrogen creams may be absorbed well enough to produce endometrial changes and withdrawal bleeding in the postmenopausal woman. Prolonged use of antibiotics may allow fungal overgrowth, and therapy should be combined with antifungal cream in such cases. Intercourse should be avoided during any treatment for vaginitis.

Reviews
1. Hurd, J. K., Jr. Vaginitis. *Med. Clin. North Am.* 63:423, 1979.
   A short review of the subject, plus management of it.
2. Felman, J. M., and Nikitas, J. A. *Trichomonas,* candidiasis and *corynebacterium vaginale* vaginitis. *N.Y. State J. Med.* 79:1563, 1979.
   Clinical and laboratory diagnosis of these organisms, plus management, are discussed.
3. Paavonen, J. Chlamydia infections. Microbiological, clinical and diagnostic aspect. *Med. Biol.* 57:135, 1979.
   A comprehensive overview of the subject, with 165 references.

Etiology
4. Andrew, D. C., et al. The role of fomites in the transmission of vaginitis. *Can. Med. Assoc. J.* 112:1181, 1975.
   They do not appear to be an important mode of transmission. Candida was the most frequent organism in a university community.
5. Thin, R. N., et al. How often are gonorrhea and genital yeast infection sexually transmitted? *Br. J. Vener. Dis.* 8:511, 1979.
   Incidence of sexual transmission is discussed.
6. Ross, C. A. Postmenopausal vaginitis. *J. Med. Microbiol.* 11:209, 1975.
   A survey of women with infected and noninfected postmenopausal vaginitis is discussed.

Pathogenesis
7. McCormack, W. M., et al. Fifteen-month follow-up study of women infected with *Chlamydia trachomatis. N. Engl. J. Med.* 300:123, 1979.
   A follow-up evaluation of this organism is presented.
8. Syverson, R. E., et al. Cellular and humoral immune status in women with chronic candida vaginitis. *Am. J. Obstet. Gynecol.* 134:624, 1979.
   Immunological disturbance is an important factor in recurrent candidiasis.
9. Miles, M. R., et al. Recurrent vaginal candidiasis. Importance of an intestinal reservoir. *J.A.M.A.* 238:1836, 1977.
   The intestinal reservoir in the pathogenesis of candida infection is stressed.

Diagnosis
10. Rubin, A. Vaginal discharge in the black pregnant patient. *S. Afr. Med. J.* 57:404, 1980.
    An evaluation of the relationship between symptomatology and diagnosis.

11. McCormack, W. M., et al. Sexually transmitted conditions among women college students. *Am. J. Obstet. Gynecol.* 139:130, 1981.
    Of 500 students, trichomonas was found in 14, gonorrhea in 2, chlamydia in 20, condylomata in 7, and herpes in 4. Gardnerella was isolated from one-third of the women.

General

12. Witchins, S. *Hemophilus vaginalis* vaginitis and gonorrhea in pregnancy. *J. Med. Soc. N.J.* 75:461, 1978.
    Importance of these infections in pregnancy is discussed.
13. Tuttle, J. P., Jr., et al. Interference of human spermatozoal motility by trichomonas vaginalis. *J. Urol.* 118:1024, 1977.
    Trichomoniasis may be a factor in infertility.
14. Hobson, D., et al. Maternal genital chlamydial infection as a cause of neonatal conjunctivitis. *Postgrad. Med. J.* 53:595, 1977.
    Chlamydial neonatal conjunctivitis may follow delivery from infected mothers.

Management

15. Malouf, M., et al. Treatment of *Hemophilus vaginalis* vaginitis. *Obstet. Gynecol.* 57:711, 1981.
    Metronidazole was effective in 90%; sulfa cream, doxycycline, and ampicillin in 47%–63%.
16. Havam, K., et al. Vulvovaginal candidiasis in pregnancy treated with clotrimazole. *Acta Obstet. Gynecol. Scand.* 57:453, 1978.
    Clotrimazole is effective therapy in candidiasis occurring during pregnancy.
17. O'Connor, B. H., and Adler, M. W. Current approaches to the diagnosis, treatment and reporting of *Trichomonas* and candidiasis. *Br. J. Vener. Dis.* 55:52, 1979.
    This article describes the current approach to the management of these conditions in clinics for sexually transmitted diseases in England and Wales.
18. Muller, M., et al. Three metronidazole-resistant strains of *Trichomonas vaginalis* from the United States. *Am. J. Obstet. Gynecol.* 138:808, 1980.
    Cure was obtained with increased dosage.
19. Milne, J. D., et al. Effect of simultaneous oral and vaginal treatment on the rate of cure and relapse in vaginal candidiasis. *Br. J. Vener. Dis.* 55:362, 1979.
    There appears to be little advantage to the use of both oral and vaginal treatment in the cure or prevention of relapses.
20. Gordon, W. E., et al. Treatment of atrophic vaginitis in postmenopausal women with micronized estradiol cream. *J. Ky. Med. Assoc.* 77:377, 1979.
    There are distinct advantages if the estrogen cream is micronized.
21. Davidson, F., and Mould, R. F. Recurrent genital candidiasis in women and the effect of intermittent prophylactic treatment. *Br. J. Vener. Dis.* 54:176, 1978.
    Prophylactic treatment improves the symptoms but does not appear to affect the return of the yeasts. The recurrences may relate to another primary underlying factor.
22. Sandler, B. Lactobacillus for vulvovaginitis. *Lancet* 2:791, 1979.
    This may be the answer to the treatment for candidiasis.

Pelvic Inflammatory Disease

Pelvic inflammatory disease (PID) is a useful clinical term and therefore widely employed. For purposes of description, however, the term is too broad and includes too wide a variety of conditions. Therefore, in this review, only those acute supracervical infections unrelated to pregnancy or surgery will be discussed.

The condition is classically divided into two groups, gonococcal and nongonococcal, depending on the presence or absence of *Neisseria gonorrhoeae*. The incidence of gonococcal salpingitis varies from 30%–80%; some 10%–17% of patients with lower genital tract gonorrhea will develop pelvic inflammatory disease. Since nongonococcal infections are not reportable, the incidence of nongonococcal salpingitis is difficult to estimate.

The overall incidence of salpingitis is rising, and this is related to the general increase in sexually transmitted infections and to increased employment of the intrauterine device (IUD). It is estimated that a half to three-quarters of a million cases are treated annually in the United States.

Bacterial cultures taken from the endocervix, from the cul-de-sac by means of culdocentesis, and from the fallopian tubes at laparoscopy indicate a polymicrobial etiology of PID. Only the presence of the gonococcus differentiates the two varieties of PID as regards endocervical cultures. There is poor correlation between endocervical and peritoneal culture, as regards the gonococcus; it varies from 6%–70% of patients studied. Tubal and cul-de-sac cultures are also not consistent. A wide variety of aerobic and anaerobic bacteria have been found, in no way dissimilar to patients with other types of pelvic infection. Thus it has been postulated that *N. gonorrhoeae* may act as a primary pathogen, followed by a secondary invasion of a mixed aerobic-anaerobic group of organisms. Several other microorganisms have been implicated in the causation of salpingitis; these include *Mycoplasma hominis*, T-mycoplasma *(Ureaplasma urealyticum)*, and *Chlamydia trachomatis*. The role of these organisms is still unclear. Actinomycosis infections have been described in association with the IUD.

The pathogenesis of nongonococcal salpingitis is unknown. The use of an IUD, especially in the never-pregnant patient, and previous gonococcal infections appear to be risk factors for the development of the condition. Gonococcal salpingitis commonly presents in the first week after menses and appears to spread along the endometrial surface to the endosalpinx. It is unclear why the gonococcus remains confined to the endocervix in some cases, while spreading to the uterus, tubes, and adjacent structures in others.

The clinical presentation is variable and not dissimilar to several other lower abdominal conditions. Symptoms include lower abdominal pain, increased vaginal discharge, fever, irregular bleeding, urinary symptoms, chills, and vomiting. Clinical findings include cervical excitation pain, elevated temperature and sedimentation rate, lower abdominal peritonism, and leucocytosis. There is little clinical difference between gonococcal and nongonococcal salpingitis, although the former may exhibit higher fevers, more discharge, and respond more readily to therapy.

The differential diagnosis includes appendicitis, endometriosis, ectopic pregnancy, and complications of ovarian cysts. Laparoscopy has shown that the clinical diagnosis is frequently incorrect. In one series, only 65% of patients clinically diagnosed as PID had the condition, 23% were normal, and 12% had other pelvic pathology.

Patients with mild cases may be treated as outpatients. Criteria for hospital admission include uncertain diagnosis, suspicion of an abscess, pregnancy, upper peritoneal signs, temperature above 38°C, and failure to respond to ambulatory therapy.

The treatment of gonococcal salpingitis is well defined, and regimens recommended by the Center for Disease Control (CDC) are highly effective. Unfortunately, because it is not possible to initially differentiate the two varieties of PID, some forms of nongonococcal salpingitis will not respond to the CDC-recommended therapy, nor are firm recommendations yet available since the therapy of nongonococcal salpingitis has not been widely studied. However, as the organisms usually found may include several species, it is now common practice, at least in hospitalized patients, to use parenteral antibiotics adequate to eradicate gonorrhea (penicillin), gram-negative bacteria (aminoglycoside), and, if there is no response in 24–48 hours, to add anaerobic cover active against *B. fragilis* (clindamycin). If *Mycoplasma* or *Chlamydia*, or both, are indeed significant pathogens in PID, tetracycline therapy also would be indicated. It is obvious that further study of adequate therapy for PID is essential.

In patients with an IUD in place removal of the device is usually required once adequate antibiotic blood levels are obtained. In mild cases, the device may be left in situ provided close observation is maintained. Bed rest and avoidance of intercourse are important adjuncts to therapy.

Surgery is not indicated for acute PID other than to exclude possible surgical emergencies, for patients unresponsive to antibiotic therapy, or for pelvic abscess formation in certain circumstances. Laparoscopy is very useful in evaluating atypical cases.

Sequelae of acute PID include adhesions, pelvic masses, chronic pain, and sterility, any or all of which may necessitate surgical intervention. The prognosis for patients with nongonococcal PID is substantially worse in terms of response to therapy and long-range sequelae. Recurrence of infection is common, usually from untreated, asymptomatic male partners. Fertility is lowered by each successive infection. A previous history of PID is common in patients with ectopic pregnancy, although data for the actual risk are not available. Good results in treatment depend on early diagnosis and rational antibiotic selection, and prevention of reinfection by means of patient education and treatment of sexual partners. At issue is the reproductive capacity of an unfortunately ever-increasing group of young women.

Review

1. Sweet, R. L. Diagnosis and treatment of acute salpingitis. *J. Reprod. Med.* 19:21, 1977.
   Excellent review with 56 references.
2. Eschenbach, D. A., and Holmes, K. K. Acute pelvic inflammatory disease: Current concepts of pathogenesis, etiology and management. *Clin. Obstet. Gynecol.* 18:35, 1975.
   Extensive review, including a section on the Fitz-Hugh–Curtis syndrome (gonococcal perihepatitis), which the authors believe is just as common with nongonococcal PID.

Bacteriology

3. Eschenbach, D. A., et al. Polymicrobial etiology of acute pelvic inflammatory disease. *N. Engl. J. Med.* 293:166, 1975.
   Mixed infections were commonly found with cul-de-sac puncture in nongonococcal PID. The most common species were B. fragilis, *peptostreptococci, and peptococci.*

4. Cunningham, F. G., et al. The bacterial pathogenesis of acute pelvic inflammatory disease. *Obstet. Gynecol.* 52:161, 1978.
The authors suggest that N. gonorrhoeae *initiates most cases of PID, but that superinfection with a mixed growth of secondary invaders precludes the recovery of gonococci.*

5. Osborne, N. G. The significance of mycoplasma in pelvic infection. *J. Reprod. Med.* 19:39, 1977.
This review concludes that the role of mycoplasma in PID, either as pathogens or synergistic contributors, remains controversial.

6. Sweet, R. L., et al. Use of laparoscopy to determine the microbiologic etiology of acute salpingitis. *Am. J. Obstet. Gynecol.* 134:68, 1979.
Cul-de-sac aspirates and simultaneous fallopian tube cultures frequently grew out differing organisms. Chlamydia *was not isolated from the tubes in this series.*

7. Chow, A. W., et al. The bacteriology of acute pelvic inflammatory disease. *Am. J. Obstet. Gynecol.* 122:876, 1975.
Cul-de-sac cultures were positive in 18 of 20 patients with PID; blood cultures were all negative.

8. Mardh, P. A., et al. Role of *Chlamydia trachomatis* infection in acute salpingitis. *N. Engl. J. Med.* 296:1377, 1977.
Implicates chlamydia as a possible cause of PID.

Etiology and Epidemiology

9. Paavonen, J., et al. *Chlamydia trachomatis* in acute salpingitis. *Br. J. Vener. Dis.* 55:203, 1979.
Of 106 patients, equal numbers (25%) grew out N. gonorrhoeae *and* C. trachomatis. *Since the organisms frequently coexist, perhaps tetracyclines should replace penicillin as first-choice therapy for gonorrhea.*

10. Treharne, J. D., et al. Antibodies to *Chlamydia trachomatis* in acute salpingitis. *Br. J. Vener. Dis.* 55:26, 1979.
High levels of chlamydial antibody in sera and cul-de-sac fluids suggested C. trachomatis *was the probable pathogen in two-thirds of 143 women with PID. This would correlate well with the high incidence of nongonococcal (50% due to chlamydia) urethritis observed in men.*

11. Ory, H. W. A review of the association between intrauterine devices and acute pelvic inflammatory disease. *J. Reprod. Med.* 20:200, 1978.
Reviews six studies and concludes that IUD use is associated with a threefold to fivefold increased risk of PID.

12. Vessey, M. P., et al. Pelvic inflammatory disease and the intrauterine device: Findings in a large cohort study. *Br. Med. J.* 282:855, 1981.
The authors postulate that chronic PID, developing gradually with an IUD in situ, leads to symptoms resulting in removal of the device.

13. Eschenbach, D. A., Harnisch, J. P., and Holmes, K. K. Pathogenesis of acute pelvic inflammatory disease: Role of contraception and other risk factors. *Am. J. Obstet. Gynecol.* 128:838, 1977.
Increased risk of gonococcal PID in non-Caucasians and relative risk of PID in IUD users were directly related to socioeconomic status.

Diagnosis, Treatment, Prognosis

14. Jacobson, L., and Westrom, L. Objectivized diagnosis of acute PID. Diagnostic and prognostic value of routine laparoscopy. *Am. J. Obstet. Gynecol.* 105:1088, 1969.
Routine laparoscopy in 905 patients was without complication, and the authors recommend it as an integral part of management.

15. Cunningham, F. G., et al. Evaluation of tetracycline or penicillin and

ampicillin for treatment of acute pelvic inflammatory disease. *N. Engl. J. Med.* 296:1380, 1977.

Center for Disease Control regimens for PID were found to be effective; however, subsequent pelvic abscess was 10 times more common in women treated for nongonococcal rather than gonococcal PID.

16. Gall, S. A., et al. Intravenous metronidazole or clindamycin with to-bramycin for therapy of pelvic infections. *Obstet. Gynecol.* 57:51, 1981.

    Use of agents active against anaerobes from the outset was highly success-ful. Metronidazole and clindamycin proved equally effective.

17. Westrom, L. Effect of acute pelvic inflammatory disease on fertility. *Am. J. Obstet. Gynecol.* 121:707, 1975.

    Tubal occlusion occurred after one attack in 12.8%, after two infections in 35.5%, and after three or more in 75%. Ectopic pregnancy was increased sixfold.

18. Falk, V. Treatment of acute nontuberculous salpingitis with antibiotics alone and in combination with glucocorticoids. *Acta Obstet. Gynecol. Scand.* 44 (Suppl. 6):3, 1965.

    The addition of steroids to the regimen did not improve results.

19. Thompson, S. E., et al. The microbiology and therapy of acute pelvic inflammatory disease in hospitalized patients. *Am. J. Obstet. Gynecol.* 136:179, 1980.

    The use of amoxacillin by mouth was compared to penicillin and genta-micin given parenterally. The cure rates were similar.

Pelvic Abscess

A pelvic abscess is a major complication of acute infection in the genital tract. The abscess may be confined to the tube (pyosalpinx), or involve tube and ovary (tuboovarian abscess), or may lie between the leaves of the broad ligament (broad ligament abscess). Purulent material may collect in the pouch of Douglas (cul-de-sac abscess) where it is usually walled off superiorly by intestinal loops and omentum, while its inferior surface dissects between rectum and vagina. A pure ovarian abscess is rare. Frequently, abscess formation is found at more than one anatomic site in the same patient since the acute infection is usually bilateral.

Rupture into the general peritoneal cavity, with diffuse peritonitis, is the major complication of a pelvic abscess. Rupture may be spontaneous or be precipitated by trauma, such as with a pelvic examination or barium enema, a fall, or an abdominal blow. If not diagnosed and correctly treated within 24–48 hours, septicemia and septic shock follow, with a resultant high mortality.

The abscess may be due to venereal disease, puerperal sepsis, an infected abortion, or may complicate pelvic surgery or be associated with an intrauterine device. On occasion, the infection may be secondary to disease in adjacent organs (appendicitis, diverticulitis).

The majority of patients are of low parity, are between 20 and 40 years old, and have a history of pelvic inflammatory disease. Low socioeconomic status is usual, but the condition may be found at any age and in any social stratum. About 2% of gynecological admissions are for pelvic abscess.

The organisms responsible for abscess formation may be exogenous pathogens, including *Neisseria gonorrhoeae,* beta-hemolytic streptococci, and rarely, *Staphylococcus aureus,* or *Mycobacterium tuberculosis.* More commonly, however, they are endogenous vaginal or bowel bacteria secondarily invading tissues damaged by surgery, delivery, or venereal disease. Endogenous anaerobes found include *Bacteroides,* peptococci, peptostreptococci, and, rarely, *Clostridia* or *Actinomyces.* The other common group of endogenous organisms are the gram-negative enteric bacilli, *Escherichia coli, Proteus, Klebsiella, Pseudomonas* and *Enterobacter.* The significance of enterococcus *(Streptococcus fecalis)* is unclear, but it too is probably an opportunistic pathogen on occasion. Most infections involve a mixed flora of anaerobic and facultative or aerobic bacteria; the role of any single species may be difficult to ascertain. Nonpathogens are also found and may play a role by lowering tissue redox potential, thus encouraging the growth of anaerobes.

The clinical presentation is characterized by severe lower abdominal pain, which may be an acute exacerbation of pain, with evidence of spreading peritonitis and with a pelvic mass no longer palpable; this is very strong evidence of intraperitoneal rupture. The clinical picture is usually sufficient to diagnose a pelvic abscess, but special investigations, including abdominal x-rays, intravenous pyelogram, pelvic sonogram, and barium enema, may add useful information or provide the diagnosis in atypical cases. Gallium scan is much less helpful in this respect. Culdocentesis and, on occasion, abdominal paracentesis yield valuable evidence of pus and of the organisms involved. This is especially helpful when intraperitoneal rupture is suspected.

The differential diagnosis includes appendicitis, diverticulitis, ectopic pregnancy, twisted ovarian cyst, and septic abortion. In this respect, serum pregnancy tests are most helpful. The physical findings of endometriosis may be very similar to those of chronic adnexal sepsis; but in the acute phase, the systemic evidence of infection provides the diagnostic clue.

Standard management is conservative. Antibiotic therapy is employed, using empiric regimes directed at the expected pathogens (usually a penicillin, an aminoglycoside, and, frequently, a drug specific for *Bacteroides fragilis*). This regimen may be modified when the results of endocervical, blood, and cul-de-sac cultures are available. Fluid and electrolyte balance are maintained with intravenous fluids and nasogastric suction. If evidence of septic shock is present, a central venous line and urinary catheter are placed, and the administration of dopamine (with or without steroids) may be necessary.

About 70% of cases respond to this regimen. Failure of conservative therapy is indicated by persistent fever, increase in the size of the pelvic mass, or spreading level of peritonism. Failure is usually evident within 48–72 hours of admission, although occasionally response may be slower. Immediate surgery is indicated if intraperitoneal rupture is suspected or if the diagnosis is uncertain. Delayed surgery is performed in patients failing to respond to conservative therapy or if the abscess "points" (usually in the posterior vaginal fornix or over the inguinal ligament).

The pointing abscess can be drained extraperitoneally via the cul-de-sac (colpotomy drainage), but this procedure may be inadequate and continued close observation is essential. More commonly, laparotomy is required, and the usual procedure is total abdominal hysterectomy with bilateral salpingo-oophorectomy. However, this is not always necessary, and in younger patients of low parity, it may be possible to conserve some reproductive tissue (especially if the lesion is unilateral). Intraoperative lavage is essential to minimize the danger of postoperative reaccumulation of subphrenic or pelvic purulent collections. Great care must be taken to avoid bowel injury. Drainage following the procedure is usually via the vaginal cuff, but occasionally flank drains are employed.

A significant proportion of patients who respond to conservative therapy require surgery at a later date for long-standing problems (such as chronic pelvic pain, menorrhagia, dyspareunia, or a persistent pelvic mass causing ureteric obstruction). Furthermore, these patients have usually now become infertile and are at risk for repeated infections, with the risk of rupture consequently ever present. Some workers therefore feel that the conservative management of pelvic abscess should be replaced by an aggressive approach, with early extirpative surgery in the acute phase. However, this opinion is not yet widely held since patients are usually young, of low parity, and because conservative therapy is successful in the majority of cases.

Review

1. McNamara, M. T., and Mead, P. B. Diagnosis and management of the pelvic abscess. *J. Reprod. Med.* 17:299, 1976.
   Compares the conservative and aggressive approach and provides an algorithm of management.

Etiology

2. Cooperman, N. R., and Ruiz, G. Clinical aspects of acute pelvic inflammatory disease: Cook County Hospital. *Am. J. Obstet. Gynecol.* 138:1026, 1980.
   Of 134 patients, 18 had a palpable, inflammatory pelvic mass.
3. Gassner, C. B., and Ballard, C. A. Pelvic abscess. A sequela of first trimester abortion. *Obstet. Gynecol.* 48:716, 1976.
   Pelvic abscess complicating therapeutic abortion may be associated with bowel injury.
4. Jafari, K., et al. Tubo-ovarian abscess in pregnancy. *Acta Obstet. Gynecol. Scand.* 56:1, 1977.
   Though rare, adnexal infection may occur during pregnancy.
5. Golde, S. H., Israel, R., and Ledger, W. J. Unilateral tuboovarian abscess: A distinct entity. *Am. J. Obstet. Gynecol.* 127:807, 1977.
   Unilateral abscess can occur with or without the presence of an IUD. Thirty-seven patients in whom unilateral adnexectomy was performed did not require any further surgery.
6. Heaton, F. C., and Ledger, W. J. Postmenopausal tuboovarian abscess. *Obstet. Gynecol.* 47:90, 1976.
   No age is exempt, although the condition is rare in the very young and in the old.
7. Ledger, W. J., et al. Adnexal abscess as a late complication of pelvic operations. *Surg. Gynecol. Obstet.* 129:973, 1969.
   Postoperative pelvic abscesses are more common with vaginal procedures, especially vaginal hysterectomy.
8. Edelman, D. A., and Berger, G. S. Contraceptive practice and tuboovarian abscess. *Am. J. Obstet. Gynecol.* 138:541, 1980.
   Proportions of women with unilateral and bilateral abscesses were similar regardless of contraceptive method.
9. Bosio, B. B., and Taylor, E. S. Bacteroides and puerperal infections. *Obstet. Gynecol.* 42:271, 1973.
   Emphasizes the importance of anaerobes in severe puerperal sepsis.

Diagnostic Aids

10. Taylor, K. J. W., et al. Accuracy of grey-scale ultrasound diagnosis of abdominal and pelvic abscesses in 220 patients. *Lancet* 1:83, 1978.
    Grey-scale ultrasound correctly diagnosed or excluded pelvic abscess in 97% of patients studied. As accurate as computerized tomography and more economical.

11. Phillips, J. C. A spectrum of radiologic abnormalities due to tubo-ovarian abscess. *Radiology* 110:307, 1974.
    Intravenous pyelogram and barium enema are often helpful in suggesting the presence of abscess in atypical cases.

Therapy

12. Mead, P. B., and Gump, D. W. Antibiotic therapy in obstetrics and gynecology. *Clin. Obstet. Gynecol.* 19:107, 1976.
    Outlines the likely pathogens and suggests antibiotics likely to succeed in the therapy of severe pelvic infection.
13. Ledger, W. J., Gassner, C. B., and Gee, C. Operative care of infections in obstetrics-gynecology. *J. Reprod. Med.* 13:128, 1974.
    Hospital- and community-acquired infections were represented equally in this report of patients requiring operative therapy for severe pelvic infections.
14. Fraser, A. C. Surgical treatment of acute pelvic sepsis. *J. Obstet. Gynaecol. Br. Commonw.* 79:560, 1972.
    English gynecologists are more conservative in their surgical approach than their American colleagues. This may be due to a less advanced degree of sepsis in their patient population.
15. Rubenstein, P. R., Mishell, D. R., and Ledger, W. J. Colpotomy drainage of pelvic abscess. *Obstet. Gynecol.* 48:142, 1976.
    The likelihood of pregnancy following colpotomy drainage when the uterus is left in place is quoted as about 10%.

Series

16. Mickal, A., and Sellmann, A. H. Management of tubo-ovarian abscess. *Clin. Obstet. Gynecol.* 12:252, 1969.
    Article discusses 741 cases, including 109 that ruptured (14.5%).
17. Collins, C. B., and Jansen, F. W. Treatment of pelvic abscess. *Clin. Obstet. Gynecol.* 2:512, 1959.
    Includes a description of ligneous cellulitis, an indurated brawny infection that must be distinguished from abscess since surgery should be avoided if possible.
18. Franklin, E. W., Hevron, J. E., and Thompson, J. D. Management of the pelvic abscess. *Clin. Obstet. Gynecol.* 16:66, 1973.
    Advocate of conservative management; also lists the criteria essential for safe colpotomy drainage.
19. Ginsburg, D. S., et al. Tubo-ovarian abscess: A retrospective review. *Am. J. Obstet. Gynecol.* 138:1055, 1980.
    Reviews 160 patients; 53% ultimately required surgery. A minimum pregnancy rate of 8% was encountered in those patients maintaining reproductive function.
20. Kaplan, A. L., Jacobs, W. M., and Ehresman, J. B. Aggressive management of pelvic abscess. *Am. J. Obstet. Gynecol.* 98:482, 1967.
    The authors advocate early surgical pelvic clearance to avoid long-term complications.

Ruptured Tuboovarian Abscess

21. Vermeeren, J., and Te Linde, R. W. Intra-abdominal rupture of pelvic abscesses. *Am. J. Obstet. Gynecol.* 68:402, 1954.
    In this classic paper, mortality was reduced from 90% to 12%.
22. Pedowitz, P., and Bloomfield, R. D. Ruptured adnexal abscess (tuboovarian) with generalized peritonitis. *Am. J. Obstet. Gynecol.* 88:721, 1964.
    The best results ever published: a mortality of 3.1%.

23. Mickal, A., Sellman, A. H., and Beebe, J. L. Ruptured tuboovarian abscess. *Am. J. Obstet. Gynecol.* 100:432, 1968.
    Ninety-three cases are described by an expert in the management of this condition.
24. Rivlin, M. E., and Hunt, J. A. Ruptured tuboovarian abscess: Is hysterectomy necessary? *Obstet. Gynecol.* 50:518, 1977.
    Suggests that, on occasion, menstrual and possibly reproductive function might be safely conserved.

Genital Tuberculosis

Infection of the genital tract with *Mycobacterium tuberculosis* is almost always secondary to a primary lesion elsewhere, usually in the lungs. Although rare in developed countries, the possibility of pelvic tuberculosis (TB) must be kept in mind, especially in foreign-born patients or in people living in conditions of poverty, overcrowding, and poor health care.

The incidence of pelvic TB varies widely, depending on the source of the estimation. For instance, in patients complaining of infertility in India, the incidence is 19%; in a similar group in the United States, this figure is under 1%. Some 10%–50% of patients with genital TB have a history of pulmonary TB or x-ray evidence of the disease. The age range for patients with the disease is between 20 and 40 in 80%–90% of cases, although it may occur in the young and after menopause.

The fallopian tubes usually bear the brunt of the hematogenous spread from the primary lesion. Less commonly, there may be direct or lymphatic spread from adjacent viscera or peritoneal surfaces. The earliest tubal lesions are generally mucosal and bilateral and may spread to the uterus and ovaries by direct extension. The endometrium is thus repeatedly reinfected from the tubes. Very rarely, the vulva and vagina may be infected, usually secondarily but possibly as a primary lesion, following trauma. In patients with genital tuberculosis, the oviducts are almost always involved. The uterus is involved in about half the cases and the ovaries in about a quarter.

The appearance of the tubes with tuberculous salpingitis varies. In severe infections they are distended with caseous material; in milder cases they are not enlarged, but small tubercles may be seen on the serosal surface. The microscopic findings in the tubes and endometrium are similar, characterized by tuberculous granulomas consisting of epithelioid cells surrounded by a zone of lymphocytes and plasma cells, together with the presence of giant cells and areas of caseating necrosis.

A family history of TB is present in some 20% of patients, while 50% have had pleurisy, peritonitis, erythema nodosum, or renal, osseous, or pulmonary TB. Up to 85% have never been pregnant, while half the remainder develop symptoms within a year of their last delivery.

Pelvic pain is the most common symptom. The pain is seldom severe unless secondary infection occurs. The pain may be worsened by coitus, exercise, and menses. Menstrual disorders, which often occur, include menorrhagia and metrorrhagia, while amenorrhea is more frequent with advanced endometrial disease. In 2% of cases postmenopausal bleeding occurs. Frequently, there is a history of poor health with weight loss, fatigue, and malaise. A diagnosis of pelvic inflammatory disease nonresponsive to antibiotics is characteristic.

There may be no abnormalities on physical examination. If abdominal involvement is present, there may be ascites with a "doughy" abdomen and irregular masses. The pelvic findings may be difficult to distinguish from those of nontuberculous pelvic inflammatory disease. However, the bilateral masses may be less tender and with a less uniform consistency. Bilateral inflammatory tuboovarian masses in a virgin provide strong presumptive evidence of genital TB.

The diagnosis depends on the demonstration of the organism or of the characteristic tubercles, usually on endometrial curettings. Direct microscopy, culture, and guinea pig inoculation of the specimens are especially valuable, not only in establishing the diagnosis, but also in ascertaining the antibiotic sensitivities of the organism. The bacteriologic results may take from 6 to 8 weeks, so therapy is usually begun on the histologic findings. In order to get the best results, curettings should be obtained from the cornua several days before a period. It must be kept in mind that other conditions cause granulomas with giant cells. These include sarcoidosis, foreign body reactions, and actinomycosis. Furthermore, since in 50% of the cases there will not be endometrial involvement, curettage will not establish the diagnosis in at least half the cases. Other diagnostic methods include culturing menstrual blood, hysterosalpingography, and laparoscopy. Unfortunately, many cases are diagnosed only at the time of laparotomy for "pelvic inflammatory disease" or tuboplasty for "blocked tubes." If the diagnosis is not then appreciated, surgery is associated with a high complication rate, including recrudescence of the infection and fistula formation.

Workup of the patient in whom the diagnosis is suspected should include a chest x-ray. It must be realized, however, that the original lesion may have healed by the time the genital lesion appears. A tuberculin skin test should also be performed, and it is very rare for a patient to have TB without a positive skin reaction. Active extragenital disease should be sought in proved cases, and this includes bacteriologic examination of sputum and urine.

The therapy of genital TB, with or without extragenital lesions, is primarily that of continuous, long-term, combined drug therapy for from 1–2 years. The usual combinations include isoniazid with ethambutol, while rifampicin has largely replaced streptomycin and para-aminosalicylic acid. If antibiotic sensitivity tests are available, the results are most helpful in choosing the optimal therapy. General therapeutic measures, including adequate diet and rest, should not be neglected. It is essential to include an experienced chest physician on the therapeutic team. Most patients may be treated on an outpatient basis. Response to therapy is monitored by repeat endometrial biopsy or curettage at 6 and 12 months, as well as by clinical observation, including pelvic examination. Long-term follow-up is essential since late recurrence is not uncommon.

Surgery is indicated if endometrial TB persists or recurs after a year of therapy, or if pelvic symptoms do not improve with long-term treatment. Further indications for surgery include persistent adnexal masses or masses increasing in size during therapy. Less commonly, surgery may be indicated for patients who do not comply with medical therapy or in patients with persistent fistulas. If genital TB is encountered unexpectedly at surgery, only biopsy should be performed since procedures performed after 3–4 months of antimicrobial therapy are technically far easier, and hence less prone to complication. For the same reason, whenever possible, surgery should be delayed until chemotherapy has been used for 3–4 months.

If surgery is necessary, patients over age 40 should have a total hysterectomy with bilateral salpingo-oophorectomy. In younger patients, if menstrual function is desired, the uterus and one or both of the ovaries may be conserved, provided they are free of TB. Drug therapy must be resumed after surgery. No attempt to preserve reproductive function should be made, nor should tuboplasty be attempted since the prognosis for further pregnancy is so poor. Only 31 cases of well-documented, successful pregnancy had been reported from 7000 cases of genital tuberculosis in the literature as of 1976. Thus, although the prognosis for cure is good, for pregnancy it is negligible. However, it is possible that newer drug regimens may offer better prospects of subsequent fertility in future patients.

Reviews

1. Schaefer, G. Female genital tuberculosis. *Clin. Obstet. Gynecol.* 19:223, 1976.
   Masterly review from a major authority.
2. Sutherland, A. M. Tuberculosis. Gynaecological tuberculosis. *Br. J. Hosp. Med.* 22:569, 1979.
   In this report 61 of 638 cases were operated on. There were no major operative complications. The author advocates pelvic clearance irrespective of age.
3. Schaefer, G. Watch for genital TB: A guide to diagnosis and treatment. *Contemp. Ob/Gyn* 17:167, 1981.
   Treatment may be by drugs, surgery, or both—depending on whether the disease is minimal or advanced.

Series

4. Hutchins, C. J. Tuberculosis of the female genital tract—a changing picture. *Br. J. Obstet. Gynaecol.* 84:534, 1977.
   In this series, most patients were in younger or older age groups. The disease often took the form of chronic infection with abscess formation.
5. Klein, T. A., Richmond, J. A., and Mishell, D. R. Pelvic tuberculosis. *Obstet. Gynecol.* 48:99, 1976.
   The majority of the patients were born outside the United States. Infertility, pelvic pain, and amenorrhea were the most common symptoms.
6. Falk, V., Ludviksson, K., and Agren, G. Genital tuberculosis. Analysis of 187 newly diagnosed cases from 47 Swedish hospitals during the ten-year period 1968 to 1977. *Am. J. Obstet. Gynecol.* 138:974, 1980.
   Analysis of 187 cases from 47 hospitals. Therapy was by chemotherapy alone in 40%, radical surgery in 38%, and conservative surgery in 8%.

Diagnosis

7. Mitchison, D., Allen, B., and Lambert, B. Selective media in the isolation of tubercle bacilli from tissues. *J. Clin. Pathol.* 25:250, 1973.
   Cultures on selective media with added antibacterial agents offer the most effective diagnostic method.
8. Ekengren, K., and Ryden, A. B. V. Roentgen diagnosis of tuberculous salpingitis. *Acta Radiol.* 34:193, 1950.
   Hysterosalpingogram is useful, although not diagnostic. Pelvic calcification or irregular filling defects along the tube should arouse suspicion.
9. Halbrecht, I. Detection of latent genital tuberculosis by culture of menstrual discharge. *Lancet* 2:447, 1947.
   This investigation is not readily available since repeated examinations by highly trained technicians are necessary.
10. Sutherland, A. M. Laparoscopy in diagnosis of pelvic tuberculosis. *Lancet* 2:95, 1979.

This author never uses laparoscopy in the diagnosis of genital TB because of the risk of bowel injury related to adhesions.

11. Padubidri, V., et al. The detection of endometrial tuberculosis in cases of infertility by uterine aspiration cytology. *Acta Cytol.* 24:319, 1980.
The combination of endometrial aspiration and biopsy is recommended as an outpatient screening technique in areas in which the rate of endometrial tuberculosis is high.

Therapy

12. Sutherland, A. M. Treatment of tuberculosis. *Br. Med. J.* 1:267, 1979.
The follow-up with the new regimens incorporating ethambutol and rifampicin is too short as yet to assess recurrence rates; such rates have been substantial with earlier regimens.

13. Altschuler, S. L., and Valenteen, J. W. Amenorrhea following rifampicin administration during oral contraceptive use. *Obstet. Gynecol.* 44:771, 1974.
Relapses are less common and toxicity less frequent and serious, although menstrual disturbance may occur.

14. East African–British Medical Research Councils. Controlled clinical trial of four short-course regimens of chemotherapy for treatment of pulmonary tuberculosis. *Lancet* 2:237, 1974.
Rifampicin, a potent bactericidal agent, has shortened the duration of therapy.

15. Tuberculosis of the female genital tract (Editorial). *Br. Med. J.* 1:260, 1978.
Drug regimens are similar to those used with pulmonary TB, but the results are less well documented.

16. Ballon, S. C., Clewell, W. H., and Lamb, E. J. Reactivation of silent pelvic tuberculosis by reconstructive tubal surgery. *Am. J. Obstet. Gynecol.* 122:991, 1975.
Beware of tubal surgery in a migrant patient from an area where TB is common.

Less Common Forms

17. La Grange, J. J. C. Postmenopausal endometrial tuberculosis. *S. Afr. Med. J.* 59:501, 1981.
Postmenopausal endometrial TB is rare. These case reports include a short review of the literature.

18. Misch, K. A., et al. Tuberculosis of the cervix: Cytology as an aid to diagnosis. *J. Clin. Pathol.* 29:313, 1976.
Two cases of tuberculous cervicitis in which epithelioid and Langhans' giant cells were noted on the Pap smear.

19. Ramos, A. D., Hibbard, L. T., and Craig, J. R. Congenital tuberculosis. *Obstet. Gynecol.* 43:61, 1974.
TB infection of placenta and endometrium is often present, although the fetus may be infected by hematogenous spread.

20. Ghattacharya, P. Hypertrophic tuberculosis of the vulva. *Obstet. Gynecol.* 51:21s, 1978.
In an ascending infection, the possibility that the husband has an active genital lesion should not be overlooked.

Pregnancy

21. O'Herlihy, C. Early successful pregnancy following tuberculous endometritis. *Acta Obstet. Gynecol. Scand.* 58:57, 1979.
Tubal patency is present in about half the cases of TB endometritis, and it

is possible that rifampicin may offer an improved outlook for fertility in these patients.

22. Nogales-Ortiz, F., Tarancon, I., and Nogales, F. F. The pathology of female genital tuberculosis. A 31-year study of 1436 cases. *Obstet. Gynecol.* 53:422, 1979.

Four cases of active female genital TB were found coexisting with intrauterine or ectopic pregnancies.

Oral contraception is the method of family planning employed by some 10 million women in the United States and 50 million worldwide. The method is highly effective, with a pregnancy rate of less than 0.2% per 100 women at the end of 1 year. There is a small but significant incidence of serious complications, so that candidates for the method must be carefully screened and all factors taken into account in deciding the risk-benefit ratio for the individual. In general, some 85% of women are suitable for oral contraception.

The combination oral steroid contraceptive ("the pill") is by far the most widely employed. The tablet contains both an estrogen and a progestogen. Also available is a progestin-only pill (minipill), but it is seldom used.

All formulations of combination pills contain varying dosages of one or the other of two synthetic estrogens. One is ethinyl estradiol; the other is ethinyl estradiol-3-methyl ether (mestranol). For clinical purposes, 35 μg of estradiol is equivalent to 50 μg of mestranol. All formulations also contain varying dosages of one or the other of five synthetic progestins. All are 19-nor-testosterone derivatives and differ in potency, with norgestrel being the most potent.

It is important to evaluate the dose and the potency of both the components of the particular product in choosing a combination pill. However, since the major, serious side effects are associated with the estrogenic component, this is the major factor to be considered. Three doses of the estrogen in general use are 35 μg, 50 μg, and 80 μg, with the middle range generally being the most suitable.

The pill acts by inhibiting the midcycle gonadotropin surge, thus preventing ovulation. The site of action is probably on the hypothalamus and on the pituitary. Further contraceptive effects occur via an alteration in the character of cervical mucus, which becomes thick, scant, and viscid, and on the endometrium, which becomes inimicable to blastocyst survival. Lastly, the motility of uterus and tubes is altered, interfering with sperm and ovum transfer. Endogenous hormones are not entirely suppressed, and their levels remain at about the levels encountered in the early follicular phase.

The general metabolic effects of the pill are similar to those found in pregnancy, although to a lesser degree. Thus there are increases in several serum protein factors, including some associated with blood coagulation and others associated with the renin-angiotensin system. Carbohydrate metabolism is affected, with a resultant decrease in glucose tolerance. Fat metabolism is altered, with an elevation of serum lipids. Some salt and water retention and a degree of weight gain is usual. Liver enzymes involved in bile excretion are also adversely affected. Progestins increase sebum production in the skin, while estrogen has an opposite effect. Melasma occurs in some instances. There does not appear to be any effect on subsequent fertility, although the return of ovulation is delayed for variable periods.

Minor pill side effects related to the estrogen component, which may respond to a progestogen-dominant pill, include leukorrhea, tender breasts, nausea, and edema. Side effects due to the progestin, which may be helped by the use of an estrogen-dominant pill, include acne, hirsutism, oily skin, psychic depression, and oligomenorrhea or amenorrhea. Most minor side effects, including breakthrough bleeding, are more marked in the first few cycles and improve thereafter. The patient should be told this when the pill is started, and, for this reason, any pill changes should be delayed until after two or three cycles.

The major serious side effects of the pill are thromboembolic disorders and other cardiovascular side effects, including myocardial infarction and cerebrovascular disease. Advancing age, obesity, diabetes, cigarette smoking, and hypertension are important risk cofactors. The pill should not be used by women over 35 who smoke.

Other serious side effects include a 2.6-fold increase in the incidence of hypertension, although this effect is usually reversible. Gallbladder disease is twice as frequent, and (rarely) benign hepatic tumors have occurred. Like all drugs, the pill may interact with other medications and this must be kept in mind. For instance, rifampin decreases oral contraceptive effectiveness.

Medical contraindications to the pill include thromboembolic, coronary, and cerebrovascular disease, or a history of these conditions. Impaired liver function, known or suspected pregnancy, undiagnosed abnormal genital bleeding, and known or suspected estrogen-dependent neoplasms or breast cancer are also contraindications.

Conditions that may be aggravated by the pill and require close observation if pill use is embarked on include uterine fibroids, epilepsy, irregular menses, hypertension, diabetes, migraine headaches, and psychic depression.

Examinations for patients on the pill should be performed every 6 months and should include history-taking, weight and blood pressure recordings, and breast and pelvic examinations, as well as a yearly Pap smear. High-risk patients should be seen more often.

The pill is usually started on day five of the menstrual period of the first pill-taking cycle. One pill is taken at the same time each day, with a 7-day interval between every 21-pill package (28-day pill packages contain 7 "blanks" and a pill is taken every day without a week's pause). Withdrawal bleeding, usually light and painless, generally occurs between courses.

If a patient has had an abortion, the pill should be started a week later, while a 2-week interval is allowed after the completion of a more advanced pregnancy. The pill is excreted in breast milk and also may suppress lactation, so it should not be used by breastfeeding mothers.

If a patient misses a pill for 2 days in a row, she should use barrier contraception for the rest of the pill course. If a patient misses two consecutive periods, pregnancy must be ruled out. Once this is done, the pill is continued and withdrawal bleeding will usually return.

After stopping the pill, while some 65% of women conceive within 3 months, about 1% have amenorrhea persisting some 6–12 months later. About 15% of these have associated galactorrhea. These patients require workup to exclude pituitary microadenoma. With therapy (clomiphene or gonadotropins) some 42% conceive.

Many clinicians advise a delay in conception after pill discontinuation, since patients who become pregnant within 1 or 2 months of the pill stoppage may have a slightly increased risk of congenital anomalies, although this finding is controversial. There is also an association between congenital abnormalities and the use of the pill in the first trimester. Progestin-estrogen withdrawal bleeding should therefore not be used as a pregnancy test.

The pill has beneficial side effects, as well as deleterious ones. Menorrhagia and dysmenorrhea are improved and benign breast disease is ameliorated. Functional ovarian cysts are less common and acne is improved. The most important benefit, however, is reliable protection from pregnancy and avoidance of mechanical intrusion on the sexual act.

The progestin-only minipill is taken daily in low doses. It is generally used for patients in whom estrogen is a risk factor, e.g., those with fibroids, hypertension, diabetes, or epilepsy. Since it does not suppress lactation, it may be given to lactating mothers. Unfortunately, irregular bleeding occurs in 70%

of patients and the pregnancy rate is 3 per 100 users per year, with an increased incidence of ectopic gestation.

The postcoital or "morning-after" pill may be used within 72 hours of unprotected intercourse to prevent normal implantation. Generally, diethylstilbestrol (25 mg), or an equivalent estrogen, is taken twice daily for 4 days. While very effective, the method has the drawback that, should pregnancy occur, the fetus has been exposed to estrogen and termination may have to be considered.

Reviews
1. Andrews, W. C. Oral contraception. *Clin. Obstet. Gynecol.* 6:3, 1979.
   There is no evidence that the pill is carcinogenic as regards breast, uterus, or ovary.
2. Mishell, D. R., Jr. Current status of oral contraceptive steroids. *Clin. Obstet. Gynecol.* 19:743, 1976.
   There is no rationale for recommending a pill-free interval.
3. Speroff, L. Which birth control pill should be prescribed? *Fertil. Steril.* 27:997, 1976.
   This author feels that breakthrough bleeding should be treated with a short course of exogenous estrogen, rather than by increasing the estrogen or progestin content of the pill.
4. Oral contraception. *ACOG Tech. Bull.* No. 41, July, 1976.
   Patient counseling is emphasized. Usually it is the "minor" side effects (weight gain, chloasma, alterations in libido) that lead to pill discontinuation.

Major Sources
5. Boston Collaborative Drug Surveillance Program. Oral contraceptives and venous thromboembolic disease, surgically confirmed gallbladder disease and breast tumors. *Lancet* 1:1397, 1973.
   The increased risk of thromboembolism is not found in postmenopausal women on estrogen replacement therapy, suggesting a dose relationship.
6. Collaborative Group for the Study of Stroke in Young Women. Oral contraceptives and stroke in young women. *J.A.M.A.* 231:718, 1975.
   Retrospective studies suggest that there is a two to three times increase, that smoking or hypertension, or both, increase risk further, and that migraine is not a factor.
7. Tietze, C. New estimates of mortality associated with fertility control. *Fam. Plann. Perspect.* 9:74, 1977.
   Compares mortality rates for various contraceptive methods, abortion, pregnancy, and childbirth.

Vascular Thrombosis, Hypertension
8. Vessey, M. P., McPherson, K., and Johnson, B. Mortality among women participating in the Oxford Family Planning Contraceptive Study. *Lancet* 2:731, 1977.
   Twofold to threefold increase in venous thrombosis and pulmonary embolism in women taking the pill.
9. Goldzieher, J. E., and Dozier, T. S. Oral contraceptives and thromboembolism: A reassessment. *Am. J. Obstet. Gynecol.* 123:878, 1975.
   Questions the validity of the relationship.
10. Green, G. R., and Sartwell, P. E. Oral contraceptive use in patients with

thromboembolism following surgery, trauma, or infection. *Am. J. Public Health* 62:680, 1972.
Pill should be discontinued 6 weeks before elective surgery.

11. Petitti, D. B., and Wingerd, J. Use of oral contraceptives, cigarette smoking, and risk of subarachnoid haemorrhage. *Lancet* 2:234, 1978.
Risk for smokers taking the pill was 21.9 times greater than for nonsmokers.

12. Meade, T. W., Greenberg, G., and Thompson, S. G. Progestogens and cardiovascular reactions associated with oral contraceptives and a comparison of the safety of 50- and 30-μg oestrogen preparations. *Br. J. Med.* 1:1157, 1980.
Low-dose pills may have negligible risks for young healthy women.

13. Slone, D., et al. Risk of myocardial infarction in relation to current and discontinued use of oral contraceptives. *N. Engl. J. Med.* 305:420, 1981.
Women currently on oral contraceptives have a threefold to fourfold increased risk. The risk persists, although at a lower level, after discontinuation and is related to the duration of use.

14. Pritchard, J. A., and Pritchard, S. A. Blood pressure response to estrogen-progestin oral contraceptive after pregnancy-induced hypertension. *Am. J. Obstet. Gynecol.* 129:733, 1977.
Previous toxemia is not a contraindication to pill use.

15. Hall, W. D., et al. Blood pressure and oral progestational agents. *Am. J. Obstet. Gynecol.* 136:344, 1980.
Progesterone-only minipill therapy (0.35 mg of norethisterone) was not associated with an increase in blood pressure after 6 to 24 months of use.

Pregnancy, Depression, Liver Disease, Amenorrhea

16. Harlap, S., and Eldor, J. Births following oral contraceptive failures. *Obstet. Gynecol.* 55:447, 1980.
There is a small but nevertheless increased risk of adverse outcome when pill use continues after conception takes place or if pregnancy occurs within a month of pill discontinuation.

17. Vessey, M. P., et al. A long-term follow-up study of women using different methods of contraception: An interim report. *J. Biosoc. Sci.* 8:373, 1976.
No increase in abnormalities noted.

18. Branham, J. Oral contraceptives and depression. *Br. Med. J.* 1:237, 1970.
Underlying cause may be a disturbance of tryptophan metabolism caused by a pill-related pyridoxine deficiency. Therapy with vitamin B_6 may be useful.

19. Vana, J., et al. Primary liver tumors and oral contraceptives: Results of survey. *J.A.M.A.* 238:2154, 1977.
Incidence in users is 3 per 100,000.

20. Campenhout, J. V., et al. Amenorrhea following use of oral contraceptives. *Fertil. Steril.* 28:728, 1977.
In this report 60% of cases had a prior history of oligomenorrhea; 38% of the galactorrheic patients had pituitary tumors.

Intrauterine Devices

The intrauterine device (IUD) is a foreign body placed in the uterus to prevent pregnancy. There are two basic categories: medicated IUDs, which carry a contraceptive agent, and nonmedicated IUDs, which do not. The majority of the over 15 million IUDs in place are nonmedicated since that category was the first to be introduced.

The mode of action of the inert (nonmedicated) devices is thought to be related to a leucocytic reaction in the endometrium; this is a sterile inflammatory reaction that creates a cytotoxic environment. The medicated devices contain copper, which also prevents implantation by a similar endometrial inflammation, or progesterone, which causes a pseudodecidual change in the endometrium inimical to implantation. The inert devices require a larger surface area of device for successful use than the medicated, which therefore have the advantage of being smaller.

Insertion is usually carried out during a menstrual period so as not to disturb a pregnancy and because the canal is then slightly dilated. No anesthesia is necessary. Careful aseptic technique by experienced personnel, prior sounding of the uterine cavity, and atraumatic fundal placement in the correct plane minimize complications. Medicated IUDs are replaced when medication is exhausted, every three years for copper (Copper 7, Copper T) and yearly for progesterone (Progestasert). Inert devices (Lippes Loop, Saf-T-Coil) do not need replacing, which is a great advantage for patients in whom motivation is limited.

The usual statistical method for comparing IUD performance is to use a life-table (Tietze-Potter), which expresses the number of "events" (pregnancy, expulsion, removal, pain, and bleeding) in one year per 100 women. Unfortunately, comparisons are greatly influenced by many factors, particularly the nature of the population studied and the health care personnel involved. In general, the IUD is highly effective in preventing pregnancy, although not quite as reliable as the hormonal contraceptives. The rate of continuation of use is similar to birth control pills and much better than traditional methods.

Problems encountered with the IUD include uterine perforation. Fundal perforations usually occur at the time of insertion. Cervical perforations occur as a result of downward displacement of the device due to uterine contractions. This mechanism is also a cause of contraception failure and of IUD expulsion. Perforation may be silent or cause pain and bleeding. Diagnosis is made after disappearance of the IUD tail by ultrasound or hysterogram or by hysteroscopy if uterine sounding does not locate the device. Copper IUDs evoke intense tissue response in the peritoneal cavity and must be removed. It is possible to leave inert devices if the IUD shape does not predispose to bowel obstruction. Removal is by laparoscopy if possible, with laparotomy if technical difficulties occur. The incidence of perforation is about 1 per 1000 but is much higher if personnel inserting it are inexperienced. All patients should have a 1- to 3-month postinsertion check and should report if they do not feel the IUD tail at the regular postmenstrual self-examination.

Expulsion is more common in nulliparous women and usually occurs in the first few months after insertion. Expulsions average 3–12 per 100 women per year. Medical removal rates, which range from 10–15, are usually the result of pain or bleeding, or both. Pain is more common with larger, stiffer devices and may be related to endometrial prostaglandin release. It is important to exclude pelvic inflammation or ectopic gestation as a cause of the pain. Excessive endometrial bleeding with the IUD may be intra-or intermenstrual. This is a common side effect and in women with borderline iron reserves will lead to anemia. The rate of loss does not decrease with time and is possibly due to the chronic endometritis set up by the device.

The pregnancy rate for users of the IUD varies from 1.8 to 2.8 per 100 women per year. Risk of pregnancy is higher if a uterine cavity measures under 6.5 cm, and if the device is inserted immediately following abortion and up to 8 weeks postpartum. Most pregnancies are intrauterine, and of these 50% will abort. These abortions are commonly septic. If pregnancy continues with the device in situ, there is an increased incidence of premature labor, amnionitis, and bleeding. Teratogenicity has not been reported. If pregnancy is diagnosed, the device should be removed if possible, and this will decrease the risk of spontaneous abortion to under 30%. The situation should also be explained to the patient, and termination may be elected, especially if the IUD cannot be retrieved. There is no increase in ectopic gestation with the IUD; thus the 1:20 ratio of ectopic to intrauterine gestations (1:200 in the general population) with the IUD indicates only the contraceptive effect of the devices. There are few reports concerning fertility after removal of the IUD.

There appears to be an increased incidence of pelvic inflammatory disease (PID) with the IUD. The incidence is 1%–2.5% overall, but in populations prone to PID, is up to 7%. Most cases are mild, but some are severe and may necessitate surgery. In all but the mild cases, the IUD should be removed; this should also be done if response to therapy is not rapid. The long-term effect on fertility has not been reported but is no doubt related to the extent of the infection. The risk of major sepsis may be compared to the risk of major thrombosis with the oral contraceptive.

The continued use of the IUD, which is in general a safe and effective contraceptive, will depend on the outcome of the debate over the incidence and importance of PID related to its use.

Reviews

1. Tatum, H. J. Intrauterine contraception. *Am. J. Obstet. Gynecol.* 112:1000, 1972.
   Fine review by developer of T*-shaped IUD (based on his belief that uterine cavity assumes* T*-shape during contraction).*
2. Perlmutter, J. F. Pregnancy and the IUD. *J. Reprod. Med.* 20:133, 1978.
   Addresses the issues of what to do when the device fails. It is noted that the contraceptive effect applies to the uterus and not the tubes and ovaries.
3. Zakin, D., Stern. W. Z., and Rosenblatt, R. Complete and partial uterine perforation and embedding following insertion of intrauterine devices: II. Diagnostic methods, prevention, and management. *Obstet. Gynecol. Surv.* 36:401, 1981.
   If IUD markers are not seen, there are four possibilities: unnoticed expulsion, pregnancy, retracted strings, or uterine perforation.
4. Ory, H. W. A review of the association between intrauterine devices and acute pelvic inflammatory disease. *J. Reprod. Med.* 20:200, 1978.
   Reviews six controlled epidemiologic studies.

Varieties of IUD

5. Keith, L., Hughey, M. J., and Berger, G. S. Experience with modern inert IUD's to date: A review and comments. *J. Reprod. Med.* 20:125, 1978.
   Reviews experience with currently used devices and explains why the Birnberg Bow, Margulies Spiral, Majzlin Spring, Dalkon Shield, Graefenberg, and Ota Rings are no longer in general use.
6. Hasson, H. M. Copper IUD's. *J. Reprod. Med.* 20:139, 1978.
   Systemic absorption of copper is of no clinical significance.
7. Pharriss, B. B. Clinical experience with the intrauterine progesterone contraceptive system. *J. Reprod. Med.* 20:155, 1978.
   Dysmenorrhea and menorrhagia are less common with the progesterone device; spotting in the first few months can be a problem, however.

Pain and Bleeding with the IUD

8. Roy, S., and Shaw, S. T., Jr. Role of prostaglandins in IUD-associated uterine bleeding—effect of a prostaglandin synthetase inhibitor (Ibuprofen). *Obstet. Gynecol.* 58:101, 1981.
   A significant reduction in menstrual blood loss as well as relieving IUD-related dysmenorrhea.

9. Westrom, L., and Bengtsson, L. P. Effect of tranexamic acid (AMCA) in menorrhagia with intrauterine contraceptive devices. A double blind study. *J. Reprod. Med.* 5:154, 1970.
   Blood loss at menses with inert IUDs was increased by 82% average and did not change with the passage of time. Antifibrinolytic drugs prevent this increase to some extent.

10. Ylikorkala, O., et al. Trophoblastic markers in women using intrauterine contraception. *Obstet. Gynecol.* 55:329, 1980.
    A subclinical abortion in women with an IUD is 7 to 10 times more common than an established pregnancy.

Pregnancy and the IUD

11. Eisinger, S. H. Second-trimester spontaneous abortion, the IUD, and infection. *Am. J. Obstet. Gynecol.* 124:393, 1976.
    Unlike the usual spontaneous abortion, infection and ruptured membranes are commonly the presenting symptoms when an IUD is associated with abortion.

12. Biggerstaff, E. D., et al. Maternal midtrimester sepsis in association with the intrauterine contraceptive device: Early histopathologic findings. *Am. J. Obstet. Gynecol.* 124:207, 1976.
    Insidious onset of a flulike syndrome, with a rapidly developing fulminant infection, and an absence of pelvic findings culminated in severe sepsis, septic shock, and maternal mortality within 72 hours.

13. Christian, C. D. Maternal deaths associated with an intrauterine device. *Am. J. Obstet. Gynecol.* 119:441, 1974.
    The majority of cases were associated with the Dalkon Shield (since withdrawn from the market), but the problem of septic abortion is prevalent with all IUDs.

14. Alvior, G. T. Pregnancy outcome with removal of intrauterine device. *Obstet. Gynecol.* 41:894, 1973.
    If the device cannot be removed and termination is refused, pregnancy must be followed very carefully for early signs of infection such as malaise, fever, chills, or bleeding.

15. Ory, H. W., and The Women's Health Study. Ectopic pregnancy and intrauterine contraceptive devices: New perspectives. *Obstet. Gynecol.* 57:137, 1981.
    Use of the IUD is probably not implicated in the recent tripling of ectopic pregnancies in the United States.

16. Hallatt, J. G. Ectopic pregnancy associated with the intrauterine device: A study of seventy cases. *Am. J. Obstet. Gynecol.* 125:754, 1976.
    If a therapeutic abortion on a patient with an IUD is performed, the products should be sent to pathology and the volume carefully noted in view of the high ectopic rate with pregnancy and a device in situ.

17. Lehfeldt, H., Tietze, C., and Gorstein, F. Ovarian pregnancy and the intrauterine device. *Am. J. Obstet. Gynecol.* 108:1005, 1970.
    Bleeding and cramping are common with the IUD and delay in diagnosis of extrauterine gestation is therefore not unusual.

Pelvic Inflammatory Disease and the IUD

18. DeSwiet, M., and Ramsey, I. D. Bacterial endocarditis after in-

sertion of intrauterine contraceptive device. *Br. Med. J.* 3:76, 1975.
Patients at risk should be given antibiotic prophylaxis.

19. Burkman, R. T., and The Women's Health Study. Association between intrauterine device and pelvic inflammatory disease. *Obstet. Gynecol.* 57:269, 1981.
Risk 1.6 times greater. Recent insertion or reinsertion increases risk, but total duration of use not a factor.

20. Dawood, M. Y., and Birnbaum, S. J. Unilateral tubo-ovarian abscess and intrauterine contraceptive device. *Obstet. Gynecol.* 46:429, 1975.
If a tubo-ovarian abscess forms with an IUD in situ, the abscess is frequently unilateral.

21. Golde, S. H., Israel, R., and Ledger, W. J. Unilateral tubo-ovarian abscess: A distinct entity. *Am. J. Obstet. Gynecol.* 127:807, 1977.
In this study 44% of all tuboovarian abscesses were unilateral, and only half of these were associated with the IUD. This finding is therefore not solely a phenomenon related to the use of the device.

22. Schiffer, M. A., et al. Actinomycosis infections associated with intrauterine contraceptive devices. *Obstet. Gynecol.* 45:67, 1975.
There appears to be a relationship between the IUD and actinomycosis infections. These are severe but unusual complications.

23. Eschenbach, D. A., Harnish, J. P., and Holmes, K. K. Pathogenesis of acute pelvic inflammatory disease: Role of contraception and other risks. *Am. J. Obstet. Gynecol.* 128:838, 1977.
The increasing incidence of pelvic inflammatory disease is related to the increased use of the IUD. These workers feel that the use of the IUD should be reconsidered.

Barrier and Chemical Contraceptives

Barrier methods of contraception, as the name implies, seek to prevent conception following coitus by interposing a mechanical and/or chemical barrier between the spermatic ejaculate and the cervical os. Displaced for a while by "modern" methods of contraception (oral contraceptives and intrauterine devices), barrier methods, which have a good reputation for safety, have had a recent surge in popularity in the face of growing concern over the harmful side effects of the modern methods. Barrier methods are nonsystemic, have no serious side effects, and can be quite effective if used properly.

One must distinguish between the theoretical-effectiveness of a birth control method and its use-effectiveness. Theoretical-effectiveness is the antifertility action of a contraceptive if used under ideal conditions without human error or negligence. Its use-effectiveness is that action achieved in real-life conditions. Effectiveness is measured in terms of failure rates by the Pregnancy Rate (PR). Pearl Index PR equals the number of pregnancies times 1200, divided by the number of women observed, times the months of exposure. In a population that does not use any contraceptive method, the PR is 80 pregnancies per 100 woman-years. The theoretical effectiveness of barrier methods is very high, with PR ranging from 1 to 7 per 100 woman-years; but, use-effectiveness varies widely with motivation and education. The PR can reach 30 per 100 woman-years.

In addition to safety and effectiveness, barrier methods also rate high on acceptability. Modern-day mechanical barriers include the condom, the diaphragm, and the cervical cap, while chemical ones are the topical spermicides.

The condom is a disposable sheath used to cover the erect penis during intercourse and collect the ejaculate. Condoms are made of latex of various colors, textures, thicknesses, and perfumes. The condom is the most widely used and available contraceptive in the world. In addition to its contraceptive role, it provides some protection against venereal disease. Its theoretical-effectiveness is very high (PR about 1 per 100 woman-years), its use-effectiveness ranges from 6–18 per 100 woman-years. Instructions given to the user will greatly increase its effectiveness. The condom must be applied before there is any contact between the penis and the vagina, with a space being left at the tip as a reservoir for the ejaculate. The penis must be withdrawn before detumescence, while the rim of the condom is held manually to prevent spillage of the semen. It should also be checked for tears. Method failure occurs when the condom breaks.

In developing countries, one disadvantage of the condom is its high cost. Some people also object to the dulling of sensations associated with its use. It has rare side effects of local irritation.

The diaphragm is a soft rubber cup with a metal-reinforced rim that is inserted into the vagina before intercourse to cover the cervix and thus prevent penetration of sperm into the uterus. It is also a receptacle for spermicidal cream or jelly and should always be used in conjunction with the spermicide.

Diaphragms range in size from 50–105 mm in diameter. Most women can be fitted with a size 70–80 mm diaphragm. The most commonly used types of diaphragms are the coil spring and flat spring for the woman with good pelvic support, and the arcing spring for the woman with poor vaginal muscle tone or cystocele.

It is essential that a diaphragm be fitted properly by trained personnel. After a pelvic exam is done, the diagonal length of the vaginal canal, from the posterior aspect of the symphysis pubis to the posterior vaginal fornix, is assessed by the examining fingers and the correct size diaphragm chosen. Alternatively, several sizes of fitting rings can be inserted and tried for determination of the correct size. The largest diaphragm that can be tolerated comfortably should be chosen. It should fit snugly between the symphysis pubis and the cul-de-sac, covering the cervix and a great part of the anterior vaginal wall. A diaphragm that is too small may slip out of place; if it's too large, it may cause discomfort or lodge itself vertically and uncover the cervix. Anatomic variations, vaginal muscle tone, pelvic surgery, and parity must be taken into account. A woman with a retroverted uterus that fills the cul-de-sac will tend to be fitted with too small a diaphragm. A postpartum woman should not be fitted until 6 weeks after delivery.

After the fitting, the user must be taught how to insert the diaphragm, not forgetting to use spermicide; how to feel the cervix to check placement; and how to remove the diaphragm. The diaphragm can be inserted up to 8 hours before intercourse, but additional spermicide should be used if more than 2 hours elapse before coitus. Adding more spermicide prior to each coital act is also recommended. The diaphragm must be left in place for at least 8 hours after intercourse, but leaving it for more than 24 hours may result in infection. An 8-hour delay is necessary before douching since douching soon after intercourse dilutes the spermicide.

The theoretical-effectiveness of the diaphragm used with spermicidal agent is high, with a PR of 3 per 100 woman-years. Use-effectiveness varies with the motivation and level of education of the user population, in practice ranging from 6–25 per 100 woman-years. Method failures occur when the diaphragm is displaced in certain coital positions or is defective.

The diaphragm is contraindicated in certain clinical conditions, such as complete uterine prolapse, severe cystocele, or rectocele.

Minor side effects are local irritation or allergic reactions. A beneficial side effect may be protection against cervical cancer, but more studies are needed on this subject.

Cervical caps are thimble-shaped cups, similar to diaphragms, that block only the cervix and are held in place by suction rather than by spring tension. Most caps are made of rigid plastic, although a newer, flexible plastic one has been introduced recently. The cap is about as effective as the diaphragm, can be used by women with poor muscle tone or prolapse who cannot use the diaphragm, and can be left in place during the entire intermenstrual period. However, because self-insertion and removal are somewhat difficult, the method is not popular. The cap cannot be used when there is cervical malformation, cervicitis, or cervical erosion. The flexible plastic cap, which is easier to use, may increase the cervical cap's popularity. Another recent development is to custom-fit a cap to a woman's cervix using dentist's compound.

Vaginal chemical contraceptives or spermicides are made of a combination of active spermicidal agents and inert base materials. The active spermicidal agents commonly used are surfactants, bactericides, and acidic salts. They are packaged in four basic forms: foams (including aerosol and tablets); creams and jellies; suppositories; and soluble films.

The spermicide is inserted high into the vagina prior to intercourse, allowing time for the spermicidal agent to disperse and block the cervix. Another full application is required if more than 1 hour elapses before coitus and prior to each coital act. No douching is permitted for at least 6 hours after the last coital act.

Vaginal chemical contraceptives are viewed as having higher failure rates (PR up to 30 per 100 woman-years) than condoms or diaphragms with jellies, but they are a readily available and widely distributed birth control method that does not require sophisticated medical intervention. When used in conjunction with condoms or diaphragms, the method is highly effective. There are no systemic effects and only occasional side effects of local irritation. It has been shown recently that vaginal contraceptives also provide some protection against venereal diseases and other vaginal infections.

Reviews
1. Tyrer, L. B., and Bradshaw, L. E. Barrier methods. *Clin. Obstet. Gynaecol.* 6:39, 1979.
   A useful summary.
2. Wortman, J. The diaphragm and other intravaginal barriers, a review. *Popul. Rep.* [H] No. 4, January, 1976.
   Everything you have always wanted to know about diaphragms.
3. Wortman, J. Vaginal contraceptives, a time for reappraisal? *Popul. Rep.* [H] No. 4, January, 1975.
   Exhaustive review.

For the Adolescent
4. Greydanus, D. E., and McAnarney, E. R. Contraception in the adolescent, current concepts for the pediatrician. *Pediatrics* 65:1, 1980.
   Overview of major methods of contraception available to the sexually active adolescent. The approach to each patient must be individualized.

Chemical Contraceptives
5. Masters, W. H., et al. In vivo evaluation of an effervescent intravaginal contraceptive insert by simulated coital activity. *Fertil. Steril.* 32:161, 1979.
   The base materials of different types of spermicide spread differently.

6. Asculai, S. S., et al. Inactivation of herpes simplex viruses by nonionic surfactants. *Antimicrob. Agents Chemother.* 13:686, 1978.
   This would be a very helpful side effect.

New Developments

7. Subir, R., et al. Comparison of metabolic and clinical effects of four oral contraceptive formulations and a contraceptive vaginal ring. *Am. J. Obstet. Gynecol.* 136:920, 1980.
   Different metabolic parameters are measured in the five user groups. Vaginal rings containing contraceptive hormones did not increase angiotensinogen, thus are unlikely to produce hypertension or other circulatory problems, which are increased in some oral contraceptive users. Data far from definitive, however.
8. Shelton, J. D., and Taylor, R. N., Jr. The Pearl Pregnancy Index reexamined: Still useful for clinical trials of contraceptives. *Am. J. Obstet. Gynecol.* 139:592, 1981.
   This paper compares the Pearl Index and life-table pregnancy rates indicating that both are useful.
9. Chvapil, M., et al. Preliminary testing of contraceptive collagen sponge. *Obstet. Gynecol.* 56:503, 1980.
   New intravaginal barriers are being developed. The collagen sponge shows great promise. Very easy to use, it can absorb more than 40 times its weight in fluid. Sponges impregnated with active spermicidal agents appear to be the most effective.
10. Richardson, A. C., and Lyon, J. B. The effect of condom use on squamous cell cervical intraepithelial neoplasia. *Am. J. Obstet. Gynecol.* 140:909, 1981.
    Condom use resulted in regression of the lesion in 136 of 139 patients; 18 had late recurrences, and 12 regressed again with further condom use.

Female Sterilization

Sterilization is the voluntary destruction of the reproductive function. It can apply either to the male or female partner, but in practice, female sterilization is performed more frequently than male sterilization.

The most frequent indication is multiparity—the woman has completed her family and wants a permanent method of contraception. Another obvious indication is the presence of any disease process in which pregnancy would endanger the patient, such as cardiac disease. Generally, any adult woman (regardless of parity or marital status) can request sterilization, but the laws governing sterilization vary from state to state, and the physician should be familiar with them. Alternatives to sterilization, failure rates, complications, and possible long-term effects of sterilization should all be discussed with the patient. It is estimated that 1% of women who have had a sterilization procedure will seek reversal of the procedure within the subsequent 5 years; the usual reason given is a change in partner.

A great variety of techniques have been used to prevent the union of the sperm and the ovum, generally by interrupting the fallopian tube. Unless there is concomitant pelvic pathology, hysterectomy is not usually considered an acceptable method of sterilization due to its potential risks and morbidity. Tubal "ligation" is a misnomer. In fact, it is a partial salpingectomy, either through a standard laparotomy incision or through a small,

2.5–3 cm, suprapubic incision (minilaparotomy); or a 3–5 cm incision through the posterior cul-de-sac (colpotomy). Both colpotomy and minilaparotomy can be done under local anesthesia. The colpotomy technique has been found to have a significantly higher infectious morbidity than the abdominal approach.

The postpartum period is very convenient for sterilization, since the fundus is near the umbilicus and the fallopian tubes are easily accessible through a mini-infraumbilical incision. In the interval procedure (sterilization done in the absence of pregnancy), the key to success is the elevation of the uterine fundus against the anterior abdominal wall. The most popular partial salpingectomy method is the Pomeroy, because of its simplicity and effectiveness (0–0.4% failure rate). A 2.5 cm midportion loop of tube is picked up and ligated at its base with absorbable suture, after which the loop is excised. The stumps are left tied together but absorption of the ligature leads to their separation after a few weeks. Many other techniques have been described: Madlener, Irving, Uchida, and so on. When using a colpotomy incision, fimbriectomy (first described by Kroener) is the procedure of choice.

The most popular approach to interval sterilization in the U.S. is laparoscopy. It is rapid; it allows visualization of the pelvic cavity; and it can be done under local anesthesia on an outpatient basis. First, the abdomen is insufflated with 2–4 liters of gas through a needle inserted in the subumbilical area. A sharp trocar is then used to introduce the laparoscope. The fallopian tube is identified, and its midportion is grasped with the forceps and destroyed by fulguration or occluded by mechanical devices.

Complications include injury to major vessels or bowels during the blind insertion of the needle or trocar; bleeding from mesosalpingeal tears during manipulation of the tubes; and bowel burns from electrical methods, especially when tubal fulgurations were first performed using unipolar electrical generators. In 1972, Rioux introduced bipolar forceps; these eliminate the need for a return electrode, since the electrons pass from one jaw of the forceps through the fallopian tube to the opposite jaw and back to the generator. The risk of burn is greatly decreased. Safety against accidental burns is also a feature of the latest electrical method, thermal coagulation. Transection or resection of a segment of tube in addition to electric coagulation does not improve the effectiveness of the procedure and increases the risk of hemorrhage. Coagulation alone is very effective if a minimum length of 3 cm of tube is destroyed by using multiple coagulation points.

In the nonelectrical or mechanical methods of laparoscopic sterilization, a special applicator is used to occlude the fallopian tube with a mechanical device, clip, or band. The spring-loaded clip designed by Hulka destroys the least amount of tissue (0.5 cm) and preserves the continuity of the utero-ovarian vascular anastomosis. It has a better potential reversibility but a higher failure rate than electrocoagulation or the Yoon band. The Yoon band, or Falope ring, is a small Silastic ring that is slipped onto the base of a loop of fallopian tube. If a tube is inadvertently transected, a ring can be applied to each stump, or they can be electrocoagulated. This method is very effective and easy to use (0.3% failure rate). If luteal pregnancies and misidentification of pelvic structures are excluded, the failure rate of the laparoscopic techniques varies from 0.9 to 6 per 1000 sterilizations. Comparisons are made difficult by lack of standardization in data collection. Results generally do not include life tables or the Pearl Index. The most serious complication of laparoscopic sterilization failure is ectopic pregnancy.

Culdoscopy, which never was very popular in the United States, is performed with the patient in the knee-chest position. The culdoscope is introduced through a puncture wound in the posterior cul-de-sac. Endometriosis, masses, or adhesions in the cul-de-sac are contraindications to the procedure. Rectal perforation is the main complication.

Many experimental methods of sterilization are now being tested. There has been a recent renewed interest in fimbrial caps. In hysteroscopic coagulation, a small endoscope is inserted via the cervix into the endometrial cavity, which is then distended by gas or liquid for proper visualization of the internal ostia. An electrode or a thermoprobe is passed into the tubal orifices, which are fulgurated at the uterotubal junction. It is a procedure fraught with technical difficulties, a high failure rate (11%–35%), and potentially life-threatening complications (uterine perforations and burns, and interstitial or cornual pregnancies following failures).

In another method, using a transcervical route via a hysteroscope, various chemicals may be instilled into the fallopian tubes. They act either by destroying the inner lining of the tube, with subsequent fibrosis (sclerosing agents), or by forming solid occluding plugs. If improved, these methods could have a future as a quick, inexpensive outpatient procedure. For the present, however, they still have a high failure rate, and many of these chemicals are very toxic, with risks of injury to structures other than the tubes if intraperitoneal or intravascular spills occur. Plugs made of Dacron, Teflon, or Silastic have been used to occlude the tubes. The plug can be withdrawn later to restore patency. Since theoretically there is no tissue damage, this could be a reversible sterilization method.

Another promising avenue for research is in immunization of the female against sperm. Animal studies have shown that local cervical secretion of antisperm antibodies can be induced. Each coital act would then serve as a booster to keep antibody titer high.

Long-term effects of sterilization are difficult to evaluate because the data published to date lack adequate controls. A poststerilization syndrome that has been described is characterized by menorrhagia, pelvic discomfort, and ovarian cyst formation. Some uncontrolled studies report very high (25%–50%) rates of menstrual disturbances. Others, using patients as their own controls and correcting for prior methods of contraception, report rates of 6% or less, the highest rates being associated with electrocautery. These problems may be related to the fact that the blood flow to the ovaries undergoes cyclic changes and is correlated with the systemic progesterone level. The mechanisms of such changes in the blood flow are unknown. Surgical sterilization seems to interfere with the vascular supply of the ovaries, especially if coagulation involving the mesosalpinx is used.

Some patients develop psychologic or sexual dysfunctions, or both, following sterilization. These problems are often related to ambivalence regarding the procedure. Furthermore, fertility is so intimately associated with femininity in many women's minds that they cannot easily relate to the loss of the reproductive function. Careful preoperative counseling is essential if these problems are to be avoided. Fortunately, most women do not regret the procedure since they need no longer fear an unwanted pregnancy.

Review

1. Soderstrom, R. M., and Yuzpe, A. A. Female sterilization. *Clin. Obstet. Gynaecol.* 6:77, 1979.
   A review of methods, with emphasis on laparoscopy.

Methods

2. Yoon, I., and Poliakoff, S. R. Laparoscopic tubal ligation: A follow-up report on the Yoon Falope ring methodology. *J. Reprod. Med.* 23:76, 1979.

A large sample showing an overall failure rate of 0.42% per 100 woman-years.

3. Laufe, L. E. Suprapubic endoscopy for interval female sterilization. *Am. J. Obstet. Gynecol.* 136:257, 1980.
   Combines minilaparotomy incision with laparoscopy. Eliminates the need for insufflation of the abdomen and the blind insertion of a sharp trocar with its attendant risks.

4. Gunning, J. E., et al. Laparoscopic tubal sterilization using thermal coagulation. *Obstet. Gynecol.* 54:509, 1979.
   The fallopian tube is withdrawn into a Teflon sheath and cauterized with special metal forceps heated by a 6-V battery.

5. Beck, P., and Gal, D. Silicone band technique for laparoscopic tubal sterilization in the gravid and nongravid patient. *Obstet. Gynecol.* 53:653, 1979.
   The Falope ring is a safe method when combined with gestation termination.

6. Oskowitz, S., et al. Experience in a series of fimbriectomies. *Fertil. Steril.* 34:320, 1980.
   High failure rate of 2.4%. Stresses the importance of adequate surgical exposure and complete removal of the fimbria.

7. Neuwirth, R. S., et al. An outpatient approach to female sterilization with methylcyanoacrylate. *Am. J. Obstet. Gynecol.* 136:951, 1980.
   Describes a small series with an 80% closure rate. The simplicity of the method warrants larger scale trials.

8. Edstrom, K. The relative risk of sterilization alone and in combination with abortion. *Bull. WHO* 52:141, 1975.
   There is no evidence that the risk of performing sterilization at the time of abortion is greater than that of exposing the patient to two separate procedures.

9. Reed, T. P., and Erb, R. A. Tubal occlusion with silicone rubber. *J. Reprod. Med.* 25:25, 1980.
   One hundred thirty-five cases: Successful in 99; one pregnancy, one uterine perforation.

Complications

10. Chi, I. C., et al. An epidemiologic study of risk factors associated with pregnancy following female sterilization. *Am. J. Obstet. Gynecol.* 136:768, 1980.
    Very good study from a large pool of international data recorded on standardized collection instruments.

11. Radwanska, E., et al. Luteal deficiency among women with normal menstrual cycles, requesting reversal of tubal sterilization. *Obstet. Gynecol.* 54:189, 1979.
    Sterilized women, by ligation or coagulation, have significantly lower midluteal progesterone levels than controls, and thus have potential infertility problems if sterilization is reversed.

12. Donnez, J., et al. Luteal function after tubal sterilization. *Obstet. Gynecol.* 54:65, 1981.
    A retarded endometrium was observed more frequently in women who underwent tubal ligation or electrocoagulation than in women who were sterilized by the Hulka clip, probably because the Hulka clip preserves the utero-ovarian artery.

13. Benjamin, L., et al. Elective sterilization in childless women. *Fertil. Steril.* 34:116, 1980.

Nulliparous women do not appear to have a higher rate of regret than parous women.

14. Grunert, G. M., Drake, T. S., and Takaki, N. K. Microsurgical reanastomosis of the fallopian tubes for reversal of sterilization. *Obstet. Gynecol.* 58:148, 1981.
    Of 63 women, 22 became pregnant and one pregnancy was ectopic.
15. Baggish, M. S., et al. Complications of laparoscopic sterilization. Comparison of 2 methods. *Obstet. Gynecol.* 54:54, 1979.
    A substantial number of patients complained of menstrual irregularity or dysmenorrhea, or both, following these sterilization procedures.

Failures

16. McClausland, A. High rate of ectopic pregnancy following laparoscopic tubal coagulation failures. Incidence and etiology. *Am. J. Obstet. Gynecol.* 136:97, 1980.
    Reviews the world literature, and theorizes the formation of a uteroperitoneal fistula following coagulation of the inner third of the tube as an etiologic factor.
17. Loeffer, F. D., and Pent, D. Pregnancy after laparoscopic sterilization. *Obstet. Gynecol.* 55:643, 1980.
    A good review of the mechanisms of sterilization failures.

Investigation of the Infertile Couple

Infertility affects 15% of reproductive-age couples in the United States. Reproductive function is the last body function established and the first body function to fail with advancing age. Moreover, many couples defer reproduction until they complete an extended education or become established in a career. It is especially frustrating for otherwise healthy men and women to find themselves unable to have children.

Infertility is a couple's problem. Of the causes of infertility, 40% can be attributed to the woman, 40% can be attributed to the man, and 20% can be attributed to both partners. Investigation of the infertile couple is directed toward establishing the cause(s) of infertility and achieving pregnancy.

Infertility is defined as the inability to conceive after 1 year of unprotected sexual intercourse. When one partner (usually the woman) requests an infertility evaluation, it should not be deferred but started immediately. Both partners should be involved in the discussions about infertility and both should be given as much information as possible to help them understand the causes of infertility. Most infertility problems are due to one of three causes: (1) failure of ovulation, (2) inadequate sperm production, or (3) abnormalities of the female genital tract. One or more of these abnormalities should be discovered early in the infertility evaluation.

Documentation of ovulation should be the first step in the infertility evaluation. Women in their reproductive prime (age 18 to 35 years) will ovulate twelve to fourteen times each year with only occasional episodes of anovulation. Women with normal ovulatory cycles have predictable menses associated with premenstrual molimina (breast fullness, decreased libido, mood changes, and uterine cramps). These changes indicate that progesterone production and progesterone withdrawal have occurred. In the absence of ovulation, the corpus luteum does not form, progesterone is not produced or withdrawn, and the manifestations of progesterone on reproductive target organs do not occur. Thus, a menstrual history is essential in evaluating the occurrence of ovulation.

Ovulation can be presumed if a biphasic shift occurs in the basal body temperature during the menstrual cycle. Again, this body change depends upon the secretion of progesterone by the corpus luteum and the action of progesterone on central nervous system thermoregulatory centers. A basal body temperature chart provides a dynamic record of reproductive-cycle events, including the length of the follicular phase of the cycle, the length of the luteal phase of the cycle, the length of the menstrual phase of the cycle, the frequency of coitus, and the temporal relationship of coitus to ovulation.

Two other methods commonly used to detect ovulation are measurement of plasma progesterone and performance of an endometrial biopsy for endometrial dating. Both of these tests are performed in the luteal phase of the reproductive cycle. Like the basal body temperature chart, measurement of plasma progesterone and histologic evaluation of the endometrium depend upon progesterone secretion by the corpus luteum to detect presumed ovulation.

If a woman is found to have ovulatory reproductive cycles, we then focus our attention on male factors, anatomic disorders in the female, and cervical causes for infertility. However, if a woman is anovulatory we concentrate on finding a cause for the anovulation. Some of the possible causes are polycystic ovarian disease, premature ovarian failure, pituitary microadenomas, nutritional amenorrhea, and congenital adrenal hyperplasia. To evaluate these endocrinopathies we measure follicle-stimulating hormone (FSH), luteinizing hormone (LH), and prolactin to establish the site of the cause (hypothalamus, pituitary gland, or ovaries); and we measure plasma androstenedione and testosterone if there is clinical evidence of androgen excess.

Evaluation of the female reproductive system can become complex indeed; but evaluation of the male reproductive system is simple because this evaluation is limited to obtaining a medical history, performing a physical examination, and examining seminal fluid. In rare instances the male evaluation includes measurement of gonadotropins, prolactin, and steroid hormones. Although the male reproductive system is equally as complex as the female reproductive system, our knowledge of male reproductive physiology is limited.

Sperm production occurs in the germinal epithelium of the seminiferous tubules. From beginning to end, the sperm maturation time is approximately 74 days. Thus, a semen analysis reflects events in sperm production that occurred 74 days before examination. Sperm production and maturation require a constant temperature, one that is maintained slightly below normal (37° C); if this temperature is increased, sperm production diminishes dramatically. The scrotum controls testicular temperature by raising the testicles against the body in cool weather or by lowering the testicles away from the body in warm weather. In men who have sedentary jobs sperm production may be altered due to increased intratesticular temperature.

In evaluating the male a careful history must be obtained to exclude known causes of oligospermia, which would include mumps orchitis, exposure to toxic chemicals, use of marihuana, and abnormalities in sexual development. On physical examination careful attention should be given to genital development and, particularly, testicular size and consistency. A soft, small testis indicates gonadal failure. We perform a semen analysis on a freshly ejaculated semen specimen that is obtained by masturbation. A period of sexual abstinence before collection of the semen specimen is not necessary as the sperm count may not reflect the functional sperm count. A normal semen specimen should have a volume of 3–5 ml and should contain greater than 20 million sperm per ml of fluid. Greater than 50% should be motile.

If the sperm count is below the normal values, it should be repeated in several weeks. If oligospermia is the sole cause of infertility, efforts should be made to identify an etiologic basis for the oligospermia and correct the cause.

When it has been established that ovulation occurs at regular, predictable intervals and the spermatogenesis and ejaculation are normal, attention is turned to finding other causes for infertility. An excellent functional test is the postcoital cervical mucus examination. For this examination the couple is asked to have intercourse late in the follicular phase of the cycle (just before ovulation), 4 to 8 hours before the examination. Endocervical mucus is aspirated from the endocervix and examined microscopically under a high-power objective. In a normal couple more than 15 motile sperm are found in each high-power field. A cervical mucus laden with neutrophiles or a tenacious cervical mucus will prohibit adequate sperm penetration.

Finally, if ovulation, spermatogenesis, and sperm penetration are normal, abnormalities in the anatomic structure of the uterus and fallopian tubes may be the cause of infertility. Radiographic examination of the uterine cavity and fallopian tubes is performed by intrauterine dye instillation (hysterosalpingogram). This examination may reveal a congenital defect in the endometrial cavity or obstruction of the fallopian tubes. If such abnormalities are found, endoscopic examination of the uterus and pelvis may lead to a precise diagnosis.

The infertility evaluation must be performed in a thorough, systematic manner. A description of the full scope of the infertility evaluation cannot be given in this short essay, but by paying attention to ovulation, spermatogenesis, and anatomic structure of the female genital tract, the physician can elicit the common causes of infertility. Above all, the infertile couple needs compassion, understanding, and information.

Normal Menstrual Cycle

1. Vanderville, R., et al. Mechanisms regulating the menstrual cycle in women. *Recent Prog. Horm. Res.* 26:63, 1970.
   A review of the function of the hypothalamic-pituitary-gonadal axis.
2. Yen, S. S. C., et al. Hormonal relationships during the menstrual cycle. *J.A.M.A.* 211:1513, 1970.
   Normal mechanism of reproductive hormone action.
3. Moghissi, K. S., Syner, F. N., and Evans, T. N. A composite picture of the menstrual cycle. *Am. J. Obstet. Gynecol.* 114:405, 1972.
   An excellent paper that establishes the relationship of the basal body temperature to plasma progesterone concentrations.

Spermatogenesis

4. Settlage, D. S. F., Motoshima, M., and Treadway, D. R. Sperm transport from the external cervical os to the fallopian tubes in women: A time and quantitation study. *Fertil. Steril.* 24:655, 1973.
   Normal sperm migration in the female genital tract.
5. MacLeod, J., and Gold, R. Z. The male factor in fertility and infertility: II. Spermatozoon counts in 1000 men of known fertility and in 1000 cases of infertile marriages. *J. Urol.* 66:436, 1951.
   The basic study from which normal values for sperm counts are derived.
6. Nelson, C. M. K., and Bunge, R. G. Semen analysis: Evidence for changing parameters for male fertility potential. *Fertil. Steril.* 25:503, 1974.
   A reevaluation of "normal" sperm counts.
7. Aggar, P. Scrotal and testicular temperature: Its relation to sperm count before and after operation for varicocele. *Fertil. Steril.* 22:286, 1971.
   Effect of temperature on spermatogenesis.

Detecting Ovulation

8. Noyes, R. W., Hertig, A. T., and Rock, J. Dating the endometrial biopsy. *Fertil. Steril.* 1:3, 1950.
   A classic—dating the endometrium.
9. Israel, R., et al. Single luteal phase serum progesterone assay as an indication of ovulation. *Am. J. Obstet. Gynecol.* 112:1043, 1972.
   Detecting ovulation by serum progesterone concentration.

Cervical Mucus Examination

10. Treadway, D. R., et al. The significance of timing for the postcoital evaluation of cervical mucus. *Am. J. Obstet. Gynecol.* 121:387, 1975.
    Use of the Sims-Huhner test.

Evaluation of the Anatomic Features of the Female Genital Tract

11. Whitelaw, M. J., Foster, T. N., and Graham, W. H. Hysterosalpingography and insufflation. *J. Reprod. Med.* 4:56, 1970.
    Methods for evaluating tubal patency.
12. Siegler, A. M. *Hysterosalpingography.* New York: Harper & Row, 1967.
    An atlas of hysterosalpingograms.
13. Israel, R., and March, C. M. Diagnostic laparoscopy: A prognostic aid in the surgical management of infertility. *Am. J. Obstet. Gynecol.* 124:969, 1976.
    Efficacy of diagnostic laparoscopy.

Infertility Due to Abnormalities in the Male Partner

Males are found to be partially or totally responsible for infertility in approximately 40% of all infertile couples. This figure emphasizes the need for evaluation of the male partner, not only in all infertile couples, but also early in the evaluation—prior to expensive and invasive diagnostic procedures. Insistence on this point is necessary as the male partners are often reluctant to undergo evaluation. There are a number of etiologic factors responsible for male infertility.

Environmental hazards to fertility include emotional stress, diet, and exposure to radiation and noxious substances. Alcohol is the most important noxious agent affecting Leydig cell function. This detrimental effect occurs in the absence of cirrhosis. Systemic diseases affecting fertility include any acute febrile illness, infectious diseases, cirrhosis, renal failure, and myotonic dystrophy. The most notable example of an infectious disease is mumps orchitis.

Testicular involvement is unilateral in about 70% of patients, with subsequent atrophy of the involved testis in about 50% of those having testicular swelling. Sterility results if the atrophy is bilateral. If atrophy does not ensue, spermatogenesis returns to normal, but this may require up to 1 year.

Endocrinopathies, such as thyroid or adrenal dysfunction, are responsible for only a very small number of infertile males with, of course, the exception of severe disease (e.g., myxedema or Addison's disease). Hypothalamic-pituitary dysfunction is the most common systemic endocrine disorder associated with testicular dysfunction. This group of disorders is due to inadequate levels of gonadotropin. As a group, they represent a small fraction of patients with infertility, but, because these disorders can be easily diagnosed and are amenable to specific therapy, it is important to diagnose them.

As genetic disorders obviously affect the whole organism, they are considered with systemic disorders. The incidence of cytogenetic abnormalities in infertile males varies from 2%–21%. The most common chromosomal abnormality associated with male infertility is Klinefelter's syndrome. Its incidence is 1 in 500 newborn males. The most common type of karyotype in this disorder is 47 XXY. The patients exhibit eunuchoid habitus; pea-size, very firm testes; azoospermia; and, frequently, gynecomastia. Plasma gonadotropin levels are markedly elevated, and testosterone levels are either normal or low.

Developmental abnormalities affecting the testes are associated with multiple etiologic factors, including genetic factors. Testicular ectopia is the most common type of developmental abnormality affecting the testes. Dubin and Amelar found 4% of a large population of infertile males to have cryptorchism. This condition must be recognized early (prior to age 6) and treated aggressively with gonadotropins, followed by surgical replacement (orchidopexy) if medical therapy is not effective.

Vascular abnormalities associated with male infertility may be due to ischemia, sometimes as a result of a hernia repair, which leads to an irreversible testicular lesion after a period of time. The most common vascular abnormality is the varicocele. This disorder is usually due to incompetency of the left, internal spermatic vein, resulting in dilatation of the pampiniform plexus of veins. The mechanism by which this causes a diminution of sperm production and sperm motility is, at present, unclear.

Faulty coital technique can prevent fertility in a surprising number of patients. Inadvertent use of lubricants, such as Vaseline, K-Y jelly, or Surgilube, may cause infertility as these are spermicidal. The optimal frequency of intercourse in couples wishing to establish a pregnancy appears to be every other day around the time of ovulation.

Impotence and premature ejaculation are associated, for obvious reasons, with male infertility. Impotence is 90% psychogenic and 10% organic. However, 50% of males with "psychogenic impotence" may have underlying organic causes, e.g., medication (such as tranquilizers and sympatholytic agents), neurologic disorders (such as paraplegia or multiple sclerosis), or endocrinopathies (the most common being diabetes mellitus).

Retrograde ejaculation (a condition in which the seminal fluid is ejaculated from the posterior urethra into the bladder cavity) may result from prostate or bladder neck surgery, or after sympathectomy or the use of ganglionic blocking agents. Diabetic neuropathy can be the cause.

Men with "unexplained infertility" have a high incidence of sperm auto-antibodies. There is currently no general agreement regarding the contribution of these antibodies to infertility.

Following a careful history and a complete physical examination (usually done by a urologist), a semen analysis is done. The specimen is collected in either a wide-mouth container (made especially for collection of semen), or in a special sheath (made by the Milex Company), which, unlike most condoms, does not contain a spermicide. The specimen is kept at body temperature by keeping it close to the body, either in the waist band of the trousers or in the wife's brassiere. The analysis is done in a reliable laboratory within 2 hours of collection. The semen analysis reflects conditions affecting spermatogenesis 45–60 days prior to its collection. For this reason, more than one semen analysis is done over a period of time, especially if the analysis is abnormal.

The International Committee of Andrology has established the following standard values for semen quality: volume, 2–6 ml; density, 40–250 million sperm/ml; motility, at least 60% of the sperm should have good, progressive motility; morphology, 60% of the sperm should have normal morphology. These values do not define the limits of fertility. For example, pregnancy rates decrease when the sperm count is below 20 million/ml.

Sperm motility is one of the most important parameters in the semen analysis. If the male has completely immotile sperm, he is sterile. Nonmotile sperm, or those with poor motility, cannot penetrate the cervical mucus.

Sperm morphology is also important. A "stress pattern" (a high percentage of tapering forms and spermatids and decreased motility) is often a clue to systemic infections, severe allergy, drug reactions, or a varicocele.

Depending on the results of the history, physical examination, and semen analysis, further evaluation may include microbiological, endocrine, immunologic, and genetic studies. Identification of etiologic factors is possible in a large majority (95%) of infertile males. Therapy is predicated upon etiologic factors, their pathophysiologic mechanisms, and availability of therapeutic modalities.

Azoospermia (absence of sperm in the ejaculate)—caused by Klinefelter's syndrome, Sertoli-cell–only syndrome, or bilateral cryptorchidism—results in sterility. No treatment is available except donor insemination of the wife.

Azoospermia associated with low fructose concentration (which comes from the seminal vesicle) may indicate blockage of the ejaculatory ducts due to an infection of the prostate or of the seminal vesicle. Appropriate antibiotic therapy may result in a restoration of fertility. When the ejaculate is azoospermic, but contains fructose, and a testicular biopsy demonstrates normal spermatogenesis, then nontuberculous, postinflammatory obstruction of the epididymis is suspected. Advances in microsurgical techniques now allow excision and reanastomosis of damaged ducts with good results.

Retrograde ejaculation can also cause azoospermia. Sympathomimetic drugs are sometimes effective in treating this condition, or sperm can be recovered from the patient's bladder and be used for artificial insemination. Surgical ligation of a varicocele results in a 70% overall improvement in the quality of spermatozoa, with a pregnancy rate of 53%.

If a patient collects a semen specimen in two sequentially numbered bottles, sperm density is greater (90% of the time) in the first portion of the ejaculate than in the second. Near the time of ovulation, the patient with a high semen volume (but with subfertile semen quality) is instructed to withdraw after the intravaginal deposition of the first portion of the ejaculate. The first fraction of ejaculate may also be used in homologous insemination (artificial insemination with husband's semen).

Clomiphene citrate increases serum immunoreactive gonadotropin-releasing hormone, gonadotropins, and testosterone in men; giving 25 to 50 mg daily, for at least 90 days, improves the semen in oligospermic (sperm count < 40 million/ml) males. However, a higher dosage may damage the seminiferous tubules.

Psychological impotence is best treated by a psychiatrist. However, as stated previously, these patients often exhibit underlying organic causes and diabetes mellitus. Perineal surgery, neurological disorders, and certain drugs should be remembered as possible causes of impotence.

Patients with hypothalamic pituitary dysfunction often respond to a regimen of human menopausal gonadotropin and human chorionic gonadotropin with complete spermatogenesis.

Reviews
1. Steinberger, E. Management of male reproductive dysfunction. *Clin. Obstet. Gynecol.* 22:187, 1979.
   Comprehensive review of disorders associated with male infertility by an authority in this field. Also addresses treatment of these disorders.
2. Magee, M. C. Psychogenic impotence: A critical review. *Urology* 15:435, 1980.
   A critical review of psychogenic impotence with emphasis on recent advances in objective evaluation of erectile function.

Physiology
3. Jenkins, A. D., et al. Physiology of the male reproductive system. *Urol. Clin. North Am.* 5:437, 1978.
   Provides background for understanding normal testicular differentiation, spermatogenesis, and capacitation.
4. Lipsett, M. B. Physiology and pathology of the Leydig cell. *N. Engl. J. Med.* 303:682, 1980.
   Excellent update on factors adversely affecting Leydig cell function.
5. Amelar, R. D., et al. Sperm motility. *Fertil. Steril.* 34:197, 1980.
   Most comprehensive and authoritative review on how sperm move and factors affecting their motility.

Etiology
6. Steinberger, E. The etiology and pathophysiology of testicular dysfunction in man. *Fertil. Steril.* 29:481, 1978.
   Correlates testicular pathophysiology with possible etiologic factors arbitrarily divided into four categories: (1) environmental, (2) systemic, (3) intratesticular, and (4) iatrogenic.

7. Zorgniotti, A. W. Testis temperature, infertility, and the varicocele paradox. *Urology* 16:7, 1980.
Provides support in favor of elevated temperature of the testis as an important factor in patients with poor semen analysis associated with varicocele.

Series

8. Dubin, L., and Amelar, R. D. Etiologic factors in 1294 consecutive cases of male infertility. *Fertil. Steril.* 22:469, 1971.
Analyzes the causes of male infertility encountered in a large referral practice by two urologists considered pioneers in the field of male infertility.
9. Montague, D. K., et al. Diagnostic evaluation, classification, and treatment of men with sexual dysfunction. *Urology* 14:545, 1979.
Reviews experience with sexual dysfunction in 165 men and provides treatment recommendations.

Management

10. Snyder, P. J. Endocrine evaluation of the infertile male. *Urol. Clin. North Am.* 5:451, 1978.
Outlines hormonal evaluation of disorders known to adversely affect spermatogenesis.
11. Jones, W. R. Immunologic infertility—fact or fiction? *Fertil. Steril.* 33:577, 1980.
Reviews current thinking on the clinical significance of antisperm antibodies and aspects of treatment in females as well as males.
12. Allag, I. S., and Alexander, N. J. Clomiphene citrate therapy for male infertility. *Urology* 14:500, 1979.
Summarizes experience with the use of clomiphene citrate to improve semen quality in 697 reported cases of male infertility.

Infertility Secondary to Tubal Factors

Approximately 15% of couples who desire pregnancy are infertile. In more than one-third of these cases, the inability to achieve successful pregnancy is related to anatomic or physiologic disorders of the fallopian tube.

The fallopian tube averages 11 cm in length. At the ovarian end is the infundibulum, the fimbria of which draw the ovum into the tube at ovulation. Ovum pickup is facilitated by the ciliary action of the ciliated cells, and the ovum draws nutrition from the tubal secretory cells. The ovum passes into the ampulla where fertilization takes place with a sperm that has undergone capacitation (ability to penetrate the ovum) during its passage through the uterus and tube. After some 72–80 hours the fertilized ovum, as a result of tubal muscular peristalsis and ciliary action, passes through the narrow isthmus and intramural portion into the uterine cavity, which is now ready for implantation.

The tubal lumen at the isthmus is about 0.5 mm, while at the junction with the ampulla, it is 2 or 3 mm. Damage due to infection is, therefore, very likely to occlude the lumen(s) and cause infertility. Furthermore, cellular damage interferes with the nutritive and ciliary tubal functions, aggravating the problem. Tubal infections commonly follow gonorrhea, which in severe cases leads to the formation of pyosalpinges, hydrosalpinges, and tubo-ovarian cysts or abscesses. Obstruction may occur in one or several sites along the tube, and the infection is commonly bilateral.

Enteric and other organisms, including anaerobes, may cause salpingitis, either following gonorrhea or complicating abortion or puerperal infections. An intrauterine device (IUD) is another important agent implicated in bacterial tubal infections.

Chlamydiae and mycoplasmas may be important causes of salpingitis, although the evidence is somewhat contradictory. Certainly, tuberculous salpingitis is uniformly accompanied by infertility, although the disease is rare in the United States.

By means of peritubal adhesions, infectious and noninfectious processes outside the tubes may close them, leading to obstruction. Examples include appendicitis, endometriosis, ruptured ovarian cysts, and abdominal or pelvic surgery (especially involving the adnexa).

Diagnosis of a possible tubal factor includes a history of sexually transmitted diseases, previous surgery, the use of an IUD, complicated pregnancy (particularly illegal abortion), and cesarean section. A previous ectopic pregnancy may have been associated with tubal disease, or the surgery may have compromised remaining tubal function. Those gynecologic symptoms suggestive of chronic pelvic inflammatory disease (PID) include menorrhagia, secondary dysmenorrhea, and deep dyspareunia.

Physical examination may be negative or may reveal a tender, fixed retroversion, adnexal tenderness, and/or masses suggestive of inflammatory disease or endometriosis. Gonococcal culture, serology and chest x-ray should be obtained routinely, and when tuberculosis is a possibility, a tuberculin skin test and endometrial biopsy should also be performed.

Tests for tubal patency include the Rubin test in which carbon dioxide insufflation of the uterus is followed by abdominal borborygmi and shoulder pain if the tubes are patent. This test is seldom used today since a hysterosalpingogram (HSG), in which radiopaque dye is injected through the cervix, provides a permanent record of the uterine cavity and the tubes. The test is monitored by fluoroscopy with the average radiation exposure being about one to two rads. The procedure is generally performed during the follicular phase of the menstrual cycle.

Probably the best, although also the most invasive, test for tubal patency is obtained by laparoscopy with concomitant insufflation of the tubes with colored solution (methylene blue). The advantage of this technique is that direct visualization of tubes and ovaries, and peritubal and periovarian adhesions can be obtained. The secretory phase is often favored for the procedure, allowing observations of the corpus luteum.

If endometriosis is noted, treatment with conservative surgery, hormonal therapy, or a combination thereof, is employed. If tuberculosis is diagnosed, fertility is highly unlikely and chemotherapy, with or without extirpative surgery, is called for.

Some patients with tubal obstruction are candidates for tubal reconstructive surgery, but as the results of the procedures vary widely, patients must be carefully screened. Work-up includes evidence of ovulation with basal body temperature recordings, and semen analysis, as well as the postcoital test, to assess the male factor. The decision must be made that neither abdominal surgery nor later pregnancy would endanger the woman's health. The degree of tubal disease and length of the tubes is crucial to success, and both HSG and laparoscopy with chromopertubation should be performed since these investigations complement one another.

Surgery is usually contraindicated in patients more than 37–40 years old because of reduced fertility. It is also contraindicated in patients with extensive PID, expecially those with recent active disease that may be reactivated by the procedure. The length of tube remaining after previous surgery is also crucial; a length of less than 3 cm is inadequate for repair.

The potential for reversal of sterilization depends on the original surgical technique in terms of the length and site of tubal damage. A good outcome may be expected if the sterilization was done with rings, clips, or the Pomeroy procedure, while only fair results follow laparoscopy electrocoagulation reversal. Fimbriectomy and Irving procedures yield poor results with tubal surgery. Each case must be judged individually, however, and laparoscopy is the definitive diagnostic procedure.

Results of tubal surgery have been greatly improved by technical advances. The introduction of microsurgery employing operating microscopes or magnifying loupes, together with fine microsurgical instruments and suture materials, have enabled accurate dissection and reanastomosis to be performed. Minimizing postoperative adhesion formation by continued tissue irrigation, atraumatic tissue handling, prophylactic antibiotics, and electrosurgery are as important as magnification in terms of satisfactory outcome. The use of steroids, stents, and postoperative hydrotubation remains controversial.

The operative procedures include fimbriolysis or salpingolysis (freeing of adhesions), reanastomosis (at various sites in the tube, commonly isthmus-isthmus), salpingoneostomy (constructing a new tubal ostium), and uterotubal implantation. The procedures generally take from 2 to 5 hours and are performed under general anesthesia.

Postoperative complications include infection and ectopic pregnancy. The incidence of the latter varies from 3%–30% and is presumably due to narrowing of the lumen at the site of surgery.

Results are best assessed by viable pregnancy rates, although comparison is difficult since the features of individual patients vary widely. In the best hands and in the best circumstances, pregnancy rates up to 60% have been reported.

Exhaustive counseling of patients prior to surgery is essential. The reasons for the request should be evaluated, and physical, emotional, and marital problems should be diagnosed and treated. Not every surgeon can emulate the outstanding results quoted in the literature and this must be explained to the patient. The risks and costs involved must be pointed out, as well as the expected outcome for the particular person. As a rule, only a minority of patients are suitable for the procedure.

Reviews
1. Pfeffer, W. H., and Wallach, E. E. When tubal factors cause infertility. *Contemp. Ob/Gyn* 15:133, 1980.
   Salpingitis isthmica nodosa, a lesion of the proximal tube (columnar cells scattered among hypertrophied smooth muscle bundles), is considered a sequel of tubal infection.
2. Reversing female sterilization. *Popul. Rep.* [C] No. 8:September, 1980.
   The patient should think of sterilization as irreversible, but the surgeon should perform it as if it were reversible.

Physiology
3. Wilhelmsson, L., Lindblom, B., and Wiqvist, N. The human uterotubal junction; contractile patterns of different smooth muscle layers and the

influence of prostaglandin E_2, prostaglandin F_{2a}, and prostaglandin I_2 in vitro. *Fertil. Steril.* 32:303, 1979.
Varying responsiveness of musculature to prostaglandins.

4. Jean, Y., et al. Fertility of a woman with nonfunctional ciliated cells in the fallopian tubes. *Fertil. Steril.* 31:349, 1979.
Neither muscular activity nor cilial beat is absolutely necessary to ovum transport.

Etiology

5. Winston, R. M. L. Why 103 women asked for reversal of sterilization. *Br. Med. J.* 2:305, 1977.
Common reasons include remarriage, death of child or husband, and mental or physical symptoms attributed to sterilization.

6. Holtz, G. Prevention of postoperative adhesions. *J. Reprod. Med.* 24:141, 1980.
Adhesions, bands of vascularized connective tissue, form when damaged or devascularized tissue reacts to blood, infection, or irritating particles.

7. Garcia, C. R., and Mastroianni, L., Jr. Microsurgery for treatment of adnexal disease. *Fertil. Steril.* 34:413, 1980.
Puerperal or postabortion sepsis is a common cause of obstruction near the uterotubal junction.

Diagnosis

8. Hutchins, C. J. Laparoscopy and hysterosalpingography in the assessment of tubal patency. *Obstet. Gynecol.* 49:325, 1977.
HSG in patients with chronic tubal infection may cause an acute exacerbation of the disease.

9. Gomel, V. Laparoscopy prior to reconstructive tubal surgery for infertility. *J. Reprod. Med.* 18:251, 1977.
Laparoscopy determines tubal length, presence of fimbria, and degree of pelvic or abdominal pathology.

Therapy

10. Siegler, A. M., and Kontopoulos, V. An analysis of macrosurgical and microsurgical techniques in the management of the tuboperitoneal factor in infertility. *Fertil. Steril.* 32:377, 1979.
Some procedures may be performed without magnification.

11. Gomel, V. Microsurgical reversal of female sterilization: A reappraisal. *Fertil. Steril.* 33:587, 1980.
In a series of 118 cases, 64% of the women went on to intrauterine pregnancy and one had an ectopic pregnancy; the mean time to pregnancy was 10 months.

12. DiZerega, G. S., and Hodgen, G. D. Prevention of postoperative tubal adhesions: Comparative study of commonly used agents. *Am. J. Obstet. Gynecol.* 136:173, 1980.
Glucocorticoids, antihistamines, anticoagulants, enzymes, dextran, intratubal stents, and prosthetic covers for the distal tube have all been tried with the single aim of minimizing adhesion formation.

13. Swolin, K. Electromicrosurgery and salpingostomy: Long term results. *Am. J. Obstet. Gynecol.* 121:418, 1974.
In 33 cases there was a 95% patency rate; 36% of the patients produced live infants, while 27% had ectopic pregnancies. Prognosis for surgery on the distal tube is variable.

14. Mettler, L., Giesel, H., and Semm, K. Treatment of female infertility due to tubal obstruction by operative laparoscopy. *Fertil. Steril.* 32:384, 1979.

Laparoscopic diagnosis and surgery were possible in one intervention in 79% of patients.

The Future
15. Wood, C., et al. Microvascular transplantation of the human fallopian tube. *Fertil. Steril.* 29:607, 1978.
    The problem of rejection has yet to be surmounted.
16. Edwards, R. G., Steptoe, P. C., and Purdy, J. M. Establishing full-term human pregnancies using cleaving embryos grown in vitro. *Br. J. Obstet. Gynaecol.* 87:737, 1980.
    Ova obtained by laparoscopy are fertilized in vitro and the embryo is reimplanted into the maternal uterus (test-tube babies).

Anovulatory Infertility

Inability to conceive is due to failure of ovulation in 10%–15% of women complaining of infertility. The frequency of anovulation may be occasional or complete; even in patients who do occasionally ovulate, however, the statistical chances for conception are greatly diminished. Ovulatory dysfunction is unusual in women with regular, predictable menstrual cycles; women with amenorrhea or dysfunctional uterine bleeding are usually anovulatory.

The detection and timing of ovulation depend on tests designed to assess the effects of hormones on target tissues or by measuring plasma hormones by radioimmunoassay. The latter method is expensive and cumbersome, the former easily available. It must be remembered, though, that the only definite proof of ovulation is pregnancy or the recovery of an ovum from the oviducts.

Basal body temperature (BBT) readings prior to ovulation are in the 97.2°–97.4° F range; after ovulation they elevate to 98° F as a result of the thermogenic action of progesterone on the thermoregulatory centers. Recording the BBT also provides information about the length of the follicular, menstrual, and luteal phases as well as the timing and frequency of intercourse. Readings should be taken immediately upon wakening, preferably with a basal body thermometer especially designed for the purpose.

Dating of the endometrium by material from an endometrial biopsy obtained 2 or 3 days prior to the expected menses provides evidence of ovulation if secretory activity is present, and provides an indication of the adequacy of the luteal phase of the cycle.

Changes in cervical mucus as regards crystallization (ferning), spinnbarkeit (capacity of cervical mucus to be drawn into threads), and viscosity may also be used in assessing hormonal status. Characteristically, under increasing estrogen stimulus the mucus is profuse, thin, watery, acellular, undergoes ferning, and can be drawn into long threads. Once progesterone is secreted, cervical mucus becomes cellular, scanty, and viscous, with absent ferning and spinnbarkeit. These changes occur over several days, and serial observations must be made in order to detect the time of ovulation. The presence of progesterone-induced changes is presumptive evidence of ovulation.

Serum progesterone concentration is the most useful, direct hormonal assay for documenting ovulation. A serum concentration greater than 5 ng/ml is consistent with ovulation. The sample is generally obtained on day 21 of the cycle.

Ovulatory cycles result from a normally functioning hypothalamic-pituitary-ovarian axis. Anovulation may result from any factor disturbing the normal endocrine-recycling events. Central to these events is the blood estrogen concentration. If estrogen fall is inadequate, follicle-stimulating hormone (FSH) may not increase. Further crucial malfunctions relate to luteinizing hormone (LH) suppression or asynchrony of LH surge due to inappropriate estrogen feedback. Finally, FSH may not stimulate follicle growth due to follicle nonreceptivity.

Central neuroendocrine failure (hypothalamic-pituitary) results in hypogonadotropic hypogonadism. Gonadotropins are depressed and estrogen activity is absent. Ovarian failure is manifested by hypergonadotropic hypogonadism with elevated gonadotropins and insufficient estrogen activity. Asynchronous gonadotropin and estrogen production results in anovulation and presents with varying clinical features. Estrogen levels are usually normal, but menstrual cycles are disrupted; FSH levels are normal; and LH levels are normal or elevated. Depending on the degree of impairment, the clinical spectrum of anovulation therefore encompasses amenorrhea, dysfunctional uterine bleeding, and infertility.

Before initiating therapy for ovulation induction, the clinician must be certain that serious disease states have been excluded. Pituitary tumors, anorexia nervosa, gonadal dysgenesis, masculinizing tumors, and adrenal and thyroid disease are all possible causes of chronic anovulation.

Therapeutic induction of ovulation cannot be achieved in women with ovarian failure. The drug most frequently used for ovulation induction is clomiphene citrate (a nonsteroidal compound related to diethylstilbestrol). Clomiphene citrate acts by reducing estrogen receptors, and this is "interpreted" by the hypothalamus as a fall in estrogen levels. The resultant rise in gonadotropin secretion induces ovulation in 80% of anovulatory women, and conception occurs in 50% of women who resume normal ovulation. Those women most likely to respond have some evidence of pituitary-ovarian function as indicated by a history of spontaneous or progesterone-induced withdrawal bleeding. The ideal candidate for clomiphene therapy is an acyclic woman with normal or elevated estrogen levels.

Because approximately 75% of clomiphene-induced pregnancies occur during the first three months of treatment, full infertility work-up need not be pursued until failure is recorded after three ovulatory cycles. The medication is started on the fifth day of a cycle following spontaneous or progestin-induced menstruation. Initially, we give 50 mg daily for 5 days; if ovulation occurs, it usually does so between days 10 and 16. We monitor ovulation by a basal body temperature recording. If ovulation does not occur, dosage is increased by 50-mg increments up to a 150 mg maximum.

Clomiphene side effects include ovarian enlargement (13%), vasomotor flushes (10%), and abdominal discomfort (5%). The incidence of multiple gestation is 5%–10%. In patients with ovarian enlargement therapy should be withheld until ovaries are normal size.

If ovulation does not occur at the 150-mg dosage, a single dose of 10,000 IU of human chorionic gonadotropin (HCG) on day 13 is added to the regimen. The HCG acts as an LH surrogate and may trigger rupture of the follicle.

Patients failing to respond to clomiphene are candidates for gonadotropin therapy. This medication is expensive, difficult to monitor, and carries a substantial complication rate. For these reasons, patients must have a complete work-up before gonadotropin therapy is begun. In particular, the uterotubal and male factors must be investigated and ovarian failure excluded. Patient counseling and instruction is essential.

Gonadotropin therapy requires only an ovary with responsive oocytes;

some 90% of patients will ovulate with it and 50%–70% will conceive. Multiple gestation is a major complication of the method, with an incidence of 20%–35%; three or more fetuses per pregnancy will occur in 5% of women. Superovulation can be kept to a minimum by withholding HCG if estrogen levels exceed 1500 pg/ml.

The second major drawback of gonadotropin treatment is the hyperstimulation syndrome. Ovarian enlargement of 5–10 cm occurs in 30% of ovulatory cycles. Because peak effects occur 4–5 days after the HCG dose, the incidence of the complication may be reduced by withholding HCG when serum estrogen exceeds 1500 pg/ml. The full picture is rare (2%), and consists of theca lutein cysts, ascites, hypovolemia, hypercoagulability, and even mortality. Ovarian rupture or hemorrhage may occur, necessitating laparotomy.

An alternative technique, helpful in diminishing the amount of gonadotropin required, is the use of clomiphene prior to administration of human menopausal gonadotropin–human chorionic gonadotropin. This method may also reduce the incidence of hyperstimulation.

Gonadotropin-releasing hormone, a hypothalamic decapeptide that has been used successfully in ovulation induction and in current research protocols, is being administered in a pulsatile fashion by pulsatile infusion pumps.

Surgery plays little or no part in the therapy of anovulation, with the occasional exception of patients with PCOD unresponsive to medical therapy who may respond to bilateral ovarian wedge resection.

Reviews

1. Taymor, M. L. Evaluation of anovulatory cycles and induction of ovulation. *Clin. Obstet. Gynecol.* 22:145, 1979.
   Includes a diagnostic flow sheet for the evaluation of amenorrhea and anovulation based on the presence or absence of bleeding in response to progesterone administration.
2. Kase, N. Anovulation. *Curr. Probl. Obstet. Gynecol.* 1:3, 1978.
   Dysfunction or disease in the hypothalamic-pituitary-ovarian axis, or imprecision in the steroid and peptide hormone signals that link these organs, leads to anovulation.

Pathogenesis

3. Harlap, S. Are there two types of postpill anovulation? *Fertil. Steril.* 31:486, 1979.
   The first entity is postulated as identical to spontaneous secondary anovulation as occurs in nonpill users, while the second type is said to occur in former pill users who were underweight.
4. Wu, Ch.h., and Mikhail, G. Plasma hormone profile in anovulation. *Fertil. Steril.* 31:258, 1979.
   The incidence of anovulatory cycles in eumenorrheic females has been estimated to be 11%.

Diagnosis

5. Morris, N. M., Underwood, L. E., and Easterling, W. Temporal relationship between basal body temperature nadir and luteinizing hormone surge in normal women. *Fertil. Steril.* 27:780, 1976.
   Ovulation probably occurs on the day prior to the first temperature elevation.
6. Buxton, C. L., and Olson, L. E. Endometrial biopsy inadvertently

taken during conception cycle. *Am. J. Obstet. Gynecol.* 105:702, 1969. *Only 2 of 26 patients aborted.*

7. Israel, R., et al. Single luteal phase serum progesterone assay as an indicator of ovulation. *Am. J. Obstet. Gynecol.* 112:1043, 1972.
Level over 3 ng/ml provided presumptive evidence of ovulation.

8. Moghissi, K. S. Prediction and detection of ovulation. *Fertil. Steril.* 34:89, 1980.
Currently no reliable method for the prediction of ovulation is available.

Pharmacologic Induction of Ovulation

9. Drake, J. S., Tredway, D. R., and Buchanan, G. C. Continued clinical experience with an increasing dosage regimen of clomiphene citrate administration. *Fertil. Steril.* 30:274, 1978.
The package insert recommends that therapy be limited to under 100 mg/day, but some 15% of clomiphene pregnancies have required higher doses; this has not increased the complication rate, although the drug is potentially hepatotoxic.

10. Shepard, M. K., Balmaceda, J. P., and Leija, C. G. Relationship of weight to successful induction of ovulation with clomiphene citrate. *Fertil. Steril.* 32:641, 1979.
There was a linear relationship between body weight and dose required to induce ovulation. In obese patients, the mechanism is thought to be due to increased estrone levels competing with the drug for hypothalamic receptor sites.

11. Hack, M., et al. Outcome of pregnancy after induced ovulation—followup of pregnancies and children born after clomiphene therapy. *J.A.M.A.* 220:1329, 1972.
The abortion rate (20%) and incidence of fetal anomalies were the same as that found in an infertile population not treated with clomiphene.

12. Klay, L. J. Clomiphene regulated ovulation for donor insemination. *Fertil. Steril.* 27:383, 1976.
Discusses timing of ovulation in irregularly ovulating women who require insemination of donor sperm.

13. Gemzell, C. A., Diczfalusy, E., and Tillinger, D. G. Clinical effects of human pituitary follicle stimulating hormone (FSH). *J. Clin. Endocrinol.* 18:333, 1958.
In the initial classic work, gonadotropins were derived from human pituitary glands removed at autopsy. Modern therapy employs gonadotropins extracted from the urine of postmenopausal females.

14. Oelsner, G., et al. The study of induction of ovulation with menotropins: Analysis of results of 1897 treatment cycles. *Fertil. Steril.* 30:538, 1978.
Estrogen levels leading to multiple ovulations are not significantly different from those preceding single ovulation.

15. Pepperell, R. J., McBain, J. C., and Healy, D. L. Ovulation induction with bromocriptine (CB 154) in patients with hyperprolactinemia. *Aust. N.Z. J. Obstet. Gynecol.* 17:181, 1977.
Some patients with normal levels of prolactin may also respond, and since therapy is relatively uncomplicated, this may become the initial approach to treatment of anovulation in the future.

16. Zarate, A., et al. Therapeutic use of gonadoliberin (follicle-stimulating hormone/luteinizing hormone–releasing hormone) in women. *Fertil. Steril.* 27:1233, 1976.
Use of gonadotropin-releasing hormone should be regarded as an investigational technique at present.

17. Menning, B. C. The emotional needs of infertile couples. *Fertil. Steril.* 34:313, 1980.
The infertile couple should be treated as a unit and involved in the plan of care. The physician must be emotionally supportive and accessible.

Surgical Induction of Ovulation

18. Judd, H. L., et al. The effects of ovarian wedge resection on circulating gonadotropin and ovarian steroid levels in patients with polycystic ovary syndrome. *J. Clin. Endocrinol. Metab.* 43:347, 1976.
Reduction of testosterone is the major change affected, suggesting that an intraovarian effect of androgen is the barrier to ovulation in PCOD.

19. Buttram, V. C., and Vaguero, C. Post-ovarian wedge resection adhesive disease. *Fertil. Steril.* 26:874, 1975.
If possible, surgery should be avoided because of the high incidence of postoperative adhesions that aggravate the infertility problem.

Complications

20. Shapiro, A. G., Thomas, T., and Epstein, M. Management of hyperstimulation syndrome. *Fertil. Steril.* 28:3, 1977.
Management centers on close control of fluid and electrolyte balance while awaiting gradual resolution with time (7 days in nonpregnant women, 10–20 days in pregnant women).

21. Ron-El, R., et al. Triplet and quadruplet pregnancies and management. *Obstet. Gynecol.* 57:459, 1981.
Iatrogenic population explosion.

Infertility Due to Cervical, Immunologic, and Luteal Phase Defects

When motile sperm are unable to traverse the cervical canal, the resulting infertility is attributed to cervical factors. The reported prevalence of infertility due to cervical factors ranges from 10%–30%.

Cervical factors are evaluated by the microscopic examination of postcoital cervical mucus obtained at midcycle. Although there are numerous variations of the postcoital test, the best known and most widely used method is the Sims-Huhner test. This test is performed 24–48 hours before ovulation and 2–12 hours after intercourse. The cervical mucus is placed on a slide, covered with a cover slip, and examined under the high-power objective of the microscope. The number of sperm and their quality of movement are recorded. The test is considered "good" when more than 20 sperm per high-power field are seen and when more than 50% of these sperm show "purposeful" motility. The test is considered "bad" when fewer than 5 sperm per high-power field are seen and the number of motile sperm falls below 50%.

The most common cause for an abnormal postcoital test is inaccurate timing. Spinnbarkeit and ferning provide insight into the nearness of ovulation. Spinnbarkeit is the capacity of mucus to be drawn into threads. There is a gradual increase in spinnbarkeit from menstruation to a peak at ovulation when cervical mucus may be drawn into threads 15 to 20 cm in length. Ferning (crystallization) is the fernlike pattern observed microscopically after cervical mucus is allowed to dry. It is an estrogen-dependent feature with maximal ferning paralleling maximal spinnbarkeit and occurring 24–48 hours before ovulation.

Although one satisfactory postcoital test result is sufficient to assume that cervical function is normal, one unsatisfactory test merely indicates the need to repeat the test. Serial abnormal postcoital tests warrrant further evaluation. If the semen analysis is normal, the evaluation focuses on coital technique and the evaluation of cervical mucus.

With regard to coital technique, patients are advised to avoid: lubricants during intercourse, postcoital douching, early withdrawal, and arising too soon after coitus.

Approximately 50% of patients with an abnormal postcoital test have abnormal cervical mucus. Of these patients about one-half have poor quality and one-half have an inadequate quantity of mucus. The quality of cervical mucus is improved in about 40% of patients by the use of diethylstilbestrol (DES) in a dosage of 0.1 mg from day 5 through 14 of the cycle. Approximately one-half of women treated with DES become pregnant. Other estrogen preparations are not as effective at these low doses, but the use of higher doses may interfere with ovulation. DES therapy increases the amount of mucus in about 50% of patients with abnormally low cervical mucus volumes. Approximately one-third of these patients become pregnant.

Antibiotics are indicated when cultures show mycoplasmas: *Mycoplasma hominis, Mycoplasma fermentans,* and *Ureaplasma urealyticum* (known as T mycoplasma). This is an empirical approach as data in this area are conflicting and remain controversial.

Another area currently viewed with skepticism and surrounded by controversy is the role of immunological factors as a cause of infertility.

The postcoital test is the only in vivo clinical test that demonstrates the existence of an immunologic incompatibility in the infertile couple. If the presence of nonmotile sperm is a recurrent feature of the postcoital test—especially if the cervical mucus is normal—immunologic factors are possible. In these cases, cross-testing is necessary. If the husband's sperm penetrate a donor's cervical mucus but not the wife's cervical mucus, and if a donor's sperm penetrate the wife's cervical mucus, the existence of a specific incompatibility between the husband's sperm and the wife's cervical mucus is concluded.

The most utilized serum tests to detect antibodies to spermatozoal antigens are: (1) the tube-slide agglutination test, formerly the Franklin-Duke's test; (2) the gelatin agglutination test, formerly the Kibrick test; and (3) Isojima's sperm immobilization test. Antisperm-antibody testing is tissue-specific rather than individual-specific since HL-A antigen and ABO blood group systems are not involved in immunologic infertility.

There is a high incidence of antisperm antibodies in the serum of both women and men with "unexplained" infertility. There is currently no general agreement regarding the contribution of these antibodies to infertility. This is due partly to poor correlation between systemic and local immunologic responsiveness and partly to varied interpretations and lack of standardization of many of the tests. There is a need for the development and application of tests of local immunologic responses to sperm.

None of the therapeutic modalities available are very effective in the treatment of immunologic infertility. Condom therapy is the predominant method in use. Presumably, this method prevents stimulation of antibody production to the antigens present in semen (spermatozoa and seminal fluid). Other modalities include immunosuppression, intrauterine insemination, and artificial insemination with washed sperm.

Luteal phase defect is an abnormal ovarian function that manifests itself by inadequate amount and/or duration of progesterone production by the corpus luteum. The corpus luteum is the major source of progesterone during the luteal phase of ovulatory cycles. Following conception the corpus luteum also persists as the major source of progesterone during the first trimester. After the tenth week of gestation, placental progesterone production alone is usually sufficient to support a normal pregnancy.

Once a controversial issue, the luteal phase defect is now generally accepted as a definite yet uncommon cause of female infertility and recurrent pregnancy wastage. The incidence of this defect is approximately 3% in a population of infertile women.

The most frequently used method to diagnose luteal phase defects is the endometrial biopsy performed 1 or 2 days prior to the succeeding menses and dated according to the criteria of Noyes, Hertig, and Rock. The patient must be recording basal body temperatures at the time the biopsy is performed. The biopsy should be in phase as determined by the date of onset of the subsequent menstrual period and the estimated date of ovulation. To make the diagnosis of a luteal phase defect, the biopsy date must be out of phase by 2 or more days in more than one menstrual cycle. The diagnosis of the luteal phase defect requires a minimum of three plasma progesterone levels during the luteal phase, but this approach is inconvenient and expensive. A single progesterone value is of little or no help in diagnosing luteal phase defects.

The luteal phase defect has multiple etiologies. These include inadequate gonadotropins in the preovulatory phase, low luteinizing hormone in the luteal phase, hyperprolactinemia, luteinized unruptured follicle, tubal ligation, postpartum and postpill menstrual cycles, and a recently reported pseudo–corpus luteum defect characterized by normal serum progesterone values.

Because the luteal phase defect manifests itself by an inadequate amount or duration of progesterone production, or both, by the corpus luteum, it stands to reason that the mainstay of treatment is substitutional progesterone therapy. This is administered as progesterone in oil, 12.5 mg given intramuscularly daily; or as progesterone vaginal suppositories, 25 mg taken twice daily, beginning 3 or 4 days after ovulation. This dosage produces serum progesterone levels compatible with those found in the luteal phase in normal cycles. Other methods of treatment depend upon the knowledge of the etiologic diagnosis, which is often difficult to determine in clinical practice. These include administration of HCG or clomiphene, or both, in patients unresponsive to progesterone. Bromocriptine appears to be therapeutic for infertile patients with luteal phase defects and elevated prolactin levels. The success rate with medical treatment of luteal phase defects is 50%–80%.

Cervical Factor

1. Blasco, L., and Wallach, E. E. When cervical factors cause infertility. *Contemp. Ob/Gyn* 15:125, 1980.
   Review of diagnostic tests and treatment modalities when abnormal interaction between sperm and cervical mucus are implicated.
2. Taylor-Robinson, D., and McCormack, W. M. The genital mycoplasmas. *N. Engl. J. Med.* 302:1003, 1980.
   Exhaustive review of subject.
3. Friberg, J. Mycoplasmas and ureaplasmas in infertility and abortion. *Fertil. Steril.* 33:351, 1980.
   Review of subject, emphasizing the role of those organisms in reproductive failure.

Immunological Factors

4. Beer, A. E., and Neaves, W. B. Antigenic status of semen from the viewpoints of the female and male. *Fertil. Steril.* 29:3, 1978.
   A detailed critical review of antisperm antibody tests.
5. Jones, W. R. Immunological infertility—fact or fiction? *Fertil. Steril.* 33:577, 1980.
   Review dealing with immunity to semen and to the zona pellucida.
6. Shulman, S., et al. Immune infertility and new approaches to treatment. *Fertil. Steril.* 29:309, 1978.
   Discusses a sperm-washing insemination method and an immunosuppression method in the management of "immunologic infertility."

Luteal Phase Defects

7. Aksel, S. Sporadic and recurrent luteal phase defects in cyclic women: Comparison with normal cycles. *Fertil. Steril.* 33:372, 1980.
   Reiterates role of hyperprolactinemia as a cause of luteal insufficiency and emphasizes appropriate procedures for making the diagnosis.
8. Rosenfield, D. L., et al. Diagnosis of luteal phase inadequacy. *Obstet. Gynecol.* 56:193, 1980.
   Emphasizes the essential need for a properly obtained endometrial biopsy for the diagnosis of luteal phase defects.
9. Wentz, A. C. Physiologic and clinical considerations in luteal phase defects. *Clin. Obstet. Gynecol.* 22:169, 1979.
   Reviews current thinking regarding pathophysiology, diagnosis, and therapy of luteal phase defects.
10. Marik, J., and Hulka, J. Luteinized unruptured follicle syndrome: Subtle cause of infertility. *Fertil. Steril.* 29:270, 1978.
    A biphasic basal body temperature graph and secretory endometrium may not necessarily be indicative of ovulation.
11. Andrews, W. C. Luteal phase defects. *Fertil. Steril.* 32:501, 1979.
    Addresses concerns about teratogenicity in substitutional progesterone therapy.
12. Noyes, R. W., et al. Dating the endometrial biopsy. *Fertil. Steril.* 1:3, 1950.
    Classic description of criteria used to date endometrial biopsies.

Half of all the teenagers in the United States are sexually active, and teenage pregnancies cost taxpayers about $8.3 billion a year in welfare and related outlays. Most teenagers say they are not ready for parenthood, yet only one out of five who does not want to fall pregnant uses any form of contraception. Two-thirds of pregnant teenage girls marry; 75% of these marriages end in divorce. Each year an estimated 200,000 teenagers contract venereal disease, and the highest rates of gonorrhea among women are in 18-year-olds. In 1975 there were 327,000 abortions performed in girls aged 15–19 and 15,000 in those aged 14 and under.

The problems resulting from adolescent sexuality are widely studied and well known; not so the means of preventing them. The attitude of society to teenage sexual activity is ambiguous and ambivalent. Empirical knowledge is inadequate, and the clinician is usually forced to rely on personal judgement and common sense in managing the adolescent patient. In order to become more effective in this area, it is vital for him to have some understanding of the nature of teenage sexuality.

Sexuality is a continuum that has its onset in infancy and continues throughout life. All children experience physical pleasure from bodily touching that can be described as sexual. Most children manipulate their genitalia, and boys are often capable of orgasm many years before they develop the capacity for ejaculation. The attitude of parents to their children's sexual curiosity and experimentation may have profound effects on their later sexual development. Parents should, therefore, be the major source of the sex education and sexual health of children. Sex should be discussed openly and frankly without embarrassment. The most important lessons, however, are taught without words and are based on the home atmosphere and attitude of the parents to the child and to each other. The loved, valued, and respected child is much more likely to be capable of loving, valuing, and respecting others, and the reverse holds true.

Puberty normally occurs between 9 and 16 years of age with the gonadal secretion of sex hormones in response to pituitary gonadotropins. The time and nature of pubertal growth are under the influence of genetic, psychologic, hormonal, and environmental factors. Over the past 50 years, there has been a trend toward earlier menarche, so that girls are capable of reproduction at a younger age. The early cycles are typically anovulatory, the interval from menarche to first ovulatory cycle varying from between three months and a year, with many exceptions to the rule. Boys, unlike girls, achieve potential fertility at the beginning rather than at the end of pubertal development.

If androgens are responsible for the sex drive in both sexes, this might explain the difference between the sexes in the time of attainment of orgasm. While both male and female have increased androgen levels at puberty, the levels in males are much higher and parallel the onset of sexual activities, including orgasm and ejaculation. By contrast, the onset of orgasm in females is not linked to androgen levels but gradually increases in incidence with time. The factors in the female are most probably societal and environmental. Estrogens, while important in priming genital tissues, do not appear to have an erotogenic effect.

Puberty is a time of deep self-absorption. Body image is of great importance, and girls are very concerned about the size of their breasts and the onset of menstruation. This is a time of further sexual awakening, and the profound nature of the sexual feeling may surprise and confuse the adolescent. In learning how to control these feelings, behavior may alter radically with periods of chaos, calm, and what may appear as irrational conduct.

The adolescent development process involves a complex series of physical, emotional, and societal changes. Final goals in the maturation process include the formation of a stable self-image, a sexual identity, and the concept of self as separate from parents. The "phase-specific tasks" of adolescence also include the enhancement of self-esteem, acceptance by the peer group, and the maturation of interpersonal relationships. Frequently, success in school, sports, and friendships outweighs sexual matters in importance to the adolescent.

It is difficult to generalize regarding sexual behavior, but during adolescence probably as many as 90% of males and 60% of females masturbate. Masturbation is normal and almost certainly beneficial, provided no feelings of guilt and worry are associated. The rate of premarital coitus among women and girls, especially white women and girls, appears to have increased. Coitus now occurs in 49% of whites and 84% of blacks by age 19. Most first sexual encounters occur at home with a partner they have known a long while and who is also an adolescent. Many teenagers are deeply ambivalent about sex, and one result of this "pleasure-guilt" attitude to sexual activity is to avoid contraceptives, the use of which would imply "premeditation."

During adolescence, strong attachments to members of the same sex are common. Mutual masturbation occurs among 6% of females, commencing at 6–10 years of age. While this behavior is transient in the majority of instances, most adult homosexuals trace the onset of their sexual preference to their adolescence.

The physician has an important role in encouraging adolescents to be responsible for their own health care. Confidentiality is essential so that the teen can speak freely and openly. It must be remembered that most adolescents learn about sexual matters from their peers and that peer group values are usually the dominant force in their lives, which explains most seemingly unreasonable behavior. Physician and parent should attempt to keep their own adolescent values out of the picture. A nonjudgmental and supportive parental attitude can spare the teenager enormous emotional stress and pain, and the physician, provided confidentiality is not breached, can provide valuable support to parent and child.

In helping the adolescent female patient overcome a particular problem, the physician should advise and educate the teenager, but the final decision should be left to her. She should be encouraged to define the situation in question and to share her needs and feelings with the significant other people in her life. It is important to help her decide what her own needs in a particular situation are and to examine, if possible, the long- and short-term alternatives available to her, as well as the likely consequences of these choices. Guidance can be given in making her choice, but it must clearly be her own choice, not that of the physician. Thereafter, the necessary actions and time sequence related to the choice should be discussed, while it is made quite clear that no decision need be final and that the physician is available for further help if needed.

An example of this approach might relate to a girl whose boyfriend is urging her to have sex in spite of her own ambivalence. The choice might lie between abstinence and use of contraception. The physician is able to help her in this choice and guide her to a rational decision with the approach outlined above.

Generally, the clinician will function best with parental knowledge, but if confidentiality is requested, treatment need not be withheld. The "mature minor rule" allows the doctor to supply full medical care if it is felt that the minor is capable of understanding the nature, extent, and consequences of the invasion of her body. Full documentation is essential.

There is confusion over sex education and education about contraception. Fears that promiscuity would result appear unfounded, but the results of education are frequently disappointing. One worker has pointed out that sexuality is now acquired long before the intellectual maturity required to handle it, and that while copulation needs no teaching, there is clearly an enormous need to teach the entire human race how to use artificial forms of contraception.

Reviews

1. Katchadourian, H. Adolescent sexuality. *Pediatr. Clin. North Am.* 27:17, 1980.
   Scholarly essay.
2. Litt, I. F., and Cohen, M. I. Adolescent sexuality. *Adv. Pediatr.* 26:119, 1979.
   The development of sexuality is intimately tied to physical development, development of intrafamilial and peer relations, cognitive function, and personality.
3. Freeman, E. W., and Rickels, K. Adolescent contraceptive use: Current status of practice and research. *Obstet. Gynecol.* 53:388, 1979.
   Only 16% of sexually active teenagers desire pregnancy.

Biology

4. Adolescent sexuality and adolescent fertility. *Lancet* 2:129, 1979.
   Discusses social and biological changes, and points out that Romeo and Juliet would have been classed as juvenile delinquents by most present-day legal codes.
5. Tanner, J. M. *Growth of Adolescence* (2nd ed.). Oxford, England: Blackwell, 1962.
   The staging of secondary sex characteristics allows the prediction of future events from present developmental status.

Statistical Sources

6. Lincoln, R., Jaffe, F., and Ambrose, L. *11 Million Teenagers.* New York: Allen Guttmacher Institute (Planned Parenthood of America), 1976.
   An important study.
7. Zelnick, M., and Kantner, J. F. Sexual and contraceptive experience of young, unmarried women in the United States, 1971 and 1976. *Fam. Plann. Perspect.* 9:55, 1977.
   Often quoted, although frequently with different conclusions.

Contraception

8. Felman, Y. M. A plea for the condom, especially for teenagers. *J.A.M.A.* 241:2517, 1979.
   An excellent method for the sexually active teenager, both as a contraceptive and as a prophylactic.
9. Tyrer, L. B., and Josimovich, J. Contraception in teenagers. *Clin. Obstet. Gynecol.* 20:651, 1977.
   Emphasizes difficulties in access to contraceptives and contraceptive education.

10. Nadelson, C. C., Notman, M. T., and Gillon, J. W. Sexual knowledge and attitudes of adolescents: Relationship to contraceptive use. *Obstet. Gynecol.* 55:341, 1980.
Expectations for responsible contraceptive planning may be at variance with the developmental stage of many sexually active adolescents.

Problems

11. Freeman, E. Abortion: Subjective attitudes and feelings. *Fam. Plann. Perspect.* 10:3, 1978.
Under 20% regretted the procedure or had strong negative feelings. Teenagers account for the majority of second trimester abortions.
12. Felice, M., et al. Follow-up observations of adolescent rape victims. *Clin. Pediatr.* 16:311, 1978.
Suspicion or knowledge of rape or incest involving a minor mandates a report to the child protection agency or police, or both.
13. McAnarney, E. R. Adolescent pregnancy—a national priority. *Am. J. Dis. Child.* 132:125, 1978.
The most common medical concern arising from adolescent sexual behavior.
14. Rosenstock, H. Recognizing the teenager who needs to be pregnant. *South. Med. J.* 73:34, 1980.
"Inadvertent pregnancy" may be a desperate escape from facing one's own personal problems.
15. Rauh, J. L., and Burket, R. L. Adolescent sexual activity and resulting gynecologic problems. *Med. Aspects Hum. Sex.* 13:56, 1979.
An estimated 50,000 to 80,000 young women are made sterile by gonorrhea every year.
16. Davidson, E. C., Jr. An analysis of adolescent health care and the role of the obstetrician-gynecologist. *Am. J. Obstet. Gynecol.* 139:845, 1981.
Many obstetrician-gynecologists were found to have negative attitudes to adolescent sexual practices. A judgmental approach may interfere with the doctor-patient relationship.

Education

17. Hein, K. Impact of mass media on adolescent sexual behavior. The chicken or the egg? *Am. J. Dis. Child.* 134:133, 1980.
The author feels that the choices regarding patterns of adolescent sexual behavior are independent of the effects of mass media.
18. Cohen, C. I., and Cohen, E. J. Health education: Panacea, pernicious or pointless? *N. Engl. J. Med.* 299:718, 1978.
Sexual behavior seems little changed by courses in sex education.

Alterations in Sexuality with Aging, Drugs, and Disease

There are certain physiological changes in sexual functioning that accompany the aging process. These are gradual and do not impede sexual expression. These involutional changes occur at different rates for different people.

In males, testosterone production decreases gradually, and there appears to be no physiologic male menopause. The testes become less firm, smaller, and do not elevate at the same degree. Seminal fluid becomes scant and ejaculatory pressure low. Penile erection is slower, and physical stimulation may be necessary; however, erection may be maintained for extended periods of time. The resolution and refractory periods after ejaculation are longer, from 12–24 hours in men over age 50.

In females, consequent to lack of estrogen, there is thinning of the vaginal mucosa, followed by atrophy of the uterus and ovaries, and involutional changes in the vagina, labia, and clitoris. Vaginal width, length, and expansive ability decrease, and vaginal lubrication is reduced. The orgasmic phase is reduced in duration and resolution is more rapid; however, women virtually never lose their capacity for orgasm.

Contrary to popular conceptions, sexual activity is the norm in older people. Three-fourths of males remain potent in their seventh decade, and a similar percentage of females remain orgasmic. Further, nongenital erotic pleasuring remains as satisfactory in later years as for the young.

Many factors influence the continuation of sexual expression in the individual. While demographic factors such as age, gender, marital status, and income are important, the most significant feature is the previous pattern of sexuality. Also important are the factors of physical and emotional health, as well as the attitudes of family, physician, and friends. An important limiting factor, especially for women, is the availability of a socially acceptable partner.

Realizing that an active sex life is healthy for the social, emotional, and physical well-being of the elderly, the physician needs to be an objective, accepting, and informed sexual counselor. Since nonacceptance of sexuality in the aged is common in the community, the clinician needs to extend counseling to the spouse, family, and relevant health care providers. For instance, provision must be made for privacy when the elderly live with their children or in institutions.

History-taking should include routine inquiry regarding sexual matters, together with education and reassurance concerning the physiologic changes of aging. With the knowledge that a wide variety of physical, emotional, and pharmaceutically induced disorders may profoundly influence sexuality, the clinician needs to diagnose and treat these problems, as well as advise the patient regarding the generally favorable outcome that can be expected. When possible, both partners should be included in the therapeutic process. The longer it has been since sexuality has ceased, the more difficult it is to resume; therefore, therapy should be prompt and vigorous.

Most elderly people cease sexual function because of psychologic and societal misconceptions, not because of aging processes or disease. As the percentage of the older age group in the population is steadily increasing, it becomes ever more important for the physician to encourage the preservation of sexuality in older men and women.

Many drugs, whether taken for social or medical reasons, have an effect on sexual function. Since male sexual failure is difficult to disguise, this effect has been widely studied. In contrast, few reports document deleterious sexual side effects of drugs in the female.

Both erection and ejaculation are under dual autonomic nervous control. In addition, satisfactory vascular, endocrine, and psychologic components are essential to sexual function. In assessing problems secondary to drug use, the underlying disease process must be taken into consideration. For instance, in one study of untreated "hypertensives," 17% complained of impotence as compared with 7% of a control group of similar age.

Drugs affecting the autonomic system are the most likely to affect sexual function, the two largest groups being the antihypertensive and psychoactive drugs. Postganglionic blockers, such as bethanidine and guanethidine, caused impotence in up to 68% of patients. Centrally acting drugs, such as methyldopa and reserpine, were somewhat better but also caused impotence in up to 26%. In sexually active patients, high-risk drugs should be avoided, using instead beta-adrenoceptor blocking agents and diuretics. Even the latter, however, have been associated with possible sexual side effects. All the major tranquillizers and phenothiazines appear to interfere with ejaculation, probably via an autonomic effect, although high prolactin levels may also play a role. The minor tranquillizers may also, rarely, interfere with sexual function, as well as the tricyclic antidepressants, which have anticholinergic properties. Once again, the extent of the problem is difficult to assess because of the underlying disease process, and in many instances, good response to the therapy may enhance sexual response.

Narcotic drugs and drugs of habituation, including alcohol, are central depressants and interfere with sexual response. Chronic addiction with poor general health may result in diminished testosterone levels. Hallucinogens may heighten sensitivity, but chronic use of marijuana can lead to impaired testosterone secretion.

Drugs acting through hormonal mechanisms include estrogens, which depress gonadotropin secretion and produce a state of secondary hypogonadism; thus, impotence is usual when estrogens are used in the therapy of prostatic carcinoma. Other drugs with antiandrogenic properties include spironolactone and glucocorticoids. The importance of hyperprolactinemia as a cause of impotence is unclear; nevertheless, drugs with an antidopaminergic action may cause increased prolactin levels and impotence, while the use of L-dopa has been shown to improve sexual function in men with parkinsonism.

The clinician must be aware of the potential sexual side effects of drugs and should avoid high-risk drugs whenever possible. Patients on therapy should be questioned regarding sexual problems, since there is a well-known disinclination to volunteer such complaints.

The range of physical and mental illness and disability that may affect sexual function is enormous. In some instances, organic sexual dysfunction is present, in others, psychosocial factors induce the dysfunction, and in a third group, sexual activity is modified as a result of physical illness. Here again, these changes have been mainly studied in the male.

Adequate sexual function requires intact vascular, neurologic, and endocrine function. Neurologic disorders, including spinal cord injury or multiple sclerosis, severely impair function, as does diabetes, the last probably via a peripheral autonomic neuropathy. Vascular disease, particularly of the pelvic arteries and veins, may compromise engorgement enough to cause impotence. Endocrine disorders influence sexuality, commonly those in which androgen levels are low as in patients on chronic hemodialysis. Thyroid, pituitary, adrenal, and ovarian disorders frequently influence sexuality adversely because of the hormonal imbalance present.

Illness or surgery involving the genitalia also causes sexual problems. These include urologic and gynecologic disorders, pelvic cancer, congenital and acquired anatomic defects, as well as sexually transmitted diseases. Procedures commonly implicated include hysterectomy, prostatectomy, castration, and radiotherapy.

Many chronic illnesses require marked sexual adjustments. These include painful conditions, such as arthritis, or the aftermath of major trauma, as well as disabling chronic respiratory disease, chronic renal failure, and chronic alcoholism. Cardiac disease, especially following myocardial infarction, frequently interferes with sexual activity.

The most common cause of sexual dysfunction is psychosocial. Physical illness normally causes marked anxiety, anger, grief, and depression, all of which frequently interfere with sexual function. This is particularly true when illness, trauma, or surgery involve change of body-image or loss of body parts with sexual connotation. For instance, mastectomy and "ostomy" patients are often left with sexual maladjustment, even though they are physiologically intact.

In managing the patient, organic and psychogenic factors must be assessed, and the impact on the family system evaluated. Counseling should be preventive whenever possible (e.g., before surgery), and should be specific and fitted to the individual. The spouse must be included, since the partner's role is crucial to therapeutic success. Treatment is generally behavioral as well as educational, informative, and psychotherapeutic, when indicated. In some instances, surgery in the form of giving the patient a penile prosthesis may be most helpful.

Aging

1. Friedeman, J. S. Factors influencing sexual expression in aging persons: A review of the literature. *J. Psychiatr. Nurs.* 16:34, 1978.
   Suggests that studies are sparse and the data equivocal.
2. Kaplan, H. S. *The New Sex Therapy.* New York: Brunner/Mazel, 1974.
   Good sexual experiences in youth lead to good experiences in old age (use it or lose it).
3. Finkle, A. L. Psychosexual problems of aging men: Urologist's viewpoint. *Urology* 13:39, 1979.
   Counseling may solve sexual problems of aging men, especially relative to threatening procedures such as prostatectomy.
4. Pfeiffer, E., Verwoerdt, A., and Wang, H. S. The natural history of sexual behavior in a biologically advantaged group of aged individuals. *J. Gerontol.* 24:193, 1969.
   There was no age group in which sexual interest or intercourse had disappeared.
5. Newman, G., and Nichols, C. R. Sexual activities and attitudes in older persons. *J.A.M.A.* 173:33, 1960.
   The first extensive longitudinal study.

Drugs

6. Editorial. Drugs and male sexual function. *Br. Med. J.* 13:883, 1979.
   Importance of male sex hormones is unclear; erections can occur in castrated men.
7. Brown, E., et al. Sexual function and affect in parkinsonian men treated with L-dopa. *Am. J. Psychiatry* 135:1552, 1978.
   Half the patients had improved sexual interest unrelated to improved locomotor function.
8. Wilson, G. T., and Lawson, D. M. Effects of alcohol on sexual arousal in women. *J. Abnorm. Psychol.* 85:489, 1976.
   As Shakespeare said, alcohol provokes the desire but takes away the performance.
9. Kolodny, R. C. Effects of alpha-methyldopa on male sexual function. *Sex. Disability* 1:223, 1978.
   Hypotensive agents may affect various aspects of male sexuality including libido, potency, and ejaculation.

Diseases

10. Jackson, G. Sexual intercourse and angina pectoris. *Br. Med. J.* 2:16, 1978.
    Beta-blockade minimized cardiovascular changes with sex such that 33 of 35 patients enjoyed pain-free intercourse.
11. Hellerstein, H. K., and Friedman, E. H. Sexual activity and the post-coronary patient. *Arch. Intern. Med.* 125:987, 1970.
    Once the patient can manage two flights of stairs comfortably intercourse may be resumed.
12. Ellenberg, M. Sexual function in diabetic patients. *Ann. Intern. Med.* 92:331, 1980.
    Impotence in diabetic men averages 50%, whereas the disease has no demonstrable effect on the female diabetic's sexuality.
13. Capone, M. A., et al. Psychosocial rehabilitation of gynecologic oncology patients. *Arch. Phys. Med. Rehabil.* 61:128, 1980.
    Counseling had a positive effect in enhancing return to normal sexual function.
14. Bors, E., and Comarr, A. E. Neurological disturbances of sexual function with special reference to 529 patients with spinal cord injury. *Urological Survey* 9–10:191, 1960.
    The incidence of psychogenic erections, reflexogenic erections, and ejaculation depends on level of cord injury.
15. Witkin, M. H. Sex therapy and mastectomy. *J. Sex Marital Ther.* 1:290, 1975.
    Preoperative and postoperative counseling, sex therapy, prostheses, and possible reconstructive surgery are important in management.
16. McGuire, L. S., Guzinski, G. M., and Holmes, K. K. Psychosexual functioning in symptomatic and asymptomatic women with and without signs of vaginitis. *Am. J. Obstet. Gynecol.* 137:600, 1980.
    The authors make the tentative suggestion that vaginal symptoms may be useful in alleviating some anxiety over sexual and marital matters.
17. Seibel, M. M., Freeman, M. G., and Graves, W. L. Carcinoma of the cervix and sexual function. *Obstet. Gynecol.* 55:484, 1980.
    Irradiated patients had significant decreases in sexual function, but a surgically treated group did not.
18. Zussman, L., et al. Sexual response after hysterectomy-oophorectomy: Recent studies and reconsideration of psychogenesis. *Am. J. Obstet. Gynecol.* 140:725, 1981.
    One in four American women reach menopause through surgery. Hormone replacement or sex therapy, or both may help the 33% to 46% who report decreased sexual response following surgery.

Female Orgasmic Dysfunction

The most common sexual problem encountered in the female is difficulty in reaching orgasm. If orgasm has never been experienced, this is called primary orgasmic dysfunction. A woman who has previously had orgasm but is now unable to, is said to have secondary orgasmic dysfunction. Secondary dysfunction may be intermittent, selective, or situational. A further distinction is drawn between those women who reach orgasm with masturbation but not with intercourse.

Female orgasmic dysfunction is reported to be present to some degree in about 50% of normal married couples. About 15% are unable to have orgasm. There appears to be little difference in incidence related to social class. Common problems include difficulty in getting and maintaining excitement, in addition to difficulty in reaching orgasm.

Normal married women also report a high incidence of "sexual difficulties," including disinterest (35%), inability to relax (47%), inconvenient time chosen by partner (31%), too little foreplay before (38%), and too little tenderness after (25%). It must be recalled that these figures quoted are for normal, happily married couples.

The two basic generalized responses to elevated levels of sexual tension are myotonia and vasocongestion. During the excitement phase of the female sexual response cycle, vasocongestion of the tissues around the vagina with intravaginal transudation result in vaginal lubrication. Further vasocongestion develops in the outer third of the vagina, creating a partial narrowing of the central lumen, while the upper part of the vagina expands and distends. The clitoris elevates and flattens on the anterior border of the symphysis. This plateau phase of response is followed by orgasm, which is characterized by the outer third of the vagina and the uterus contracting rhythmically. (Another interpretation is that it is the pubococcygeus muscle that undergoes the orgasmic contractions.) Finally, the resolution phase, with disappearance of myotonia and vasocongestion, follows. This is rapid if orgasm has occurred but is slow and leaves residual sexual tension if orgasm has not been achieved.

Sociocultural deprivation and ignorance, rather than psychiatric or medical illness, are thought to constitute the etiologic background for most sexual dysfunction. Sex is a physiologic function often interfered with by myths and taboos. There is never an uninvolved partner in a sexual problem, and usually it is the relationship that is the patient. For instance, male potency problems, such as premature ejaculation, may be the cause of female orgasmic difficulties.

Sexual problems often stem from repressive social and religious attitudes, faulty parental unbringing, and poor experiential learning. Frequently, performance anxiety, fear of failure, and "spectatoring" aggravate the situation. Often, the sexual problem is only part of a larger marital dysfunction such that resentment and hostility interfere with the sexual relationship. Communication between the partners may be poor or absent, and lack of communication is a major source of sexual difficulties.

The primary-care physician can deal with many patients with orgasmic difficulties; however, some should be referred for more intensive therapy. A careful general and sexual history with a full physical and pelvic examination provides the clinician with the basic information required to triage the patient. The presence of severe anxiety, depression, or psychosis would suggest psychiatric referral. A finding of major marital disharmony might result in referral for marital therapy. Abnormal medical, surgical, or gynecologic findings would indicate the relevant referrals. Clearly, the expertise of the individual physician influences the incidence of referral. When in doubt, the doctor can commence therapy and be guided in future management by the response.

Many sexual concerns can be handled by giving the client permission to engage or not engage in certain sexual behaviors. Reassurance from a professional that there is nothing wrong or bad about what they are or are not doing is most helpful, as, too, is the information that similar concerns are common and are shared by many other people.

While it is possible to be effective while seeing only one member of a couple, it is preferable to see both. Commonly, one or two half-hour meetings a week can be set aside to interview and counsel the couple. Every effort must be made to remain nonjudgmental and not to be premature or hasty in advising or reassuring the couple regarding specific problems.

A major role of the clinician is that of education. Misconceptions, myths, bad sexual experiences, and faulty information need to be discussed and factual information provided. The physician, by providing support and specific information, may also prevent many sexual concerns. For instance, he can give careful and thorough counseling prior to surgical interventions such as hysterectomy or mastectomy that are not infrequently followed by sexual dysfunction.

In dealing with problems related to the female orgasm, it is important to identify and treat dysfunction such as premature ejaculation in the partner. Certain diseases including thyroid dysfunction, diabetes, or neurologic or vascular disorders must be excluded during the workup, as, too, must physical causes of dyspareunia. Depressive illness and the use of many drugs have profound sexual implications and must be kept in mind during the evaluation.

In counseling the couple, the importance of foreplay, the desire of most women to be courted, and advice regarding the time, place, and form of sexual contact are outlined. If the problem is one of orgasm by clitoral stimulation only, rather than with intercourse, it may be possible to get the patient to accept the situation as a normal response. If not, continuation of manual or vibrator masturbation by the partner or patient during intercourse may be used as a "bridging" technique until, by experiential learning, orgasm may occur during coitus. In general, better clitoral contact and stimulation are obtained in the female superior position, rather than in the more generally used "missionary" position.

The prognosis for the patient with orgasmic difficulty is not easy to predict since reported studies differ in definitions, length and type of therapy, interpretation of cure, and length of follow-up. In general, it would appear that these problems are neither easy nor impossible to cure. The primary-care physician has an important role in screening patients, taking into account physical as well as psychopathologic problems. All treatment modalities should be considered, including education, desensitization, sexual skill training, and behavioral modification. It is as essential for the clinician to remain current in new developments in sexual medicine as in any other field.

When simple advice and information are insufficient, behavioral modification can be employed. The use of sensate focus exercises, which are directed away from the genitals and toward the many other sources of sexual pleasure, such as holding, kissing, and massaging, can be suggested. The use of lubrication jellies and vibrators, as well as using various positions during intercourse, may be very helpful. Techniques of masturbation, genital touching, and oral-genital sexuality may be discussed, and exercises for the pubococcygeus muscles taught and practiced. There should be a continual emphasis on bettering the couple's communication skills at all levels, including the sexual. Many practitioners may not be comfortable in, or may lack the experience or background for, supervising therapy of this nature, so may wish to refer the patient. If there is no response to therapy, it may be that the sexual problem has a neurotic or characterologic basis, and referral for psychotherapy may be necessary.

Reviews

1. Pion, R. J., and Reich, L. A. Management of sexual disorders. *J. Reprod. Med.* 20:56, 1978.

Cognition (thinking) and affects (feeling) are highlighted in this learning and behavior-oriented approach.

2. Kilmann, P. R. The treatment of primary and secondary orgasmic dysfunction: A methodological review of the literature since 1970. *J. Sex Marital Ther.* 4:155, 1978.
Points out major methodologic deficiencies in the studies reviewed.

3. O'Connor, J. F. Effectiveness of psychological treatment of human sexual dysfunction. *Clin. Obstet. Gynecol.* 19:449, 1976.
Reviews behavioral and group therapy, hypnosis, psychotherapy, and rapid treatment techniques.

Physiology, Incidence, Etiology

4. Masters, W., and Johnson, V. *Human Sexual Response.* Boston: Little, Brown, 1966.
The classic reference—unfortunately difficult reading.

5. Masters, W., and Johnson, V. *Human Sexual Inadequacy.* Boston: Little, Brown, 1970.
Equally classic—just as difficult to read.

6. Frank, E., Anderson, C., and Rubinstein, D. Frequency of sexual dysfunction in "normal" couples. *N. Engl. J. Med.* 299:111, 1978.
Suggests that there is an epidemic of sexual dysfunction and unhappiness.

7. Gambrell, R. D., Jr., et al. Changes in sexual drives of patients on oral contraceptives. *J. Reprod. Med.* 17:165, 1976.
While it seems likely that highly progestogenic pills would possibly lead to a loss of libido, removal of pregnancy fears has a reverse effect, hence no consistent findings emerge.

8. Andreasen, N. C. Sexual problems and affective disorders. *Med. Aspects Hum. Sex.* 15:134, 1981.
Sexual disinterest in depression and elevated or misdirected sexuality in manic states frequently cause marital problems.

9. Johnson, S. R., et al. Factors influencing lesbian gynecologic care: A preliminary study. *Am. J. Obstet. Gynecol.* 140:20, 1981.
It is estimated that 5% of the general population are lesbians. In this study of 117 female homosexuals, many expressed concern about physicians' negative attitudes to homosexuals.

10. Wells, C. G., Lucas, M. J., and Meyer, K. Jr. Unrealistic expectations of orgasm. *Med. Aspects Hum. Sex.* 14:53, 1980.
Modern woman is expected to be assertive, independent, and multiorgasmic. This alteration from traditional dependency, passivity, asexuality, and nurturing is replete with conflict and fear for the woman.

Management

11. Burchell, R. C. Coital positions. *Med. Aspects Hum. Sex.* 9:51, 1975.
Variety is the spice of love.

12. Kegel, A. Sexual function of the pubococcygeus muscle. *West. J. Surg. Obstet. Gynecol.* 60:521, 1952.
Regular pelvic floor exercises appear to increase vaginal perception and sensation during genital intercourse.

13. Riley, A. J., and Riley, E. J. A controlled study to evaluate directed masturbation in the management of primary orgasmic failure in women. *Br. J. Psychiatry* 133:404, 1978.
In this study 85% of patients became coitally orgasmic as compared with 47% treated with sensate focus and supportive counseling only.

14. Witkin, M. H. Procedures to enhance female coital response. *Med. Aspects Hum. Sex.* 14:87, 1980.
   Anxiety and "spectatoring" (the woman detaches herself from her experience to monitor her own performance and responsiveness) are significant barriers to sexual satisfaction.

Problems of Orgasmic Response in the Male

Erection results from distension of vascular spaces in the penis; parasympathetic cholinergic fibers and adequate blood supply are critical factors at this stage. The term used for failure to achieve or sustain erection is *erectile impotence.* The next phase is contraction of the vasa deferentia, prostate, and seminal vesicles, which is under sympathetic adrenergic control. Semen enters the bulbous urethra and ejaculation follows, inevitably and immediately. The parasympathetic reflex that produces ejaculation causes rhythmic contraction of the bulbocavernosus muscles, expelling the semen. The bladder neck is tightly closed by a sympathetic reflex at the same time, thus preventing retrograde intravesical flow. Failure of this stage is referred to as *ejaculatory failure.*

Impotence, the inability of a male to achieve and maintain an erection sufficient for vaginal penetration and intercourse, may be primary or secondary. The latter always follows a period of normal erectile function. Situational impotence is experienced by all men, at one time or another, and is commonly associated with fatigue, stress, and alcohol. The incidence of persistent impotence is about 1 per 1000 at age 20 years and gradually rises to 7% in men 75 years of age or older.

An estimated 90% of cases are caused by psychological factors. Sexual and nonsexual problems related to spouse, family, work, and finances may engender anxiety or depression, with serious adverse effects on libido and sexual function. Sometimes a sexual dysfunction in the partner is the underlying causative factor.

Modern research suggests that organic causes are much more common than were once thought. For instance, endocrine disorders (such as hypogonadism, hypothyroidism and hyperthyroidism, and hyperprolactinemia) have been associated with impotence. Neurologic and vascular diseases, as well as many drugs, also interfere with the penile erection and ejaculatory reflexes.

Diagnosis depends on taking a careful history with particular reference to physical factors such as diabetes, alcoholism, and drugs. A detailed psychosexual history is taken, and evidence of depressive illness must be sought. A history of nocturnal and waking erections, as well as erections following tactile stimulation, may suggest psychologic impotence, while a slowly progressive decline in erectile function suggests organic causes. The marital relationship should also be assessed, with both partners if possible.

The physical examination should include vascular and neurologic assessment, as well as assessment of testicular volume and secondary sexual characteristics. Anxieties regarding penile size may be assuaged at this time.

Special investigations, such as a glucose tolerance test, will be suggested by the clinical situation. If hypogonadism is suspected, measurements of serum testosterone, gonadotropins, and prolactin should be obtained. Should facilities be available, nocturnal penile tumescence studies are most helpful in distinguishing organic from psychogenic causes.

Management should include medical, surgical, psychiatric, sexual, and marital counseling, tailored to the individual patient. It is important to keep in mind that psychogenic factors aggravate many organic problems and should not be neglected in therapy.

Defective sexual skills due to ignorance or misinformation and obsessive concerns over sexual performance are common and require correction through education and counseling. Behavioral alterations directed at removing performance anxiety include the use of self-stimulation, sensate focus exercises, and techniques such as "stuffing" (in which the flaccid penis is literally stuffed into the vagina with no requirement for actual intercourse).

Drug therapy is indicated only for specific reasons, such as injections of testosterone for patients with clinical and biochemical evidence of hypogonadism or bromocriptine in some impotent men with hyperprolactinemia. The place of androgens in normal men remains highly controversial, and it must be realized that exogenous androgens inhibit spermatogenesis, may elevate cholesterol, and may cause polycythemia and cholestatic jaundice.

Prosthetic surgery may be considered if psychologic treatment fails and in some cases of organic impotence. Sexual counseling of both partners, with careful psychological screening preoperatively, is essential for a successful outcome.

The prognosis is worse if significant depression and poor libido are present. A stable marital/sexual relationship is critical. Success rates of 69% for secondary and 59% for primary impotence have been reported.

Premature ejaculation is probably the most frequent sexual disorder. There is no known common physical cause, and, in fact, early orgasm is essentially natural, especially in the younger male. Delay of ejaculation is, therefore, probably a culturally induced expectation requiring a positive effort on the part of the male participant. While definition is difficult, ejaculation during foreplay or immediately prior to penetration clearly fits the diagnosis. Once intromission has occurred, the number of thrusts, partner satisfaction, and period of time in the vagina are arbitrary diagnostic criteria used in attempts at defining the problem. Incidence of the disorder is independent of education, race, marital status, or occupation. It occurs in good and bad marriages, as well as in men with or without psychiatric problems.

The causes appear to be multiple and probably function through a common mechanism of increased anxiety and muscular tension. Faulty learning via initial sexual experiences with furtive masturbation, backseat intercourse, and impatient prostitutes may lead to rapid ejaculation becoming a conditioned reflex to sexual stimuli. In the marital context, the symptom may be used as a weapon by either partner to serve destructive functions in the transactional relationship of the couple. Not infrequently, the complaint may be secondary to a masked female sexual dysfunction.

Sexual counseling of the couple is usually highly successful. Careful history taking for both remote and recent factors contributing to the condition, together with information and education, is combined with behavioral techniques aimed at extending voluntary control over the ejaculatory reflex. These include vaginal containment without thrusting (to acclimate the penis) and the "stop and go" technique (in which intercourse is interrupted to allow arousal to diminish). Another valuable technique is firm squeezing of the glans penis to end excitement intermittently.

Retarded ejaculation is a relatively rare disorder and is psychologic in origin. Management is based to some extent on use of a reversal of the behavioral techniques employed for premature ejaculation, as well as using those techniques employed for the female with the essentially similar complaint, "failure to reach orgasm."

Review
1. Burger, H., and Rose, N. Sexual impotence. *Med. J. Aust.* 2:24, 1979.
   Helpful summary.
2. Smith, A. D. Causes and classification of impotence. *Urol. Clin. N. Am.* 8:87, 1981.
   Recent studies indicate that male impotence may be of truly psychogenic origin in as little as 38% of cases.

Diagnosis
3. Shrom, S. H., Lief, H. I., and Wein, A. J. Clinical profile of experience with 130 consecutive cases of impotent men. *Urology* 13:511, 1979.
   Obtaining an adequate erection with failure to maintain it is virtually diagnostic of functional impotence.
4. Karacan, I., et al. Nocturnal penile tumescence and diagnosis in diabetic impotence. *Am. J. Psychiatry* 135:191, 1978.
   Three nights of recording penile measurements are essential, as well as waking the patient to confirm that the erection is sufficiently rigid for vaginal penetration.
5. Malvar, R., Baron, T., and Clark, S. S. Assessment of potency with the Doppler flowmeter. *Urology* 2:396, 1973.
   Blood flow studies and penile blood pressure recordings may be used in assessing neurovascular mechanisms of erectile capacity.
6. Jevtich, M. J. Penile body temperature as screening test for penile arterial obstruction in impotence. *Urology* 17:2, 1981.
   A differential of 3 degrees between intraurethral and sublingual temperatures is thought to be significant.
7. Spark, R. F., White, R. A., and Connolly, P. B. Impotence is not always psychogenic. Newer insights into hypothalamic-pituitary-gonadal dysfunction. *J.A.M.A.* 243:750, 1980.
   Screening serum testosterone levels of 105 consecutive patients with impotence showed that 37 had disorders of the hypothalamic-pituitary-gonadal axis.
8. Deutsch, S., and Sherman, L. Previously unrecognized diabetes mellitus in sexually impotent men. *J.A.M.A.* 244:2430, 1980.
   Seven of 58 men (12.5%) with secondary impotence were found to have diabetes.
9. Miller, J. B., Howards, S. S., and McLeod, R. M. Serum prolactin in organic and psychogenic impotence. *J. Urol.* 123:862, 1980.
   Impotence did not seem to be related to hyperprolactinemia in the absence of pituitary disease.

Management
10. Lundberg, P. O., and Wide, L. Sexual function in males with pituitary tumors. *Fertil. Steril.* 29:175, 1978.
    Absent libido-potency was related to low testosterone levels, not hyperprolactinemia. Administration of testosterone yielded good results.
11. Scott, F. B., Fishman, I. J., and Light, J. K. An inflatable penile prosthesis for treatment of diabetic impotence. *Ann. Intern. Med.* 92:340, 1980.
    In this report on 50 patients, there was a 95% success rate, and the infection incidence was under 2%.

12. Bommer, J., et al. Improved sexual function in male haemodialysis patients on bromocriptine. *Lancet* 2:496, 1979.
   Bromocriptine, a dopaminergic agonist, reduced prolactin levels and improved sexual function; severe side effects (e.g., hypotension) were common. Testosterone levels were not taken.

13. Small, M. P., Carrion, H. M., and Gordon, J. A. Small-Carrion penile prosthesis, new implant for management of impotence. *Urology* 5:479, 1975.
   Paired silicone rubber rods are implanted in the corpora.

14. Annon, J. S. *The Behavioral Treatment of Sexual Problems.* Honolulu: Enabling Systems, 1974.
   It is what you do with what you have, rather than what you have that counts.

15. Schiavi, R. C. Psychological treatment of erectile disorders in diabetic patients. *Ann. Intern. Med.* 92:337, 1980.
   Psychological and organic factors may interact.

Premature Ejaculation

16. Weis, H. D. The physiology of human penile erection. *Ann. Intern. Med.* 76:793, 1972.
   Parasympathetic fibers (nervi erigentes) act on the vascular spaces, their action being mediated by acetylcholine.

17. Derogatis, L. R. Etiologic factors in premature ejaculation. *Med. Aspects Hum. Sex.* 14:32, 1980.
   Never occurs during solitary masturbation.

18. Cooper, A. J. Causes of premature ejaculation. *Med. Aspects Hum. Sex.* 15:76A, 1981.
   Causes of premature ejaculation include organic factors, interpersonal conflicts, habituation to rapid ejaculation, or faulty sexual techniques. However, anxiety is the most significant underlying cause.

Dyspareunia and Vaginismus

Dyspareunia is defined as pain associated with coitus. It may be of organic or psychologic origin. However, even if the basic cause is organic, the discomfort frequently results in a particular pattern of behavior that may persist even after the basic cause is dealt with. The sexual problem must, therefore, be treated together with the underlying physical condition.

Dyspareunia is generally divided into two categories: superficial dyspareunia, in which the pain is perceived at or near the introitus; and deep dyspareunia, when the pain is perceived as deep in the vagina or lower abdomen.

The physical causes of superficial pain on entry include inflammatory disease of the vulva, vagina, and bladder, such as any of the forms of vulvovaginitis, urethritis, trigonitis, and Bartholinitis. Postoperative tender or contracted scars, especially those following episiotomy or vaginal repair surgery, are common causes. In the older woman, lack of estrogen or vulvar dystrophy frequently lead to discontinuation of intercourse because of pain. In the younger patient, a rigid hymen or developmental anomaly of the vagina are obvious etiologic factors. Traumatic factors include errors in sexual technique, such as an absence of foreplay, leading to poor lubrication, or conversely, overzealous clitoral stimulation. Foreign bodies, including coital aids, are occasional causes of dyspareunia, as too, is anal intercourse without sufficient prelubrication. Contraceptive chemicals, feminine sprays, and vaginal douches are also possible causes as a result of vaginitis medicamentosa.

The physical causes of deeply situated coital pain are often less obvious and more difficult to diagnose or differentiate from psychologic causes. In most instances, endometriosis or pelvic inflammatory disease cause the symptom as a result of inflammation, adhesions, and endometriotic or inflammatory adnexal masses. The pain that may follow pelvic surgery can be due to adhesions, scarring, or because an ovary has been sutured to the vaginal cuff. Radiation therapy and radical pelvic surgery or pelvic neoplasms may cause sufficient anatomic distortion as to cause dyspareunia and even apareunia (absent intercourse). While a retrodisplaced uterus is a frequently encountered normal variation, on occasion an ovary displaced to the cul-de-sac, or a tender retroflexed uterine fundus may lead to "deep thrust" dyspareunia. Uterine prolapse, especially if of major degree, also impairs sexual function and may cause coital pain. Cervical lacerations and scars can also be significant etiologic factors.

The "pelvic congestion syndrome" may be a common cause of deep dyspareunia. These patients complain of a vague ache in the lower abdomen and pelvic region after intercourse and frequently also have minor menstrual irregularities and dysmenorrhea. Physical findings are negative or the uterus may be somewhat enlarged, boggy, tender, and retroflexed. It is thought that the syndrome results from an inadequate sexual response, resulting in chronic pelvic congestion. In cases coming to surgery, pelvic varicosities and broad ligament edema are sometimes encountered. However, since no abnormal histopathologic findings are present, many gynecologists do not accept the syndrome as a diagnostic entity.

Of patients with long-standing dyspareunia 60%–70% have no identifiable organic factors present. The psychologic factors involved may be specifically sexual, such as fear, disinterest, ignorance, and anxiety. They may involve the relationship with the partner, who may himself have a sexual dysfunction, or toward whom the patient may have feelings of hostility. There is on occasion a history of a previous negative experience, such as rape or a homosexual encounter. As a rule, many factors coexist in the individual patient, and other symptoms such as anorgasmia are present.

Dyspareunia occurs in from 4%–40% of gynecologic patients. It may be primary or secondary (following previously painless coitus), complete or specific (only in particular circumstances). There are often multiple associated symptoms, including dysmenorrhea, pelvic and abdominal pain, menstrual irregularity, problems with contraception, infertility, depression, and tension headaches.

The incidence of the various etiologic factors varies. It is likely that some 30% of cases have an organic basis, 30% an interpersonal (relationship) problem, and 40% an intrapersonal (intrapsychic) etiology. Commonly, more than one factor is present in the individual patient.

The diagnosis is dependent on the history, with particular reference to the site and duration of pain, and on physical examination, when different maneuvers should be employed to reproduce the same kind of pain the patient feels during coitus. Special investigations may be helpful in certain circumstances, in particular, laparoscopy, which may be essential in establishing the diagnosis of minimal endometriosis or confirming the absence of genital pathology.

The organic and psychologic components of the problem having been identified, therapy is directed toward ameliorating these factors. The patient and, if possible, her partner should be educated and reassured regarding the nature and prognosis of the problem. Organic disease is dealt with by standard pharmacologic or surgical methods, as for instance in the therapy of atrophic vaginitis with estrogen, or endometriosis with danazol or surgery. When indicated, marital/sexual therapy should be offered, with particular emphasis on the couple's communication skills or lack thereof, sensate focus exercises, relaxation, and masturbatory techniques.

Specific behavioral techniques include changes in coital position, Kegel's pelvic floor exercises, and vaginal self-dilation with lubricated fingers and graduated dilators. Specific surgical procedures indicated for introital dyspareunia include excision of painful scars with resuture in the transverse plane or hymenotomy for the unruptured or inadequately ruptured hymen. Plastic surgical procedures to the vulva or vagina (perineoplasty, vaginoplasty), or both, may be required to correct congenital or surgically acquired disorders not amenable to progressive self-dilation.

Specific surgical procedures for deep dyspareunia unresponsive to standard therapy include ventral suspension of the retroverted uterus with ovaries prolapsed in the cul-de-sac, or hysterectomy in a few carefully selected patients with disabling symptomatology who have no wish for conception. In patients with postoperative adhesions or with ovaries trapped in the cul-de-sac, lysis of adhesions and removal or resuspension of the ovaries may be indicated.

All surgical procedures also require psychologic/marital/sexual therapy as indicated in order to obtain best results. In general, prognosis is good, with some 60%–90% of patients responding to treatment. The best results are generally obtained in patients with organic disorders, the worst in those with interpersonal problems.

Prophylaxis, as always, is superior to therapy. Use of midline rather than mediolateral episiotomy has markedly diminished the incidence of episiotomy pain. Posterior vaginal wall repair procedures, once associated with a 30% incidence of dyspareunia, are now performed only for symptomatic rectocele and great care is taken to avoid introital stenosis. Unfortunately, because sex education and premarital examination and counseling have yet to extend to even a minority of women, ignorance of sexual technique or physiology is still widespread.

Vaginismus is defined as an involuntary reflex spasm of the perineal and levator ani muscles surrounding the outer third of the vagina in response to attempts at vaginal penetration. Vaginismus and dyspareunia are linked symptoms: each may cause the other. A vicious cycle, involving fear of pain with coitus and resultant anxiety, is set up. Sexual response may or may not be present. Psychogenic factors predominate but an organic etiology with resulting dyspareunia must also be sought.

Management is the same as for patients with dyspareunia, with special emphasis on the pelvic assessment; this is not only diagnostic but should be used as an important educational tool in instructing the patient regarding home self-dilation and pelvic floor exercises. Results are excellent, with success rates of 80%–100%. Examination under anesthesia or hymenotomy is not helpful in the absence of organic factors.

Review

1. Fordney, D. S. Dyspareunia and vaginismus. *Clin. Obstet. Gynecol.* 21:205, 1978.

Contains detailed descriptions of Kegel's pubococcygeus exercises and of vaginal self-dilation procedures.

Dyspareunia

2. Lamont, J. A. Female dyspareunia. *Am. J. Obstet. Gynecol.* 136:282, 1980.
   This article covers a series of 230 women, of whom 78 refused treatment. The patients who refused treatment were mostly from the groups in whom interpersonal and intrapersonal problems were thought to be the major etiologic factors.
3. Woodruff, J. D., Genadry, R., and Poliakoff, S. Treatment of dyspareunia and vaginal outlet distortions by perineoplasty. *Obstet. Gynecol.* 57:750, 1981.
   Gives causes, technique, results in 42 cases.
4. Munsick, R. A. Introital operations for dyspareunia. *Clin. Obstet. Gynecol.* 23:243, 1980.
   Contains detailed description of the O'Donnell operation for the relief of relative hypospadias potentiated by inadequate rupture of the hymen, causing chronic inflammation of the lower part of the urinary tract with dyspareunia and recurrent cystitis ("honeymoon cystitis").
5. Batts, J. A., Jr. Deep thrust dyspareunia. *Med. Aspects Hum. Sex.* 12:107, 1978.
   The author advocates prophylactic suture of the adnexa to the round ligaments in the lateral position at the time of hysterectomy, thus keeping the ovaries out of the cul-de-sac.
6. Huffmann, J. W. Uterine displacement as a cause of dyspareunia. *Med. Aspects Hum. Sex.* 10:62, 1976.
   The clinician must determine whether the pain is due to the retroflexion per se, or due to the pathology holding the uterus in retroflexion, e.g., endometriosis or chronically inflamed adnexa.
7. Allen, W. M., and Masters, W. H. Traumatic laceration of uterine support: The clinical syndrome and the operative treatment. *Am. J. Obstet. Gynecol.* 70:500, 1955.
   The authors feel that broad and sacrouterine ligament lacerations following pelvic trauma or childbirth may cause severe dyspareunia and will then require surgical correction.
8. Grillo, L., and Grillo, D. Management of dyspareunia secondary to hymenal remnants. *Obstet. Gynecol.* 56:510, 1980.
   Surgical removal followed by sexual therapy and progressive vaginal dilatation.

Vaginismus

9. Lamont, J. A. Vaginismus. *Am. J. Obstet. Gynecol.* 131:632, 1978.
   In this series of 80 patients, physical factors were responsible for the vaginismus in 24; during therapy 15 male partners experienced situational impotence.
10. Fertel, N. Vaginismus: A review. *J. Sex Marital Ther.* 3:113, 1977.
   Analytic theories suggest that fear and anxiety are etiologic factors. Behavioral theories suggest that the fear and anxiety are learned or conditioned dysfunctions reactive to painful and stressful coital experiences.
11. Fuchs, K. Therapy of vaginismus by hypnotic desensitization. *Am. J. Obstet. Gynecol.* 137:1, 1980.
   A combination of hypnosis, systematic desensitization, and the use of graded Hegar dilators cured 53 of 54 cases.

Rape

Rape is coitus or attempted coitus by force, or the threat of force, with a woman without her consent. Rape is not a medical diagnosis and establishing whether rape occurred is a legal, not a medical, task. Nevertheless, the medical attendant has the responsibility, in addition to the purely medical management, of also establishing whether intercourse has occurred and of collecting legal evidence, safeguarding the legal records, and protecting the chain of evidence.

Rape is the fastest growing of the crimes of violence, with an incidence of over 52,000 cases annually; furthermore, only a minority report the incident to the police. Changing public attitudes and the introduction of rape crisis centers, as well as increasing efforts at bringing rapists to justice make it imperative that doctors alter their previous reluctance to care for the victims of sexual assault. Adequate instruction in the medical, psychologic, and legal requirements of these patients, together with knowledgeable assistants and a careful protocol of management, will result in a better medical and legal outcome.

Rape victims are usually young, single females, the majority not using an ongoing form of birth control. Unfortunately, though understandably, about a third of patients change clothes, bathe, or douche before presenting themselves for examination.

Some victims may be pregnant and others may have had recent intercourse with consent. Race of victims and assailants varies; in one series, race was concordant in 55%, discordant in 8%, and unrecorded in the remainder. Assailants may be single or multiple, and coercive force is common, frequently with the threat of the use of weapons. Children are commonly molested by adults known to them rather than by strangers, although the opposite holds true for mature women. Rapes usually occur late at night, during weekends, often in the victim's or assailant's home, and in automobiles as well as in dwellings. About a third of victims suffer from multiple types of sexual assault, particularly rectal or oral penetration.

Rapists vary, although the pattern of rape is similar for the individual and can be used in identification. Rape is a sexual expression of conflict and the struggle for power involving violence and hostility. Often the rapist is seeking reassurance of virility and denying feelings of inadequacy. Because the act itself is unsatisfying to the rapist and will be repeated, the recidivism rate from prison is 57%. Rehabilitation programs may improve this unsatisfactory situation.

The psychological response to rape is an acute stress reaction to a life-threatening situation. Specific symptomatology may be expected. There is first an early phase of disorganization in lifestyle, characterized by physical symptoms and feelings of fear. Two to three weeks later a second phase of reorganization and coping begins with changes in lifestyle, phobic reactions, and motor activity being commonly encountered. For instance, it is common for the victim to change her accommodations. The "rape trauma syndrome" may be minimized by crisis counseling, close follow-up, reassurance, and support. The emotional state of the victim at the time of presentation may be very misleading. In one series, 73% were described as being calm, while the remainder varied from depressed to hysterical. The "silent" reaction does not imply that no problem exists; rather, it represents a method of coping no different, even if less obvious, than depression or hysteria.

The majority of victims present themselves for medical examination within 24 hours. Although some may not wish to use police services at first, this attitude may change, and all cases should be managed in similar fashion. Prior to the taking of a history and physical examination, consent forms specific for particular procedures should be completed. These include permission for photographs, special tests, and release of information to the relevant authorities. Documentation should be typed or at least legibly written, specimens must be clearly marked, and a "chain of evidence" form be used so that all people handling evidentiary material are identified.

History-taking includes a menstrual and contraceptive history and record of time of last coitus prior to assault. The circumstances of the assault are recorded, especially as regards injuries, penetration, ejaculation, extragenital acts, ingestion of drugs or alcohol, and whether clothes have been changed or a bath taken or douche used since the attack.

Physical examination for evidence of genital or extragenital trauma, with attention to hymenal and anal status, includes assessment of clothing and the presence of hair or stains on it. Pelvic examination is performed, with an unlubricated speculum, to check for discharges, blood, and lacerations, and for the collection of samples. Bimanual examination with particular reference to uterine size and pelvic hematomas completes the physical assessment.

The lab samples gathered include vaginal saline samples for sperm and for acid phosphatase. Pap, Gram's stain, and gonorrhea (GC) cultures are obtained, and, when applicable, rectal and oral GC cultures are also taken. Blood is drawn for serology, and when indicated, for alcohol and drug screen. Urine is sent for a pregnancy test and on occasion for drug screen. Pubic hair is combed and sent together with clipped samples of patient's pubic hair.

Treatment is directed first at injuries; if serious, liberal use of consultation, including radiology, is called for. Emotional care is essential, and the assistance of such personnel as psychiatric social workers, rape crisis center representatives, or specially trained nurses is most helpful.

Although the incidence of sexually transmitted disease is low, follow-up is usually poor, so antibiotic prophylaxis is commonly given. Therapy should be adequate to eradicate GC and incubating syphilis. If there is a risk of pregnancy, prophylaxis should be offered, although here again the incidence is low. Therapy must be given within 72 hours and consists of estrogen in high doses (example, Premarin 40 mg, three times a day for 3 days). Patients must be adequately counseled regarding the nausea and vomiting commonly encountered with the medication. All victims should be offered pregnancy termination should pregnancy result from the assault.

Physical follow-up is essential to assess healing of injuries and for pregnancy and venereal disease surveillance. No less important is emotional support and follow-up. Since the majority of victims fail to keep follow-up appointments, whenever possible the services of rape crisis centers or social and psychiatric workers should be employed to keep the patient in touch with the health services available.

In practice, the examining physician's testimony is only required in about 5% of cases. A well-performed and well-documented examination speaks for itself and may preclude the necessity for a court appearance and, if it does become necessary, will make such an appearance comfortable and nontraumatic.

Series and Review

1. Hicks, D. J. Rape: Sexual assault. *Am. J. Obstet. Gynecol.* 137:931, 1980. *The report from a Miami rape treatment center is based on the manage-*

ment of over 5000 victims. *Few suffered serious physical injuries, but all suffered psychologic trauma and required medical care and psychologic counseling to minimize the adverse effects of the assault.*
2. Soules, M. R., et al. The spectrum of alleged rape. *J. Reprod. Med.* 20:33, 1978.
   Prospective series of 110 victims, of whom only 6% returned for follow-up by appointment, an experience similar to that of other reports.
3. Evrard, J. R., and Gold, E. M. Epidemiology and management of sexual assault victims. *Obstet. Gynecol.* 53:381, 1979.
   Experience with 126 victims indicated the need for the integration of trained health and legal personnel, a protocol to satisfy the physical, psychologic, and evidentiary requirements of the patient, and an adequate follow-up system.

The Rapist
4. Burgess, A. W., and Groth, A. N. Address at the Workshop for Victimology. Fresno, Calif., May, 1976.
   Rape, although a sexual offense, is mainly concerned with anger, rage, revenge, power, and punishment. Sex is used as a weapon, and there is seldom sexual gratification to the assailant.
5. Groth, A. N., and Burgess, A. W. Sexual dysfunction during rape. *N. Engl. J. Med.* 297:764, 1977.
   Interviews with convicted rapists and victims suggest that 34% of rapists manifest sexual dysfunction. Impotence and retarded ejaculation were the most common forms of dysfunction reported.

The Victim
6. Massey, J. B., et al. Management of sexually assaulted females. *Obstet. Gynecol.* 38:29, 1971.
   Male victims are relatively uncommon.
7. Hayman, C. R., and Lanza, C. Sexual assault on women and girls. *Am. J. Obstet. Gynecol.* 109:480, 1970.
   Most victims are young and single, and a significant number have been raped before.
8. Finkelhor, D., and Yllo, K. *Forced Sex in Marriage: A Preliminary Report.* Family Violence Research Program, Department of Sociology, University of New Hampshire, January 7, 1980.
   Estimates of marital rape range from 400,000 to 2,000,000 per year. These assaults are almost never reported.
9. Seltzer, V. L., Hassman, H., and Bigelow, B. Abnormal Papanicolaou smears found in victims of sexual assault. *J. Reprod. Med.* 20:233, 1978.
   Of 116 women undergoing treatment for rape 4 were found to have abnormal Pap smears.

Psychology
10. Burgess, A. W., and Holmstrom, L. L. Rape trauma syndrome. *Am. J. Psychiatry* 131:9, 1974.
    Two stages are described: an immediate, acute phase with emotional responses that are expressed or controlled and are a response to a life-threatening situation; a long-term phase of reorganization, with changes in life style, phobic reactions, and dreams and nightmares.
11. Bohmer, C., and Blumburg, A. Twice traumatized—the rape victim and the court. *Judicature* 58:391, 1975.

The concept of the second traumatic event, the court appearance in this case, should not be allowed to also apply to the victim's medical management.

Statutory Rape

12. Schiff, A. R. Attending the child "rape" victim. *South. Med. J.* 72:906, 1979.
    Rarely was the assailant not known to the victim. Sexual intercourse was uncommon because of anatomic disproportion. Counseling of parents was essential.
13. McCary, J. L. Prevalent sexual myths. *Med. Aspects Hum. Sex.* 12:109, 1978.
    Pedophilia is often more traumatic to parents than to the child, and the reaction of the parents may be more harmful than the experience itself.
14. Walters, D. R. *Physical and Sexual Abuse of Children, Causes and Treatment.* Bloomington: Indiana University Press, 1975.
    Treatment of the entire family is essential, especially if incest is a factor. Therapy is frequently not wanted, and the family may choose to "forget it," since the problem is so difficult to face.
15. Peters, J. J. The Philadelphia rape victim study. Presented at the First International Symposium of Victimology, Jerusalem, September, 1973.
    Few studies exist on the long-term effects of sexual assault in childhood. In this study of assaulted children, it was noted that as adults, relationships frequently were either not established or proved to be unstable. Other studies have also indicated that child assailants were often themselves assaulted as children.

Laboratory Evidence

16. Soules, M. R., et al. The forensic laboratory evaluation of evidence in alleged rape. *Am. J. Obstet. Gynecol.* 130:143, 1978.
    Serial vaginal samples taken after intercourse from 15 volunteers revealed no instances of pubic hair transfer; acid phosphatase was absent in 50% by 9 hours, and sperm was present up to 72 hours in 50%.
17. Halbert, D. R., and Jones, D. E. D. Medical management of the sexually assaulted woman. *J. Reprod. Med.* 20:265, 1978.
    Details the evidentiary material required, lists supplies necessary for a "rape tray," and provides examples of a detailed patient consent form as well as a laboratory chain-of-evidence form.
18. Rupp, J. C. Sperm survival and prostatic acid phosphatase activity in victims of sexual assault. *J. Forensic Sci. Soc.* 12:363, 1972.
    Clothing samples should be retained in sealed plastic bags if they reveal tears or stains. The stains may retain sperm, acid phosphatase, and ABO antigens for months.

Medical Management

19. Hayman, C. R., and Lanza, C. Sexual assault on women and girls. *Am. J. Obstet. Gynecol.* 109:480, 1971.
    The risk of pregnancy from an isolated act of intercourse is around 1%. The incidence of pregnancy after rape is therefore very low.
20. Schroeter, A. L., et al. Therapy for incubating syphilis—effectiveness of gonorrhea treatment. *J.A.M.A.* 218:711, 1971.
    Recommended penicillin therapy for gonorrhea will also abort incubating syphilis.

21. Hayman, C. R., et al. Rape in the District of Columbia. *Am. J. Obstet. Gynccol.* 113:91, 1972.
   Under 1% of rape victims die but over 10% suffer severe physical or psychological damage.
22. Lippes, J., Malik, T., and Tatum, H. J. Postcoital Copper T. Proceedings of American Association of Planned Parenthood Physicians, Los Angeles, Calif., April, 1975.
   Postcoital insertions of the Copper T prevented pregnancy in every one of 97 patients.

Medical taxonomists subdivide amenorrhea (failure to menstruate) into primary amenorrhea and secondary amenorrhea. Women with primary amenorrhea have never menstruated; women with secondary amenorrhea have menstruated at least once. From this subclassification of amenorrhea, we assume that primary amenorrhea represents a more serious disorder of the reproductive system than secondary amenorrhea, but this assumption is not always correct. By established definition, a young woman who has not menstruated by the age of 18 or a young woman who has failed to establish breast development and menstruation by the age of 16 has primary amenorrhea.

Three conditions are necessary for menstruation. First, the pituitary gland must secrete gonadotropins in sufficient quantity to stimulate ovarian follicles. Second, the ovary must contain follicles, and these follicles must possess the enzymatic machinery necessary for synthesis and secretion of estradiol-17β (E_2). Finally, the genital tract must be patent from the endometrium to the vaginal introitus to allow egression of menstrual blood. A disorder in any one of these three systems will result in primary amenorrhea.

From the time of birth until the time of puberty, the pituitary gland secretes only small quantities of follicle-stimulating hormone (FSH) and luteinizing hormone (LH). At the time of puberty, the hypothalamic-pituitary axis is turned on by unknown mechanisms. Hypogonadotropic-hypogonadism is a rare cause of primary amenorrhea, but it must be considered in the evaluation of this disorder. Measurement of FSH and LH is the first diagnostic step in the evaluation of primary amenorrhea when it is obvious from physical examination that no obstruction to the genital outflow tract exists. Hypogonadotropic-hypogonadism is found in Kallman's syndrome (anosmia, sexual infantilism, and primary amenorrhea), Prader-Willi syndrome (hyperphagia, morbid obesity, mental retardation, and sexual infantilism), and anorexia nervosa.

Some girls develop anorexia nervosa before puberty begins or during the pubertal process before menarche occurs. These girls can establish ovulatory menstrual cycles by overcoming their aversion to food and fear of obesity. Although girls with Kallman's syndrome and Prader-Willi syndrome will never establish cyclic gonadotropic secretion, sexual maturation and induction of ovulation (and pregnancy) can be stimulated by administration of exogenous hormones.

Lack of ovarian follicles (gonadal dysgenesis) and failure of ovarian synthesis and secretion of E_2 are more serious causes of primary amenorrhea. Sexual maturation can be induced by administration of exogenous steroid hormones, but ovulation cannot be induced. Thus premature ovarian failure from any cause precludes pregnancy. Most women with primary gonadal failure or inability to secrete E_2 have a partial or complete deletion of one of the X chromosomes or an autosomal recessive disorder. However, some chemotherapeutic agents (notably the alkylating agents used for treating childhood neoplasms) will induce gonadal failure if given before or during puberty.

In the sequence of maturational events that occur with puberty, breast development is dependent upon gonadal estrogen production, while sexual hair growth is dependent upon adrenal and gonadal androgen production. If sexual hair appears in the absence of breast development, androgen production is occurring (although it may be abnormal), while estrogen production is either absent or inadequate to stimulate breast growth. When both breast development and sexual hair growth fail to occur, an enzymatic defect in steroidogenesis that prevents synthesis of androgens and estrogens is the most likely cause.

Any discussion of primary amenorrhea due to gonadal failure would be incomplete without mention of congenital and acquired androgen-excess disorders and polycystic ovarian disease. Severe forms of congenital adrenal hyperplasia (CAH) with excess androgen production rarely escape notice during early childhood. However, some of the less severe forms of CAH may attenuate breast development and delay menarche so as to present a picture of ovarian failure. Also, acquired syndromes of androgen excess (adrenal and ovarian androgen-secreting tumors) will prevent normal breast development and delay menarche.

These latter forms of menstrual delay can usually be distinguished from gonadal failure by physical examination and measurement of pituitary gonadotropins. Young women with delayed menarche due to androgen excess have full sexual hair growth, excess body hair, and acne. Young women with polycystic ovarian disease will manifest full breast development, with an abundance of endocervical mucus. (Paradoxically, these women have estrogen excess.) In disorders of ovarian failure or lack of steroid biosynthesis plasma concentrations of pituitary gonadotropins exceed the normal limits and fall within the range found in menopausal women. In those women with androgen-excess disorders or polycystic ovarian disease, plasma gonadotropin concentrations (specifically FSH) are in the normal range.

Finally, women with obstruction of the genital outflow tract, extending anywhere from the endometrium to the vaginal introitus, will present with primary amenorrhea. Women with genital tract obstruction can be readily distinguished from women with pituitary or gonadal failure because the former have normal secondary sexual development (i.e., full breast development and sexual hair growth), whereas those with impaired pituitary or ovarian function will fail to have normal secondary sexual development. In some young women an imperforate hymen is the sole point of genital tract obstruction. A simple hymenotomy relieves the obstruction and restores fertility. In some young women there is congenital absence of the uterus and vagina (Rokitansky-Kuster-Hauser syndrome). In these women reproduction is permanently impaired, and sexual function is impossible until a vaginal vault is created. Anomalies of the urinary tract (unilateral renal agenesis, horseshoe kidney, pelvic kidney) may coexist with genital tract anomalies; therefore, evaluation of the upper and lower urinary tract is indicated.

We recommend that women with vaginal agenesis undergo a vaginal construction operation in their mid-teens. If surgical treatment is delayed until these women become sexually active or contemplate marriage, psychosexual problems can develop that will handicap their subsequent sexual development. These sexual difficulties can be avoided by performing early surgery.

Primary amenorrhea results from one of three major disorders of the reproductive-endocrine system. These are: (1) pituitary or gonadal failure, (2) defects in sex steroidogenesis, or (3) an anatomic defect of the reproductive tract. We set our therapeutic objectives to establish secondary sexual development in young women with sexual infantilism and to establish a functional vagina or patent genital tract in young women with anatomic defects. Consideration must be given to future fertility when counseling women with primary amenorrhea.

Amenorrhea of Central Nervous System Origin

1. Tagatz, G., et al. Hypogonadotropic hypogonadism associated with anosmia in the female. *N. Engl. J. Med.* 282:1326, 1970.
   A review of Kallman syndrome as a cause of primary amenorrhea.

2. Warren, M. P., and Vande Wiele, R. L. Clinical and metabolic features of anorexia nervosa. *Am. J. Obstet. Gynecol.* 117:435, 1973.
   A comprehensive review of anorexia nervosa.
3. Franks, S., et al. Incidence and significance of hyperprolactinemia in women with amenorrhea. *Clin. Endocrinol.* 4:597, 1975.
   Pituitary microadenomas as a cause of primary and secondary amenorrhea.
4. Rubin, D., et al. Isolated deficiency of follicle-stimulating hormone. *N. Engl. J. Med.* 287:1313, 1972.
   A rare cause of primary amenorrhea.
5. Goldenberg, R. L., et al. Gonadotropins in women with amenorrhea: The use of plasma follicle stimulating hormone to differentiate women with and without ovarian follicles. *Am. J. Obstet. Gynecol.* 116:1003, 1973.
   A simple diagnostic method of distinguishing amenorrhea of central origin from amenorrhea of ovarian origin.

Amenorrhea of Ovarian Origin

6. Prader, A., and Anders, G. J. Zur genetik der kongenitalen Lypoidhyperplasie der Nebenieren. *Helv. Paediatr. Acta* 17:285, 1962.
   Original description of the Prader-Willi syndrome.
7. Frisch, R. E., and Revelle, R. Height and weight at menarche and a hypothesis of critical body weight and adolescent events. *Science* 169:397, 1970.
   Body weight must be considered in the evaluation of primary amenorrhea.
8. Turner, H. H. A syndrome of infantilism, congenital webbed neck and cubitus valgus. *Endocrinology* 23:566, 1938.
   The original description of Turner's syndrome.
9. Bates, G. W., and Cleland, W. C. Arrest of follicular maturation following busulfan therapy. (Unpublished data.)
   A prepubertal girl treated with busulfan for chronic granulocytic leukemia developed sexual infantilism due to follicular arrest.
10. Goldsmith, O., Soloman, D. H., and Horton, R. Hypogonadism and mineralocorticoid excess: The 17-hydroxylase deficiency syndrome. *N. Engl. J. Med.* 277:673, 1967.
    A major enzymatic deficiency that results in sexual infantilism and primary amenorrhea.
11. Bongiovanni, A. M., and Root, A. W. The adrenogenital syndrome. *N. Engl. J. Med.* 268:1283, 1342, 1391, 1963.
    A major review of congenital adrenal hyperplasia.
12. Goldzieher, J. W., and Green, J. A. The polycystic ovary: I. Clinical and histologic features. *J. Clin. Endocrinol. Metab.* 22:325, 1962.
    Primary amenorrhea occurs in 15% of women with polycystic ovarian disease.
13. Griffin, J. E., et al. Congenital absence of the vagina. *Ann. Intern. Med.* 85:224, 1976.
    A clear review of syndromes of vaginal agenesis.
14. Fore, S. R., et al. Urologic and genital anomalies in patients with congenital absence of the vagina. *Obstet. Gynecol.* 46:410, 1975.
    Congenital anomalies associated with vaginal absence.
15. Geary, W. L., and Weed, J. C. Congenital atresia of the uterine cervix. *Obstet. Gynecol.* 42:213, 1973.
    A rare cause of primary amenorrhea.
16. Polishuk, W. Z., and Sharf, M. Primary amenorrhea due to intrauterine adhesions. *Gynaecologia* (Basel) 154:181, 1962.
    Intrauterine adhesions are a rather frequent cause of secondary amenorrhea but rarely cause primary amenorrhea.

Secondary Amenorrhea

A diagnosis of secondary amenorrhea (in the absence of pregnancy) is made when no menses have occurred for a period of 6 months when cycles have always been regular, or a period of 12 months when cycles have been irregular. The division of amenorrhea into primary amenorrhea (never menstruated) and secondary amenorrhea (cessation of menstruation) implies that primary amenorrhea is a more serious condition than secondary amenorrhea. This division is arbitrary, however, and the implication is not necessarily true.

In evaluating women with secondary amenorrhea, consider functional causes first. Pregnancy is the most common cause of secondary amenorrhea, but this consideration may be overlooked, especially in women with a lifelong history of menstrual irregularity and in women approaching menopause. Thus, pregnancy should be excluded as a cause before administering drugs to produce withdrawal uterine bleeding.

Secondary amenorrhea is more common at the extreme ends of a woman's reproductive life. During the early postmenarchal years and the late perimenopausal years, when ovulation is infrequent, there may be long intervals of absent menses.

Any disruption of the hypothalamic-pituitary-ovarian axis or of the functional integrity of the endometrium is manifested by secondary amenorrhea. The following "examples" illustrate some of the causes of secondary amenorrhea.

Hypothalamic dysfunction occurs in anorexia nervosa, simple weight loss, anxiety reactions, psychotropic drug therapy, and marijuana use. In anorexia nervosa and simple weight loss, hypothalamic release of gonadotropin releasing hormone (GnRH) is disrupted such that the pituitary secretory pattern of follicle-stimulating hormone (FSH) and luteinizing hormone (LH) reverts to a prepubertal pattern. Ovulation and menstruation cease. In cases of anorexia nervosa and simple weight loss, restoration of body weight to ideal adult levels causes the return of ovulation and cyclic menstruation in most women. Tricyclic antidepressants and pheothiazines suppress gonadotropin secretion and stimulate prolactin secretion. Thus, amenorrhea and galactorrhea may develop in women who use these drugs for long periods of time. Marijuana acts in the hypothalamus to suppress GnRH secretion; anovulation and amenorrhea result. When amenorrhea is drug-induced or related to marijuana use, discontinuation of the causal agent restores cyclic reproductive function.

Pituitary failure and pituitary microadenomas lead the list of pituitary causes of secondary amenorrhea. Pituitary failure may be idiopathic (Simmonds' disease) or it may result from pituitary necrosis following a massive postpartum hemorrhage (Sheehan's syndrome). In both of these conditions, pituitary failure may be complete (loss of gonadal, thyroid, and adrenal function) or partial. When partial pituitary failure occurs, loss of gonadotropin secretion is the first sign of pituitary failure, and this sign is manifested by secondary amenorrhea.

Interest in pituitary disease has focused recently on pituitary microadenomas, especially prolactin-secreting pituitary microadenomas. Over the past decade these tumors have been recognized with increasing frequency, although it is uncertain that the incidence has increased. Prolactin-secreting pituitary microadenomas present with subtle alterations of menstrual function and progress to secondary amenorrhea with galactorrhea. They are found both in nulliparous women and in women who have had children. The etiology of a prolactin-secreting microadenoma is obscure, but most respond favorably to bromocriptine therapy.

The most frequent cause of secondary amenorrhea is polycystic ovarian disease (PCOD). PCOD is characterized by anovulation, amenorrhea, androgen excess, and infertility. Commonly, women with PCOD are obese, but the disorder is found in slender women as well. Women with PCOD demonstrate signs of androgen and estrogen excess. They tend to have large breasts, abundant endocervical mucus, and endometrial hyperplasia (signs of estrogen excess); they have acne as well as increased hair growth on the face, lower abdomen, thighs, and chest (signs of androgen excess). When samples of blood are obtained from these women for the purpose of measuring gonadotropin and steroid hormones, they usually have normal concentrations of FSH but increased concentrations of LH. Androstenedione, a weak androgen of adrenal and ovarian origin, is increased. Testosterone, a potent androgen of adrenal, ovarian, and extraglandular origin, may be normal. Estrone, a weak estrogen, is found in increased concentrations in women with PCOD despite the fact that estradiol-17β, a potent estrogen secreted by the ovarian follicle, is reduced. In women with PCOD, estrone is derived from the extraglandular aromatization of androstenedione. Thus, the paradox of signs of androgen excess and estrogen excess is explained by the extraglandular aromatization of increased circulating androstenedione.

Premature ovarian failure is often an unsuspected cause of secondary amenorrhea. Unlike PCOD, a condition of estrogen excess, premature ovarian failure is a condition of estrogen deficiency; women with premature ovarian failure complain of breast atrophy, hot flashes, vaginal dryness, and decreased libido.

Failure of the endometrium to respond to sex-steroid stimulation is a rare cause of secondary amenorrhea. Tuberculous endometritis was a cause of endometrial failure in the past, but it is rarely encountered today. Endometrial fibrosis and intrauterine synechiae (Asherman's syndrome) following endometrial curettage is being recognized with increased frequency. If, in the course of performing an endometrial curettage, the endometrium is denuded below the basal level, the endometrium will fail to regenerate. It will be permanently scarred and menstruation will cease.

An evaluation of secondary amenorrhea calls for identification of that part of the hypothalamic-pituitary-gonadal axis that is dysfunctional. The menstrual history is a valuable diagnostic tool. A history of cyclic, predictable menses indicates an acquired ovulatory dysfunction; a history of irregular, unpredictable menses from the time of puberty may suggest a chromosomal defect or an underlying endocrine disorder. The physician should attempt to ascertain whether the secondary amenorrhea is associated with estrogen deficiency or estrogen excess. In conditions of estrogen deficiency, women experience breast atrophy, vaginal dryness, hot flashes, and loss of libido. In conditions of estrogen excess, women experience breast enlargement, increased vaginal secretion, and episodic, heavy vaginal bleeding.

On physical examination, careful attention should be given to the sex-steroid target tissues. These are the hair follicles, breasts, clitoris, vaginal endocervix, and uterus. Excessive androgen production is manifested by excessive terminal hair growth, and in the event of testosterone excess, clitoral enlargement. Excessive estrogen production is manifested by tubular breasts, large nipples and areolae, excessive vaginal rugation, and abundant endocervical mucus secretion. Conversely, estrogen deficiency is manifested by breast atrophy, a smooth vagina, and a dry endocervix.

Interpretation of plasma gonadotropin (FSH and LH) concentration leads to establishing an etiology for secondary amenorrhea. In cases of hypothalamic and pituitary failure, the gonadotropins are abnormally low (prepubertal) or are in the low range of normal. When the secondary amenorrhea results from anorexia nervosa or simple weight loss, gonadotropins are abnormally low and the FSH concentration exceeds LH concentration, as is found in prepubertal girls. In cases of PCOD, FSH is in the normal adult range, but the concentration of LH is elevated above that normally found in the follicular phase of the cycle. Finally, in ovarian failure (premature menopause) the gonadotropins are elevated to menopausal levels.

Measurement of prolactin is a useful adjunct for the diagnosis of secondary amenorrhea when a woman has galactorrhea or when no other cause is immediately apparent. A chromosomal karyotype can be important in establishing the cause to be premature ovarian failure.

Women who have secondary amenorrhea in the face of estrogen excess or adequate estrogen production will have withdrawal uterine bleeding after a progestin has been administered and withdrawn. Estrogens stimulate endometrial growth; progesterone and progestins convert a proliferative endometrium into a secretory endometrium; withdrawal of progestins from an estrogen-stimulated endometrium causes endometrial sloughing (withdrawal bleeding). The progestin withdrawal test is an excellent method for determining estrogen production and endometrial integrity. When no uterine bleeding occurs following progestin withdrawal, either the endometrium has not been adequately stimulated by estrogens or the endometrium is absent.

Although the progestin withdrawal test is often used to evaluate estrogen production, examination of the endocervix for the presence or absence of endocervical mucus can serve the same purpose. We have not seen a woman with endocervical mucus (excluding women with Asherman's syndrome) who does not respond to progestin withdrawal.

Secondary amenorrhea is not a disease. Secondary amenorrhea is a symptom of disruption of the cyclic endocrine events in the hypothalamic-pituitary-ovarian axis, or a symptom of inadequate endometrium. Diagnosis should be aimed at localizing the area of endocrine system that is dysfunctional. Therapy should be directed toward restoring the cyclic events within the hypothalamic-pituitary-ovarian axis.

Hypothalamic Amenorrhea

1. Drossman, D. A., Ontjes, D. A., and Heizer, W. D. Anorexia nervosa. *Gastroenterology* 77:1115, 1979.
   An excellent review article of the endocrine pathology and psychopathology of anorexia nervosa.
2. Vigersky, R. A., et al. Hypothalamic dysfunction in secondary amenorrhea associated with simple weight loss. *N. Engl. J. Med.* 297:1141, 1977.
   A detailed investigation of the hypothalamic alterations associated with weight loss.
3. Bates, G. W., Whitworth, N. S., and Bates, S. R. Effects of body weight control on reproductive function. *Fertil. Steril.* 35:248, 1981.
   An evaluation of 17 women with unexplained infertility due to control of body weight below ideal limits.
4. Besch, N. F., et al. The effect of marihuana (delta-9-tetrahydrocannabinol) on the secretion of luteinizing hormone in the ovariectomized rhesus monkey. *Am. J. Obstet. Gynecol.* 128:635, 1977.
   Marijuana suppresses LH-GnRH secretion in the hypothalamus.
5. Asch, R. H., et al. Effects of Δ9-Tetrahydrocannabinol during the follicular phase of the Rhesus monkey. *J. Clin. Endocrinol. Metab.* 52:50, 1981.

An animal study that describes the mechanism of action of marijuana in inhibiting ovulation.

Pituitary Origin of Amenorrhea

6. Sheehan, H. L. Simmonds' disease due to postpartum necrosis of the anterior pituitary gland. *Q. J. Med.* 8:277, 1939.
Original description of postpartum pituitary necrosis.
7. Kleinberg, D. L., Noll, G. L., and Frantz, A. G. Galactorrhea: A study of 235 cases, including 48 with pituitary tumors. *N. Engl. J. Med.* 296:589, 1977.
In-depth review of the pathophysiology of amenorrhea-galactorrhea syndromes.
8. Varga, L., Wenner, R., and del Pozo, E. Treatment of galactorrhea-amenorrhea syndrome with Br-ergocriptine (CB154): Restoration of ovulatory function and fertility. *Am. J. Obstet. Gynecol.* 117:75, 1973.
Method for medical management of prolactin-secreting pituitary microadenomas.
9. Hardy, J. Transsphenoidal microsurgery of the normal and pathological pituitary. *Clin. Neurosurg.* 16:185, 1969.
Original description of the surgical method of management of the pituitary microadenoma.

Ovarian Causes of Secondary Amenorrhea

10. Siiteri, P. K., and MacDonald, P. C. Role of Extraglandular Estrogen in Human Endocrinology. In R. A. Geyer, E. B. Astwood, and R. O. Greep (Eds.), *Handbook of Physiology*, Section 7, *Endocrinology.* Washington, D. C.: American Physiological Society, 1973.
Mechanisms for estrogen excess in conditions associated with androgen excess.
11. Rebar, R., et al. Characterization of the inappropriate gonadotropin secretion in polycystic ovary syndrome. *J. Clin. Invest.* 57:1320, 1976.
The role of LH excess in the etiology of polycystic ovarian disease.
12. Jones, G. S., and De-Moraes-Ruehsen, M. A new syndrome of amenorrhea in association with hypergonadotropism and apparently normal ovarian follicular apparatus. *Am. J. Obstet. Gynecol.* 104:597, 1969.
The resistant-ovary syndrome—a cause of premature ovarian failure.

Intrauterine Adhesions

13. Klein, S. M., and Garcia, C. R. Asherman's syndrome: A critique and current review. *Fertil. Steril.* 24:722, 1973.
A review of the causes of and treatment for intrauterine synechiae.

Diagnosis of Secondary Amenorrhea

14. Kletzky, O. A., et al. Classification of secondary amenorrhea based on distinct hormonal patterns. *J. Clin. Endocrinol. Metab.* 41:660, 1975.
Utilization of plasma hormone concentrations for evaluation of women with secondary amenorrhea.
15. Kletzky, O. A., et al. Clinical categorization of patients with secondary amenorrhea using progesterone-induced uterine bleeding and measurement of serum gonadotropin levels. *Am. J. Obstet. Gynecol.* 121:695, 1975.
A method for evaluating estrogenic action on the endometrium.

Precocious Puberty

The prepubertal child, from the time of birth until the initiation of sexual maturation, can respond to tropic hormones and sex steroids. The gonads, if properly stimulated by tropic hormones (human chorionic gonadotropin [HCG], follicle-stimulating hormone [FSH], and luteinizing hormone [LH]), will secrete androgens and estrogens; secondary–sex organ growth (breasts, uterus, penis, and sexual hair) can be stimulated by these sex steroids. The neuroendocrine mechanism that holds sexual maturation in abeyance until the appropriate time is unknown, as is the mechanism that initiates puberty.

Sexual development at puberty progresses in a predictable way. In the female, breast budding (thelarche) occurs first, followed by sexual hair growth (adrenarche), and then menarche. In the male, testicular enlargement is the first sign of puberty, followed by sexual hair growth and penile enlargement. Any deviation from this predictable sequence suggests abnormal pubertal development.

When faced with a child with precocious sexual development, the physician should ask which hormone(s) is responsible for stimulating which part of sexual development. For example, if a female child presents with pubic hair growth in the absence of breast budding, an extragonadal source of androgens is suggested; or if a female child has breast development in the absence of pubic hair growth, an exogenous source of estrogens or an estrogen-producing ovarian tumor is suggested. If a male child has pubic hair growth in the absence of testicular enlargement, an extragonadal source of androgens is suggested. On the other hand, if sexual maturation proceeds in a physiologic manner, either pituitary gonadotropin secretion is normal but advanced, or there is an ectopic source of gonadotropins (hepatic tumors, gonadal tumors). Thus a carefully obtained history, a complete physical examination, and selected laboratory studies are necessary to distinguish benign causes of precocious puberty from serious, even fatal, causes.

Less than 1% of children will develop signs of puberty before the age of 8 in girls and 9 in boys. In some of these children there will be a family history of early sexual development, but most have no familial history of early maturation or signs of organic disease. The condition may occur in infancy, in which case it is associated with electroencephalographic abnormalities. In such cases in boys, testicular enlargement precedes other signs of maturation and is followed by sexual hair growth, penile enlargment, muscular development, and sexual arousal. In girls, breast development occurs first and is followed by sexual hair growth, menarche, and the occurrence of regular menses. Pituitary gonadotropin secretion in these children is normal, and subsequent reproductive function is normal.

Children with idiopathic precocious puberty experience accelerated long bone growth in association with their advanced sexual development and are larger than their peers. However, their adult height is below average because of early epiphyseal closure.

Congenital adrenal hyperplasia (CAH) is a common cause of premature androgen secretion. This is an autosomal recessive disorder that has a wide spectrum of severity. The most severe forms of CAH that affect girls are recognized at birth as syndromes of congenital genital ambiguity. In girls treatment can be initiated soon after birth. In boys, however, the disorder may go unrecognized until early childhood when sexual hair appears, penile enlargement begins, and a muscular body habitus develops. Because the adrenal gland is the source of androgen excess in these children, breast development will not occur in girls and testicular enlargement does not occur in boys.

21-hydroxylase deficiency is the common form of CAH. To a much lesser extent, 11β-hydroxylase and 3β-ol dehydrogenase cause CAH. To establish the diagnosis of CAH, measure 24-hour urinary excretion of pregnanetriol and 17-ketosteroids. These metabolities of adrenal androgens are elevated in 21-hydroxylase deficiency and will revert to normal levels once glucocorticoids are administered. If the condition goes untreated for a prolonged time, short stature may result. There is no alteration in subsequent sexual development or reproductive function once suppression by glucocorticoids is begun.

Virilizing adrenal neoplasms are rare in children. Most often they are found in association with Cushing's syndrome. As in CAH urinary concentration of adrenal androgen metabolites is increased in adrenal neoplasms, but, unlike CAH, the concentration of androgen metabolites cannot be suppressed by administering glucocorticoids. Surgical excision of the adrenal tumor is the treatment.

Midline central nervous system (CNS) tumors may cause precocious puberty by impinging upon the hypothalamus to stimulate release of gonadotropin releasing hormone. Craniopharyngiomas and hamartomas are the most common CNS tumors that activate the hypothalamic-pituitary axis. Other CNS conditions associated with precocious puberty are the McCune-Albright syndrome (polyostotic fibrous dysplasia), characterized by long bone cysts and café-au-lait spots; and von Recklinghausen's disease (neurofibromatosis), characterized by café-au-lait spots and subcutaneous neurofibromas.

Tumors that secrete human chorionic gonadotropin (HCG) can cause precocious puberty. The HCG from these tumors stimulates the gonads directly, causing them to secrete sex steroids. The most serious of these tumors is the hepatoma.

An often-overlooked cause of precocious puberty is exposure to exogenous sex steroids, particularly estrogens. Skin creams and lotions contain estrogens that are readily absorbed. Estrogen therapy for vulvar agglutination in girls and ingestion of oral contraceptive tablets can cause premature thelarche in girls and boys.

One transient phenomenon of puberty in males is the development of gynecomastia. Unilateral or partial bilateral breast enlargement in early puberty is a common event. This results from the increased estrogen relative to testosterone that is produced in early puberty. Thoughtful reassurance is adequate treatment as the gynecomastia regresses with advancing pubertal development.

Idiopathic premature thelarche in girls is also a benign, self-limited disorder. A source of exogenous estrogen should be sought and, if found, eliminated. Otherwise, no therapy is warranted.

Normal Puberty

1. Tanner, J. M. *Growth at Adolescence* (2nd ed.). Oxford: Blackwell Scientific Publications, 1962.
   A classic text on the normal events occurring in boys and girls at puberty.
2. Zacharias, L. W., Rand, M., and Westman, R. J. Age at menarche. *N. Engl. J. Med.* 280:868, 1969.
   A study of the age of menarche in American girls.
3. Marshall, W. A., and Tanner, J. M. Variations in the pattern of pubertal changes in boys. *Arch. Dis. Child.* 45:13, 1970.

A longitudinal study of the development stages in sexual maturation in boys.

4. Grumbach, M. M. Onset of Puberty. In S. R. Berenberg (Ed.), *Puberty.* Leiden: H. E. Stenfert Kroese, 1975.
   Discusses normal pubertal development.

Abnormal Pubertal Development

5. Bates, G. W. Disorders of puberty. *Comtemp. Ob/Gyn* (In press).
   A review of abnormal sexual maturation.
6. Grumbach, M. M., Van Wyck, J. J. Disorders of Sex Differentiation. In R. H. Williams (Ed.), *Textbook of Endocrinology* (5th ed.). Philadelphia: Saunders, 1974.
   A comprehensive review of abnormal sexual development, including congenital adrenal hyperplasia.
7. Cohen, H. N., et al. Clinical value of adrenal androgen measurement in the diagnosis of delayed puberty. *Lancet* 1:689, 1981.
   A description of a diagnostic test to distinguish delayed puberty from pubertal failure.
8. Money, J., and Clopper, R. R., Jr. Psychosocial and psychosexual aspects of errors of pubertal onset and development. *Hum. Biol.* 46:173, 1974.
   Discussion of the psychologic aspects of precocious and delayed puberty.
9. Siurjonsdottir, T. H., and Hayes, A. B. Precocious puberty: A report of 96 cases. *Am. J. Dis. Child.* 115:309, 1968.
   A study elucidating the many causes of precocious puberty.
10. Cook, C. D., McArthur, J. W., and Berenberg, W. Pseudoprecocious puberty in girls as a result of estrogen ingestion. *N. Engl. J. Med.* 248:671, 1953.
    Exogenous estrogen—an often-overlooked cause of precocious puberty.
11. Eberlien, W. A., et al. Ovarian tumors and cysts associated with sexual precocity. *J. Pediatr.* 57:484, 1960.
    Functional ovarian tumors that secrete estrogen can cause pseudoprecocious puberty.
12. McArthur, J. W., et al. Sexual precocity attributable to ectopic gonadotropin secretion by hepatoblastoma. *Am. J. Med.* 54:390, 1973.
    Effect of ectopic gonadotropin on gonadal function.
13. Benedict, P. H. Sex precocity and polyostotic fibrous dysplasia. *Am. J. Dis. Child.* 3:429, 1966.
    A review of the McCune-Albright syndrome.
14. Banna, M. Craniopharyngioma in children. *J. Pediatr.* 83:781, 1973.
    Effects of midline, benign central nervous system tumors on sexual development.

Hirsutism and Virilization

In evaluating androgen excess syndromes, a clear distinction must be made between hirsutism and virilization. Hirsutism is excessive hair growth on body surfaces where hair growth ordinarily does not occur. Virilization includes excessive hair growth, but in addition the female takes on masculine features. The initial sign of virilization is clitoral enlargement. This is followed by breast atrophy, recession of temporal hair, deepening of the voice, and remodeling of the body contours into masculine configuration. In evaluating women with the complaint of hirsutism, search must be made for signs of virilization. In their absence, a functional condition such as acquired mild to moderate adrenal hyperplasia or polycystic ovarian disease is usually the cause of androgen excess. When virilization is found, the woman either has a severe form of adrenal hyperplasia or polycystic ovarian disease, or she may have a testosterone-secreting adrenal or ovarian neoplasm. Under these circumstances, a diligent search must be made for a testosterone-secreting tumor.

Congenital adrenal hyperplasia results from an enzymatic defect in the synthesis of glucocorticoids and mineralocorticoids. The most common defect is a 21-hydroxylase deficiency; next in frequency of occurrence is an 11β-hydroxylase deficiency. These disorders have an autosomal recessive inheritance pattern, with varying degrees of penetrance. The defect is usually incomplete and varying degrees of severity may occur.

If the adrenal enzymatic defect is severe, signs of androgen excess will be evident at birth; the female child presents with genital ambiguity manifested by clitoral enlargement and labial fusion. In the male the signs may not be evident at birth, but precocious puberty occurs in these children. If the hydroxylase defect is mild, there may be no evidence of congenital adrenal hyperplasia until the time of puberty. With puberty, in girls, increased adrenal steroidogenesis may produce a clinical picture of menstrual irregularities, hirsutism, acne, and mild virilization.

It is difficult clinically to distinguish ovarian-androgen excess from adrenal-androgen excess on initial examination. However, if the disorder had its beginning at the time of puberty and breast development is delayed or subnormal, the most likely source of the androgen excess is the adrenal gland. On the other hand, if breast development occurs earlier than the expected time and there is full breast development, the probable cause is polycystic ovarian disease.

Acquired adrenal hyperplasia may present as a syndrome of androgen excess. However, it is more commonly found as a feature of Cushing's syndrome; the signs of obesity, plethora, red striae, diabetes, and the tendency to bruise easily suggest the diagnosis. In some cases, inappropriate secretion of adrenocorticotropic hormone (ACTH) by the pituitary or from ectopic sources causes the adrenal hyperplasia (Cushing's disease). Rarely will adrenal neoplasms secrete androgens in excess. In these conditions, the diurnal variation of cortisol secretion is lost.

Polycystic ovarian disease, Stein-Leventhal syndrome, and ovarian stromal hyperplasia are the most common causes of ovarian androgen excess. Although the names given these disorders are different, they may represent a spectrum of varying degrees of the same clinical entity. Clinically, women with ovarian androgen-excess disorders present with menstrual irregularity or amenorrhea, acne, hirsutism, infertility, and mild virilization. Paradoxically, estrogen excess may be a concomitant feature and is manifested by excessive endocervical mucus production, breast enlargement, and heavy vaginal bleeding resulting from endometrial hyperplasia.

P. K. Siiteri and P. C. MacDonald have described the mechanism whereby androstenedione and testosterone are metabolized to estrone and estradiol by aromatization in peripheral tissues. In these syndromes of androgen excess, estrogen excess will be a side effect. There is continued debate as to whether the polycystic ovarian syndrome is primarily a disorder of steroid synthesis within the gonad or excessive ovarian stimulation by the neuroendocrine axis. In a mechanism proposed by Yen and associates, polycystic ovarian disease is a self-perpetuating disorder in that continued production of ovarian steroids results in continued tonic secretion of luteinizing hormone (LH) by the pituitary gland. Thus, with increased production of ovarian steroids, there is increased secretion of LH, and the disorder continues unabated until there is some interruption in this cycle.

Obesity is a frequent feature of polycystic ovarian disease. If the obesity begins before puberty, the syndrome of polycystic ovarian disease may begin immediately with puberty. On the other hand, if obesity occurs later in life, polycystic ovarian disease may begin at that time. An explanation for the association between polycystic ovarian disease and obesity is the positive correlation that exists between the extraglandular aromatization of androgens to estrogens and increasing body weight.

To evaluate syndromes of androgen excess, begin with the assumption that the androgen excess is ovarian in origin. The initial laboratory evaluation includes measurement of plasma follicle-stimulating hormone (FSH), LH, prolactin, androstenedione (A), and testosterone (T). In conditions of ovarian androgen excess, LH is frequently elevated while FSH is in the normal to low normal range. The androgens A and T are mildly elevated, with A being elevated to the greatest degree; T is usually at the upper limits of normal. One of the many schemes for the evaluation of androgen-excess syndrome is the measurement of 24-hour urinary ketosteroids. In polycystic ovarian disease, 17-ketosteroid excretion may be mildly increased. If the laboratory picture suggests polycystic ovarian disease, a short trial of pituitary suppression by the administration of oral contraceptive steroids or a progestin will result in suppression of LH and ovarian androgen biosynthesis. The laboratory studies should then be repeated 6 weeks after the pituitary suppression has begun.

If the history suggests adrenal hyperplasia, then in addition to the measurement of plasma gonadotropins and androgens, dehydroepiandrosterone (DHEA) should be measured and a 24-hour urine for measurement of 17-ketosteroids and pregnanetriol collected. If adrenal hyperplasia is the problem, these steroids and their metabolites will be elevated. A short course of prednisone therapy, 5 mg twice a day, will result in suppression of DHEA and a subsequent reduction in pregnanetriol excretion and 17-ketosteroid excretion.

In utilizing the simplistic diagnostic scheme for the evaluation of androgen-excess syndromes, the physician must be careful not to overlook an adrenal adenoma or an ovarian neoplasm. When there are signs of Cushing's syndrome, rapid progression of hirsutism, or virilization, a neoplastic source for the androgen excess must be sought.

Androgen Production and Metabolism

1. Abraham, G. E. Ovarian and adrenal contribution to peripheral androgens during the menstrual cycle. *J. Clin. Endocrinol. Metab.* 39:340, 1974.
   Normal plasma androgen concentrations is reproductive-age women.
2. Horton, R., and Tait, J. F. Androstenedione production and interconversion rates measured in peripheral blood and studies on the possible sites of its conversion to testosterone. *J. Clin. Invest.* 45:301, 1966.
   Mechanism for extraglandular testosterone production.
3. Vermeulen, A., et al. Capacity of testosterone-binding globulin in human plasma and influence of specific binding of testosterone on its metabolic clearance rate. *J. Clin. Endocrinol. Metab.* 29:1470, 1969.
   Androgens are bound to testosterone-binding globulin. The free, not bound, testosterone stimulates excessive hair growth and produces virilization.

4. Siiteri, P. K., and MacDonald, P. C. Role of Extraglandular Estrogen in Human Endocrinology. In R. A. Geyer, E. B. Astwood, and R. O. Greep (Eds.), *Handbook of Physiology, Section 7, Endrocrinology.* Washington, D.C.: American Physiological Society, 1973.
   Mechanism for estrogen excess in conditions associated with androgen excess.

Congenital Adrenal Hyperplasia
5. Bongiovanni, A. M., and Root, A. W. The adrenogenital syndrome. *N. Engl. J. Med.* 268:1283, 1342, 1391, 1963.
   A comprehensive review of the subject.
6. Givens, J. R., et al. Adrenal function in hirsutism: I. Diurnal change and response of plasma androstenedione, testosterone. 17-hydroxy-progesterone, cortisol, LH and FSH to dexamethasone and ½ unit of ACTH. *J. Clin, Endocrinol. Metab.* 40:988, 1975.
   Basis for dexamethasone therapy in adrenal hyperplasia.
7. Judd, H. L., et al. Correlation of the effects of dexamethasone administration on urinary 17-ketosteroids and serum androgen levels in patients with hirsutism. *Am. J. Obstet. Gynecol.* 128:408, 1977.
   The effect of dexamethasone in hirsute women.
8. Werk, E. E., Sholiton, L. J., and Kalejs, L. Testosterone-secreting adrenal adenoma under gonadotropin control. *N. Engl. J. Med.* 277:399, 1967.
   Report of an androgen-producing adrenal tumor.

Polycystic Ovarian Disease
9. Stein, I. F., and Leventhal, M. L. Amenorrhea associated with bilateral polycystic ovaries. *Am. J. Obstet. Gynecol.* 29:181, 1935.
   The original description of polycystic ovarian disease.
10. Judd, H. L. Endocrinology of polycystic ovarian disease. *Clin. Obstet. Gynecol.* 21:99, 1978.
    A contemporary review of polycystic ovarian disease.
11. Goldzieher, J. W., and Axelrod, L. R. Clinical and biochemical features of polycystic ovarian disease. *Fertil. Steril.* 14:631, 1963.
    A descriptive analysis of polycystic ovarian disease.
12. DeVane, G. W., et al. Circulating gonadotropins, estrogens, and androgens in polycystic ovarian disease. *Am. J. Obstet. Gynecol.* 121:496, 1975.
    A detailed study of hormones in polycystic ovarian disease.
13. Yen, S. S. C., Chaney, C., and Judd, H. L. Functional Aberrations of the Hypothalamic-Pituitary System in Polycystic Ovary Syndrome: A Consideration of the Pathogenesis. In V. H. T. James, M. Serio, and G. Guisti (Eds.), *The Endocrine Function of the Human Ovary.* New York: Academic Press, 1976.
    A consideration of the pathogenesis of polycystic ovary disease.
14. Bates, G. W., and Whitworth, N. S. Effect of body weight reduction on plasma androgens in obese, infertile women. (Unpublished data, 1980.)
    Weight reduction in obese women reduces plasma androgens to normal and restores fertility.
15. Easterling, W. E., Jr., Talbert, L. M., and Potter, D. H. Serum testosterone levels in the polycystic ovary syndrome. *Am. J. Obstet. Gynecol.* 120:385, 1974.
    A study of testosterone concentrations in the plasma of women with polycystic ovary syndrome.
16. Givens, J. R., et al. Dynamics of suppression and recovery of plasma

FSH, LH, androstenedione, and testosterone in polycystic ovarian disease using an oral contraceptive. *J. Clin. Endocrinol. Metab.* 38:727, 1974.
The basis for therapy of polycystic ovarian disease with oral contraceptives.

Androgen Excess Disorders in Childhood

17. Bates, G. W. Hirsutism and androgen excess problems in childhood and adolescence. *Pediatr. Clin. North Am.* 28:513, 1981.
A comprehensive review of pediatric androgen excess disorders with discussions of treatment.

Dysfunctional Uterine Bleeding

Cyclic menstruation is the culmination of a series of hormonal interactions on the endometrium. In the course of a normal ovulatory cycle, follicle-stimulating hormone (FSH) stimulates an ovarian follicle to mature. The stimulated ovarian follicle begins secreting increasing quantities of estradiol-17β (E_2). E_2 has negative feedback upon the pituitary secretion of FSH and suppresses further secretion of FSH; E_2 has positive feedback upon the pituitary secretion of luteinizing hormone (LH) and stimulates LH secretion. When the rising plasma concentration of E_2 reaches the critical peak necessary to induce ovulation, an LH surge occurs and ovulation follows. These events constitute the follicular phase of the reproductive cycle and usually occur during the first 14 days of a 28-day cycle.

In response to increasing ovarian E_2 secretion, the endometrium undergoes proliferation; the stroma thickens and becomes compact; and the endometrial glands increase in number and length. If estrogen secretion continued, unopposed by the action of progesterone, the endometrium would continue to proliferate and thicken until eventually it would outgrow its blood supply and slough away from the myometrium. This endometrial sloughing could be focal, resulting in frequent episodes of vaginal spotting, or the endometrial sloughing could be extensive, resulting in frank menorrhagia.

In the normal ovulatory cycle, however, ovulation is followed by the formation of a corpus luteum at the site of the ovarian follicle, and the corpus luteum begins secreting progesterone (P) within 24 hours of ovulation. P acts upon the endometrium to suppress the mitogenic action of E_2 and converts the proliferative endometrium into a secretory endometrium. The straight, narrow endometrial glands become tortuous and dilated; the thick, compact endometrial stroma becomes edematous. Under the influence of P, the endometrium is prepared for implantation of a fertilized ovum.

If fertilization and implantation of the ovum do not occur, the corpus luteum fails approximately 12 days after it is formed. With corpus luteal failure, E_2 and P are withdrawn from the endometrium and menstruation begins. A new cycle is initiated.

The normal reproductive cycle is repeated ten to thirteen times a year in nonpregnant, sexually mature women. The repetitive nature of the cycle depends upon cyclic changes in the two pituitary gonadotropins, FSH and LH, and the two ovarian steroid hormones, E_2 and P. If any one of these four hormones becomes tonically elevated or suppressed, anovulation results.

Uterine bleeding that is acyclic and associated with anovulation is dysfunctional uterine bleeding. Moreover, dysfunctional uterine bleeding should respond to appropriate steroid hormone therapy.

Examples of times of or conditions in which anovulation due to tonic gonadotropin or steroid hormone secretion occurs are: (1) puberty, (2) climacteric, (3) anorexia nervosa, (4) polycystic ovarian disease, (5) pregnancy, and (6) obesity. At the time of puberty, the cyclic hormonal interactions are not fully established; E_2 secretion is continuous; and irregular uterine bleeding occurs. In the climacteric, FSH and LH become tonically elevated; E_2 secretion becomes tonic; ovulation fails; and irregular uterine bleeding occurs. In women with anorexia nervosa, FSH and LH secretion become tonically low; the ovarian follicles are not stimulated; E_2 secretion is deficient; the endometrium is not stimulated; and amenorrhea results. In polycystic ovarian disease, LH and estrone are tonically elevated; the endometrium is chronically stimulated by estrogens; ovulation fails; and the endometrium sloughs at irregular intervals. In pregnancy, P is tonically elevated; gonadotropins are suppressed; the endometrium is maintained in a secretory state; and menstruation does not occur. In association with obesity, estrone production becomes tonic and LH is tonically elevated (as in polycystic ovarian disease); the endometrium is chronically stimulated with estrogens; and irregular uterine bleeding results. In evaluating anovulation, it should first be asked which hormone(s) is tonically elevated or suppressed, then how the cyclic interactions between gonadotropins and sex steroids can be restored.

The most common causes of dysfunctional uterine bleeding are puberty, perimenopause, obesity, and polycystic ovarian disease. In each of these conditions, the endometrium is stimulated by estrogens without the suppressive action of P and without the withdrawal of P that initiates cyclic bleeding. Thus the treatment of dysfunctional uterine bleeding is directed at the endometrium by suppressing the action of unopposed estrogens.

Before therapy for dysfunctional uterine bleeding can be undertaken, organic disease of the uterus, cervix, or endometrium must be excluded. In the young, adolescent girl, it would be unusual to find an organic disease of the reproductive tract, but organic disease is not unusual in the sexually mature woman. Since chronic estrogen stimulation of the endometrium is often associated with endometrial polyps and endometrial hyperplasia, a dilation and curettage (D and C) should be considered as part of the diagnostic evaluation.

Once an organic cause for irregular uterine bleeding has been excluded, a regimen of medical therapy directed toward suppressing chronic estrogen stimulation and restoring cyclic interactions between the pituitary gland and ovaries is begun. For a woman actively bleeding, medroxyprogesterone acetace (MPA), 10 mg twice daily for 5 days, is administered. MPA is a potent progestin and, like progesterone, will convert a proliferative endometrium into a secretory endometrium. When the MPA is discontinued, withdrawal uterine bleeding will follow. A woman who is treated with MPA should be forewarned of the withdrawal bleeding; otherwise she will think that the treatment has been a failure. After the dysfunctional bleeding has been controlled by MPA therapy, the physician should establish an etiology for the bleeding and develop a long-term therapeutic plan.

Adolescent girls can be reassured that the problem is self-limiting and will remit spontaneously when ovulatory cycles are established. Likewise, perimenopausal women can be reassured that irregular bleeding will subside with menopause (although other hormonal management may be required). Obese women of all ages should be encouraged to reduce their body weight to near-ideal size. Spontaneous resumption of ovulatory cycles often follows weight reduction. Polycystic ovarian disease, especially in nonobese women, tends to be chronic and requires long-term medical management in accordance with the patient's treatment goals. If control of irregular bleeding is the desired therapeutic goal, chronic ovarian suppression with a progestin-dominant oral contraceptive agent will control the bleeding and suppress the excess androgen secretion associated with polycystic ovarian disease. If fertility is the desired goal, ovulation-induction with clomiphene citrate is indicated.

Dysfunctional uterine bleeding results from loss of normal cyclic interaction between the pituitary gonadotropins and ovarian E_2 and P. An organic cause for the bleeding must be excluded before medical therapy is instituted.

Normal Menstrual Cycle

1. Speroff, L. Regulation of the Menstrual Cycle. In L. Speroff, R. H. Glass, and N. G. Kase (Eds.), *Clinical Gynecologic Endocrinology and Infertility* (2nd ed.). Baltimore: Williams & Wilkins, 1978.
   A comprehensive, clear presentation of the endocrine events of the normal menstrual cycle.
2. Judd, H. L., and Yen, S. C. C. Serum androstenedione and testosterone levels during the menstrual cycle. *J. Clin. Endocrinol. Metab.* 38:475, 1973.
   A description of the changes in plasma androgens during the normal menstrual cycle.
3. Treloar, A. E., et al. Variation of human menstrual cycle through reproductive life. *Int. J. Fertil.* 12:77, 1967.
   An account of the expected variation in cycle length during the reproductive years.
4. Sherman, B. W., and Korenman, S. G. Hormonal characteristics of the human menstrual cycle throughout reproductive life. *J. Clin. Invest.* 55:699, 1975.
   A longitudinal study of the dynamics of gonadotropin and sex-steroid hormones during the reproductive years.

Variations in Gonadotropin and Steroid Hormone Secretion

5. Noyes, R. W., Hertig, A. T., and Rock, J. Dating the endometrial biopsy. *Fertil. Steril.* 1:3, 1950.
   The classic description of the dynamic events in endometrial maturation.
6. Boyar, R. M., et al. Synchronization of augmented luteinizing hormone secretion with sleep during puberty. *N. Engl. J. Med.* 287:582, 1972.
   A classic paper on the secretory pattern of gonadotropins in children during the pubertal transition.
7. Fraser, I. S., et al. Pituitary gonadotropins and ovarian function in adolescent dysfunctional uterine bleeding. *J. Clin. Endocrinol. Metab.* 37:407, 1973.
   Describes the steady-state plasma hormonal concentrations associated with puberty.
8. Boyar, R. M., et al. Anorexia nervosa: Immaturity of the 24-hour luteinizing hormone secretory pattern. *N. Engl. J. Med.* 291:861, 1974.
   In this disorder, the pituitary gonadotropin secretory pattern reverts to a prepubertal state.
9. Sherman, B. M., West, J. H., and Korenman, S. G. The menopausal transition: Analysis of LH, FSH, estradiol, and progesterone concentrations during menstrual cycles in older women. *J. Clin. Endocrinol. Metab.* 42:629, 1976.

An analysis of the gradual hormonal changes occurring in the late reproductive years.

10. Grodin, J. M., Siiteri, P. K., and MacDonald, P. C. Source of estrogen production in postmenopausal women. *J. Clin. Endocrinol. Metab.* 36:207, 1973.
    Discusses the mechanism for estrogen production in menopausal women.

Management of Dysfunctional Uterine Bleeding

11. Givens, J. R., et al. Dynamics of suppression and recovery of plasma FSH, LH, androstenedione, and testosterone in polycystic ovarian disease using an oral contraceptive. *J. Clin. Endocrinol. Metab.* 38:727, 1974.
    Mechanism of action of oral contraceptives in treatment of dysfunctional uterine bleeding and the rationale for their use.

12. Kase, N. G. Dysfunctional Uterine Bleeding. In L. Speroff, R. H. Glass, and N. G. Kase (Eds.), *Clinical Gynecologic Endocrinology and Infertility* (2nd ed.). Baltimore: Williams & Wilkins, 1978.
    An overview of the clinical problem and suggestions for therapy.

The Menopause

While the age of onset of menarche has declined over the past two centuries, the age of menopause has remained constant at approximately age 50 years. Moreover, the life expectancy for women has increased to 78 years, thereby extending the length of the menopausal years and increasing the number of menopausal women. Menopause is intertwined with aging to such an extent that difficulties arise in trying to separate those events due to ovarian failure from those events due to advancing age.

At the time of birth a girl child is endowed with approximately 2 million primordial ovarian follicles. She draws upon this endowment during her reproductive years until the time of menopause when approximately 5,000 follicles remain. The remaining residual follicles require an increasing concentration of follicle-stimulating hormone (FSH) to induce follicle maturation.

Endocrine changes in the pituitary-ovarian axis begin approximately a decade before a woman has her last menstrual period. The first detectable change in pituitary-ovarian function is a gradual rise in the basal plasma FSH concentration. Despite the subtle chemical changes that herald menopause, there are few associated clinical features. As menopause nears, the plasma FSH continues to increase until it exceeds the plasma concentration of luteinizing hormone (LH). During the prime reproductive years the basal plasma concentration of LH is 2.5 times greater than FSH. As residual ovarian follicles become refractory to gonadotropin stimulation, estradiol-17β (E_2) production by the theca cells decreases and thus decreases the negative feedback upon the hypothalamic-pituitary secretory mechanism.

The physiologic changes that occur in pituitary-ovarian function with approaching menopause require nearly 10 years from beginning to end. Following surgical castration of ovulating women, the rise in gonadotropins from a premenopausal level to a menopausal level occurs in 1 month or less. The symptoms that occur with gradual estrogen withdrawal and excess gonadotropin secretion can be produced immediately by surgical castration.

Despite ovarian failure at menopause, the menopausal woman continues to produce estrogen by the aromatization of adrenal androstenedione to estrone. Estrone is the postmenopausal estrogen, the principle behind which was established by MacDonald, Siiteri, and co-workers. Prior to ovarian failure, androstenedione is secreted in equal amounts (1.5 mg/day) by the adrenal glands and the ovaries. During the reproductive years a woman metabolizes approximately 1.5% of the androstenedione to estrone by aromatization. This metabolic pathway accounts for a daily production of estrone of approximately 40 μg per day. Following menopause the ovarian secretion of androstenedione becomes nil, but, remarkably, the extent of aromatization increases from 1.5% to 3%, so that the net production of estrone remains unchanged. Advancing age accounts for this increase in aromatization, but other factors (e.g., obesity and liver disease) can further increase this extraglandular estrogen production.

Judd and colleagues measured the peripheral and ovarian venous concentrations of androgens and estrogens in postmenopausal women. They report that ovaries of menopausal women continue to secrete androstenedione and testosterone as well as small amounts of estrone and estradiol. Because the ovarian blood flow is reduced at menopause, Siiteri argues that the ovarian contribution to steroid production is exceedingly small.

The symptoms of menopause are hot flushes, vaginal dryness, dyspareunia, and mood changes. Hot flushes herald menopause, being the first recognized symptom. The pathophysiology of the hot flush is poorly understood, but most investigators acknowledge that the hot flush accompanies estrogen withdrawal. Prepubertal girls who have not been exposed to estrogen do not experience hot flushes; young women with gonadal dysgenesis who have never been exposed to estrogen do not experience hot flushes. Yet, once a person is exposed to estrogens (either by endogenous production or exogenous administration) and has that source of estrogen withdrawn, that person will experience hot flushes. This occurs in both men and women.

Casper, Yen, and Wilkes demonstrated that each hot flush episode in a woman is followed by a pulsatile release of pituitary LH. The initiating event of this pulsatile LH secretion is unknown.

Prolonged estrogen deprivation results in atrophy of estrogen-dependent target issues. The breasts lose their turgor; the vaginal epithelium becomes smooth and thin; the cervix ceases secretion of large amounts of cervical mucus. These atrophic changes result in vaginal dryness and dyspareunia, and some women lose their sense of feminine identity. Estrogen replacement reverses these atrophic changes to variable degrees in symptomatic menopausal women. Some women achieve complete restoration of tissue function while others achieve only partial recovery of function.

Menopausal women complain of mood changes and emotional instability in their early menopausal years. Depression, despondency, lack of self-interest, and lack of interest in other family members are frustrating changes for women who formerly led active, adjusted lives. For lack of a physiologic explanation, these complaints have been attributed to an "empty nest syndrome" or a sense of loss of self-worth due to reproductive failure.

Recent advances in the understanding of estrogen metabolism may offer some basis for an understanding of the mood disturbances that accompany menopause. When radiolabeled estradiol is infused into normal volunteers, part is metabolized by 16α-hydroxylation, resulting in the formation of estriol; and part is metabolized by 2-hydroxylation, resulting in the formation of 2-hydroxyestradiol. The latter compound is named a catechol estrogen because of the identical structure of the "A-ring" of the steroid nucleus and the catechol ring of the catecholamine neurotransmitters. Catechol estrogens are formed in high concentrations in the hypothalamus; moreover, these estrogen metabolites compete with the neurotransmitters for the metabolizing enzyme, catechol-O-methyltransferase. Thus the important chemical link existing between estrogens and catecholamine neurotransmitters may play an important role in central nervous system function.

Beyond the age of 20 years, bone resorption increases modestly throughout life in normal individuals. With normal formation and increased resorption, bone density gradually decreases in the normal population. All patients with osteoporosis appear to have an increased rate of resorption, regardless of the cause. Albright and associates first suggested an association between osteoporosis and the menopause. In men and women who show gonadal failure at puberty, osteoporosis is almost a universal finding by age 30. Estrogens do not seem to stimulate bone formation, but they may inhibit bone resorption.

Meema and Meema found that castrated women have significantly less bone mass than premenopausal women of the same average age. They found that untreated postmenopausal women demonstrated a significant loss in bone mass, while estrogen-treated postmenopausal women showed no such loss.

Aitkin and colleagues made prospective studies of bone mass in women who had undergone oophorectomy for benign conditions. Untreated women lost bone at an accelerated rate in the 2 years following oophorectomy, while those women who received estrogen replacement (mestranol) showed no acceleration of bone resorption. When estrogen replacement therapy was initiated within 3 years of oophorectomy, bone mass increased. However, when estrogen replacement was delayed for 6 years beyond surgical castration, estrogen replacement had no effect on bone mass.

Daniell reported an epidemiologic analysis of women that links osteoporosis with a slender body habitus (< 110% of ideal body weight) and smoking. From these data the author suggests estrogen deficiency as a cause of osteoporosis. On the basis of available data the use of estrogens appears warranted in women at high risk for osteoporosis. These are slender (< 110% of ideal body weight) Caucasian women who smoke. Moreover, women with premature ovarian failure and those undergoing surgical menopause may benefit from estrogen replacement to retard bone demineralization.

In younger life, myocardial infarction occurs more frequently in men than in women. In the age range of 25–35, the sex ratio (male to female) is approximately 7:1. By age 80 the ratio becomes equal. This disparity in the risk of cardiovascular disease is attributed to the protective effects of estrogen during the premenopausal years. Epidemiologic data to support such a relationship are lacking. Such variables as life style, smoking, presence of hypertension, and stress are more likely causal factors in the risk of cardiovascular disease. The administration of estrogen as prophylactic protection against cardiovascular disease is unwarranted.

Menopause is an inevitable fact of life for women who live beyond the age of 50. Moreover, with the extended life expectancy of women in modern society, the number of menopausal women in our population will continue to increase. Definite alterations in endocrine physiology occur in the decade preceding actual menopause and continue for the remainder of a woman's life. Only 25% of menopausal women experience the overt symptoms (i.e., mood changes, hot flushes, and genital atrophy) of menopause; an equal number experience the insidious effects on bone density. Clearly, estrogen replacement alleviates the hot flush, restores estrogen target tissues, and enhances a return of psychologic well-being. Further, estrogen appears to retard the process of bone demineralization. Yet, our current understanding of the immediate and remote effects of hypergonadotropism and estrogen deprivation is inadequate to enable physicians to make categorical recommendations concerning hormonal replacement therapy.

Physiology of the Menopause

1. Sherman, B. M., and Korenman, S. G. Hormonal characteristics of the human menstrual cycle throughout reproductive life. *J. Clin. Invest.* 55:699, 1976.
   A cross-sectional study of the effects of aging on the menstrual cycle.
2. Aksel, S., et al. Vasomotor-symptoms, serum estrogens, and gonadotropins in surgical menopause. *Am. J. Obstet. Gynecol.* 126:165, 1976.
   The effects of surgical castration in premenopausal women.
3. Siiteri, P. K., and MacDonald, P. C. Role of Extraglandular Estrogen in Human Endocrinology. In R. A. Geyer, E. B. Astwood, and R. O. Greep (Eds.), *Handbook of Physiology, Section 7, Endocrinology.* Washington, D.C.: The American Physiological Society, 1973.
   A comprehensive review of extraglandular estrogen metabolism.
4. Grodin, J. M., Siiteri, P. K., and MacDonald, P. C. Source of estrogen production in postmenopausal women. *J. Clin. Endocrinol. Metab.* 36:207, 1973.
   The physiology of estrogen production after menopause.
5. Judd, H. L., et al. Endocrine function of the postmenopausal ovary; concentrations of androgens and estrogens in ovarian and peripheral vein blood. *J. Clin. Endocrinol. Metab.* 39:1020, 1974.
   A study of ovarian steroidogenesis in postmenopausal women.
6. Siiteri, P. K. Post Menopausal-Estrogen Production. In P. A. VanKeep and C. Lauritzen (Eds.), *Ageing and Estrogens.* New York: Karger, 1973. Vol. 2.
   Discusses mechanisms of steroidogenesis in postmenopausal women.
7. Fishman, J., Boyar, R. M., and Hellman, L. Influence of body weight on estradiol metabolism in young women. *J. Clin. Endocrinol. Metab.* 41:989, 1975.
   Body weight modulates estrogen metabolism in premenopausal and postmenopausal women.

Vasomotor Symptoms

8. Casper, R. F., Yen, S. S. C., and Wilkes, M. M. Menopausal flushes: A neuroendocrine link with pulsatile luteinizing hormone secretion. *Science* 205:823, 1979.
   A classic paper on the relationship between gonadotropin secretion and the hot flush.
9. Bates, G. W. On the nature of the hot flush. *Clin. Obstet. Gynecol.* 24:231, 1981.
   A review of the mechanisms of the hot flush.
10. Ball, P., et al. Interactions between estrogens and catechol amines: III. Studies on the methylation of catechol estrogens, catechol amines, and other catechols by the catechol-O-methyltransferase of the human liver. *J. Clin. Endocrinol. Metab.* 34:736, 1972.
    Discusses interactions of estrogens and catecholamines that are relevant to menopause.

Osteoporosis

11. Albright, F., Smith, P. H., and Richardson, A. M. Postmenopausal osteoporosis: Its clinical features. *J.A.M.A.* 116:2645, 1941.

Original description of the relationship of menopause and osteoporosis.
12. Meema, S., and Meema, H. E. Menopausal bone loss and estrogen replacement. *Isr. J. Med. Sci.* 12:601, 1976.
   Classic paper on the effect of estrogen in reducing bone loss.
13. Aitken, J., et al. Prevention of bone loss following oophorectomy in premenopausal women. A retrospective assessment of the effects of oophorectomy and a prospective controlled trial of the effects of oophorectomy and a prospective controlled trial of the effects of mestranol therapy. *Isr. J. Med. Sci.* 12:607, 1976.
   Effects of estrogen in preventing bone loss.
14. Daniell, H. W. Osteoporosis of the slender smoker. *Arch. Intern. Med.* 136:298, 1976.
   A classic paper describing the effects of smoking and body habitus on bone metabolism.

Treatment of the Menopause
15. Bates, G. W., Ruvinsky, E. D., and Thompson, S. W. Medical management of the menopause. *J. Miss. State Med. Assoc.* 22:113, 1981.
   A paper that presents modern methods of management for menopausal women.
16. Riddick, D. H. Hormonal management of the climacteric. *Female Patient* 6:15, 1981.
   Another contemporary discussion of medical management of the menopausal woman.

Gonadal Dysgenesis

Gonadal dysgenesis is characterized by sex chromosomal abnormalities, gonadal maldevelopment, abnormal sexual development, and somatic abnormalities. It is classically divided into three types: Turner's syndrome, mixed gonadal dysgenesis, and pure gonadal dysgenesis.

The principal features of Turner's syndrome are primary amenorrhea, sexual infantilism, nonfunctional streak gonads, and short stature. Somatic anomalies are common and include shield chest, webbing of the neck, cubitus valgus, coarctation of the aorta, and renal abnormalities. The etiologic basis for Turner's syndrome is the complete or partial deletion of the X chromosome or structural abnormality of the X chromosome. The 45X is the most frequent karyotype, although mosaics are also common and usually less severely affected. Most patients are sterile, although a small number may spontaneously menstruate and 58 pregnancies have been reported in women with a mosaic form of Turner's syndrome.

The most common presentation of mixed gonadal dysgenesis is that of ambiguous genitalia at birth, yet a wide range of phenotypes from normal female to normal male are possible. Although various abnormal karyotypes occur, XO/XY mosaicism is the most common. There is always some Y chromosomal component. A streak gonad on one side and a testis on the contralateral side is the usual gonadal presentation. Most of these infants are raised as females and removal of the dysgenetic gonads is indicated as soon as possible to prevent unwanted virilization and the development of gonadal tumors, especially gonadoblastomas.

The category of pure gonadal dysgenesis refers to those patients who are phenotypic females and have streak gonads, sexual infantilism, and a normal XX or XY karyotype. These individuals comprise one-third of patients with streak gonads. In both forms environmental damage to the gonad during embryogenesis has been postulated; however, there is evidence to suggest an autosomal recessive inheritance in the XX form, and X-linked recessive inheritance in the XY form. Patients with the XY karyotype may show variable degrees of müllerian regression, resulting in abnormalities of the uterus and vagina. Moreover, they are at high risk for the development of gonadoblastomas.

Regardless of the particular type of gonadal dysgenesis, the treatment is basically the same for all patients. First, adequate counseling must be provided for those patients who have difficulty adjusting emotionally to their situation. Second, hormonal therapy should be instituted at the appropriate age to induce secondary sexual characteristics and menses. Finally, patients who have a Y chromosomal component must undergo surgical removal of their gonads to prevent the occurrence of gonadal tumors.

As girls with Turner's syndrome show signs of sexual infantilism, we direct our therapy to stimulating growth of the secondary sexual organs. In the female, breast development is the first event in sexual maturation, and breast development is a manifestation of estrogen secretion. Vaginal maturation, uterine enlargement, and endometrial growth are concomitant events resulting from estrogen secretion. To simulate the normal pubertal process, we administer conjugated equine estrogens, 1.25 mg twice daily, and continue the regimen until uterine bleeding occurs. (This corresponds to menarche in a normal adolescent.) Breast growth, sexual hair growth, and uterine enlargement parallel that in normal puberty. Once uterine bleeding occurs, we change the hormonal regimen to conjugated equine estrogens, 1.25 mg once a day, for 25 days each month and add medroxyprogesterone acetate (MPA), 10 mg daily, from day 16 through 25 of the hormonal cycle. The addition of MPA produces rounding of the breasts and cyclic withdrawal bleeding.

We do not advocate the use of synthetic estrogens or combination oral contraceptives for initiating sexual development in girls with gonadal dysgenesis. The former produce abnormal development of the nipple, and the latter does not promote full breast development.

In those individuals who have a Y chromosome, we perform a gonadectomy in the midteen years (ages 15–17) to prevent a subsequent gonadoblastoma. As these tumors arise only after adolescence we do not believe that surgical removal during childhood is indicated.

General
1. McDonough, P. G., and Byrd, J. R. Gonadal dysgenesis. *Clin. Obstet. Gynecol.* 20:565, 1977.
   An excellent general review of the forms of gonadal dysgenesis, including work-up and treatment.
2. Simpson, J. L. Genes, chromosomes, and reproductive failure. *Fertil. Steril.* 33:107, 1980.
   Outstanding discussion of the genetic mechanisms of sexual differentiation.

Turner's Syndrome
3. Palmer, C. G., and Reichmann, A. Chromosomal and clinical findings in 110 females with Turner's syndrome. *Hum. Genet.* 35:35, 1976.

A study comparing abnormal karyotypes in patients with Turner's syndrome and the incidence of somatic anomalies.

4. Reyes, F. I., Koh, K. S., and Faiman, C. Fertility in women with gonadal dysgenesis. *Am. J. Obstet. Gynecol.* 126:668, 1976.
   Comprehensive review of the reproductive history of patients with Turner's syndrome.

5. Litvak, A. S., et al. The association of significant renal anomalies with Turner's syndrome. *J. Urol.* 120:671, 1978.
   An excellent study and literature review detailing renal anomalies in Turner's syndrome.

Mixed Gonadal Dysgenesis

6. Donahoe, P. K., Crawford, J. D., and Hendren, W. H. Mixed gonadal dysgenesis, pathogenesis, and management. *J. Pediatr. Surg.* 14:287, 1979.
   Case studies with an excellent discussion of the genetics, pathophysiology, and management of mixed gonadal dysgenesis.

Pure Gonadal Dysgenesis

7. Edman, C. D., et al. Embryonic testicular regression, a clinical spectrum of XY agonadal individuals. *Obstet. Gynecol.* 49:208, 1977.
   Case presentations with hormonal profiles and discussion of embryogenesis and possible etiologies.

8. Coulam, C. B. Testicular regression syndrome. *Obstet. Gynecol.* 53:44, 1979.
   Excellent review of embryogenesis and interesting proposals for revised terminology in this area.

9. German, J., Simpson, J. L., and Chaganti, R. S. K. Genetically determined sex-reversal in 46 XY humans. *Science* 202:53, 1978.
   Very interesting discussion on the possible existence of a new gene controlling testicular differentiation.

Gonadal Tumors in Gonadal Dysgenesis

10. Manuel, M., Katayama, K. P., and Jones, H. W. The age of occurrence of gonadal tumors in intersex patients with a Y chromosome. *Am. J. Obstet. Gynecol.* 124:293, 1976.
    A study of the age-related incidence of gonadal tumors in patients with gonadal dysgenesis and other intersex states.

Testicular Feminization

Testicular feminization syndrome is characterized by an XY karyotype, bilateral functional testes, female external genitalia, a blind vagina, and no müllerian derivatives. At birth these genotypic males are assigned a female gender and are raised as females during childhood and adolescence. It is estimated that this disorder occurs in 1 in 60,000 males, and despite its rarity, understanding this fascinating disorder makes clear the mechanisms of androgen action.

In males testosterone (T) is secreted by the Leydig cells of the testes, bound to testosterone-estrogen–binding globulin, and transported to androgen-dependent tissues. A small fraction of the bound T disassociates and diffuses across the cell membrane of androgen-dependent cells. Within the cytosol, T is reduced to a more potent androgen, dihydrotestosterone (DHT). DHT is bound to a cytosolic androgen receptor and carried into the nucleus of the cell where androgen action takes place. In testicular feminization syndrome, the androgen-dependent cells lack a cytosolic receptor for DHT.

During fetal life the Sertoli cells and Leydig cells of the fetal testes secrete müllerian duct–inhibiting factor (MDIF) and testosterone, respectively. MDIF inhibits the müllerian ducts to suppress development of the fallopian tubes, uterus, and upper vagina; T stimulates development of the wolffian ducts, phallus, and scrotum.

In testicular feminization syndrome the fetal testes function in a normal fashion to secrete MDIF and T. Thus, there are no female internal genitalia, but, since there is no cytosolic receptor for DHT within androgen-dependent cells, the phallus and scrotum fail to develop. The external genitalia then are female.

At the time of puberty the testes enlarge and secrete testosterone as expected, but again there is no androgen action and the genitalia remain female. Moreover, the sexual hair follicles require DHT for their function, and because of the lack of androgen action, axillary and pubic hair do not appear at puberty. Lack of sexual hair (but not lack of scalp hair) is a distinguishing feature of this disorder and may be the clue that leads to the correct diagnosis.

As the testes are capable of normal testosterone secretion at puberty and thereafter in these people, plasma testosterone concentration is within or exceeds the normal male range. Testosterone is the substrate for estradiol-17β (E_2) in men and women. In this disorder a fraction of T is aromatized to E_2 in extraglandular sites, and this E_2, in the absence of T action, stimulates full breast development.

Thus, at the time of puberty, female gender identity in these genotypic males is preserved because of the development of breasts and the appearance of other female contours. However, because of the lack of a uterus, menstruation never occurs and these women present to the gynecologist for evaluation of primary amenorrhea.

The diagnosis can be made on clinical grounds. Absence of sexual hair, absence of a uterus and vagina, and inguinal gonads suggest the diagnosis. Confirmation is made by finding an XY karyotype, plasma T in the male range, normal FSH, and elevated LH. A positive diagnosis is made by demonstrating lack of a cytosolic receptor for DHT in androgen-dependent tissues.

After puberty is complete the testes should be removed since they are prone to undergo neoplastic change; inguinal hernias, if present, should be repaired; a vaginoplasty should be performed to facilitate normal sexual function. Once the testes have been removed, estrogen replacement therapy is required to sustain estrogen-dependent tissues and to prevent postcastration hot flashes.

Mechanisms of Sexual Differentiation

1. Jost, A. Problems of fetal endocrinology: The gonadal and hypophysial hormones. *Recent Prog. Horm. Res.* 8:379, 1953.
   A review of the classic studies performed by Jost on the role of the gonad in sexual differentiation.

2. Jost, A., et al. Studies on sex differentiation in mammals. *Recent Prog. Horm. Res.* 29:1, 1973.
   An updated review by Jost on his discoveries.

3. Wilson, J. D. Recent studies on the mechanism of action of testosterone. *N. Engl. J. Med.* 287:1284, 1972.
A review of the cellular action of testosterone.
4. Wilson, J. D. Testosterone uptake by the urogenital tract of the rabbit embryo. *Endocrinology* 92:1192, 1973.
Studies on the action of testosterone in the fetus.
5. Siiteri, P. K., and Wilson, J. D. Testosterone formation and metabolism during male sexual differentiation in the human embryo. *J. Clin. Endocrinol. Metab.* 38:113, 1974.
A correlation of fetal development with a 5-α reductase activity.
6. Josso, N. Permeability of membranes to the müllerian-inhibiting substance synthesized by the human fetal testes *in vitro:* A clue to its biochemical nature. *J. Clin. Endocrinol. Metab.* 34:265, 1972.
A study of müllerian-inhibiting factor.

Biochemical Studies in Testicular Feminization

7. Southern, A. T., et al. Plasma concentration and biosynthesis of testosterone in the syndrome of feminizing testes. *J. Clin. Endocrinol. Metab.* 25:518, 1965.
Testosterone secretion, metabolism, and action.
8. Judd, H. L., et al. Androgen and gonadotropin dynamics in testicular feminization. *J. Clin. Endocrinol. Metab.* 34:229, 1972.
Pituitary-gonadal action in testicular feminization.
9. Rosenfield, R. L. Androgens and androgen responsiveness in the feminizing testes syndrome: Comparison of complete and incomplete forms. *J. Clin. Endocrinol. Metab.* 32:625, 1971.
There are incomplete variations of testicular feminization as well as the complete form.
10. Wilson, J. D., et al. Familial incomplete male pseudohermaphroditism, Type I. Evidence of androgen resistance and variable clinical manifestations in a family with the Reifenstein syndrome. *N. Engl. J. Med.* 290:1097, 1974.
Studies on an incomplete form of testicular feminization.

Vulvar Dystrophies and Atypias

Dystrophies of the vulva are chronic disorders of epithelial growth that result in alterations of the surface appearance and architecture. The changes seen may be localized or diffuse, thickened or thinned. White or red color changes may be evident. The two basic forms are hyperplastic dystrophy and lichen sclerosus. When both are present simultaneously, a mixed dystrophy is present. Because diagnosis is based entirely on histology, biopsy is mandatory.

Cellular atypia may exist in the squamous epithelium with or without a vulvar dystrophy present. Mild, moderate, or severe categories are recognized, depending on the extent of the change. When these cellular changes involve the epithelium totally, carcinoma in situ is present. Once again, the gross appearance is variable and diagnosis is dependent on biopsy.

The major microscopic features of hyperplastic dystrophy include epithelial thickening (hyperplasia), thickening of the keratin layer (hyperkeratosis), elongation and widening of the epithelial rete ridges (acanthosis), the retention of nuclear material in the keratin layer (parakeratosis), and varying degrees of chronic inflammation within the dermis. On gross examination, the lesions may be small or extensive. White patches, a red appearance, fissures, and excoriations from scratching may be present.

Most patients are in the 20–50-year-old age group. Frequently, there is a history of contact irritation such as that due to clothes washed with a new laundry detergent or the use of hygiene sprays. Tight clothing and synthetic underwear, by increasing local conditions of heat and moisture, may be factors. As with all dystrophies, pruritus is the most prominent symptom.

Whatever the cause, therapy with topical corticosteroids is highly effective. General measures include therapy of vaginitis, if present, the use of loose cotton underwear, and hygienic measures directed toward keeping the vulva clean and dry. The itch-scratch cycle, which so aggravates the condition, may respond to the use of crotamiton (Eurax) cream in conjunction with the steroid.

Lichen sclerosus is usually a disease of postmenopausal women, although it may occur in children and young adults. The etiology is unknown. The skin surface is dry, rough, and has been likened to parchment or cigarette paper, although the appearance may be diffuse, macular, pale, or wet. Fissures, cracks, and ecchymoses are common. Identical lesions can appear elsewhere on the body. As the condition progresses, the labia minora are taken up into the majora, adhesions bury the clitoris, and the introitus shrinks in diameter (kraurosis).

Microscopically, thinning, with loss of epithelial folds (rete ridges), is seen in varying degrees. The dermis beneath the squamous epithelium has an acellular homogeneous appearance. An inflammatory infiltrate is frequently present at the lower margin of this dermal area. On occasion, hyperkeratosis or parakeratosis may be present.

Treatment consists of application of topical 2% testosterone propionate ointment two or three times daily for at least 4 weeks, and thereafter once or twice weekly as maintenance therapy. Side effects of therapy sometimes encountered are clitoral enlargement and increased libido, but these seldom require cessation of treatment. In most instances, clinical response is satisfactory.

Islands of epithelial hyperplasia (hyperplastic dystrophy) may be interspersed between areas of lichen sclerosus; this is then termed a *mixed dystrophy*. Some 27%–35% of patients with lichen sclerosus may exhibit such areas of squamous hyperplasia. The entities are treated in the usual manner, individually (either at the same time or in sequence), and response is as for the individual lesions.

The incidence of malignant change with a chronic vulvar dystrophy is small, probably 1%–5% over many years. The incidence with lichen sclerosus is practically nil, and malignant change is most likely to occur in those cases of hyperplastic dystrophy (pure or mixed) in which epithelial atypia (dysplasia) is also present. In all instances, however, these patients require close observation, with multiple biopsies of the vulva at regular intervals.

Cellular atypias are encountered with viral infections and hyperplastic dystrophies, as well as with many other local stimuli. There is no definitive gross alteration, although whitish, red, or pigmented areas may be seen. The cytologic changes in mild atypia include enlarged hyperchromatic nuclei, while there is coarse chromatin clumping in moderate atypia. In the moderate form, the increased cellularity and cellular disarray is confined to the inner two-thirds of the epithelium. In severe atypia, more than two-thirds is involved; cells of the parabasal type are found near the surface; and chromatin clumping is moderately coarse and irregular. Carcinoma in situ is characterized by full-thickness cellular disorientation (with the exception of the most superficial keratinized layers) with giant cells, multinucleated cells, individual cell keratinization, corps ronds formation (pale halo of cytoplasm around a pyknotic nucleus), abnormal mitoses, and squamous "pearls" at the tips of the rete pegs. Parakeratosis and hyperkeratosis may be present, and there is usually an inflammatory response in the dermis.

Diagnostic biopsy is aided by the use of a nuclear stain, 1% toluidine blue. The dye is applied, allowed to set, and decolorized with 1% acetic acid. The nonulcerated areas that remain blue are probably parakeratotic and, thus, atypical. While helpful, there is an unfortunately high false-positive and false-negative rate.

The progression of vulvar atypia, or carcinoma in situ, to invasive vulval carcinoma has not been demonstrated anywhere near as clearly as has that of the cervical dysplasias. Conservatism should, therefore, be the rule, and individualization of therapy is most important. In mild cases, elimination of pruritus and removal of the causative agent, if possible, may be sufficient. Wide local excision is called for with marked atypias.

Carcinoma in situ occurs in a much younger age group (the median age is between 30 and 40) than invasive cancer and is encountered far more frequently. Itching, a lump, bleeding, and pain are the most common symptoms. The lesions may be pink, white, red, or brown, and often are slightly elevated. Diagnosis is via biopsy, aided by toluidine blue staining or colposcopy, or both. Cytology is rarely helpful. Since cervical, vaginal, or perineal epithelial neoplasms may coexist in up to 25% of cases, workup should include screening for these possibly associated lesions.

Therapy is basically surgical, with wide local excision of unifocal areas; if the margins are uninvolved, results are good. Extensive, confluent multicentric lesions require "skinning" vulvectomy, with primary closure or skin grafting. Lesions of the inner vulva that are not hyperkeratotic may respond to a 6-week course of 5-fluorouracil cream, although painful sloughing may require hospitalization. A success rate of 50% has been claimed. In all patients, careful follow-up of the entire area and lower genital tract is mandatory.

Carcinoma in situ and Paget's disease are classified as intraepithelial neoplasms of the vulva. The latter is a disease of older women and is characterized by moist, reddish lesions diagnosed by the presence of the pathognomonic Paget cells (large cells with a clear vacuolated cytoplasm), which may be associated with an underlying adenocarcinoma. Treatment of the condition is by wide local excision, or modified vulvectomy, after excluding associated carcinoma by thorough preoperative assessment.

Reviews

1. International Society for the Study of Vulvar Disease. New nomenclature for vulvar disease. *Obstet. Gynecol.* 47:122, 1976.
   Older terms deleted from use include lichen sclerosus et atrophicus, leukoplakia, kraurosis vulvae, neurodermatitis, *and* hyperplastic vulvitis.
2. Kaufman, R. H., and Gardner, H. L. Vulvar dystrophies. *Clin. Obstet. Gynecol.* 21:1081, 1978.
   Excellent review.
3. Buscema, J., et al. Carcinoma in situ of the vulva. *Obstet. Gynecol.* 55:225, 1980.
   The specific term carcinoma in situ *has replaced earlier nomenclature, including* Bowen's disease *and* erythroplasia of Queyrat.
4. Breen, J. L., Smith, C. I., and Gregori, C. A. Extramammary Paget's disease. *Clin. Obstet. Gynecol.* 21:1107, 1978.
   A composite evaluation of 98 cases.

Dystrophies

5. Kaufman, R. H. Hyperplastic dystrophy. *J. Reprod. Med.* 17:137, 1976.
   Administration of estrogens is worthless since the dystrophies are unrelated to estrogen deficiency.
6. Friedrich, E. G., Jr. Lichen sclerosus. *J. Reprod. Med.* 17:147, 1976.
   Local testosterone therapy arrests the dystrophic agglutination process.
7. Jasionowski, E. A., and Jasionowski, P. A. Further observations on the effect of topical progesterone on vulvar disease. *Am. J. Obstet. Gynecol.* 134:565, 1979.
   Good results in all varieties of dystrophy, but there were only 11 patients in the series.

Atypias

8. Broen, E., and Ostergard, D. Toluidine blue and colposcopy for screening and delineating vulvar neoplasia. *Obstet. Gynecol.* 38:5, 1971.
   The Keyes' dermal punch is a useful instrument for obtaining the biopsies from the areas delineated.
9. Wilkinson, E. J., Friedrich, E. G., Jr., and Fu, Y. S. Multicentric nature of vulvar carcinoma in situ. *Obstet. Gynecol.* 58:69, 1981.
   A comparison of multicentric and confluent lesions.
10. Baggish, M. S., and Dorsey, J. H. CO_2 laser for the treatment of vulvar carcinoma in situ. *Obstet. Gynecol.* 57:371, 1981.
    One-third of 35 patients treated were under 30 years of age. Treatment was successful and left no scarring.

Vulvar Carcinoma

Invasive cancer of the vulva is the fourth most common primary pelvic cancer, occurring in from 3%–4% of pelvic cancer cases. It is usually seen in women in their mid to late sixties, although a group of younger patients are

also seen in whom the disease has followed sexually transmitted granulomatous vulval infections (including granuloma inguinale or neglected condylomata accuminata).

The significance of the vulval dystrophies and atypias in the genesis of
invasive epidermoid cancer has already been covered in the previous essay.
In addition, an appreciable number of vulvar carcinomas have followed radiotherapy for cervical cancers. It is not uncommon to find multiple primary
neoplasms (invasive or preinvasive) of the cervix, vagina, anus, and vulva.
These lesions may occur synchronously or metachronously. This association of malignant change in an embryologically similar area of squamous
epithelium suggests the possible action of a carcinogenic factor or a predisposed area, and at present, the most likely possible etiologic agent appears to
be the type II herpes virus.

Ninety percent of vulvar carcinomas are squamous; 5% are melanomas.
Sarcoma, adenocarcinoma (usually of Bartholin's glands or with Paget's disease), basal cell carcinoma, and lymphoma comprise the remainder. The
location of the lesion is labial in 70% and clitoral in 13% of cases. The urethra
and perineum may also be the site of the tumor.

Spread is by contiguity to adjoining structures. Growth is slow, but many
patients are reluctant to see a physician, and perineum, anus, vagina, and
even pubic bone may be involved in neglected cases. Lymphatic spread is
almost always predictable and constant, first to inguinal nodes, then femoral
nodes, and later to pelvic and paraaortic nodes. Drainage to the contralateral
groin nodes occurs, especially in tumors situated near the midline.

Vulval cancer is staged by clinical criteria based chiefly on pelvic examination. Stage I cases have a tumor less than 2 cm in diameter confined to the
vulva. Stage II cases have a tumor more than 2 cm in diameter confined to
the vulva. Groin nodes are not suspicious in either stage I or II. Stage III is
characterized by spread to urethra, vagina, perineum, or anus, and/or suspicious groin nodes. Stage IV is diagnosed when bladder, rectum, or upper
urethral mucosa are infiltrated or there is bony fixation or distant metastasis.

The clinical picture is usually pruritus or pain associated with a lump
or ulcer. A bloody discharge may be present. Diagnosis is made by taking a
biopsy specimen from the edge of the lesion. Toluidine blue or colposcopy
may be of assistance in directing the biopsy as outlined in the previous chapter. Once the diagnosis has been made, workup includes chest x-ray, intravenous pyelogram, cervical Pap smear, cystoscopy, and/or proctoscopy as
indicated by the site of the lesion. If pelvic lymph node involvement is suspected, lymphangiography and CAT scan may be helpful, especially if needle
biopsy of suspicious nodes is available to the clinician.

Obesity, hypertension, diabetes, previous syphilitic infection, and arte-
riosclerosis are common in these patients, which, together with their advanced age, complicates therapy. Nevertheless, the majority of patients are
sufficiently healthy for definitive therapy, which is generally surgical since
radiotherapy and chemotherapy are relatively unsuccessful in the treatment
of vulvar cancer.

The standard surgical therapy is radical vulvectomy and bilateral inguinal and femoral lymphadenectomy. The procedure removes the tumor with
lymphatics and nodes en bloc. If the deepest femoral node in the femoral
canal (Cloquet's) is shown by frozen section to be involved by tumor, a deep
pelvic node dissection may then be performed, removing the external iliac,
obturator, and hypogastric nodes. Because a large amount of skin and subcutaneous tissue are excised, the postoperative course tends to be prolonged,

with a high incidence of wound necrosis requiring secondary closure or skin grafting.

Since radical surgery can produce serious sexual dysfunction, especially in younger patients, as well as lymphedema of the lower limbs, surgery may be modified in selected cases. Thus, more conservative surgery may be employed in patients with microinvasive disease with minimal invasion. In some patients with more advanced disease, exenterative surgery may be required in addition to the standard procedure, for instance, when rectal mucosa is involved.

The use of radiotherapy has been limited, not by tumor resistance, but by the relative sensitivity of the vulvar tissues. Nevertheless, the use of megavoltage therapy is being reevaluated since some success has been obtained in advanced disease in which preoperative therapy has shrunk the tumor enough for surgery to be feasible and occasionally less radical. Other applications of radiation therapy include external beam treatment of involved deep pelvic nodes or local implantations of radium needles for tumor recurrences not amenable to surgical removal. When radiotherapy is used as the only modality for inoperable cases, the central tumor and the groin and pelvic nodes must be treated.

The size of the tumor is not always a good guide to the presence of groin metastasis (10% of lesions less than 2 cm have nodal involvement), and clinical assessment of lymph node involvement is incorrect in 13%–39% of cases. If the tumor is confined to the vulva, an 86% corrected 5-year survival may be expected; if superficial nodes are positive, this rate falls to 55%; if deep nodes are positive, the rate falls to 12.5%–50%.

At the present time, a degree of individualization in therapy appears to be possible without compromising the good results obtained in the past.

Reviews

1. Green, T. H., Jr. Carcinoma of the vulva. A reassessment. *Obstet. Gynecol.* 52:462, 1978.
   No instance of deep pelvic node involvement in the absence of superficial inguinofemoral node involvement.

2. Choo, Y. C., and Morley, G. W. Double primary epidermoid carcinoma of the vulva and cervix. *Gynecol. Oncol.* 9:324, 1980.
   In this series, 20.8% of patients with vulvar carcinoma had a second primary tumor. This paper also reviews the incidences previously reported in the literature.

Etiology

3. Friedrich, E. G., Jr., Wilkinson, E. J., and Fu, Y. S. Carcinoma in situ of the vulva: A continuing challenge. *Am. J. Obstet. Gynecol.* 136:830, 1980.
   Of 50 cases, 30% had a previous or concomitant vulval viral infection, 60% were associated with another sexually transmitted disease, and 30% had abnormal epithelium of the cervix or vagina, or both.

4. Hay, D. M., and Cole, F. M. Post-granulomatous carcinoma of the vulva. *Am. J. Obstet. Gynecol.* 107:479, 1970.
   Report from Jamaica where granulomatous sexually transmitted vulval disease is common.

5. Powell, L. C., Jr. Condyloma acuminatum: Recent advances in development, carcinogenesis, and treatment. *Clin. Obstet. Gynecol.* 21:1061, 1978.

Condyloma of the vulva coexists with or precedes vulvar cancer in up to 16% of cases.

Pathology

6. Buscema, J., Stern, J., and Woodruff, J. D. The significance of the histologic alterations adjacent to invasive vulvar carcinoma. *Am. J. Obstet. Gynecol.* 137:902, 1980.
   In situ changes were found in less than 20% of cases. Vulvar and cervical neoplasia appear to be different biologically and histopathologically.
7. Selim, M. A., and Lankerani, M. R. Verrucous carcinoma of the vulva. *J. Reprod. Med.* 22:93, 1979.
   In this review of the literature, there are 11 vulvar, 4 vaginal, and 6 cervical cases described. These tumors can generally be considered microinvasive carcinomas.
8. Curry, S. T., Wharton, J. T., and Rutledge, F. Positive lymph nodes in vulvar squamous carcinoma. *Gynecol. Oncol.* 9:63, 1980.
   Decreased survival if there are more than three positive nodes or if there are bilateral positive nodes.

Series

9. Iverson, T., et al. Squamous cell carcinoma of the vulva: A review of 424 patients, 1956–1974. *Gynecol. Oncol.* 9:271, 1980.
   Positive nodes in 10.5% of those with stage I lesions, 29.8% with stage II, 66% with stage III, and 100% with stage IV.
10. Buscema, J., Stern, J. L., and Woodruff, J. D. Early invasive carcinoma of the vulva. *Am. J. Obstet. Gynecol.* 140:563, 1981.
    A series of 58 cases illustrating problems associated with less than radical procedures based on unclear histopathologic diagnostic information.
11. Iversen, T., Abeler, V., and Aalders, J. Individualized treatment of stage I carcinoma of the vulva. *Obstet. Gynecol.* 57:85, 1981.
    Analyzes 117 cases. In the authors' opinion, treatment for most stage I cases should be hemivulvectomy with ipsilateral inguinal lymphadenectomy.

Treatment

12. Barnes, A. E., et al. Microinvasive carcinoma of the vulva: A clinicopathologic evaluation. *Obstet. Gynecol.* 56:234, 1980.
    Most cases can be treated by conservative surgery. Confluent infiltration or vascular invasion necessitates radical surgery.
13. DiSaia, P. J., Creasman, W. T., and Rich, W. M. An alternate approach to early cancer of the vulva. *Am. J. Obstet. Gynecol.* 133:825, 1979.
    A sampling of superficial inguinal nodes is utilized as a guide to therapy to avoid unnecessary mutilating surgery.
14. Calame, R. J. Pelvic relaxation as a complication of the radical vulvectomy. *Obstet. Gynecol.* 55:716, 1980.
    Complicated 17% of 58 cases; the author recommends preventive or reconstructive procedures during the primary operation.
15. Deppe, G., Cohen, C. J., and Bruckner, H. W. Chemotherapy of squamous cell carcinoma of the vulva: A review. *Gynecol. Oncol.* 7:345, 1979.
    Responses occurred only with regimens containing bleomycin and methotrexate.
16. Buchler, D. A., et al. Treatment of recurrent carcinoma of the vulva. *Gynecol. Oncol.* 8:180, 1979.

Report of 29 patients treated with either surgery or irradiation. Palliation was adequate in the majority, and 2 patients survived.

Other Vulvar Malignancies

17. Chung, A. F., Woodruff, J. M., and Lewis, J. L., Jr. Malignant melanoma of the vulva: A report of 44 cases. *Obstet. Gynecol.* 45:638, 1975.
    Enlargement or pruritis of a junctional nevus suggests the diagnosis. When confined to the vulva, there is 80% survival with radical surgery.

18. Dennefors, B., and Bergman, B. Primary carcinoma of the Bartholin gland. *Acta Obstet. Gynecol. Scand.* 59:95, 1980.
    Biopsy is indicated if necrotic material drains, if induration is present, or if healing is slow after drainage or marsupialization of a Bartholin cyst or abscess. Lesions are adenocarcinoma in 46% and squamous cell carcinoma in 40% of cases. Therapy is radical surgery.

19. Breen, J. E., et al. Basal cell carcinoma of the vulva. *Obstet. Gynecol.* 46:122, 1975.
    This type is locally invasive and requires wide local excision or simple vulvectomy.

20. DiSaia, P. J., Rutledge, F., and Smith, J. P. Sarcoma of the vulva: Report of 12 patients. *Obstet. Gynecol.* 38:180, 1971.
    Treatment of these rare tumors is radical surgery. Patients with rhabdomyosarcoma usually have a poor prognosis, while those with leiomyosarcoma often show prolonged survival.

Cervical Dysplasia

The junction between the squamous epithelium lining the ectocervix, and the columnar epithelium lining the endocervix, is called the squamocolumnar junction or transitional zone (TZ). Before puberty the junction is well out on the ectocervix (ectopy), while in the menopausal woman the junction is well into the cervical canal. The process by which the junction moves from its original to its final site is under hormonal influence, possibly by means of changes in vaginal pH. The replacement of the more fragile red columnar glandular epithelium by the more resistant pink squamous epithelium is called squamous metaplasia. The significance of these observations is that all grades of cervical neoplasia originate in the TZ. Normal epithelial maturation proceeds outward from the basal cells on the basement membrane and minor lesions involve this zone only.

All grades of abnormal epithelial maturation evidence abnormalities in DNA content or chromosome number. Various degrees of cytologic and histologic dedifferentiation are seen and cytologic cervical smears (Pap smears) as well as cervical biopsies are graded according to the degree and extent of the cellular abnormalities. Size, configuration, denseness of chromatin, mitoses, pleomorphism, and percentage of abnormal cells form the basis of the cytologic and histologic grade of the lesions. If the undifferentiated neoplastic cells extend through the full thickness of the epithelium but the basement membrane is not penetrated, the lesion is called carcinoma in situ (CIS).

Mild, moderate, and severe cervical dysplasia, together with CIS, represent stages along a continuum of preinvasive lesions of the epithelium of the uterine cervix. These lesions differ in the degree of cellular abnormalities seen and in the thickness of the epithelium involved. An alternative terminology, gaining in popularity, employs the term *cervical intraepithelial neoplasia* (CIN), such that CIN I equals mild, CIN II equals moderate, and CIN III represents severe dysplasia and carcinoma in situ. It is vital to clear understanding that in none of these lesions is the basement membrane breached (although glandular involvement is common) and that these lesions, although they may progress to invasion, are as yet not invasive and fall into Stage 0 of invasive cervical cancer. Unlike invasive cancer, these lesions are reversible or may arrest, and this is especially true of the earlier changes seen in CIN I and CIN II. Unfortunately, it is not possible to predict the behavior of the lesion in the individual patient other than in terms of percentage probabilities. Furthermore, the natural course may be modified by biopsy, drugs, and possibly trauma. For instance, in one series, CIS disappeared in 25%, persisted in 60%, and progressed to questionable or definite invasion in 15%.

The etiology of cervical precancer and cancer appears to involve an increased receptivity of the adolescent cervix to oncogenic initiation; thus, engaging in coitus first at an early age, with a high rate of venereal disease, is common in these patients. Sperm and a venereally transmitted virus (herpes simplex II) have been proposed as mutagens in this cancer.

Cervical cytology is basic to the diagnosis of dysplasia. A properly taken Pap smear should sample the endocervix and ectocervix. False-negative rates vary from 2%–22%; repetition of smears over a period of time improves these rates of pickup markedly. Historically, Pap test results were reported as being class I–V, with class I being negative; class II, inflammation; and classes III, IV, and V, increasing grades of dysplasia. At present, reporting is as for histology, i.e., negative to CIS. The prevalence of dysplasia by cytology varies from 5–65 per 1000, depending on the population group being screened.

Cervical cytology is a screening process only; definitive diagnosis requires tissue sampling. The colposcope delineates the extent of the cervical lesion and directs biopsy to the worst areas. If colposcopy is unavailable, biopsy of areas nonstaining with iodine (Schiller's test) may be employed, but frequently cone biopsy becomes necessary. Cone biopsy is also required if colposcopic examination is unsatisfactory. (Colposcopy is deemed unsatisfactory if the entire TZ cannot be seen, or if the colposcopic biopsy reveals a lesser grade of disease than the smear, or if the endocervical curettage [ECC] is positive.) Cone biopsy is used for therapy as well as diagnosis.

The treatment of CIN must be individualized according to the extent and grade of the lesion, the age and parity of the patient, the presence or absence of pregnancy, and the desire for future childbearing. The patient's suitability for surgery, her reliability in regard to regular follow-up, and the cost of therapy must also be taken into account.

In general, less extensive lesions and those of lesser severity are treated by local outpatient methods such as eradication of infections known to cause inflammatory cellular atypia (trichomonas), cryosurgery, electrocautery, excisional biopsy, and laser therapy. More severe and more extensive lesions are usually treated by cone biopsy and, on occasion, especially if other indications exist in patients who have completed their families, by hysterectomy. A concomitant pregnancy presents a problem, and if possible, treatment is postponed until after pregnancy, though cone biopsy may be performed during pregnancy if necessary. In recent years, the more extensive lesions and those of greater severity have also been treated by the nonextirpative methods mentioned, and this appears to be a continuing trend, which is probably safe, provided meticulous follow-up is employed.

Reviews

1. Briggs, R. M. Dysplasia and early neoplasia of the uterine cervix: A review. *Obstet. Gynecol. Surv.* 34:70, 1979.
   Comprehensive survey with 209 references.
2. Koss, L. G. Dysplasia: A real concept or a misnomer. *Obstet. Gynecol.* 51:374, 1978.
   The author states that it is the size, the location, and the presence or absence of invasion of the lesion that counts as a guide to treatment, rather than the histologic grade.

Etiology

3. Reagan, J. W., Ng, A. B., and Wentz, W. G. Concepts of genesis and development in early cervical neoplasia. *Obstet. Gynecol. Surv.* 24:860, 1969.
   It is postulated that a stimulus, usually a chemical carcinogen, "initiates" a potentially neoplastic state, which is then "promoted" by the same or other stimuli into a second stage, with morphologic alterations visible in the epidermis. The young cervix appears to be particularly susceptible to this "initiation-promotion" process.
4. Kessler, I. I. On the etiology and prevention of cervical cancer—a status report. *Obstet. Gynecol. Surv.* 34:790, 1979.
   Summarizes the evidence implicating genital herpes virus (HSV-2) as a factor in the etiology of cervical cancer.
5. Kurman, R. J., et al. Immunoperoxidase localization of papillomavirus antigens in cervical dysplasia and vulvar condylomas. *Am. J. Obstet. Gynecol.* 140:931, 1981.
   Papillomavirus antigens were present in 48% of patients with CIN and in 50% of women with vulvar condylomas.

Epidemiology

6. Stern, E. Epidemiology of dysplasia. *Obstet. Gynecol. Surv.* 24:711, 1969.
   In a middle-class, middle-aged, white population, the prevalence of dysplasia was 5.4 per 1000.
7. Feldman, M. J., et al. Abnormal cervical cytology in the teen-ager: A continuing problem. *Am. J. Obstet. Gynecol.* 126:418, 1976.
   The prevalence of dysplasia in a population of teenagers was 65 per 1000.

Pathogenesis

8. Reagan, J. W., Siedemann, I. L., and Saracusa, Y. Cellular morphology of carcinoma in situ and dysplasia or atypical hyperplasia of uterine cervix cancer. *Cancer* 6:224, 1953.
   Classic paper introducing the use of the term dysplasia *for lesions not as extensive as carcinoma in situ but with the capacity to progress to cancer.*
9. Wied, G. L. An international agreement on histological terminology for lesions of the uterine cervix. (Editorial.) *Acta Cytol.* (Baltimore) 6:235, 1962.
   CIS was defined as an epithelium in which throughout its thickness, no differentiation takes place. Unfortunately, the definition of differentiation was not provided.
10. Richart, R. M. Cervical intraepithelial neoplasia. *Pathol. Annu.* 8:301, 1973.
    The author argues that the division of CIN into two diseases, dysplasia

and CIS, is unwarranted. He notes that the cells contain abnormal chromosome numbers, and this aneuploid state persists through the spectrum of CIN, any level of which is capable of proceeding to invasion.

11. Richart, R. M., and Barron, B. A. A follow-up study of patients with cervical dysplasia. *Am. J. Obstet. Gynecol.* 105:386, 1969.
The mean time required to transit from dysplasia to CIS, taking all dysplasias together, was 4 years.

Diagnosis

12. Garite, T. J., and Feldman, M. J. An evaluation of cytologic sampling techniques. A comparative study. *Acta Cytol.* (Baltimore) 22:83, 1978.
The best yield for cervical cytologic diagnosis of dysplasia was obtained by studying two samples: one obtained by using an ectocervical spatula and the other an endocervical sample obtained with a cotton tipped applicator.

13. Urcuyo, R., Rome, R. M., and Nelson, J. H., Jr. Some observations on the value of endocervical curettage performed as an integral part of colposcopic examination of patients with abnormal cervical cytology. *Am. J. Obstet. Gynecol.* 128:787, 1977.
Although colposcopically directed cervical biopsy is considered adequate if the entire transformation zone is seen, most workers nevertheless routinely take an endocervical tissue sample lest disease in the canal be overlooked.

14. McDonnell, J. M., et al. Colposcopy in pregnancy. A twelve year review. *Br. J. Obstet. Gynaecol.* 88:414, 1981.
Cone biopsy was not performed in any of 195 patients and no cases of invasive cancer were missed.

15. Fidler, H. K., Boyes, D. A., and Worth, A. J. Cervical cancer detection in British Columbia: A progressive report. *J. Obstet. Gynaecol. Br. Commonw.* 75:392, 1968.
Pioneers in mass Pap screening to detect cervical cancer and precancer. Women most in need of screening are the least likely to come forward, and screening programs must seek out these high-risk groups.

Treatment

16. Javaheri, G., Balin, M., and Meltzer, R. M. Role of cryosurgery in the treatment of intraepithelial neoplasia of the uterine cervix. *Obstet. Gynecol.* 58:83, 1981.
Comparison with cone, hysterectomy, and electrocautery. Cryosurgery proved effective provided precise diagnosis was established by colposcopic biopsy.

17. Kolstad, P., and Klem, V. Long term follow-up of 1121 cases of carcinoma-in-situ. *Obstet. Gynecol.* 48:125, 1976.
In patients treated by conization and also in those treated by hysterectomy, around 1% developed invasive carcinoma and 2%, recurrent CIS. Follow-up was from 5–25 years and mortality from invasive cancer was 0.5%.

18. Chanen, W. Electrocoagulation diathermy treatment of cervical intraepithelial neoplasia. *Obstet. Gynecol. Surv.* 34:829, 1979.
General anesthesia was necessary, but the cure rate was 94.8%, and there were no instances of invasive carcinoma in the 812 cases treated.

19. Masterson, B. J., et al. The carbon dioxide laser in cervical intraepithelial neoplasia: A five-year experience in treating 230 patients. *Am. J. Obstet. Gynecol.* 139:565, 1981.
The 230 patients treated with a 90% success rate.

20. Jones, H. W., III, and Buller, R. E. The treatment of cervical intraepithelial neoplasia by cone biopsy. *Am. J. Obstet. Gynecol.* 137:882, 1980.

Problems sometimes encountered with cone biopsy include postoperative hemorrhage, nonclear surgical margins, and adverse effects on future fertility. Advantages include definitive histologic diagnosis and retention of fertility in most instances.

21. Averette, H. E., et al. Cervical conization in pregnancy. Analysis of 180 operations. *Am. J. Obstet. Gynecol.* 106:543, 1970.
    Blood transfusion was required for 17 patients.
22. Townsend, D. E., et al. Invasive cancer following outpatient evaluation and therapy for cervical disease. *Obstet. Gynecol.* 57:145, 1981.
    This report analyzes 66 cases. The authors suggest a minimum of two negative smears or one negative smear and colposcopy before therapy for a "cervical erosion" with hot or cold cautery.

Carcinoma of the Cervix

In the United States, cervical cancer is second only to corpus cancer as the most common gynecologic malignancy. It is second only to ovarian cancer as the most common cause of death from gynecologic malignancy. For the year 1980, it was estimated that 16,000 cases would be diagnosed, with 7400 deaths.

Epidemiologically, early sexual exposure appears to be the most significant factor in predisposing to cervical cancer. The socioeconomic factors of low income, frequent intercourse with multiple partners, pregnancy at an early age, multiple pregnancies, and high infection rates are important risk factors. The disease is common in prostitutes and rare in nuns.

It is thought that invasive cervical cancer is usually preceded by cervical intraepithelial neoplasia, although it seems likely that some carcinomas are invasive from the onset. Supporting this concept is the finding that the average age of patients is in the midforties, 10 years older than the average age of patients with carcinoma in situ. The intraepithelial lesion becomes invasive when the basement membrane is broken through with cancer cells invading the stroma.

Adenocarcinomas constitute only 5% of cervical cancers. The remaining 95% are epidermoid, of which 65% are large-cell nonkeratinizing, 23% are large-cell keratinizing, and 17% are small cell.

The growth may be exophytic, infiltrating, or ulcerating. Tumor extension occurs by contiguity down the vagina, into the parametrium, myometrium, and into bladder and rectum. Lymphatic spread is through the pelvic lymphatic chain to the paracervical, obturator, and hypogastric nodes. In advanced disease, common iliac, paraaortic, inguinal, and scalene nodes may be involved. Hematogenous spread is rare.

Cervical cancer is staged according to the FIGO (International Federation of Gynecology and Obstetrics) classification. Stage I lesions are confined to the cervix, with microinvasive (early stromal invasion) being designated as Ia and the remainder as Ib (occult cancer is marked "occ."). In stage IIa the cancer involves the upper vagina, and in stage IIb there is parametrial involvement. In stage IIIa the tumor involves the lower vagina, and in stage IIIb there is extension to the pelvic wall and/or hydronephrosis or a nonfunctioning kidney. In stage IVa growth has involved adjacent organs (bladder, rectum), and stage IVb indicates distant spread.

The incidence of involved regional nodes is directly related to the bulk of the tumor. Stage I shows 15% nodal involvement, stage II 25%, stage III 50%, and stage IV 66%.

Clinically, cervical cancer may present with intermenstrual, postcoital, or postmenopausal bleeding. Vaginal discharge is a later symptom and then may be serosanguinous or purulent. Pain is a symptom of late disease, representing visceral or neurologic involvement.

Physical examination usually reveals a hard, indurated, friable cervical lesion. Rectovaginal examination for extension of growth in the parametrium and uterosacral ligaments is an essential part of the physical assessment.

Diagnosis in patients with a gross lesion is by cervical punch biopsy. Colposcopy and cone biopsy are reserved for patients with abnormal cytology and no gross lesion. There is a high incidence of negative Pap smears with invasive cancer, since much of the tumor may be necrotic. Cytology should therefore not be relied on to exclude invasion.

Staging work-up of the patient once diagnosis is confirmed by histology should include blood chemistry, hematology, chest x-ray, and pyelogram. A cystoscopy and sigmoidoscopy are also usually performed. Lymphangiography is used by some, but others feel that this study is unreliable and do not use it.

The treatment plan for each patient should be determined by the gynecologic oncologist and radiotherapist in consultation. In general, most patients are treated by radiotherapy, although surgery is applicable to the treatment of early disease and in certain cases may be combined with radiotherapy. The surgical and radiotherapeutic procedures, along with their complications, are further discussed in the essays on radical surgery and radiotherapy.

Some controversy exists as regards the depth of penetration at which microinvasion should be regarded as frank invasion. A commonly accepted limiting depth is 3 mm from the base of the epithelium. If lymphatics or vessels contain tumor cells, the lesion is always regarded as frankly invasive as too are multifocal lesions.

The treatment of microinvasive disease is also controversial. Some feel that simple total hysterectomy is sufficient; others feel that a radical hysterectomy, with or without pelvic lymphadenectomy, should be performed. In patients unfit for surgery, radiotherapy is employed.

In stage Ib and in some early stage II cases, radical (Wertheim) hysterectomy with pelvic lymphadenectomy is favored in young patients since ovarian function is conserved and the vaginal mucosa remains fully functional. In general, however, irradiation is applicable to more cases than surgery since many patients are old, obese, or in poor health. In all other stages, radiotherapy is the treatment of choice. Intracavitary and intravaginal radiation are combined with external irradiation to treat the tumor, parametria, and draining lymph nodes.

Surgical staging prior to radiotherapy, employing extraperitoneal lymph node sampling, has been increasingly employed in recent years. In particular, the finding of cancer in the paraaortic nodes results in alterations of standard radiotherapy. Unfortunately, little improvement in prognosis has been proved following paraaortic irradiation, and it is to be hoped that diagnosis based on lymph node needle biopsy, whole body scanning, and lymphangiography may preclude the need for diagnostic surgery.

Follow-up visits after therapy should be made at least every 2 months, since most recurrent disease occurs within the first 2 years. At each visit, history and physical examination with Pap smear are obtained. At 6-month intervals, intravenous urography and chest x-rays are performed. Other investigations are ordered when suggested by the clinical findings.

Persistent or recurrent disease may be centrally situated, in the lymph nodes, or widespread. Symptoms include pain, discharge, bleeding, leg edema, and weight loss. It is often difficult on clinical grounds to distinguish recurrence from radionecrosis. Tissue biopsy should be obtained to confirm the diagnosis if at all possible; this may require surgical exploration.

Management is difficult. A few selected cases of central persistence or recurrence may be cured by surgery, including exenterative procedures, and radiation may be used for local recurrences outside the field of previous therapy. Chemotherapy may be employed, but results have been disappointing. Unfortunately, most recurrences are suitable for palliative management only. Pain relief, employing neurosurgical procedures when necessary, is an important aspect of therapy.

Occasionally, the patient with cervical cancer is pregnant, and management depends on the extent of the tumor and the duration of the pregnancy. Prior to 24 weeks, the pregnancy may be disregarded and treatment with external irradiation commenced. Abortion generally follows in 4 to 5 weeks, allowing internal therapy to be employed, or if not, hysterotomy can be performed. In some pregnancies over 24 weeks, fetal viability may be awaited, followed by cesarean delivery and initiation of therapy. Surgery may be chosen in place of irradiation, as in the nonpregnant woman.

The results in the treatment of cervical cancer are most closely related to the stage of the disease. Survival rates decrease with advanced stages (stage I, 90% or more; stage II, 60%–80%; stage III, 35%–45%; stage IV, 14%). The overall cure rate for all stages is generally about 50%–60%.

Reviews

1. Fennell, R. H. Microinvasive carcinoma of the uterine cervix. *Obstet. Gynecol. Surv.* 33:406, 1978.
   Incidence of nodal metastases is not well established.
2. Delgado, G. Stage Ib squamous cancer of the cervix: The choice of treatment. *Obstet. Gynecol. Surv.* 33:174, 1978.
   Five-year survival of stage Ib patients with positive lymph nodes is about 60%.
3. Benedet, J. L., et al. Radical hysterectomy in the treatment of cervical cancer. *Am. J. Obstet. Gynecol.* 137:254, 1980.
   Discusses the indications for radical hysterectomy and lymphadenectomy.

Epidemiology

4. Henson, D., and Tarone, R. An epidemiologic study of cancer of the cervix, vagina, and vulva based on the Third National Cancer Survey in the United States. *Am. J. Obstet. Gynecol.* 129:525, 1977.
   This article discusses the theory of multicentric origins of squamous cancers of the lower genital tract to explain the coexistence of these tumors in some patients relative to the findings of the survey.
5. Sebastian, J. A., Leeb, B. O., and See, R. Cancer of the cervix: A sexually transmitted disease; cytologic screening in a prostitute population. *Am. J. Obstet. Gynecol.* 131:620, 1978.
   Separating two epidemiologic factors provided further evidence of the importance of age at first coitus as aginst frequent intercourse with multiple partners.

Diagnostic Evaluation

6. Photopulos, G. J., et al. Computerized tomography applied to gynecologic oncology. *Am. J. Obstet. Gynecol.* 135:381, 1979.
   Valuable in evaluating pelvic wall and paraaortic regions for treatment planning.

7. Lagasse, L. D., et al. Pretreatment lymphangiography and operative evaluation in carcinoma of the cervix. *Am. J. Obstet. Gynecol.* 134:219, 1979.
   Lymphangiogram was unreliable.
8. Kademian, M. T., and Bosch, A. Staging laparotomy and survival in carcinoma of the uterine cervix. *Acta Radiol.* 16:314, 1977.
   Analysis of three large series indicated that pretreatment staging laparotomy did not improve survival.
9. Averette, H. E., et al. Staging of cervical cancer. *Clin. Obstet. Gynecol.* 18:215, 1975.
   There was an overall difference of 36.2% between clinical and surgical staging. However, by convention, all cases remain in their original clinical stage for comparative data, although treatment may be altered appropriately.

Series

10. Sedlis, A., et al. Microinvasive carcinoma of uterine cervix: Clinical-pathologic study. *Am. J. Obstet. Gynecol.* 133:64, 1979.
    A study of 265 cases from the 19 institutions of the Gynecologic Oncology Group (GOG).
11. Currie, D. W. Operative treatment of carcinoma of the cervix. *J. Obstet. Gynaecol. Br. Commonw.* 78:385, 1971.
    Radical hysterectomy entails removal of the parametria, uterosacral tissues, upper third of the vagina, and paracolpos together with the uterus.
12. Kottmeier, H. L. Ten year end results, radiological treatment of carcinoma of the cervix. *Acta Obstet. Gynecol. Scand.* 41:195, 1962.
    In this article 1891 cases were treated with primary radiotherapy.
13. Hiilesmaa, V. K., et al. Carcinoma of the uterine cervix stage III: A report of 311 cases. *Gynecol. Oncol.* 12:99, 1981.
    Survival rates were better in the older age groups.
14. Symmonds, R. E., Pratt, J. H., and Webb, M. J. Exenterative operations: Experience with 198 patients. *Am. J. Obstet. Gynecol.* 121:907, 1975.
    In addition to radical hysterectomy and lymphadenectomy, the bladder or rectum, or both, may be removed (anterior, posterior, or total exenteration).
15. McCall, M. L. The radical vaginal operative approach in the treatment of carcinoma of the cervix. *Am. J. Obstet. Gynecol.* 78:712, 1959.
    The Schauta procedure is seldom employed in the United States, although it is used to some extent in Europe.
16. Prempree, T., Patanaphan, V., and Scott, R. M. Radiation management of carcinoma of the cervical stump. *Cancer* 43:1262, 1979.
    The survival rates were the same as in patients with an intact uterus.

Special Problems

17. Thompson, J. D., Caputo, T. A., and Franklin, E. W., III. The surgical management of invasive cancer of the cervix in pregnancy. *Am. J. Obstet. Gynecol.* 121:853, 1975.
    Of 42 patients, 9 were treated by irradiation, 33 with primary surgery.
18. Green, T. H., Jr., and Morse, W. J., Jr. Management of invasive cervical cancer following inadvertent simple hysterectomy. *Obstet. Gynecol.* 33:763, 1969.
    Simple hysterectomy is inadequate therapy for invasive cervical cancer. In managing patients who have undergone "cut through" hysterectomy, cure rates ranging from 40%–65% may be obtained if adequate therapy is given within four months of surgery.

19. Jobson, V. W., Girtanner, R. E., and Averette, H. E. Therapy and survival of early invasive carcinoma of the cervix uteri with metastases to the pelvic nodes. *Surg. Obstet. Gynecol.* 151:27, 1980.
Patients with occult nodal metastases at radical surgery should receive postoperative irradiation.
20. Kanbour, A. I., Klionsky, B., and Murphy, A. I. Carcinoma of the vagina following cervical cancer. *Cancer* 34:1838, 1974.
Three possible causes are a residual lesion, multicentricity, and a new tumor.
21. Shingleton, H. M., et al. Adenocarcinoma of the cervix. I. Clinical evaluation and pathologic features. *Am. J. Obstet. Gynecol.* 139:799, 1981.
This series of 137 cases suggests that adenocarcinoma does not differ in clinical behavior or prognosis from squamous carcinoma of the cervix.
22. Lu, T., Macasaet, M. A., and Nelson, J. H., Jr. The barrel-shaped cervical carcinoma. *Am. J. Obstet. Gynecol.* 124:596, 1976.
In these patients, the technical problems of irradiation are such that a limited extrafascial hysterectomy is frequently necessary after the completion of radiation therapy.

Recurrent Disease
23. Keettel, W. C., Van Voorhis, L. W., and Latourette, H. B. Management of recurrent carcinoma of the cervix. *Am. J. Obstet. Gynecol.* 102:671, 1968.
It is frequently difficult to draw a distinction between persistent and recurrent disease.
24. Lifshitz, S., Debacker, L. J., and Buchsbaum, H. J. Subarachnoid phenol block for pain relief in gynecologic malignancy. *Obstet. Gynecol.* 48:316, 1976.
Relief of intractable pain.

Endometrial Hyperplasia

The endometrium of the uterus is a target organ responsive to the ovarian hormones. Abnormalities of ovarian hormone secretion, frequently secondary to hypothalamic-pituitary dysfunction, result in abnormal maturation of the endometrium. The most common disorders are related to anovulation with prolonged unopposed estrogen secretion. The glands, stroma, and vessels comprising the endometrium become hyperplastic; and a continuum of histologic changes appears, which in some instances undergoes atypical (dysplastic) changes and may culminate in endometrial adenocarcinoma, i.e., these endometrial hyperplasias, once atypical changes are evident, must be regarded as cancer precursors.

The earliest change, cystic hyperplasia, shows an increased number of normal-sized and dilated glands separated by hyperplastic stroma ("swiss-cheese endometrium"). As in normal proliferative endometrium, the glandular cells are tall columnar with basal nuclei. Grossly, multiple cysts may be seen. In the absence of adenomatous change, malignancy does not occur.

Adenomatous hyperplasia shows projections and outpouchings of the increased number of glands. The gland cells are tall columnar, with basal enlarged nuclei. The stroma is moderately abundant. Grossly, there may be little change or the endometrium may be thickened and polypoid.

Atypical adenomatous hyperplasia shows glands that are closely related but separated by a definite stroma. Infoldings and outpouchings of the glands are evident. Gland cells are large columnar with basophilic cytoplasm. Nuclei are enlarged, basal, or intermediately located with granular chromatin.

Adenocarcinoma in situ is characterized by numerous glands separated by limited amounts of stroma, with foci of back-to-back glands where there is no separating stroma. The glandular epithelium is low columnar with enlarged oval nuclei, basal or intermediate in location.

The lesions may be focal or widespread. Frequently, the various types of precursors may be encountered in the same specimen. Squamous metaplasia or acanthosis (replacement of glandular cells by squamous cells) may be present. This change is found in normal endometrium but is more common (9.8%) in hyperplastic endometrium. This metaplastic squamous epithelium is capable of undergoing the same dysplastic and invasive changes as that of the cervical, vaginal, or vulvar squamous epithelium.

The incidence of the hyperplasias is not known. The mean age for cystic hyperplasia is 44, that for atypical hyperplasia is 55, contrasted to that for adenocarcinoma, which is 60.

Assessing the risk for cancer in one series, 14.6% of patients with persisting cystic hyperplasia, 26.5% with persisting adenomatous hyperplasia, 75% with persisting atypical hyperplasia, and all patients with in situ lesions, if untreated, eventually develop frank cancer.

The metabolic hormonal background is similar for patients with hyperplasias and carcinoma. Risk factors include advancing age; obesity; anovulatory, dysfunctional uterine bleeding; hypertension; nulliparity; and diabetes.

The evidence favoring unopposed, prolonged estrogen effect in the causation of endometrial hyperplasia and carcinoma is overwhelming. Patients with estrogen-producing ovarian tumors have a 5% incidence of endometrial carcinoma. Patients with polycystic ovarian disease have a high incidence of hyperplasia and carcinoma of the endometrium. Some patients receiving estrogen preparations, including sequential oral contraceptives, have developed atypical hyperplasia and carcinoma. Adenocarcinoma has developed in some patients with gonadal dysgenesis who were treated with estrogen therapy.

The clinical picture is usually one of menstrual irregularities associated with anovulation or of postmenopausal bleeding. Infertility is another common presenting feature. Many patients are without symptoms—the diagnosis being made in the course of routine endometrial sampling of menopausal patients on estrogen therapy. There are no characteristic findings on physical examination other than those described when identifying patients at higher risk for the condition.

The diagnosis of endometrial hyperplasia is dependent on the performance of fractional dilatation and curettage in symptomatic patients who are at risk for endometrial cancer. Endometrial biopsies and Vabra uterine aspiration are techniques used in patients at low risk or as screening procedures for patients receiving estrogen therapy. Endometrial cytologic screening is of value in screening for endometrial cancer if persons skilled in cytology are available, but cytology is relatively ineffective in the diagnosis of cancer precursors.

The management of endometrial hyperplasia must be individualized. The patient's age, desire for children, and the nature of the lesion are important factors that may modify therapy. If possible, the underlying cause of the lesion should be removed. Usually this entails cessation or modification of exogenous estrogen therapy, or rarely, the removal of an ovarian tumor.

In older patients with atypical hyperplasia or carcinoma in situ, hysterectomy provides definitive therapy. If surgery is not possible for medical reasons, progesterone therapy may be an alternative. However, although progesterone may reverse the precursor changes, very close observation for potential malignant change is essential. If the lesion is cystic or adenomatous hyperplasia without atypical changes, a 3–6-month observation period after curettage is in order since in many cases the endometrium may revert to normal. Should the lesions persist or advance, treatment is as outlined above.

Younger patients desirous of children should be treated by removal of the cause and induction of ovulation whenever possible. If attempts at ovulation induction fail over a period of 3–6 months and hyperplasia persists, progesterone therapy, followed by further attempts at ovulation induction, should be attempted. Cystic and adenomatous hyperplasia appear more easily reversible than the more advanced lesions. If atypical hyperplasia or carcinoma in situ are present and response to conservative therapy is not rapid, hysterectomy may be necessary.

Those patients in whom the adenomatous lesion also contains dysplastic squamous epithelium may require hysterectomy should the squamous change progress to squamous carcinoma in situ. This should prevent the potential development of an adenosquamous carcinoma.

Endometrial cancer is now the most common pelvic malignancy and the incidence appears to be increasing. Adequate management of precursor lesions and careful follow-up of menopausal patients on hormone therapy should decrease the incidence of invasion. Clearly, however, what is needed is an outpatient screening technique equivalent to the Pap smear. Cytologic techniques such as the Isaacs cell sampler and histologic techniques such as Vabra aspiration are currently available, and in skilled hands provide results comparable to cervical cancer screening methods. Screening for precursor and invasive endometrial lesions should be part of the routine examination in high-risk patients.

Reviews

1. Gusberg, S. B. Precursors of corpus carcinoma estrogens and adenomatous hyperplasia. *Am. J. Obstet. Gynecol.* 54:905, 1947.
   A classic paper.
2. Gusberg, S. B., and Kaplan, A. L. Precursors of corpus cancer. *Am. J. Obstet. Gynecol.* 87:662, 1963.
   Dr. Gusberg reported that 12% of cases of adenomatous hyperplasia progress to cancer.
3. Davies, J. L., et al. A review of the risk factors for endometrial carcinoma. *Obstet. Gynecol. Surv.* 36:107, 1981.
   Reviews the more prominent papers on constitutional factors and estrogen therapy.

Etiology

4. McDonald, T. W., Malkasian, G. D., and Gaffey, T. A. Endometrial cancer associated with feminizing ovarian tumor and polycystic ovarian disease. *Obstet. Gynecol.* 49:654, 1977.
   Endometrial cancer associated with a coexistent endogenous estrogen stimulus is usually low-grade, low-stage, and superficial, with a good prognosis.
5. Rosenwaks, Z., et al. Endometrial pathology and estrogens. *Obstet. Gynecol.* 53:403, 1979.
   A study of 46 hypogonadal patients on estrogen-progesterone replacement

therapy. Progesterone did not completely prevent endometrial abnormalities, since there were 6 cystic hyperplasias and 1 adenocarcinoma.

6. MacDonald, P. C., and Siiteri, P. K. The relationship between the extraglandular production of estrogen and the occurrence of endometrial neoplasia. *Gynecol. Oncol.* 2:259, 1974.
An increased availability of the precursor hormone, androstenedione, or an increased capacity for the extraglandular conversion of androstenedione to estrone was demonstrated in older obese women, the same population at high risk for endometrial neoplasia.

7. Wagner, D., Richart, R. M., and Terner, J. Y. Deoxyribonucleic acid content of presumed precursors of endometrial carcinoma. *Cancer* 20:2067, 1967.
Of 16 cases of hyperplasia, 2 showed an aneuploid DNA distribution, the pattern found with invasive cancer. This finding suggests a more precise method of evaluation.

8. Jelovsek, F. R., et al. Risk of exogenous estrogen therapy and endometrial cancer. *Am. J. Obstet. Gynecol.* 137:85, 1980.
The overall risk was 2.38 times as high as in nonusers. The risk was confined to stage I, grade 1 lesions that carried a 94.7% survival rate.

Diagnosis

9. Hutton, J. D., et al. Endometrial assessment with Isaacs cell sampler. *Br. Med. J.* 1:947, 1978.
There was a 95% correlation between the histologic and cytologic diagnosis.

10. Hibbard, L. T., and Schwinn, L. E. Diagnosis by endometrial jet washings. *Am. J. Obstet. Gynecol.* 111:1039, 1971.
The Gravlee jet washer has a somewhat large cannula, which may necessitate dilatation of the cervix.

11. Studd, J. W. W., et al. Value of cytology for detecting endometrial abnormalities in climacteric women receiving hormone replacement therapy. *Br. Med. J.* 1:846, 1979.
The Vabra aspiration technique, which employs a suction apparatus, provides histologic samples of high diagnostic accuracy. By comparison, in this study, the Isaacs cell sampler was found to yield unsatisfactory results.

12. Koss, L. G., et al. Screening of asymptomatic women for endometrial cancer. *Obstet. Gynecol.* 57:681, 1981.
Preliminary study using cytologic and histologic techniques. Major risk factors were obesity and exogenous estrogens.

13. Greenwood, S. M., and Wright, D. J. Evaluation of the office endometrial biopsy in the detection of endometrial carcinoma and atypical hyperplasia. *Cancer* 43:1474, 1979.
A useful diagnostic tool. In this series, 5% of patients in whom insufficient material was obtained had positive findings at hysterectomy.

Management

14. Chamlian, D. L., and Taylor, H. B. Endometrial hyperplasia in young women. *Am. J. Obstet. Gynecol.* 36:659, 1970.
Of 97 patients treated, 20 had term pregnancies, 40 had hysterectomies within 16 years of diagnosis, and 14 developed adenocarcinoma within 1–14 years of diagnosis.

15. Wentz, W. B. Treatment of persistent endometrial hyperplasia. *Am. J. Obstet. Gynecol.* 96:999, 1966.

Progesterone converts an actively growing and dividing tissue to a nonactive, highly differentiated state.

16. Kistner, R. W., Lewis, J. L., and Steiner, G. J. Effects of clomiphene citrate on endometrial hyperplasia in the premenopausal female. *Cancer* 19:115, 1966.
   Therapeutic effects are temporary.
17. Whitehead, M. I., et al. Progestogen modification of endometrial histology in menopausal women. *Br. Med. J.* 2:1643, 1978.
   The addition of a progestogen to unopposed estrogen therapy in menopausal women reduced the incidence of hyperplasia from 32% (high-dose estrogen) or 16% (low-dose estrogen) to 5%.

Endometrial Carcinoma

Cancer of the endometrium of the uterine corpus is the most common malignancy of the female genital organs in the United States, with an estimated 38,000 new cases and 3200 new cancer deaths per year (1980). The disease is most common in women in their sixties or seventies. Nulliparity, obesity, hypertension, and diabetes are frequently associated findings. Conditions that predispose to the disease appear to be those in which chronic hyperestrinism (characterized by chronic anovulation with dysfunctional bleeding) is present. These predisposing factors are discussed in further detail in the preceding essay on endometrial hyperplasia.

The histologic types include adenocarcinoma (70%), adenoacanthoma (24%), and adenosquamous carcinoma (4%). Papillary, mucinous, and clear-cell carcinomas comprise the remainder. The gross appearance is that of a fungating, friable tumor mass with areas of necrosis and hemorrhage.

The tumors are graded according to Broder's classification. Grade 1 lesions have glands quite similar to normal endometrium (i.e., well differentiated). Grade 2 and 3 lesions exhibit increasing degrees of dedifferentiation, with the least differentiated forms comprising only sheets of neoplastic cells.

Lymphatic spread occurs to the pelvic nodes, and dissemination can also take place via the infundibulopelvic lymphatics to common iliac and aortic glands, bypassing the pelvic nodes.

Local dissemination into the myometrium and extension to the uterine isthmus and cervix, as well as metastasis to the tubes and ovaries, occurs frequently. Distant metastases pass along lymphatic chains to supraclavicular and inguinal nodes and also are blood-spread, particularly to the lungs.

Clinical staging of the disease is based primarily on bimanual pelvic examination and fractional dilatation and curettage. Stage 0 is adenocarcinoma in situ. Stage Ia is growth confined to the corpus; Ib is similar but differs in that the uterine cavity is more than 8 cm in length. Stage I is further subdivided into three grades according to the histologic degree of differentiation. Stage II carcinoma involves the cervix as well as the corpus. Stage III growth has involved the adnexa, vagina, or bowel serosa, but has not extended beyond the true pelvis. In stage IV, the tumor has extended beyond the pelvis or involves bladder or rectal mucosa.

The clinical presentation is commonly postmenopausal bleeding. Persistent or irregular perimenopausal bleeding is another common symptom. Vaginal discharge is a nonspecific feature, and pain is present only with advanced disease. The typical patient at risk has already been described.

The clinical examination is generally unhelpful, although the uterus may be enlarged on occasion. Pap smear fails to diagnose abnormal cells in 50% of cases, so it is not very helpful. Office techniques for sampling endometrium are reliable in about 80% of cases, but the definitive diagnostic and staging procedure is fractional (endocervix sampled before endometrium) dilatation and curettage. This should be performed in all patients with postmenopausal bleeding or when there is a real suspicion of the diagnosis.

Generally, tumors deeply invading the myometrium are relatively anaplastic and lymphatic nodal involvement is much more likely. These features, together with advanced staging, are important adverse prognostic findings. Uterine size, although included in staging, does not appear to be a significant prognostic index.

Management of stage I, grade 1 and 2 lesions, is by total abdominal hysterectomy with bilateral salpingo-oophorectomy (TAH-BSO). If pathologic examination reveals penetration deeper than one-third of the myometrium, or if undiagnosed cervical involvement is found, postoperative radiotherapy to the whole pelvis of about 4000 rads is indicated since the risk of nodal involvement in these circumstances is about 30%.

Since recurrence in the vaginal vault occurs in 5%–10% of patients treated with surgery alone, and since this incidence is halved by adjunctive radiation, many clinicians employ radiotherapy, usually in the form of vaginal radium, either before or after surgery.

Stage II lesions, or poorly differentiated stage I lesions, require more extensive therapy, with combined surgery and radiation. Preoperative total pelvic irradiation consists of 4000 to 4500 rads with radium insertion to reach 3500 rads to point A (a dosage reference point placed 2 cm above and 2 cm lateral to the internal os. A second reference site, point B, indicates the pelvic side wall, and is calculated in a similar fashion, but with 5 cm intervals). TAH-BSO is carried out 1–6 weeks after completion of the radiotherapy. An alternative treatment is the same as for cervical cancer: radical hysterectomy and pelvic lymphadenectomy. With this approach, postoperative irradiation (5000 rads) is given only if nodes are positive.

Therapy of recurrent vaginal lesions is by local radium, employing vaginal cylinders or radium needles. Whole pelvis irradiation may be combined with this local radium, and this modality is the primary therapy of pelvic lymph node recurrence.

Progestins are used in the management of disseminated disease in the form of Depo-Provera (medroxyprogesterone acetate) injections, 500–1000 mg weekly. Megace (megestrol acetate) is an oral agent equally efficacious, given in a dose of 80–160 mg daily. Pulmonary lesions respond best (30%–35%); well-differentiated lesions respond better (50%) than do the poorly differentiated (15%); and responders survive longer than nonresponders.

Chemotherapy for this tumor is not well documented, but adriamycin appears to be an active agent. In general, the overall response rate appears to be under 25%.

Cure rates for the disease are 85%–90% in stage I, 50%–65% in stage II, 30% in stage III, and under 10% in stage IV. Fortunately, most cases present in stage I (76%), so that the overall prognosis is relatively favorable.

Review

1. Boronow, R. C. Endometrial cancer. *Obstet. Gynecol.* 47:630, 1976. *Not a benign disease.*

Diagnosis

2. Edinger, D. D., Jr., Watring, W. G., and Anderson, B. Hysterography as a diagnostic technique in endometrial carcinoma. *Clin. Obstet. Gynecol.* 22:729, 1979.
Filling the uterus (but not the tubes) with a radiopaque dye provided information about the extent and the degree of myometrial penetration.
3. Joelsson, I., Levine, R. U., and Moberger, G. Hysteroscopy as an adjunct in determining the extent of carcinoma of the endometrium. *Am. J. Obstet. Gynecol.* 111:696, 1971.
May indicate cervical involvement or be useful when D and C is negative, but the high intrauterine pressure required may cause spill of tumor cells into the tubes and so should not be used routinely.
4. Douglas, B., MacDonald, J. S., and Baker, J. W. Lymphography in carcinoma of the uterus. *Clin. Radiol.* 23:286, 1972.
Interpretation is difficult, but helpful if used with fine needle–lymph node aspiration for cytologic study.
5. Crissman, J. D., et al. Endometrial carcinoma in women 40 years of age or younger. *Obstet. Gynecol.* 57:699, 1981.
Occurred in 2.9% of endometrial cancer cases in the study community. Six (19%) of 32 patients in this series had coexisting ovarian neoplasms.

Treatment

6. Piver, M. S., et al. A prospective trial comparing hysterectomy, hysterectomy plus vaginal radium, and uterine radium plus hysterectomy in stage I endometrial carcinoma. *Obstet. Gynecol.* 54:85, 1979.
No statistical difference in the survival rates of the three groups.
7. Hernandez, W., et al. Stage II endometrial carcinoma. Two modalities of treatment. *Am. J. Obstet. Gynecol.* 131:171, 1978.
Radiation plus surgery was more effective than radiation alone.
8. Kneale, B. L. G. The current status of surgery for endometrial carcinoma: Facts and fantasy. *Aust. N.Z. J. Surg.* 49:327, 1979.
Cervical suturing and vaginal cuff removal are ineffective in the prevention of vaginal cuff recurrences.
9. Masubuchi, S., Fujimoto, I., and Masubuchi, K. Lymph node metastasis and prognosis of endometrial carcinoma. *Gynecol. Oncol.* 7:36, 1979.
Of 112 patients treated with radical surgery, nodal metastasis occurred in 10 (8.9%), of whom only 4 showed clearance of the cancer.
10. Fletcher, G. H. Clinical dose-response curves of human malignant epithelial tumors. *Br. J. Radiol.* 46:541, 1973.
This article showed that administering 5000 rads in 5 weeks to involved pelvic nodes eliminates 90% of microscopic spread and 50% of gross disease.
11. Deppe, G., et al. Chemotherapy of advanced and recurrent endometrial carcinoma with cyclophosphamide, doxorubicin, 5-fluorouracil, and megestrol acetate. *Am. J. Obstet. Gynecol.* 140:313, 1981.
Mean duration of survival for responders (13 of 29) was 11 months.
12. Cohen, C. J., Deppe, G., and Bruckner, H. W. Treatment of advanced adenocarcinoma of the endometrium with melphalan, 5-fluorouracil, and medroxyprogesterone acetate. *Obstet. Gynecol.* 50:415, 1977.
There was an objective response in 6 of 7 patients, but the gestagen may have been the active agent.

Pathology, Prognosis

13. Goplerud, D. R., and Belgrad, R. The importance of histologic grade in stage II endometrial carcinoma. *Surg. Gynecol. Obstet.* 148:406, 1979.

Tumor grade has the same prognostic significance in the more advanced stages.

14. Henriksen, E. The lymphatic dissemination in endometrial carcinoma. A study of 188 necropsies. *Am. J. Obstet. Gynecol.* 123:570, 1975.
    Pattern of lymphatic spread is less predictable than with cervical cancer.
15. Salazar, O. M., et al. Adenosquamous carcinoma of the endometrium: Entity with an inherent poor prognosis? *Cancer* 40:119, 1977.
    Authors did not find that this cancer is either increasing in incidence or has a poorer prognosis than pure adenocarcinoma.
16. Malkasian, G. D., Jr. Carcinoma of the endometrium: Effect of stage and grade on survival. *Cancer* 41:996, 1978.
    No relationship between depth of uterine cavity and survival. Author suggests that distinction between stage Ia and Ib disease is unnecessary.
17. Creasman, W. T., et al. Adenocarcinoma of the endometrium: Its metastatic lymph node potential. *Gynecol. Oncol.* 4:239, 1976.
    In this article 36% of grade 3 lesions had pelvic node metastases and 28% also had aortic node metastases.
18. Cheung, A. Y. C. Prognostic significance of negative hysterectomy specimen following intracavitary irradiation in stage I endometrial carcinoma. *Br. J. Obstet. Gynaecol.* 88:548, 1981.
    If residual tumor was present, relapse was 19.2%; if absent, it was 3.8%.

Uterine Sarcoma

Sarcomas may arise from the endometrial stroma, the myometrium, or in a leiomyoma. They are rare, highly malignant tumors, with generally poor prognosis and account for about 3% of all malignancies of the corpus. With rare exceptions (sarcoma botryoides), they present in the fifth and sixth decades of life. They differ from epithelial tumors in that vascular metastasis is common and early, particularly to the lung, liver, and brain.

The uterus is the site of a variety of mesenchymal tumors of widely differing histopathologic patterns and clinical behavior. These tumors are classified on their histologic appearance according to whether they contain a single sarcomatous element, in which case the term *pure* is used, or more than one element, in which case the term *mixed* is used. If the tumor contains cells derived from tissue normally present in the uterus, it is a homologous tumor; if tissue not normally present in the uterus is found (e.g., bone, cartilage, and so on), it is a heterologous growth. When an epithelial tumor (generally adenocarcinoma) is found together with a homologous or heterologous sarcoma, it is called a homologous or heterologous mixed müllerian (mesodermal) tumor. Some tumors consist of totally undifferentiated cells and are referred to as unclassified sarcomas. The last group in the classification is the very rare malignant lymphoma.

In the management of all patients with uterine sarcomas, a careful metastatic survey is required in the pretreatment work-up since metastasis to liver, lung, and bone are common. In deciding on the pelvic extent of the tumor, sonography and CAT scans as well as intravenous pyelogram and barium enema are usually indicated.

There is no official clinical staging of uterine sarcomas, but they may be staged in a manner equivalent to that used for endometrial carcinoma. While the extent of the disease is the most important prognostic feature, the histologic grade and degree of mitotic activity are also important. Worsening atypia or high mitotic counts are associated with a poor outcome.

Included in the group of pure homologous sarcomas are the leiomyosarcoma, endometrial stromal sarcoma, and endometrial stromatosis (endolymphatic stromal myosis).

Leimyosarcoma is the most common of the uterine sarcomas (50%–70%). Differentiating it from a benign cellular leiomyoma is difficult, so that figures for both incidence and prognosis vary with the diagnostic criteria employed. The tumor is generally bosselated, lobulated, bulky, and involves the uterine wall. The cells show great variation in size and nuclear stain, and mitoses are numerous and may be abnormal. Malignancy and survival correlate with the mitotic number; when there are greater than 10 mitoses per 10 high power fields, the prognosis is very poor.

Leiomyomas are usually multiple, while the leiomyosarcoma is a solitary tumor. The incidence of malignant degeneration in a preexisting fibroid is very low, probably in the range of 0.18%–0.24%. The clinical picture is generally one of irregular vaginal bleeding in a woman aged between 40 and 60 years. A pelvic mass is usually present, and a cervical ulcer or polypoid growth may be found. A history of rapid growth of a previously noted fibroid is most uncommon.

Management includes work-up for distant metastases. Fractional curettage is indicated but may not always provide the diagnosis. Therapy is basically surgical, with total abdominal hysterectomy and bilateral salpingo-oophorectomy. The place of preoperative radiation is uncertain but it may be helpful. Chemotherapy is also of potential benefit; reports of the successful use of adriamycin or VAC (vincristine, actinomycin, and cyclophosphamide) have appeared in the literature. Survival in the absence of invasion is good (80%–90%), but once invasion has occurred, death is almost invariable.

Endometrial stromal sarcomas form a polypoid or diffuse mass in the endometrial cavity, protruding through the cervix in 20% of cases. These sarcomas are rare but very malignant, the degree of malignancy being related to mitotic number. Vaginal bleeding and pelvic pain are the usual symptoms, and surgery is the keystone of therapy. Radiotherapy before or after surgery is probably worthwhile.

Endometrial stromatosis is an indolent tumor microscopically characterized by stromal cells pushing into the myometrium. There is no cellular atypia and mitoses are few. However, local recurrences may follow surgery and lung metastases have occurred. Prognosis is usually excellent following removal of the uterus and adnexa, which is the standard therapy. Recurrent and metastatic lesions should be treated surgically or with radiotherapy. Since those tumors that spread do so chiefly by local extension, some workers feel that radical hysterectomy with pelvic lymphadenectomy should be used for those patients with a low mitotic count and no metastases.

The mixed mesodermal tumors account for about 30% of uterine sarcomas. They contain mixtures of malignant epithelial and malignant stromal elements. Homologous mixed müllerian tumors with sarcomatous and carcinomatous components are often called "carcinosarcomas." Prognosis is uniformly poor, irrespective of tumor type, with 5-year survival rates in the 20% range.

Predisposing factors are similar to those in endometrial cancer as regards obesity, hypertension, and age, with almost all cases being postmenopausal. A history of prior pelvic radiation may be significant. Bleeding, pain, discharge, and anorexia are common symptoms. Generally, a pelvic mass is present, and curettage provides the diagnosis in 75% of cases.

The tumors form large polypoid masses arising from the uterine lining;

some polyps may prolapse through the cervix. Hemorrhage is frequent. The basic cellular structure consists of fusiform cells, while the common heterologous elements include muscle, bone, and cartilage sarcomas. Epithelial elements include adenocarcinoma and rarely, squamous carcinoma.

Treatment usually consists of total abdominal hysterectomy and adnexal removal, together with radiotherapy. Multiple-drug chemotherapy is used as a supplement. Prognosis is better if the tumor is limited to the uterus (43%) but falls to 5% when spread is present. Since recurrence is generally in the pelvic cavity, more aggressive therapy in the form of radical surgery with pelvic lymphadenectomy may be warranted in selected cases.

Review

1. Cavanagh, D., Praphat, H., and Ruffolo, E. H. Sarcomas of the uterus. *Obstet. Gynecol. Annu.* 8:413, 1979.
   The 5-year survival for patients with leiomyosarcoma is about 40% and is better than for other sarcomas in which the range is 0%–35%.
2. Aaro, L. A., Symmonds, R. E., and Dockerty, M. B. Sarcoma of the uterus: A clinical and pathological study of 177 cases. *Am. J. Obstet. Gynecol.* 94:101, 1966.
   Includes 3 cases of malignant lymphoma (lymphosarcoma).
3. Teufel, G., et al. Sarcomas of the female genitalia. Therapy and prognosis. *Path. Res. Pract.* 169:173, 1980.
   Experience with therapy of 216 sarcomas of the female genitalia.

Classification

4. Ober, W. B., and Tovell, H. M. M. Mesenchymal sarcomas of the uterus. *Am. J. Obstet. Gynecol.* 77:246, 1959.
   It is often difficult histologically to separate benign from malignant mesenchymal neoplasma.
5. Kempson, R. L., and Bari, W. Uterine sarcomas. Classification, diagnosis and prognosis. *Hum. Pathol.* 1:331, 1970.
   Modification of Ober's classification that is histogenetically correct and clinically applicable.

Pure Sarcomas

6. Vardi, J. R., and Tovell, M. M. Leiomyosarcoma of the uterus: Clinicopathologic study. *Obstet. Gynecol.* 56:428, 1980.
   Retrospective study of 32 cases, with review of the literature.
7. Benjamin, R. S., Wiernik, P. H., and Bachur, N. R. Adriamycin: A new effective agent in the therapy of disseminated sarcomas. *Med. Pediatr. Oncol.* 1:63, 1975.
   The most important ECG sign of cardiac toxicity is low voltage. In addition to nonspecific ECG changes, dose-related cardiomyopathy can occur.
8. Norris, H. J., and Taylor, H. B. Mesenchymal tumors of the uterus: I. A clinical and pathologic study of 53 endometrial stromal tumors. *Cancer* 19:755, 1966.
   The authors set a dividing line between the mitotic activity of stromal sarcoma and stromatosis at 10 mitoses per 10 high-power fields.
9. Hart, W. R., and Yoonessi, M. Endometrial stromatosis of the uterus. *Obstet. Gynecol.* 49:393, 1977.
   Also called stromatous endometriosis or endolymphatic stromal myosis.
10. Dallenbach-Hellweg, G. The stromal and myogenic sarcomas of the uterus. *Path. Res. Pract.* 169:127, 1980.

Stromal sarcomas of the uterus generally originate as homologous tumors from endometrial stromal cells with fixed potentialities.

11. Grosfeld, J. L., Smith, J. P., and Clatworthy, J. R. Pelvic rhabdomyosarcoma in infants and children. *Urology* 107:673, 1972.
Botryoid sarcomas may contain heterologous elements and are then mesodermal mixed tumors.

Mixed Sarcomas

12. Disaia, P. J., Castro, J. R., and Rutledge, F. N. Mixed mesodermal sarcoma of the uterus. *Am. J. Roentgenol. Radium Ther. Nucl. Med.* 117:632, 1973.
Best results were obtained when surgery and radiotherapy were combined.

13. Perez, C. A., et al. Effects of irradiation on mixed müllerian tumors of the uterus. *Cancer* 43:1274, 1979.
This report on 54 patients suggests the use of 6000 rads to the whole pelvis; lymphatic and hematogenous metastases were seen in about 75% of cases.

14. Smith, J. P., et al. Combined irradiation and chemotherapy for sarcoma of the pelvis in females. *Am. J. Roentgenol. Radium Ther. Nucl. Med.* 123:571, 1975.
Chemotherapy is the logical treatment in view of the early and widespread dissemination of most sarcomas.

15. Marmion, P. J., Goldfarb, P. M., and Youngkin, T. P. Uterine sarcoma following adjuvant radiotherapy for rectal carcinoma. *J. Surg. Oncol.* 17:63, 1981.
There is a well-documented association of uterine sarcoma—especially mixed mesodermal sarcoma—with antecedent radiotherapy.

Benign Ovarian Neoplasms

Nonneoplastic functional ovarian cysts are the most common adnexal masses encountered in the reproductive years. Their significance lies in differentiating them from more serious ovarian or tubal lesions.

Follicular and corpus luteum cysts are rarely larger than 6 cm in diameter, are unilateral, and are freely mobile. There may be menstrual abnormalities. Uncommonly, hemorrhage, torsion, or rupture of a cyst may lead to evidence of an acute abdomen. Observation, or a short course of oral contraceptive pills, is usually followed by disappearance of the cysts, which are dependent on gonadotropin stimulation.

Theca-lutein cysts are usually large and bilateral. They result from high levels of chorionic gonadotropins commonly due to trophoblastic disease. They may also follow the use of ovulation-inducing agents such as clomiphene. Involution occurs when the hormonal stimulus is removed.

Most ovarian neoplasms (70%) are derived from the coelomic germinal surface epithelium. This epithelium is of paramesonephric (müllerian) origin, so these tumors contain epithelium similar to that lining adult müllerian structures (endocervix, endometrium, endosalpinx) and are named mucinous, endometrioid, or serous neoplasms, respectively.

Serous cystadenomas account for 25% of benign ovarian tumors. In general, these neoplasms occur in the reproductive years. They may occur as unilateral, unilocular cysts called simple cystomas, but serous cystadenomas are usually multilocular and bilateral in 15%, and may have papillary excrescences. The papillary cystadenoma is the most likely to undergo malignant change. Symptoms are dependent on size and whether accidents, such as rupture or torsion, occur. They are treated by conservative surgery in young adults and by removal of the uterus and adnexa in older women.

Mucinous cystadenomas are multilocular tumors containing a thick mucinous substance secreted by the columnar epithelium lining the cyst. They are usually unilateral and can become very large. Papillary excrescences may develop and increase the malignant potential. Rupture of the cyst may lead to pseudomyxoma peritonei, a rare but serious condition complicated by extensive adhesions with bowel obstruction. The clinical picture and management of the mucinous cystadenomas are similar to those for the serous tumors.

The remaining benign epithelial tumors are uncommon. Endometrioid and mesonephroid (clear cell) cysts are included in this category and are extremely rare. The Brenner tumor, composed of nests of epithelial cells in a fibrous stroma, accounts for 1% of ovarian tumors. Usually found in postmenopausal women, the malignant potential is low. The tumor may also occur in conjunction with mucinous or dermoid cysts. Management is usually removal of the uterus and adnexa because of the patient's age group.

Some 20% of primary ovarian neoplasms are derived from the germ cell. The benign cystic teratoma (dermoid), the most common tumor of young women, is second only to the serous tumors in frequency in all age groups. The tumor may contain tissues derived from all three germ layers, although ectodermal elements (particularly sebaceous fluid and hair) usually predominate. In 15%, functional or nonfunctional thyroid tissue may be present (struma ovarii). The tumor is mobile and may lie anterior to the uterus. Malignant change is rare. Symptoms are uncommon, unless a complication (usually torsion) occurs. Management is generally by conservative surgery with ovarian cystectomy and bisection of the opposite ovary, since 15% are bilateral. In older patients, removal of the uterus and adnexa should be performed.

Some 5% of primary ovarian neoplasms are derived from sexually undifferentiated mesenchymal tissue. The fibroma, a connective tissue tumor composed of fibroblasts and collagen, is relatively common and accounts for 20% of solid ovarian tumors. The tumors are solid, vary greatly in size, and are bilateral in 10% of patients. Generally symptomless, or if large, exerting pressure effects, some 75% have a degree of ascites while 3% exhibit Meigs' syndrome (hydrothorax with ascites). The average age at diagnosis is 48 years; therapy is usually hysterectomy with removal of the adnexa, although malignant change is rare. Other supporting tissue tumors (such as myxoma, lipoma, hemangioma, and so on) are occasionally seen, but all are rare.

A further 5% of ovarian tumors are derived from specialized gonadal stroma (sexually differentiated mesenchymal tissue). These are "functioning" tumors capable of producing estrogen (granulose-theca cell) or androgen (Sertoli-Leydig cell) or both (gynandroblastoma). The majority of these tumors are potentially malignant, however, and therefore are not regarded as benign tumors.

Generally, most ovarian neoplasms are clinically silent other than for pressure symptoms such as urinary frequency, constipation, and pelvic heaviness. Very large tumors cause abdominal swelling and discomfort and might be confused with pregnancy. Pain may occur due to stretching of the ovarian capsule or as the result of torsion, rupture, or intracystic hemor-rhage. If the tumors are functional, menstrual abnormalities may occur.

On physical examination, it will be noted that most ovarian tumors lie behind the uterus or have ascended into the abdomen, although dermoids may be anteriorly placed. Benign tumors tend to be unilateral, cystic, mov-able, and symmetrical; and there is no ascites. By contrast, malignant growths are usually bilateral, solid, fixed, and nodular, and there is ascites.

Diagnostic evaluation should include chest and abdominal x-ray, as well as an intravenous pyelogram. Further investigations depend on the indi-vidual case and may include bowel x-rays, sonography, and laparoscopy.

Women aged 15–45 years with clinically benign ovarian cysts under 6 cm in diameter may be observed monthly for a short while, but premenarchal and postmenopausal females are at high risk for malignancy and early di-agnosis is essential.

Laparotomy is performed as soon as diagnostic procedures are completed. Features of benign disease include a unilateral, freely mobile, smooth cyst with no ascitic fluid, and smooth peritoneal surfaces. If there is any doubt, frozen sections should be obtained.

In older patients, even with benign neoplasms, total abdominal hys-terectomy with bilateral salpingo-oophorectomy is the treatment of choice. In younger patients, conservative surgery is the rule for benign disease. Ovar-ian cystectomy or unilateral salpingo-oophorectomy, with great care to establish the absence of disease in the remaining ovary, is the usual proce-dure. Since the lesions are benign, the prognosis is excellent.

Functional Cysts

1. Spanos, W. J. Preoperative hormonal therapy of cystic adnexal masses. *Am. J. Obstet. Gynecol.* 116:551, 1973.
   All patients in whom a cyst persisted for 6 weeks while they were on oral contraceptives did not have functional cysts.
2. Hensleigh, P. A., and Woodruff, J. D. Differential maternal-fetal re-sponse to androgenizing luteoma or hyperreactio luteinalis. *Obstet. Gynecol. Surv.* 33:262, 1978.
   Pregnancy luteoma is a benign hyperplastic thecal luteinization that re-gresses postpartum.

Neoplasms Derived from Coelomic Epithelium

3. Woodruff, J. D., and Novak, E. R. Papillary serous tumors of the ovary. *Am. J. Obstet. Gynecol.* 67:1112, 1954.
   One-fourth of papillary serous cystadenomas contain microscopic calco-spherites, psammoma bodies, which may show up on x-ray.
4. Woodruff, J. D., Bie, L. S., and Sherman, R. J. Mucinous tumors of the ovary. *Obstet. Gynecol.* 16:699, 1960.
   Malignancy occurs in 5%–10% of primarily benign mucinous cysts.
5. Sandenbergh, H. A., and Woodruff, J. D. Histogenesis of pseudomyxoma peritonei: Review of nine cases. *Obstet. Gynecol.* 49:339, 1977.
   Mortality is high in mucinous ascites even with benign histology.
6. Rome, R. M., et al. Functioning ovarian tumors in postmenopausal women. *Obstet. Gynecol.* 57:705, 1981.
   Many epithelial tumors of the ovary, whether benign or malignant, secrete hormones and should therefore be identified as functioning or endocrine tumors.

7. Yoonessi, M., and Abell, M. R. Brenner tumors of the ovary. *Obstet. Gynecol.* 54:90, 1979.
Of 24 cases 3 were malignant.

Neoplasms Derived from Germ Cells

8. Malkasian, G. D., Jr., Dockerty, M. B., and Symmonds, R. E. Benign cystic teratomas. *Obstet. Gynecol.* 29:719, 1967.
Teeth are present in nearly 50% of the teratomas and can be visualized on x-ray.
9. Curling, O. M., Potsides, P. N., and Hudson, C. N. Malignant change in benign cystic teratoma of the ovary. *Br. J. Obstet. Gynaecol.* 86:399, 1979.
Malignant change occurs in about 1% of these teratomas—usually in women in the postmenopausal age group—and especially in the rare solid dermoid with yolk sac elements.
10. Kempers, R. D., et al. Struma ovarii-ascitic, hyperthyroid, and asymptomatic syndromes. *Ann. Intern. Med.* 72:883, 1970.
The term struma ovarii *is used when thyroid is the predominant tissue in a dermoid.*
11. Stern, J. L., et al. Spontaneous rupture of benign cystic teratomas. *Obstet. Gynecol.* 57:363, 1981.
The incidence, etiology, and pathology of this complication are discussed, and four cases are presented.
12. Pantoja, E., et al. Complications of dermoid tumors of the ovary. *Obstet. Gynecol.* 45:89, 1975.
Of 253 dermoids studied, rupture occurred in 3, torsion of the pedicle in 24, and malignancy in 9.

Neoplasms Derived from Nonspecific Mesenchyme

13. Dockerty, M. B., and Masson, J. C. Ovarian fibroma: A clinical and pathological study of 283 cases. *Am. J. Obstet. Gynecol.* 47:741, 1944.
The ovarian fibroma is not easily distinguishable from the thecoma clinically or histologically.
14. Meigs, J. V. Fibroma of the ovary with ascites and hydrothorax—Meigs' syndrome. *Am. J. Obstet. Gynecol.* 67:962, 1954.
Occurs in under 5% of fibromas.

Diagnosis

15. DeLand, M., et al. Ultrasonography in the diagnosis of tumors of the ovary. *Surg. Gynecol. Obstet.* 148:346, 1979.
Ultrasonography differentiated ovarian from other pelvic tumors in 90% of patients.
16. Laing, F. C., et al. Dermoid cysts of the ovary: Their ultrasonographic appearances. *Obstet. Gynecol.* 57:99, 1981.
There was a wide variation in appearance. The typical picture of an echogenic focus with acoustic shadowing in a mainly cystic mass was seen in only 33% of the cases.
17. McGowan, L., Bunnag, B., and Arias, L. B. Peritoneal fluid cytology associated with benign neoplastic ovarian tumors in women. *Am. J. Obstet. Gynecol.* 113:961, 1972.
Culdocentesis provided cell samples sufficient for accurate cytologic diagnosis.
18. Barber, H. R. K., and Graber, E. A. The PMPO syndrome (postmenopausal palpable ovary syndrome). *Obstet. Gynecol.* 38:921, 1971.
A palpable ovary in the postmenopausal woman requires investigation to exclude cancer.

Management
19. Blum, M., and Meidan, A. Late results of conservative operations for bilateral benign ovarian tumors. *Int. Surg.* 61:561, 1976.
    Conservation of ovarian tissue is important in younger patients.
20. Novak, E. R., Lambrou, C. D., and Woodruff, J. D. Ovarian tumors in pregnancy. An ovarian tumor registry review. *Obstet. Gynecol.* 46:401, 1975.
    This article discusses 100 cases, of which 10 were dermoids.

Ovarian Carcinoma

Cancer of the ovary is the third most common gynecologic malignancy. Each year 17,000 new cases are diagnosed in the United States, with 11,200 deaths. Mortality from ovarian cancer is greater than that from cervical and endometrial cancer combined. One of seventy (1.4%) females will develop ovarian malignancy and the incidence is increasing.

The disease is more common in whites than in nonwhites and in industrialized countries (with the puzzling exception of Japan) than in non-developed areas. The mean age at onset is 62 years and the mean age at death is 63 years.

Women with breast cancer have twice the standard risk of developing a primary ovarian cancer and both diseases may be linked with spinsterdom, infertility, or late pregnancy. A familial risk of ovarian cancer is also well recognized.

Ovarian cancer is classified histologically into epithelial, gonadal stromal, and germ cell tumors. Of the epithelial tumors, some 10%–35% are serous, 5%–10% are mucinous, 15%–20% are endometrioid, and 4%–6% are clear cell. Gonadal stromal tumors (granulosa cell, Sertoli-Leydig cell) comprise some 5%–10%. Of the germ cell tumors, dysgerminoma (1%–2%), embryonal teratoma (1%–2%), and malignant dermoids (1%–2%) are the most common. Metastatic tumors (4%–8%) are generally derived from the bowel, breast, or thyroid.

Epithelial tumors are further differentiated into borderline and malignant. Borderline growths display nuclear abnormalities and cellular stratification but lack stromal invasion.

Ovarian growths generally develop within the ovarian substance, are often cystic, and secrete seromucinous fluid. Spread is by local infiltration through the capsule with intraperitoneal extension or implantation. Lymphatic spread occurs in a mode similar to that of the uterine carcinomas, while hematogenous spread is rarely seen clinically. Transdiaphragmatic dispersion is common.

Staging of ovarian cancer is based on findings at laparotomy. Stage Ia growth is limited to one ovary; stage Ib is involvement of both ovaries. Both of these categories are further designated (i), if the external surface is unbreached and without tumor, or (ii), if the capsule is ruptured or has tumor on the surface. Stage Ic is Ia or Ib with ascites present or positive peritoneal washings.

Stage IIa is growth on one or both ovaries with extension to the uterus or tubes, or both; stage IIb is extension to other pelvic tissues. If either of these groups has ascites or positive washings, it is stage IIc.

Stage III growth involves metastases outside the pelvis and/or positive retroperitoneal nodes or extension to small bowel or omentum.

Stage IV implies distant metastases, including liver parenchyma or lung. A special category is allocated to unexplored cases thought to be ovarian carcinoma.

There are no symptoms of early ovarian cancer. The usual complaints of abdominal swelling, pain, and a mass are symptoms of advanced disease. Nonspecific gastrointestinal disorders such as dyspepsia, mild anorexia, flatulence, and vague abdominal discomfort are common. In some instances, the tumor may exhibit endocrine activity, resulting in menstrual abnormality, but this is rare.

Pelvic examination may indicate the presence of bilateral firm, fixed, nontender adnexal masses. Bilateral tumors occur in 70% of ovarian cancers versus 5% in benign lesions. Firm nodules palpated in the cul-de-sac may indicate peritoneal seeding with tumor. Ascites and a right-sided pleural effusion are common findings in advanced disease.

A diagnostic work-up including gastrointestinal series and intravenous pyelogram should be carried out. Paracentesis and lymphangiogram, laparoscopy, CAT scan, and sonography may be indicated in some instances. Exploratory laparotomy is indicated in any pelvic mass encountered after menopause or in the very young. Pelvic masses in the reproductive years require exploration if they are larger than 8–10 cm, if they enlarge while under observation, or when definite diagnosis of a cause such as fibroids cannot be made.

Certain rare germ cell tumors produce substances that may be useful for diagnosis or for monitoring therapy. For instance, the endodermal sinus tumor produces alphafetoprotein and the ovarian choriocarcinoma produces chorionic gonadotropin. Unfortunately, no specific serum tumor markers for the more common forms of ovarian carcinoma have yet been identified.

The cornerstone of treatment is surgery. Preoperative bowel preparation is advisable. An adequate midline incision is used and every attempt is made to avoid rupture of the tumor during removal. A total abdominal hysterectomy with bilateral salpingo-oophorectomy is the standard operation. Many surgeons also routinely perform omentectomy. In young patients with low-grade, unilateral, and encapsulated tumors, conservative surgery may be considered. Peritoneal washings or ascitic fluid are sent for cytology, and biopsies are taken from the pelvic peritoneum, right diaphragm, paracolic gutters, and any suspicious areas. The pelvic and aortic nodes are palpated and biopsied if suspicious. Extensive procedures should not be employed in advanced cases if significant residual tumor will still be left behind. However, if tumor debulking can be safely achieved, adjuvant therapy is more likely to be successful.

Chemotherapy is generally used following operation in patients with or without residual disease and has generally replaced radiotherapy, with the exception of its use for radiosensitive tumors such as the dysgerminoma. Single or combination agents may be used, the former generally being employed for early disease. The use of cytotoxic agents, radiation, and intraperitoneal isotopes is further discussed in the chapters related to these treatment modalities.

Second-look operation is the term applied to repeat laparotomy in patients who have completed cytotoxic treatment without evidence of disease and are being considered for cessation of chemotherapy. Termination of therapy is desirable because of the risk of leukemia that is associated with long-term chemotherapy. The staging technique is the same as for the initial operative procedure.

Problems to be palliated in advanced ovarian cancer include ascites, pleural effusions, intestinal or urinary tract obstruction, and bowel fistula. Repeated paracentesis, nasogastric intestinal decompression, total parenteral nutrition, and conservative bypass surgery all play a role in managing these difficult situations.

The prognosis varies; approximately 70% of stage I and 50% of stage II patients survive 5 years. However, as some 60%–70% are either stage III or IV at the time of initial diagnosis, there is only a 15%–25% 5-year survival overall. The cause of death is usually related to diminished immunocompetence (resulting in severe sepsis) and malnutrition (associated with bowel obstruction).

The germ cell tumors include the dysgerminoma, which is a tumor similar to the seminoma of the testis. Only 5%–10% are bilateral, and in young patients conservative therapy is acceptable. In advanced disease, complete pelvic surgery with postoperative radiation to pelvic and aortic nodes is necessary. Germ cell cancers derived from teratomas (embryonal) and from extraembryonic tissues (endodermal sinus, choriocarcinoma) are highly malignant, have a poor prognosis, and require complete surgery and aggressive chemotherapy.

Gonadal stromal malignancies include granulosa and Sertoli–Leydig cell cancers that are usually unilateral with low-grade malignancy and recurrence typically confined to the pelvis. Late recurrences are common. Early disease in young patients may be treated conservatively.

The gonadoblastoma is composed of both germ cell and gonadal stromal cell tumors in varying combinations. Most patients are intersexual and 90% are chromatin-negative. The malignant potential is determined by the germ cell tumor present. Generally, bilateral gonadectomy is indicated.

Review

1. Barber, H. R. K. Ovarian cancer: Part I. *CA* 29:341, 1979.
   Ovarian cancer must be ruled out in women over 40 with gastrointestinal symptoms that cannot be definitely diagnosed.
2. Barber, H. R. K. Ovarian cancer: Part II. *CA* 30:2, 1980.
   The author feels that when a hysterectomy is indicated in a patient over 40 years of age, bilateral salpingo-oophorectomy should also be advised as prophylaxis against ovarian cancer.

Diagnosis

3. Watring, W. G., Edinger, D. D., Jr., and Anderson, B. Screening and diagnosis in ovarian cancer. *Clin. Obstet. Gynecol.* 22:745, 1979.
   In suspected ovarian cancer, radiologic examination of the gastrointestinal tract is important, since gastrointestinal tumors frequently metastasize to the ovaries.

Pathology

4. Morrow, C. P. Classification and characteristics of ovarian cancer. *Clin. Obstet. Gynecol.* 22:925, 1979.
   Classification is based on the presumed cell of origin, i.e., a histogenetic classification.
5. Mandell, G. L., et al. Ovarian cancer: A solid tumor with evidence of normal cellular immune function but abnormal B cell function. *Am. J. Med.* 66:621, 1979.
   B lymphocytes mediate the humoral arm of the immune response; in this investigation, T cell (cellular immunity) function was normal while B cell function was abnormal in patients with ovarian cancer.

Staging

6. Greer, B. E., Rutledge, R. N., and Gallager, H. S. Staging or restaging laparotomy in early-stage epithelial cancer of the ovary. *Clin. Obstet. Gynecol.* 23:293, 1980.
   Prognosis is poor if tumor is present at a second-look procedure.
7. Knapp, R. C., and Riedman, E. A. Aortic lymph node metastases in early ovarian cancer. *Am. J. Obstet. Gynecol.* 119:1013, 1974.
   Of 26 patients with stage I disease 5 had aortic metastases (19%).
8. Mangioni, C., et al. Indications, advantages, and limits of laparoscopy in ovarian cancer. *Gynecol. Oncol.* 7:47, 1979.
   Valuable check of clinically nonfollowable intraperitoneal disease and for inspection of the subphrenic areas, but it does not diagnose retroperitoneal spread.

Management

9. Wijnen, J. A., and Rosenshein, N. B. Surgery in ovarian cancer. *Arch. Surg.* 115:863, 1980.
   Debulking procedures, reexploration, and adjuvant therapy may cause "remissions" but have not improved survival.
10. Ballon, S. C. Immunotherapy and immune diagnosis of ovarian cancer. *Clin. Obstet. Gynecol.* 22:993, 1979.
    Immunotherapeutic agents have not been shown to have specific antitumor activity, although enhanced immunologic reactivity has been demonstrated.
11. Williams, T. J., Symmonds, R. E., and Litwak, O. Management of unilateral and encapsulated ovarian cancer in young women. *Gynecol. Oncol.* 1:143, 1973.
    Reoperation and definitive surgery should be considered after childbearing is complete because of late recurrences (2 out of 33 cases in this series).
12. Creasman, W. T., et al. Germ cell malignancies of the ovary. *Obstet. Gynecol.* 53:226, 1979.
    Combining surgery, chemotherapy, and, in some cases, radiotherapy, resulted in an 89% 2-year survival in 26 patients.
13. Bjorkholm, E., and Pettersson, F. Granulosa-cell and theca-cell tumors: The clinical picture and long-term outcome for the Radiumhemmet series. *Acta Obstet. Gynecol. Scand.* 59:361, 1980.
    There were 263 patients, 8% of the ovarian neoplasms treated at the Radiumhemmet. Associated endometrial cancer was present in 11% of the women.
14. Berek, J. S., Griffiths, T., and Leventhal, J. M. Laparoscopy for second-look evaluation in ovarian cancer. *Obstet. Gynecol.* 58:192, 1981.
    Repetitive laparoscopy permitted early detection of recurrence. Major complications (14%) were much reduced by preceding needle laparoscopy.
15. Castaldo, T. W., et al. Intestinal operations in patients with ovarian carcinoma. *Am. J. Obstet. Gynecol.* 139:80, 1981.
    The authors attempt to define indications for resection or bypass from an analysis of 42 cases.
16. De Palo, G., et al. Restaging of patients with ovarian carcinoma. *Obstet. Gynecol.* 57:96, 1981.
    Positive findings on peritoneoscopy in conjunction with lymphography were found in 11 of 34 patients with no clinical evidence of disease, and in 25 of 30 with clinically evident disease.

Prognosis

17. Ozols, R. F., et al. Advanced ovarian cancer. Correlations of histologic grade with response to therapy and survival. *Cancer* 45:572, 1980.

Cytologic and histologic grading of ovarian cancer correlates with re-sponse to chemotherapy and survival.
18. Russell, P., and Merkur, H. Proliferating ovarian "epithelial" tumors: A clinico-pathological analysis of 144 cases. *Aust. N.Z. J. Obstet. Gynaecol.* 19:45, 1979.
Borderline epithelial tumors may be managed by conservative surgery in young patients, provided histologic grade and clinical stage are favorable.

Surgery

Three procedures specific to pelvic malignancies will be reviewed in this essay. These are radical hysterectomy, pelvic exenteration, and staging laparotomy.

Radical hysterectomy (Wertheim) is generally reserved for patients with cervical carcinoma stage Ib and perhaps early IIa who are free of medical contraindications to surgery. Further indications include certain endometrial stage II cancers, some vaginal cancers, and patients with cervical cancer unresponsive to radiotherapy in whom surgery is technically feasible.

Results with surgery or radiotherapy in stage I cervical cancer are essentially comparable. However, surgery allows the ovaries to be conserved and does not adversely affect vaginal function, important advantages for the younger patient.

The operative approach is also undertaken when radiotherapy is contraindicated because of pelvic inflammatory disease or large fibroids. Surgery may also be the treatment of choice for the bulky endocervical lesion (together with irradiation) and for pregnant patients with early disease.

Preoperative work-up is as for the patient with cervical cancer as well as preparation for major surgery. At laparotomy, the decision is made as to whether surgery is feasible. If biopsy and frozen section of the paraaortic nodes reveal tumor, the procedure is terminated; opinion is divided as to whether the presence of positive pelvic nodes should alter the approach or whether the procedure should still be completed.

Wertheim hysterectomy includes total abdominal hysterectomy, excision of the upper one-third to one-half of the vagina, the uterosacral ligaments, and the paracervical and paravaginal tissues out to the pelvic sidewalls. Pelvic lymphadenectomy is nearly always combined with the removal of the pelvic nodes to the aortic bifurcation. Nodes removed include the obturator, hypogastric, and external iliac groups. The adnexa are removed in older patients or in patients in whom adjunctive radiotherapy is employed.

Operative mortality is low (0.3%–1.7%), but urinary complications are not infrequent, since a major portion of the endopelvic fascia is removed and the bladder and ureters are extensively dissected. The most common problems are those of voiding dysfunction and loss of vesical sensation. Rarer, but major, urinary problems are those of vesicovaginal or ureterovaginal fistulas (0.7%–1.6%), which are especially common in patients who have also been treated with radiotherapy.

Another, not uncommon, surgical complication is the formation of lymphocysts (3%–24%). Fortunately, these generally regress, although some may require drainage, especially if infected. Other complications are those found with any major surgery and all are more common in patients treated with radiotherapy. For this reason, most surgeons prefer to avoid irradiation preoperatively and only employ the modality postoperatively if positive pelvic nodes are encountered.

Pelvic exenteration is seldom used as primary therapy. When the operation is performed it is almost always employed for recurrence after radiation therapy, generally of cervical cancer. For the procedure to be feasible, it is essential that the tumor is considered completely resectable. This decision is based on the clinical evaluation and operative findings. In general, a swollen leg or sciatic nerve pain is indicative of inoperable disease. Metastasis to common iliac or aortic nodes or outside the pelvis also indicates disease too extensive for resection.

For those few patients with operable central recurrence, anterior or total exenterations are usually employed, depending on the site of disease. Posterior exenteration is seldom carried out alone since urinary fistulas frequently occur as complications of this operation.

Exenteration involves removal of the pelvic lymph nodes, the internal genitalia, and the vagina. Since bladder and often rectum are also removed, urinary and fecal diversions become necessary. These generally take the form of ileal or colon conduits with sigmoid colostomy. A neovagina may also be constructed at the same time or at a later procedure.

Several operative techniques have been developed for the management of the large defect in the pelvic floor and the open pelvic cavity that otherwise predispose to pelvic hematoma, abscess, bowel obstruction, or even evisceration. The other major complications of the procedure involve problems with the urinary anastomoses, especially if irradiated tissues have been utilized.

The operative mortality is about 3%–14% and the overall survival rate is about 25%–40%. In view of the formidable nature of the procedure, it should be reserved for those patients who have the physical and psychological resources to cope with the therapy. Exenteration is not considered a suitable means of palliation.

Exploratory celiotomy for surgical staging is generally accepted for ovarian cancer and is becoming a fairly common procedure for endometrial carcinoma. However, in these conditions, surgery is generally the primary treatment modality; thus, the performance of a laparotomy is seldom in question. Since cervical cancer is usually treated by radiotherapy, staging laparotomy implies the possibility of "unnecessary surgery" and the operation is therefore highly controversial.

The concept of surgical staging to better evaluate the extent of the cervical disease is based on the finding that in patients who come to surgery, clinical staging is incorrect in over one-third of cases.

The procedure is directed primarily at biopsy of the common iliac and aortic lymph nodes. In addition, the pelvic and abdominal cavities are inspected and perirectal or perivesical biopsies are obtained if indicated. Surgery delays definitive therapy an average of about 8 days, and there is an operative mortality of about 1%.

In the event that common iliac or aortic nodes are positive, as occurs in some 20% of patients, routine radiation fields will not encompass the disease process and inevitable failure of standard therapy will follow. Therefore, treatment should be modified to include the involved areas if this is technically possible.

In order to justify the procedure, treatment modifications should be shown to increase survival. In practice, the major modification is that of extended field radiation, generally some 4500 rads to the paraaortic area in addition to standard pelvic irradiation. The additional therapy seems unsuitable as a routine prophylactic measure since there is a definite complication rate, related in particular to small bowel problems. These complications of therapy have, however, been much reduced by the use of an extraperitoneal approach to node sampling. Surgical staging for cervical cancer is still a clinical investigation rather than a routine procedure because there are as yet no data to support an increase in survival, since patients with positive aortic nodes often also have uncontrolled pelvic disease or metastasis elsewhere, resulting in a uniformly poor prognosis.

The development of nonoperative lymph node sampling techniques may obviate the need for surgery in many instances. Furthermore, the place of routine extended-field paraaortic radiation may require reevaluation, since a recent study utilizing this approach reported increased survival in patients with stage IIb disease compared to standard therapy, without a marked increase in radiation complications.

Radical Hysterectomy

1. Webb, M. J., and Symmonds, R. E. Wertheim hysterectomy: A reappraisal. *Obstet. Gynecol.* 54:140, 1979.
   In 610 cases, there was an 86% 5-year survival for vaginal cancer, 78% for cervix cancer, and 55% for endometrial cancer. In cervix cancer cases, positive lymph nodes lowered survival from 83% to 57%.
2. Piver, M. S., Rutledge, F., and Smith, J. P. Five classes of extended hysterectomy for women with cervical cancer. *Obstet. Gynecol.* 44:265, 1974.
   Operative modifications tailored to the individual patient.
3. Abdulhayoglu, G., et al. Selective radiation therapy in stage IB uterine cervical carcinoma following radical pelvic surgery. *Gynecol. Oncol.* 10:84, 1980.
   Suggests the use of postoperative irradiation even with negative nodes, in patients with nondifferentiated lesions, or when there is involvement of the outer one-third of the cervical stroma or vascular invasion.
4. Forney, J. P. The effect of radical hysterectomy on bladder physiology. *Am. J. Obstet. Gynecol.* 138:374, 1980.
   Suggests that autonomic denervation is responsible for the changes in bladder function.
5. Macasaet, M. A., Lu, T., and Nelson, J. H., Jr. Ureterovaginal fistula as a complication of radical pelvic surgery. *Am. J. Obstet. Gynecol.* 124:757, 1976.
   Discusses prevention and management.

Exenteration

6. Rutledge, F. N., et al. Pelvic exenteration: Analysis of 296 patients. *Am. J. Obstet. Gynecol.* 129:881, 1977.
   Case selection, status of lymph nodes, and complications of surgery are the vital factors relating to the procedure.
7. Creasman, W. T., and Rutledge, F. Is positive pelvic lymphadenopathy a contraindication to radical surgery in recurrent cervical carcinoma? *Gynecol. Oncol.* 2:482, 1974.
   Survival with exenteration in the presence of positive nodes varies between 0 and 20%.
8. McGraw, J. B., et al. Vaginal reconstruction with gracilis myocutaneous flaps. *Plast. Reconstruct. Surg.* 58:176, 1976.
   The rotated gracilis muscles, together with an omental pedicle graft, fill in the emptied pelvic space and provide a functional vagina.
9. Fallon, B., et al. Urologic complications of pelvic exenteration for gynecologic malignancy. *J. Urol.* 122:158, 1979.
   Of 43 cases, 9 had urinary infection or calculi and 9 had problems related to the urinary diversion, requiring a second procedure, from which 2 of these died. Advantages of the ileal and colon conduits are discussed.

10. Magrina, J. F., and Masterson, B. J. Vaginal reconstruction in gynecological oncology: A review of techniques. *Obstet. Gynecol. Surg.* 36:1, 1981.
    Restoration of vaginal function has a strong impact on ultimate rehabilitation.

Staging Laparotomy

11. Wharton, J. T., et al. Preirradiation celiotomy and extended field irradiation for invasive carcinoma of the cervix. *Obstet. Gynecol.* 49:333, 1977.
    In 120 patients there were 2 postoperative deaths. Of 24 patients with positive aortic nodes, 3 survived over 2 years; 10 of the 24 had serious radiation complications, which caused death in 5.
12. Piver, S. M., Barlow, J. J., and Krishnamsetty, R. Five-year survival (with no evidence of disease) in patients with biopsy-confirmed aortic node metastasis from cervical carcinoma. *Am. J. Obstet. Gynecol.* 139:575, 1981.
    The intestinal complication rate with radiation was 10% when 4400 to 5000 rads were administered. The five-year survival was 9.6% in this 31 case series.
13. Kademian, M. T., and Bosch, A. The value of staging laparotomy in cervical cancer. *Am. J. Obstet. Gynecol.* 136:264, 1980.
    Suggests that inability to control pelvic disease causes most treatment failures and that chances of controlling aortic disease are small; hence, staging surgery is not justifiable and may increase radiation complications.
14. Buchsbaum, H. J. Extrapelvic lymph node metastases in cervical carcinoma. *Am. J. Obstet. Gynecol.* 133:814, 1979.
    In 150 patients there was 1 postoperative death; 6 of 32 patients with positive aortic nodes survived over 2 years. The author advocates pretreatment celiotomy for advanced pelvic cervical carcinoma.
15. Jaques, P. F., et al. CT-assisted pelvic and abdominal aspiration biopsies in gynecological malignancy. *Radiology* 128:651, 1978.
    It is possible that transperitoneal percutaneous lymph node aspiration, directed by CT scan, ultrasound, lymphangiography, or fluoroscopy may replace operative lymph node sampling in most cases.
16. Belinson, J. L., et al. Fine-needle aspiration cytology in the management of gynecologic cancer. *Am. J. Obstet. Gynecol.* 139:148, 1981.
    There were 90 cases, with two false negative biopsies, one false positive biopsy and no complications. The technique was used for diagnosis and follow-up.

Radiation Therapy

Radiotherapy is widely employed in the treatment of gynecologic cancer. Irradiation may be employed as the only therapy or may be combined with surgery, chemotherapy, or immunotherapy. Treatment may be delivered to the tumor from radioactive isotopes, such as radium or cesium, placed locally in the uterine or vaginal cavities, or both, or it may be administered from an external source. External irradiation is usually given with supervoltage machines that have replaced the earlier orthovoltage instruments. Frequently, local and external therapy are combined, the former administering the major radiation dosage to the tumor and the latter being directed toward the draining lymph nodes. Radiation therapy dosage is calculated in rads, which are the units of absorbed dose. Using computer techniques, dosimetry can be accurately calculated so that too much radiation to normal tissues is avoided, while cancericidal doses are administered to the tumor and lymph nodes. Normal tissues that are rapidly dividing, such as the epithelial tissues of the urinary and intestinal tracts, are less able to tolerate radiation than are the more stable tissues such as those of the vagina and cervix.

Tumors differ in their radiosensitivity, frequently sharing this property with that of the parent tissue. Sensitivity is dependent on the histology, clinical variety, tumor bed, and oxygen tension. An anoxic tumor is radioresistant as is frequently seen in large or recurrent tumors with inadequate blood supply. However, radiosensitivity is not the same as radiocurability, since a relatively resistant tumor, well localized, may be cured, while a widespread radiosensitive tumor can usually be controlled only locally.

Tolerance to radiation depends on several factors. These include the total dose administered, the period of time over which the dose is given, and the volume of tissue irradiated. Tolerance is better when dosage is fractionated and spread over a longer time period and when smaller, rather than larger, areas are treated. These factors must be included in planning a radiotherapeutic treatment plan.

The intensity of radiation from a source varies inversely as the square of the distance from the source. For instance, in treating a cervical tumor, the dose rate at 1 cm from the radium source is nine times that at 3 cm from the source. In this way, the sensitive bladder and rectal tissues receive doses well within their individual safety margins (3500 and 3000 rads, respectively), while 15,000 rads or more may be delivered at the tumor site.

Radiation sources are placed in systems designed to fit in the uterine and vaginal cavities. These systems include the uterine applicator (called the tandem) and the vaginal applicators (called colpostats), which may be inserted with or without general anesthesia. Vaginal packing and a keel keep the systems stable and in place. Localization films are then taken to ascertain position and to calculate isodose curves for various areas in the pelvis. The actual radioactive sources are inserted thereafter if application is satisfactory. This technique, called afterloading, minimizes personnel exposure. Generally sources are left in situ 48–72 hours, and insertions are carried out 2–4 weeks apart. In treating cervical cancer, two applications are usually employed and these are given before, during, or after a concomitant course of external therapy.

Computerized dosimetry is used in balancing dosage from external and internal sources. External therapy is generally delivered from mega-voltage instruments in doses fractionated over several weeks. The radiation is delivered to measured areas called portal-of-entry fields. The shape and size of ports vary with the lesion to be treated. In treating the whole pelvis, these are generally 15–18 cm by 15–18 cm. Radiosensitive tissues may be protected during external beam therapy with lead screens. For instance, a 4 cm central shield protecting the bladder and rectum may be employed during whole pelvis irradiation. In treating cervical cancer, generally some 4000 to 6000 rads are administered to the lymph nodes. This dose is fractionated such that the total treatment time is 6–7 weeks.

Therapeutic levels of radiotherapy damage cell nuclei and cause an obliterative endarteritis. These effects on normal tissue result in complications that are closely related to dosage. It is the complication rate, rather than the cure rate, that places limits on radiation dosage. Local applications tend to cause focal injuries, while external therapy produces a more uniformly irradiated field.

The older orthovoltage therapy (200 kv) caused marked skin and subcutaneous tissue reactions, as well as a pronounced systemic effect. Supervoltage x-ray therapy (10,000 kv) or cobalt-60 beam therapy (1000 kv) cause little skin or systemic reaction since the penetration is so much greater. However, the depth dose is such that more damage is caused to deeper visceral tissues.

Early side effects of radiotherapy include cystitis and proctosigmoiditis, both of which usually respond to symptomatic treatment. Bone marrow suppression and radiation sickness are rarely encountered. An important early complication is the occasional occurrence of acute pelvic sepsis, which necessitates termination of therapy until the infection is cleared.

The late complications are far more difficult to deal with and are related to the ischemic and necrotizing effects of excessive ionizing radiation. They may occur months or years after the completion of therapy. Large bowel complications involving the rectum and sigmoid may cause hemorrhage, ulceration, fistulas, or stricture. Milder forms may respond to conservative measures, while the more severe will require defunctioning colostomy.

Small bowel problems occur particularly where previous surgery has fixed loops by adhesions or where small bowel remains relatively immobile, as at the terminal ileum. Enteritis, subacute obstruction, hemorrhage, ulceration, and perforation may occur. These complications are more common where irradiation has been extended to the upper abdomen. Management is difficult and may involve surgery with resection or bypass procedures.

Urinary tract problems related to the bladder and ureters include cystitis, ulceration, hemorrhage, stenosis, and fistula formation. If conservative measures are unsuccessful, surgical diversion of the urinary stream may be necessary.

The vagina responds to radiation with epithelial atrophy, erosions, and adhesion formation. Later, there may be stenosis and even complete vaginal obliteration. These changes can be partially prevented by the use of hormones, dilators, and, most importantly, continuation of intercourse as soon as possible after therapy. The cervix also commonly becomes stenotic with, on occasion, retention of secretions in the uterine cavity, thus leading to a pyometra that will require drainage. The most serious of the local complications, although fortunately rare, is complete vault necrosis, often with associated urinary or fecal fistulas.

In the management of complications following radiotherapy, it is vital to keep in mind the poor healing powers of irradiated tissue. Frequently there is difficulty in differentiating recurrence from radiation injury and in performing diagnostic procedures, especially biopsies. Great care must be taken to avoid perforation or fistula formation. Should surgery become necessary, the poor healing and poor infection-resistant properties of irradiated tissue must be allowed for in the therapeutic plan.

Complications associated with radiation therapy are fortunately uncommon and occur chiefly in patients in whom increased dosage is used as a calculated risk in attempting cure of advanced disease. The incidence of complications with standard regimens in early cases is low and the cure rate excellent when disease is localized.

Treatment should be individualized, and a management team including a gynecologic oncologist, a chemotherapist, and a radiotherapist should arrive at a treatment plan following accurate staging of the disease. This plan should be reviewed at intervals for response to therapy and the occurrence of complications that might necessitate a change in management.

Radiotherapy is the major modality of treatment for cervical cancer. In endometrial cancer, radiotherapy is commonly used in conjunction with surgery. Ovarian cancer is now more frequently managed by surgery and chemotherapy, with radiotherapy used only for particularly radiosensitive tumors such as the dysgerminoma. Vaginal cancer is commonly managed by radiotherapy, often in conjunction with surgery. While recurrent cancer may be treated with radiation therapy, previous treatment will often limit the dosage that can be employed such that the therapy is only palliative, as in the prevention or therapy of hemorrhage or the relief of pain. Further details on irradiation of pelvic cancer can be found in the essays relating to the individual malignancies.

Reviews
1. Brady, L. W. Radiation therapy in gynecologic cancer: Future prospects. *Clin. Obstet. Gynecol.* 18:125, 1975.
   Reviews treatment programs for endometrial, cervical, and ovarian cancer.
2. Bloomer, W. D., and Hellman, S. Normal tissue responses to radiation therapy. *N. Engl. J. Med.* 293:80, 1975.
   Therapeutic ratio is the ratio between the lethal tumor dose and tissue tolerance.

Cervical Cancer
3. Adcock, L. L. Radical hysterectomy preceded by pelvic irradiation. *Gynecol Oncol.* 8:152, 1979.
   The authors found an unacceptable incidence of urinary tract complications when full irradiation was followed by radical hysterectomy.
4. Durrance, F. Y., and Fletcher, G. H. Computer calculations of dose contribution to regional lymphatics from gynecological radium insertions. *Radiology* 91:140, 1968.
   Discusses sophisticated dosimetry.
5. Hintz, B. L., et al. Systemic absorption of conjugated estrogenic cream by the irradiated vagina. *Gynecol. Oncol.* 12:75, 1981.
   Absorption was comparable to that of nonirradiated controls.

Endometrial Cancer
6. Baker, H. W., et al. Stage I adenocarcinoma of the endometrium. A clinical and histopathological study of 65 cases treated with preoperative radium. *Obstet. Gynecol.* 54:146, 1979.
   Authors recommend preoperative irradiation for stage Ia lesions.
7. Morrow, C. P., Disaia, P. J., and Townsend, D. E. Current management of endometrial carcinoma. *Obstet. Gynecol.* 42:399, 1973.
   Authors recommend primary hysterectomy, and radiation therapy postoperatively only when appropriate.
8. Graham, J. B. The value of preoperative or postoperative treatment by radium for carcinoma of the uterine body. *Surg. Gynecol. Obstet.* 132:855, 1971.
   A controversial topic.
9. Gilbert, H. A., et al. The value of radiation therapy in uterine sarcoma. *Obstet. Gynecol.* 45:84, 1975.
   While radiation therapy is seldom successful, a few long-term survivals have followed radiotherapy alone or in combination with surgery.

Ovarian Cancer
10. Eltringham, J. R. Radiation therapy for ovarian carcinoma. *Clin. Obstet. Gynecol.* 22:967, 1979.

Extensive review concludes that data regarding postoperative irradiation are inadequate for evaluation.

11. Rosenshein, N. B., Leichner, P. K., and Vogelsang, G. Radiocolloids in the treatment of ovarian cancer. *Obstet. Gynecol. Surv.* 34:708, 1979.
    Results of treatment with radioactive gold and radioactive phosphorus given intraperitoneally are reviewed, and it is concluded that no proof of efficacy exists in the literature.

12. Lucraft, H. H. A review of thirty-three cases of ovarian dysgerminoma emphasizing the role of radiotherapy. *Clin. Radiol.* 30:585, 1979.
    A rare, malignant germ cell tumor of children and young adults that is distinguished by marked radiosensitivity and a high cure rate.

Vaginal and Vulvar Cancer

13. Hilgers, R. D. Squamous cell carcinoma of the vagina. *Surg. Clin. North Am.* 58:25, 1958.
    Radiotherapy is the major modality of treatment, with an overall 5-year survival of 46%–52%.

14. Fleming, P., et al. Description of an afterloading ^{192}Ir interstitial-intracavitary technique in the treatment of carcinoma of the vagina. *Obstet. Gynecol.* 55:525, 1980.
    A variety of vaginal applicators including ovoids, cylinders, and interstitial needles are available for local irradiation to supplement external therapy.

15. Tak, W. K. Interstitial therapy in gynecological cancer. *Gynecol. Oncol.* 6:429, 1978.
    Interstitial insertion of radium needles is suitable for many gynecologic tumors when residual tumor is left after external irradiation and when no adequate cavity exists for radium application.

16. Acosta, A. A., et al. Preoperative radiation therapy in the management of squamous cell carcinoma of the vulva: Preliminary report. *Am. J. Obstet. Gynecol.* 132:198, 1978.
    Generally, radiotherapy has little role to play in the management of vulval cancer, although some workers (as in this report) would disagree.

Complications

17. Cuthbertson, A. M. The treatment of fistulas following irradiation damage. *Aust. N.Z. J. Surg.* 50:124, 1980.
    Successful repair requires carefully planned procedures, using nonirradiated tissue to close the defect.

18. Martimbeau, P. W., Kjorstad, K. E., and Kolstad, P. Stage Ib carcinoma of the cervix, the Norwegian Radium Hospital, 1968–1970: Results of treatment and major complications. *Am. J. Obstet. Gynecol.* 131:389, 1978.
    Severe lymphedema occurred in 5% of their patients.

19. Lee, M. S., et al. Late effects of para-aortic irradiation in carcinoma of the uterine cervix and endometrium. *Radiology* 135:771, 1980.
    Using the extraperitoneal approach for diagnostic lymph node biopsy lessens the incidence of small bowel complications.

20. Ballon, S. C., et al. Survival after extraperitoneal pelvic and paraaortic lymphadenectomy and radiation therapy in cervical carcinoma. *Obstet. Gynecol.* 57:90, 1981.
    There was a 23% actuarial survival of patients with paraaortic metastases; however, these results require longer follow-up for confirmation.

21. Muram, D., et al. Postradiation ureteral obstruction: A reappraisal. *Am. J. Obstet. Gynecol.* 139:289, 1981.

Differentiating periureteral radiation fibrosis from recurrent carcinoma may require laparotomy in some cases.

22. Blythe, J. G. Cervical bacterial flora in patients with gynecologic malignancies. *Am. J. Obstet. Gynecol.* 131:438, 1978.

Irradiation of the pelvis in the presence of pelvic inflammatory disease, parametritis, or pyometra can be catastrophic.

Chemotherapy in Gynecologic Cancer

Chemotherapy has been employed as an effective treatment modality for gynecologic cancer for over two decades. Very little information, however, is available on the less common gynecologic cancers. This review is concerned with general principles and with the three common gynecologic cancers: ovarian, endometrial, and cervical carcinoma.

The use of drugs to treat cancer depends upon a metabolic attack on the neoplastic cell. Since there are no well-defined unique metabolic steps in the neoplastic cell to which this attack can be directed, adverse effects on normal tissue are predictable. Minimizing these effects on normal tissue requires the application of two observations: (1) in general neoplastic cells require longer to reproduce themselves; (2) drugs may have additive antineoplastic effects and differing adverse effects on normal tissue. The first observation suggests that chemotherapy should be administered in cycles, with intervals timed to permit normal tissue recovery. Such recovery is usually best reflected clinically by return of leukocytes and platelets to normal levels. Since normal tissue should recover more rapidly than neoplastic tissue, successive cycles of chemotherapy should stepwise reduce the size of the neoplastic cell population while avoiding cumulative effects on normal tissue. The second observation suggests that combination chemotherapy will permit a greater antineoplastic effect at only slightly greater toxicity. In fact, experience has shown that combinations of active drugs in general achieve a greater frequency of tumor reduction with longer-lasting responses and a greater impact on patient survival.

If this rationale to the use of chemotherapy is followed, a knowledge of active drugs is important. For each particular gynecologic cancer, active drugs will be discussed. Results are discussed in terms of response and survival. Response rate is defined as the sum of complete and partial response rates. A complete response is total disappearance of all evidence of gross disease for 1 or more months. A partial response is a 50% or greater reduction in the size of each measurable lesion for 1 or more months. Survival refers to the median time from initiation of therapy to either death or the patient's being lost to follow-up.

Proper management of patients on chemotherapy necessitates a knowledge of adverse effects. The major concern is myelosuppression. No course of therapy should be initiated if the leukocyte count is less than 3000/mcl or the platelet count less than 100,000/mcl. In the case of leukopenia, maximum suppression of granulocytes occurs 1–3 weeks after therapy; if the resultant granulocyte count is less than 1000/mcl, the result is a greater risk of infection, particularly with gram-negative rods (most commonly, *Escherichia coli*, *Klebsiella* species, and *Pseudomonas aeruginosa*). Fever may be the only manifestation and demands immediate cultures and broad-spectrum antibiotic combinations, including a cephalosporin, an aminoglycoside, and a synthetic penicillin with antipseudomonas activity. Delay to await culture results may result in a mortality exceeding 50%. Continuation of antibiotics until recovery of granulocytes is essential. In the case of thrombocytopenia, similar timing of platelet nadir should be expected. A count of less than 20,000/mcl demands prophylactic platelet transfusion, while a count of less than 50,000/mcl requires platelet transfusion only if hemorrhage occurs. Other common adverse effects include nausea and vomiting, alopecia, and immunosuppression. Important additional adverse effects to remember include: the leukemogenic effect of the alkylating agents, hemorrhagic cystitis with cyclophosphamide, cardiotoxicity with adriamycin, and nephrotoxicity and ototoxicity with cis-platinum.

The most common use of chemotherapy in gynecologic cancer is to treat ovarian adenocarcinoma. As a result of the relatively advanced stage of most ovarian adenocarcinomas at the time of presentation, most studies concern the treatment of advanced stage III or IV disease. Drugs possessing antineoplastic activity in ovarian carcinoma include the alkylating agents, adriamycin, mitomycin-C, hexamethylmelamine, cis-platinum, methotrexate, 5-fluorouracil, and vinblastine. Standard therapy for the treatment of such cases has consisted of an alkylating agent alone, with alkeran (phenylalanine mustard, melphalan), 0.2 mg/kg/day for 5 days every 4–6 weeks, being the most commonly used regimen. Such therapy has been reported to yield a response rate of 12%–54% (average 30%), with a median duration of 7 months and a median survival of 9 to 12 months. Only half the responders will achieve a complete response.

Recently, studies of combination chemotherapy using other active drugs with alkylating agents have yielded results that appear to be superior to those achieved with alkylating agents alone. A four-drug combination of hexamethylmelamine, cyclophosphamide, methotrexate, and 5-fluorouracil achieved a 76% response rate (33% complete response) and a 29-month median survival in patients with advanced stage III or IV disease, results that were significantly better than those seen in a concomitantly treated, randomized control arm using alkeran alone. Other drug combinations that also appear to possess some advantage include adriamycin plus cyclophosphamide and the same two drugs plus cis-dichlorodiamine platinum (II) (cis-platinum).

The exact role and type of chemotherapy indicated in earlier stage ovarian adenocarcinoma are not entirely clear. For patients with stage III disease that can be significantly bulk-reduced surgically, chemotherapy would appear to enhance survival to a greater degree than is seen with bulkier disease. Among patients with still earlier stage I and II disease, the value of adjuvant therapy with drugs has not been conclusively demonstrated. Most practitioners, however, employ single alkylating agents to treat at least high-risk patients (those with capsular penetration, high-grade neoplasms, positive peritoneal cytology, or spread to the pelvis).

The use of chemotherapy in squamous cell carcinoma of the cervix has been less extensively evaluated than is the case with its use in ovarian adenocarcinoma. All studies to date deal with advanced or recurrent disease and not with chemotherapy as an adjuvant treatment. Several single drugs have been shown to have moderate activity in achieving objective regressions in such patients. No highly active agent was identified, however, until a trial of cis-platinum in patients not previously given chemotherapy achieved a 50% response rate (11 responses in 22 patients). The optimum dose and schedule of the drug are not known, but a regimen of 50 mg/m^2 given intravenously every 3 weeks was employed in this particular study. Responses were relatively brief (6 months median) and survival short (9 months median).

While combination chemotherapy does not currently appear to offer an advantage in this disease, one regimen of mitomycin-C, vincristine, and bleomycin did yield a 60% response rate and represents an alternative to cis-platinum.

Trials of chemotherapy in endometrial carcinoma have received even less attention than is the case with its use with cervical carcinoma. Only one definitely active drug has been identified to date. Adriamycin, in two separate trials as a single agent, achieved 19% and 38% objective response rates. Median survival was only 7 months, but in the latter trial employing a larger dose of the drug (60 mg/m^2 given intravenously every 3 weeks), 25% of the patients achieved a complete response with a median survival of 14 months. Other drugs that have been evaluated include cyclophosphamide, 5-fluorouracil, cis-platinum, and piperazinedione; none of these appear to be significantly active. Attempts to employ combination chemotherapy have thus far not improved on the adriamycin response rate.

Only anecdotal data are available on the treatment of most other gynecologic cancers with chemotherapy. These include nonsquamous cervical carcinoma, rare ovarian neoplasms, and vulvar and vaginal carcinomas. In the case of uterine sarcoma, some data suggest that adriamycin is moderately active in the treatment of leiomyosarcomas (28% response rate) but only minimally active in mixed mesodermal tumors (12% response rate).

In summary, the role of chemotherapy as an effective treatment in ovarian adenocarcinoma is well established. Efforts now are directed to further refinement of therapy with long-term control as a realistic goal, even for patients with advanced disease. Much more work is needed in squamous cell carcinoma of the cervix and endometrial carcinoma to identify highly active drugs other than cis-platinum and adriamycin so that logical combinations can be built and, hence, results improved. For the less common neoplasms, only minimal data are available, and no firm recommendations can be made.

General

1. DeVita, V., Jr., et al. Perspectives and research in gynecologic oncology. *Cancer* 38:509, 1976.
   Excellent review of the status of chemotherapy in gynecologic cancer as of 1976.
2. DeVita, V., Jr., and Schein, P. The use of drugs in combination for the treatment of cancer. *N. Engl. J. Med.* 288:948, 1973.
   Excellent article on rationale for combination chemotherapy.
3. Morton, D. L., et al. Recent advances in oncology. *Ann. Int. Med.* 77:431, 1972.
   This older article has an excellent section on cell kinetics and cancer chemotherapy.

Adenocarcinoma of the Ovary

4. Tobias, J., and Griffiths, T. Management of ovarian carcinoma: Current concepts and future prospects. *N. Engl. J. Med.* 294:818, 1976.
   This excellent review article concisely records the state of the art of the treatment of ovarian carcinoma as of 1976. The roles of surgery and radiation are described. Chemotherapy at this time consisted of single alkylating agents with no proved advantage to drug combinations.
5. Messerschmidt, G., Hoover, R., and Young, R. Gynecologic cancer treatment: Risk factors for therapeutically induced neoplasia. *Cancer* 48:442, 1981.
   The authors summarize a number of risk factors associated with surgery,

radiation, and chemotherapy. With regard to acute leukemia after alkylating agents, the authors note a significant increase in incidence (9.3-fold) which is even greater (66.7-fold) in those patients on alkylating agents for 2 or more years. The disease developed an average of 41.5 months after initiation of chemotherapy.

6. Thigpen, T., et al. Cis-dichlorodiamine platinum (II) in the treatment of gynecologic malignancies: Phase II trials by the gynecologic oncology group. *Cancer Treat. Rep.* 63:1549, 1979.
   Cis-platinum is the only drug with significant activity in patients who have failed on alkylating agents. This article describes 10 responses among 34 patients with advanced ovarian carcinoma resistant to alkeran and thus confirms cis-platinum as a valuable drug in this disease.

7. Young, R., et al. Advanced ovarian adenocarcinoma: A prospective clinical trial of melphalan (L-PAM) versus combination chemotherapy. *N. Engl. J. Med.* 299:1261, 1978.
   This study documents that the four-drug combination (76% response rate vs 54% for alkeran; 33% complete response vs 16% for alkeran; and 29-month survival vs 17 months for alkeran) is significantly superior to the single alkylating agent.

8. Omura, G., et al. A randomized trial of melphalan versus melphalan plus hexamethylmelamine versus adriamycin plus cyclophosphamide in advanced ovarian adenocarcinoma. *Proc. AACR-ASCO* 20:358, 1979.
   This trial reports on a complete response rate with each combination that is twice that of alkeran alone (34% vs 17%). Complete responders lived significantly longer than other patients.

9. Ehrlich, C., et al. Response, second-look status and survival in stage III–IV epithelial ovarian cancer treated with cis-dichlorodiamine platinum (II) (cis-platinum), adriamycin (ADR), and cyclophosphamide (CTX). *Proc. AACR-ASCO* 21:423, 1980.
   This combination yielded a 79% response rate (41% complete response) with a median survival for complete responders that exceeds 2 years.

10. Edmonson, J., et al. Different chemotherapeutic sensitivities and host factors affecting prognosis in advanced ovarian carcinoma versus minimal residual disease. *Cancer Treat. Rep.* 63:241, 1979.
    This study demonstrates that, in patients with minimal residual disease after surgical debulking of stage III ovarian carcinoma, combination chemotherapy gives a better survival rate than single alkylating agents.

11. Hreshchyshyn, M., et al. The role of adjuvant therapy in stage I ovarian cancer. *Am. J. Obstet. Gynecol.* 138:139, 1980.
    The relapse rate in stage I ovarian carcinoma treated with adjuvant alkeran was 6% as compared to 17% for those receiving no adjuvant therapy and 30% for those receiving pelvic radiation.

Squamous Cell Carcinoma of the Cervix

12. Thigpen, T., et al. Cis-platinum in treatment of advanced or recurrent squamous cell carcinoma of the cervix: A phase II study of the gynecologic oncology group. *Cancer* 48:899, 1981.
    The authors report a 50% response rate for squamous cell carcinoma of the cervix to cis-platinum if the patients have had no prior chemotherapy. Thus, cis-platinum is the single most active drug to date in squamous cell carcinoma of the cervix.

13. Baker, L., et al. Mitomycin C, vincristine, and bleomycin therapy for advanced cervical cancer. *Obstet. Gynecol.* 52:146, 1978.
    The authors report response rates as high as 60% in cervical carcinoma with this three-drug combination.

14. Thigpen, T. et al. Chemotherapy in the management of advanced or recurrent cervical and endometrial carcinoma. *Cancer* 48:658, 1981.
    The authors provide an overview of chemotherapy in cervical and endometrial carcinoma. The data are current for 1981 and represent the best available information on these topics.

Endometrial Carcinoma
15. Thigpen, T., et al. Phase II trial of adriamycin in the treatment of advanced or recurrent endometrial carcinoma: A gynecologic oncology group study. *Cancer Treat. Rep.* 63:21, 1979.
    The authors report a 37% response rate (25% complete response) in advanced or recurrent endometrial carcinoma. No other agent or drug combination exceeds these results.

INDEX

Index